STANDARD LOAN

Applied Respiratory Physiology

Applied Respiratory Physiology

2nd Edition

J. F. NUNN

M.D., Ph.D., F.F.A., R.C.S. (Eng.)

Head of Division of Anaesthesia, Medical Research Council Clinical Research Centre; Honorary Consultant Anaesthetist, Northwick Park Hospital, Middlesex. Formerly Professor of Anaesthesia, University of Leeds.

BUTTERWORTHS
LONDON–BOSTON
Sydney–Wellington–Durban–Toronto

First edition 1969
Reprinted 1971
Reprinted 1971
Reprinted 1972
Reprinted 1975
Second edition 1977
Reprinted 1978
Reprinted 1981

© Butterworth & Co (Publishers) Ltd 1977

Library of Congress Cataloging in Publication Data

Nunn, John Francis.
Applied respiratory physiology.

First ed. published in 1969 under title: Applied respiratory physiology with special reference to anaesthesia.

Bibliography: p. 473
Includes index.
1. Respiration. 2. Anesthesia. I. Title.

[DNLM: 1. Respiration. WF102 N972a]
QP121.N75 1977 612.2'024'617 76-54340
ISBN 0-407-00060-7

Printed in England by the Whitefriars Press Ltd., London and Tonbridge

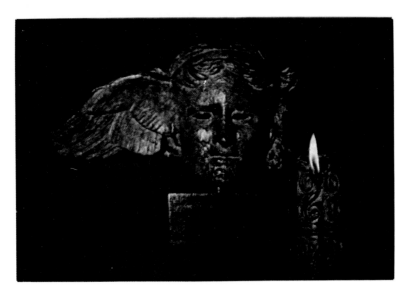

Hypnos and the Flame
(original photograph courtesy of Dr John W. Severinghaus)

[facing p. v

Foreword to the First Edition

A FLAME FOR HYPNOS

The lighted candle respires and we call it flame. The body respires and we call it life. Neither flame nor life are substance, but process. The flame is as different from the wick and wax as life from the body, as gravitation from the falling apple, or love from a hormone. Newton taught science to have faith in processes as well as substances—to compute, predict and depend upon an irrational attraction. Caught up in enlightenment, man began to regard himself as a part of nature, a subject for investigation. The web of self-knowledge, woven so slowly between process and substance, still weaves physiology, the process, and anatomy, the substance, into the whole cloth of clinical medicine. Within this multihued fabric, the warp fibres of process shine most clearly in the newest patterns, among which must be numbered anaesthesiology. The tailors who wove the sciences into the clinical practice of anaesthetics are men of our time such as Ralph Waters and Chauncey Leake who knit together respiratory physiology and pharmacology to cloak the first medical school Department of Anesthesiology, at Wisconsin, scarecely 45 years ago. Both of them still delight in watching the fashion parade they set in motion. Their partnership lasted only five years, but anaesthesiology and respiratory physiology remain as intimately interwoven as any pair of clinical and basic sciences. In this volume stands the evidence: references to more than 100 anaesthetists who have substantially contributed to respiratory physiology and John Francis Nunn's superb text which, for the first time, comprehensively binds the two together.

Man's interest in his own reaction to his environment constituted a further leap of the intellect. From substance to process to self-examination, and then full circle to the processes of interaction. 1969 may be considered the centenary of environmental or applied physiology. One hundred years ago Paul Bert, in a series of lectures to the Academie de Science in Paris, proposed to investigate the role of the low partial pressure of oxygen upon the distress experienced at high altitudes. Applying Dalton's law of partial pressures to physiology for the first time, he thus launched his monumental research of the barometric pressure, surely the cornerstone of applied physiology. The demands of military aviation during World War II generated a quantum jump of interest in applied physiology, exemplified by the founding 21 years ago of the *Journal of Applied Physiology*. This youngster, having just come of age, provides well over 100 references in Nunn's text, many of them written by anaesthetists. Anaesthesia may justly claim its birthright share of *Applied Respiratory Physiology*. Three years hence will be celebrated the bicentenary of N_2O, noting that Joseph Priestley reported N_2O two years before O_2!

And what of the god of sleep, patron of anaesthesia? The centuries themselves number more than 21 since Hypnos wrapped his cloak of sleep over Hellas. Now before Hypnos, the artisan, is set the respiring flame—that he may, by knowing the process, better the art.

San Francisco   JOHN W. SEVERINGHAUS

Preface to the Second Edition

Important advances in pure and applied respiratory physiology have required the production of a new edition.

Most sections have been revised, many have been expanded and there are new sections on subjects which have undergone rapid development since the first edition. For example, the chapter on control of breathing has undergone most extensive revision with hardly a paragraph remaining unchanged. Sections on pulmonary oedema, pulmonary oxygen toxicity, airway closure and the therapeutic use of oxygen have been greatly expanded. There are no new chapters but entirely new sections include non-respiratory functions of the lung, time dependence of pulmonary elastic behaviour, changes in lung volume associated with anaesthesia, the use of positive end-expiratory pressure, techniques of weaning from artificial ventilation, the role of 2,3-diphosphoglycerate and cytochrome P-450. Some 350 new references have been included. Happily a few sections have been omitted since their content is now too familiar to warrant the detailed exposition which seemed appropriate in 1969.

Applied Respiratory Physiology now covers a wider field with greater emphasis on pulmonary disease and special circumstances such as high altitude and exercise. Since 1969, the author has been heavily involved in intensive therapy and this has greatly influenced the content of the book.

The second edition will span the transitional phase for the adoption of Systeme Internationale Units. It has been necessary, therefore, to use both traditional and SI units throughout the text and in all the diagrams. Where greater precision is not essential, I have rounded off conversions to two significant figures to avoid smothering the reader in endless digits which have no real physiological significance. I have, for example, tended to take 1 kilopascal as equivalent to 10 centimetres of water where this simplification is justified by the context.

Once again it is a pleasure to acknowledge the help of so many friends and colleagues who have acquainted me with the latest developments in their fields and have, in many cases, kindly criticized the manuscript. I am especially grateful to Dr J. W. Severinghaus; Dr T. F. Hornbein; Dr S. H. Ngai; Dr R. A. Mitchell; Dr J. B. West; Dr K. Rehder; Dr M. J. Purves; Dr V. S. Bakhle; Professor M. K. Sykes; Professor D. G. McDowall; Dr S. S. Brown; Dr R. S. Cormack; Dr J. S. Milledge; Dr M. J. Halsey; Dr J. G. Jones; Dr G. H. Hulands; Mrs J. E. Sturrock; Mrs M. Berry and Mrs B. Minty. I am especially indebted to Dr N. A. Staub for permission to reproduce his magnificent colour photographs and to Dr E. R. Weibel and Dr A. P. Fishman for their superb electron micrographs. Dr Charles Norris submitted a most valuable critique of the first edition.

Preface to the First Edition

Clinicians in many branches of medicine find that their work demands an extensive knowledge of respiratory physiology. This applies particularly to anaesthetists working in the operating theatre or in the intensive care unit. It is unfortunately common experience that respiratory physiology learned in the pre-clinical years proves to be an incomplete preparation for the clinical field. Indeed, the emphasis of the pre-clinical course seems, in many cases, to be out of tune with the practical problems to be faced after qualification and specialization. Much that is taught does not apply to man in the clinical environment while, on the other hand, a great many physiological problems highly relevant to the survival of patients find no place in the curriculum. It is to be hoped that new approaches to the teaching of medicine may overcome this dichotomy and that, in particular, much will be gained from the integration of physiology with clinical teaching.

This book is designed to bridge the gap between pure respiratory physiology and the treatment of patients. It is neither a primer of respiratory physiology, nor is it a practical manual for use in the wards and operating theatres. It has two aims. Firstly, I have tried to explain those aspects of respiratory physiology which seem most relevant to patient care, particularly in the field of anaesthesia. Secondly, I have brought together in review those studies which seem to me to be most relevant to clinical work. Inevitably there has been a preference for studies of man and particular stress has been laid on those functions in which man appears to differ from laboratory animals. There is an unashamed emphasis on anaesthesia because I am an anaesthetist. However, the work in this speciality spreads freely into the territory of our neighbours.

References have been a problem. It is clearly impracticable to quote every work which deserves mention. In general I have cited the most informative and the most accessible works, but this rule has been broken on numerous occasions when the distinction of prior discovery calls for recognition. Reviews are freely cited since a book of this length can include only a fraction of the relevant material. I must apologize to the writers of multi-author papers. No one likes to be cited as a colleague, but considerations of space have precluded naming more than three authors for any paper.

Chapters are designed to be read separately and this has required some repetition. There are also frequent cross-references between the chapters. The principles of methods of measurement are considered together at the end of each chapter or section.

In spite of optimistic hopes, the book has taken six years to write. Its form, however, has evolved over the last twelve years from a series of lectures and tutorials given at the Royal College of Surgeons, the Royal Postgraduate Medical School, the University of Leeds and in numerous institutions in Europe and the United States which I have been privileged to visit. Blackboard sketches have gradually taken the form of the figures which appear in this book.

The greater part of this book is distilled from the work of teachers and colleagues. Professor W. Melville Arnott and Professor K. W. Donald introduced me to the study of clinical respiratory physiology and I worked under the late Professor Ronald Woolmer for a further six years. My debt to them is very great. I have also had the good fortune to work in close contact with many gifted colleagues who have not hesitated to share the fruits of their experience. The list of references will indicate how much I have learned from Dr John Severinghaus, Professor Moran Campbell, Dr John Butler and Dr John West. For my own studies, I acknowledge with gratitude the part played by a long series of research fellows and assistants. Some fifteen are cited herein and they come from eleven different countries. Figures 2, 3, 6, 11 and 15 [Figures 3, 12, 21 and 24 in the second edition] which are clearly not my blackboard sketches, were drawn by Mr H. Grayshon Lumby. I have had unstinted help from librarians, Miss M. P. Russell, Mr W. R. LeFanu and Miss E. M. Reed. Numerous colleagues have given invaluable help in reading and criticizing the manuscript.

Finally I must thank my wife who has not only borne the inevitable preoccupation of a husband writing a book but has also carried the burden of the paper work and prepared the manuscript.

J.F.N.

Contents

Chapter 1 Physical and Morphological Features of Gas Exchange and Non-respiratory Functions of the Lung

The Gas Laws
Lung Volumes and Capacities
Relation of Pulmonary Structure to Function
Non-respiratory Functions of the Lung

A knowledge of physics is more important to the understanding of the respiratory system than of any other system of the body. Not only gas transfer, but also ventilation and perfusion of the lungs occur largely in response to physical forces, with vital processes playing a less conspicuous role than is the case, for example, in brain, heart or kidney. It will therefore be clear that much of this book is concerned with physics, and it seems best to start with a brief review of those aspects which are most relevant to the behaviour of gases in the respiratory system. This is followed by an account of the structural aspects of the lungs, which is the only valid starting point for a consideration of function.

Physical quantities and units of measurement are perennial sources of confusion in respiratory physiology. Apart from any inherent difficulty, we suffer from an unnecessary duplication of units, particularly those of pressure. Appendices A and B are intended to resolve some of these difficulties but they need not be read by those readers who have already obtained a grasp of the subject.

THE GAS LAWS

Certain physical attributes of gases are customarily presented under the general heading of the gas laws. These are of fundamental importance in respiratory physiology.

Boyle's law describes the inverse relationship between the volume and absolute pressure of a perfect gas at constant temperature:

$$PV = K \qquad \qquad \dots (1)$$

where P represents pressure and V represents volume. At temperatures near their boiling point, gases deviate from Boyle's law. At room temperature, the deviation is negligible for oxygen and nitrogen and is of little practical importance for carbon dioxide or nitrous oxide. Anaesthetic vapours show substantial deviations.

1

Charles' law describes the direct relationship between the volume and absolute temperature of a perfect gas at constant pressure:

$$V = KT \qquad \qquad \dots (2)$$

where T represents the absolute temperature. There are appreciable deviations at temperatures immediately above the boiling point of gases. Equations (1) and (2) may be combined as follows:

$$PV = RT \qquad \qquad \dots (3)$$

where R is the universal gas constant, which is the same for all perfect gases and has the value of 8·1314 joules/degree kelvin/mole. From this it may be derived that the mole volume of all perfect gases is 22·4 litres at STPD. Carbon dioxide and nitrous oxide deviate from the behaviour of perfect gases to the extent of having mole volumes of 22·2 litres at STPD.

Van der Waals' equation is an attempt to improve the accuracy of equation (3) in the case of non-perfect gases. It makes allowance for the finite space occupied by gas molecules and the forces which exist between them. The Van der Waals equation includes two additional constants:

$$(P + a/V^2)(V - b) = RT \qquad \qquad \dots (4)$$

where a corrects for the attraction between molecules and b corrects for the volume occupied by molecules. This expression is of particular interest to anaesthetists since the constants for anaesthetic gases are related to their anaesthetic potency (Wulf and Featherstone, 1957).

An alternative method of correction for non-ideality is to express equation (3) in the following form:

$$PV/RT = Z \qquad \qquad \dots (5)$$

For a perfect gas, Z equals unity. For a particular gas at a particular temperature and pressure, the non-ideality may be expressed as the special value for Z (usually less than unity) which may be obtained from tables.

Since Z has a special value for each gas at each temperature and pressure, useful tables of Z values are necessarily very cumbersome. It is therefore much more convenient to replace Z with a power series as follows:

$$PV/RT = 1 + B/V + C/V^2 + . \qquad \qquad \dots (6)$$

The constants B, C, etc., are known as virial coefficients and vary only with temperature for a particular gas. Compilations are therefore simplified and the serious student is referred to Dymond and Smith (1969) or to Kaye and Laby (1966) which is more generally available but less complete. Values for B may be positive or negative and it is seldom necessary to use more than the one coefficient.

Adiabatic heating.   A great deal of respiratory physiology can fortunately be understood without much knowledge of thermodynamics. However, a recurrent problem is the heating which occurs when a gas is compressed. This effect is sufficiently large to be a readily detectable source of error in such techniques as the body plethysmograph (page 6), and the use of a large rigid container as a simulator for the paralysed thorax.

Henry's law describes the solution of gases in liquids with which they do not react. It does not apply to vapours which, in the liquid state, are infinitely miscible with the solvent (e.g. ether in olive oil) (Nunn, 1960b). The general principle of Henry's law is simple enough. The number of molecules of gas dissolving in the solvent is directly proportional to the partial pressure of the gas at the surface of the liquid, and the constant of proportionality is an expression of the solubility of the gas in the liquid. This is a constant for a particular gas and a particular liquid at a particular temperature but usually falls with rising temperature.

For many people, confusion arises from the multiplicity of units which are used. For example, when considering oxygen dissolved in blood, it has been customary to consider the amount of gas dissolved in units of vols per cent (ml of gas (STPD) per 100 ml blood) and the pressure in mm Hg. Solubility is then expressed as: vols per cent/mm Hg, the value for oxygen in blood at 37° C being 0·003. However, for carbon dioxide in blood, we tend to use units of mmol/l of carbon dioxide per mm Hg. The units are then: mmol l^{-1} mm Hg^{-1}, the value for carbon dioxide in blood at 37° C being 0·03. Both vols per cent and mmol/l are valid measurements of the quantity (mass or number of molecules) of the gas in solution and are interchangeable with the appropriate conversion factor.

Physicists are more inclined to express solubility in terms of the *Bunsen coefficient*. For this, the amount of gas in solution is expressed in terms of volume of gas (STPD) per unit volume of solvent (i.e. one-hundredth of the amount expressed as vols per cent and the pressure is expressed in atmospheres).

Biologists, on the other hand, prefer to use a related term—the *Ostwald coefficient*. This is the volume of gas dissolved, expressed as its volume under the conditions of temperature and pressure at which solution took place. It might be thought that this would vary with the pressure in the gas phase, but this is not so. If the pressure is doubled, according to Henry's law, twice as many molecules of gas dissolve. However, according to Boyle's law, they would occupy half the volume at double the pressure. Therefore, if Henry's and Boyle's laws are obeyed, the Ostwald coefficient will be independent of changes in pressure at which solution occurs. It will differ from the Bunsen coefficient only because the gas volume is expressed as the volume it would occupy at the temperature of the experiment rather than at 0° C. Conversion is thus in accord with Charles' law and the two coefficients will be identical at 0° C. This should not be confused with the fact that, like the Bunsen coefficient, the Ostwald coefficient falls with rising temperature.

The partition coefficient is the ratio of the number of molecules of gas in one phase to the number of molecules of gas in another phase when equilibrium between the two has been attained. If one phase is gas and another a liquid, the liquid/gas partition coefficient will be identical to the Ostwald coefficient. Partition coefficients are also used to describe partitioning between two media (e.g. oil/water, brain/blood, etc.). At the time of writing, it is too early to say when SI units will come into general use for expression of solubility (*see* Appendix A). The coherent unit is millimole litre^{-1} kilopascal^{-1}.

Graham's law of diffusion governs the influence of molecular weight on the diffusion of a gas through a gas mixture. Diffusion rates through orifices or through porous plates are inversely proportional to the square root of the molecular weight. This factor is only of importance in the gaseous part of the pathway between ambient air and the tissues, and is of limited importance in the whole process of 'diffusion' as understood by the respiratory physiologist.

Dalton's law of partial pressure states that, in a mixture of gases, each gas exerts the pressure which it would exert if it occupied the volume alone. This pressure is known as the partial pressure (or tension) and the sum of the partial pressures equals the total pressure of the mixture. Thus, in a mixture of 5 per cent CO_2 in oxygen at a total pressure of 101 kPa (760 mm Hg), the carbon dioxide exerts a partial pressure of $5/100 \times 101 = 5·05$ kPa (38 mm Hg). In general terms:

$$P_{CO_2} = F_{CO_2} \times P_B*$$

(Note that fractional concentration is expressed as a fraction and not as a percentage: per cent concentration = F x 100.)

In the alveolar gas at sea level, there is about 6·2 per cent water vapour, which exerts a partial pressure of 6·3 kPa (47 mm Hg). The available pressure for other gases is therefore $(P_B - 6·3)$ kPa or $(P_B - 47)$ mm Hg, an expression which recurs frequently in the following pages.

Tension is synonymous with partial pressure and is applied particularly to gases dissolved in a liquid such as blood. Molecules of gases dissolved in liquids have a tendency to escape, but net loss may be prevented by exposing the liquid to a gas mixture in which the tension of the gas exactly balances the escape tendency. The two phases are then said to be in equilibrium and the tension of the gas in the liquid is considered equal to that of the tension of the gas in the gas mixture with which it is in equilibrium. Thus a blood P_{CO_2} of 5·3 kPa (40 mm Hg) means that there would be no net exchange of carbon dioxide if the blood were exposed to a gas mixture which had a P_{CO_2} of 5·3 kPa (40 mm Hg). Directly or indirectly this forms the basis of all methods of measurement of blood P_{CO_2} and P_{O_2} (pages 372 and 441).

It is not the intention to discourse on physics any more than is necessary for the understanding of what follows in the rest of this book. Physics as applied to respiratory physiology and anaesthesia has been presented in *Physics for the Anaesthetist* (MacIntosh, Mushin and Epstein, 1958) and *Physics Applied to Anaesthesia* (Hill, 1972), which will also serve as an introduction to more advanced reading such as *The Physics of Gases*, by Radford (1964).

LUNG VOLUMES AND CAPACITIES

The lung volume is considered in relation to three volumes which are relatively fixed for a particular patient under particular conditions.

1. *Total lung capacity* (TLC), which is the volume of gas in the lungs at the end of a maximal inspiration.
2. *Functional residual capacity* (FRC), which is the volume of gas in the lungs at the end of a normal expiration. In the unconscious patient, the FRC is defined as the volume of gas in the lungs when there is no inspiratory or expiratory muscle tone and when the alveolar pressure equals the ambient pressure.
3. *Residual volume* (RV), which is the volume of gas in the lungs at the end of a maximal expiration.

* Abbreviations and symbols are listed in Appendix C.

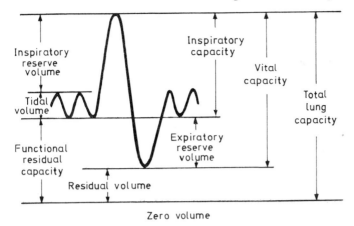

Zero volume

Figure 1. Static lung volumes. The 'spirometer curve' indicates the lung volumes which can be measured by simple spirometry. These are the tidal volume, inspiratory reserve volume, expiratory reserve volume, inspiratory capacity and vital capacity. The residual volume cannot be measured by observation of a simple spirometer trace and it is therefore impossible to measure the functional residual capacity or the total lung capacity without further elaboration of methods. Dynamic measurements of maximal breathing capacity and forced expiratory volume are discussed at the end of Chapter 4

Within this framework, there is no difficulty in defining inspiratory and expiratory reserve volumes, tidal volume, vital capacity and inspiratory capacity. This is best shown diagrammatically (*Figure 1*).

The total lung capacity is reached when the force developed by the inspiratory muscles is exactly balanced by forces opposing and resisting expansion. *Expiratory* muscles are contracting strongly at the end of a maximal inspiration. Inspiratory capacity may be limited either by weakness of contraction of inspiratory muscles or by diminished mobility of the lungs, chest wall or diaphragm.

There has been doubt about the precise factors governing the residual volume but it is clearly determined by the balance between the force exerted by the expiratory muscles and the resistance to decrease in volume provided by lungs, chest wall and diaphragm.

The functional residual capacity is usually considered to be dependent upon the balance of elastic forces and is considered in detail in Chapter 3. It is altered by changes in posture, alveolar pressure (relative to ambient) and development in tone of either inspiratory or expiratory muscles. It is also altered by changes in abdominal pressure (e.g. due to pregnancy) or by changes in elasticity of lungs or chest wall. Thus destruction of lung tissue in emphysema causes loss of elastic recoil and increase in functional residual capacity. It has recently been shown that anaesthesia is generally associated with a decrease in FRC and this is considered in some detail on pages 67 *et seq.*

Principles of measurement of lung volumes

Tidal volume, vital capacity, inspiratory capacity, inspiratory reserve volume and expiratory reserve volume can all be measured by simple spirometry without the necessity of using a spirometer designed for high frequency response or low inertia. Of these measurements, only the tidal volume has any significance in the unconscious patient.

Total lung volume, functional residual capacity and residual volume all contain a fraction (the residual volume) which cannot be measured by simple spirometry. However, if one is measured, the others can be easily derived since the volumes which relate them can be measured by simple spirometry. Measurement of FRC can be made by one of three techniques. The first method is to wash the nitrogen out of the lungs by several minutes of oxygen breathing with measurement of the total quantity of nitrogen eliminated. Thus if 4 litres of nitrogen are eliminated and the initial alveolar nitrogen concentration was 80 per cent it follows that the initial volume of the lung was 5 litres. The second method uses the wash-in of a tracer gas such as helium. If 50 ml of helium is introduced into the lungs and the helium concentration is then found to be 1 per cent it follows that the volume of the lung is 5 litres. In practice, the patient's alveolar gas is allowed to equilibrate with gas in a closed-circuit spirometer circuit which contains a known concentration of helium. The resultant fall in helium concentration is a function of the FRC in relation to the volume of the spirometer circuit. It is possible to avoid the necessity of measuring the volume of the spirometer circuit by the following routine:

1. Prime the spirometer circuit with helium to give a helium concentration of He_1.
2. Draw a known volume of gas (V) into the spirometer and after equilibration note the new reduced helium concentration He_2.
3. Allow the patient's alveolar gas to equilibrate with the spirometer and after equilibration note the final helium concentration He_3.

The following expression indicates the FRC:

$$V \cdot He_1(He_2 - He_3)/He_3(He_1 - He_2)$$

appropriate corrections being made for apparatus dead space and for temperature. FRC is normally expressed under conditions of body temperature and pressure, saturated with water vapour (BTPS).

Helium concentrations are usually measured with a catharometer and corrections are required for the presence of anaesthetic vapours. Anaesthesia with or without paralysis requires considerable modifications of technique but the problems are not insuperable (Hewlett et al., 1974a).

The third method of measurement of functional residual capacity uses the body plethysmograph making use of Boyle's law (DuBois et al., 1956). The subject is confined within a gas-tight box so that changes in the volume of his body may be readily determined as a change in either the gas volume or pressure within the box. He then adjusts his lung volume to FRC, purses his lips around a tube leading to a manometer and attempts to breathe against the occluded airway. This is rather like a Valsalva or Müller manoeuvre except that occlusion is not at the glottis but within the external breathing apparatus at a point distal to the manometer. Changes in alveolar pressure are recorded during the obstructed breathing together with the changes in lung volume which result from the pressure changes. The lung volume changes are measured as changes in whole body volume which are considered to be the same as lung volume changes under these conditions. These data permit calculation of the lung volume and the method is both accurate and convenient. Clearly there are formidable difficulties in applying this technique to anaesthetized patients, but it has been used under these conditions in the important study by Westbrook et al. (1973) considered in Chapter 3.

RELATION OF PULMONARY STRUCTURE TO FUNCTION

This section is not intended as an exposition of lung structure but is rather an account of those structural features which are directly relevant to an understanding of function. During recent years there has been a regrettable tendency for pulmonary structure and function to be pursued as separate subjects. It is now generally realized that a full understanding of function is not possible without a morphological background.

An excellent introduction to pulmonary structure in relation to function has been written by Staub (1971). There are major reviews by Krahl (1964) and Weibel (1964, 1973). Source books are *The Lung* (Miller, 1947), *The Human Lung* (von Hayek, 1960), *The Human Pulmonary Circulation* (Harris and Heath, 1962) and *Morphometry of the Human Lung* (Weibel, 1963). The Ciba Foundation held a symposium on *Pulmonary Structure and Function,* published under the editorship of de Reuck and O'Connor in 1962.

The air passages

Simplified accounts of lung function distinguish sharply between conducting air passages and areas in which gas exchange takes place. In fact, no such sharp demarcation occurs and the air passages gradually change their character showing a transition from the trachea to the alveoli, with the role of conduction gradually giving way to the role of gas exchange. *Table 1* traces the essential structural features progressively down the respiratory tract. The different levels are indicated as generations, with the trachea as the first, the main bronchi as the second, and so on down to the alveolar sacs as the twenty-third. It may be assumed that the passages of each generation bifurcate so that the number of passages in any one generation is twice that in the previous generation. In fact, there are many situations in which clear-cut bifurcation does not occur and trifurcation or lateral branching may be seen. Nevertheless, consideration of air passages in generations *as if* bifurcation occurred at each generation is very helpful and the numbers of air passages at each generation so calculated do, in fact, accord very closely with the numbers actually observed in the lungs.

Table 1 gives only the mean values for the number of generations down to each level. Thus, for example, it shows the transition from terminal bronchi to bronchioles occurring after the eleventh generation. In fact the transition may occur anywhere between the ninth and fourteenth generations.

Trachea

The trachea has a mean diameter of 1·8 cm and length of 11 cm. It is supported by U-shaped cartilages which are joined posteriorly by smooth muscle

Table 1. STRUCTURAL CHARACTERISTICS OF THE AIR PASSAGES (AFTER WEIBEL, 1963)

	Generation (mean)	Number	Mean diameter (mm)	Area supplied	Cartilage	Muscle	Nutrition	Emplacement	Epithelium
Trachea	0	1	18	Both lungs	U-shaped	Links open end of cartilage			
Main bronchi	1	2	13	Individual lungs					
Lobar bronchi	2 → 3	4 → 8	7 → 5	Lobes	Irregular shaped and helical plates	Helical bands	From the bronchial circulation	Within connective tissue sheath alongside arterial vessels	Columnar ciliated
Segmental bronchi	4	16	4	Segments					
Small bronchi	5 → 11	32 → 2 000	3 → 1	Secondary lobules					
Bronchioles Terminal bronchioles	12 → 16	4 000 → 65 000	1 → 0·5			Strong helical muscle bands		Embedded directly in the lung parenchyma	Cuboidal
Respiratory bronchioles	17 → 19	130 000 → 500 000	0·5	Primary lobules	Absent	Muscle bands between alveoli	From the pulmonary circulation		Cuboidal to flat between the alveoli
Alveolar ducts	20 → 22	1 000 000 → 4 000 000	0·3	Alveoli		Thin bands in alveolar septa		Forms the lung parenchyma	Alveolar epithelium
Alveolar sacs	23	8 000 000	0·3						

bands. In spite of the cartilaginous support, the trachea is fairly easy to occlude by external pressure of the order of 5–7 kPa (50–70 cm H_2O)*. For part of its length, the trachea is not subjected to intrathoracic pressure changes but it is subject to pressures arising in the neck as, for example, due to haematoma formation after thyroidectomy. The mucosa is columnar ciliated epithelium containing numerous mucus-secreting goblet cells. The cilia beat in a co-ordinated manner causing an upward stream of mucus and foreign bodies. Cilial beat is rendered ineffective by clinical concentrations of anaesthetics (Nunn et al., 1974) and also by drying, which is very prone to occur when patients breathe dry gas through a tracheostomy.

Main, lobar and segmental bronchi (first to fourth generations)

The trachea bifurcates asymmetrically, with the right bronchus being wider than the left and leaving the long axis of the trachea at a smaller angle. It is thus more likely to receive foreign bodies, extra long endotracheal tubes, etc. Main, lobar and segmental bronchi have firm cartilaginous support in their walls, U-shaped in the main bronchi but in the form of irregular shaped and helical plates lower down. Where the cartilage is in the form of irregular plates, the bronchial muscle takes the form of helical bands which form a geodesic network extending down to the lowest limits of the air passages. The bronchial epithelium is similar to that in the trachea although the height of the cells gradually diminishes in the more peripheral passages until it becomes cuboidal in the bronchioles. Bronchi in this group are sufficiently regular in pattern to be named.

Bronchi of the first to fourth generations are subjected to the full effect of changes in intrathoracic pressure and will collapse when the intrathoracic pressure exceeds the intraluminar pressure by about 5 kPa (50 cm H_2O)*. This occurs in the larger bronchi during a forced expiration since the greater part of the alveolar-to-mouth pressure difference is taken up in the segmental bronchi under these circumstances. Therefore the intraluminar pressure within the larger bronchi remains well below the intrathoracic pressure, particularly in patients with emphysema (Macklem, Fraser and Bates, 1963; Macklem and Wilson, 1965). Collapse of the larger bronchi limits the peak expiratory flow rate in the normal subject and gives rise to the brassy note of a 'voluntary wheeze' produced in this way.

Small bronchi (fifth to eleventh generations)

The small bronchi extend through about seven generations with their diameter progressively falling from 3·5 to 1 mm. Since their number approximately doubles with each generation, the *total* cross-sectional area increases markedly with each generation to a value (at the eleventh generation) of about seven times the total cross-sectional area at the level of the lobar bronchi.

Down to the level of the smallest true bronchi, air passages lie with branches of the pulmonary artery in a sheath containing pulmonary lymphatics which

* 1 kilopascal (1 kPa) is approximately equal to 10 centimetres of water (10 cm H_2O).

may be distended by oedema fluid (*Plates 1 and 2*). They are not directly attached to the lung parenchyma and thus are not subjected to direct traction. They are nevertheless subject to intrathoracic pressure and if the extramural pressure is substantially above the intraluminar pressure, collapse will occur. It now seems likely that this does not occur to any great extent in the small bronchi since the resistance to air flow between alveoli and small bronchi is now known to be less than had formerly been deduced from study of post-mortem lungs which had been fixed without inflation. It is now believed that during a forced expiration, the intraluminar pressure in the small bronchi rapidly rises to more than 80 per cent of the alveolar pressure. This pressure is sufficient to withstand the collapsing tendency of the high extramural intrathoracic pressure.

Secondary lobule.   The area of lung supplied by a small bronchus immediately before transformation to a bronchiole is sometimes referred to as a secondary lobule, each of which has a volume of about 2 ml and is defined by connective tissue septa.

Bronchioles (twelfth to sixteenth generations)

An important change occurs at about the eleventh generation where the diameter is of the order of 1 mm. Cartilage disappears from the wall of the air passages at this level, and structural rigidity ceases to be the principal factor in maintaining patency. Fortunately, at this level the air passages leave their fibrous sheath and come to be embedded directly in the lung parenchyma. Elastic recoil of the alveolar septa is then able to hold the air passags open like the guy ropes of a bell tent. The calibre of airways below the eleventh generation is, therefore, mainly influenced by lung volume, since the forces acting to hold their lumina open are stronger at high lung volume. The calibre of the bronchioles is,

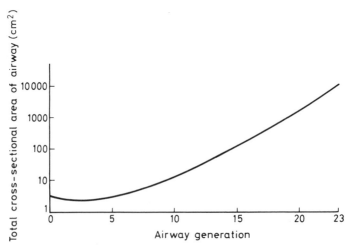

Figure 2. The total cross-sectional area of the air passages at different generations of the airways. Note that the minimal cross-sectional area is at generation 3 (lobar to segmental bronchi). The total cross-sectional area becomes very large in the smaller air passages. It approaches a square metre in the alveolar ducts. (Redrawn from data of Weibel, 1964)

however, less influenced by intrathoracic pressure than is the case in the bronchi.

In succeeding generations, the number of bronchioles increases far more rapidly than the calibre diminishes. Therefore the *total* cross-sectional area increases until, in the terminal bronchioles, it is about 30 times the area at the level of the large bronchi (*Figure 2*). It is therefore hardly surprising that the resistance to flow offered by the smaller air passages (less than 2 mm diam.) is only about one-tenth of total flow resistance (Macklem and Mead, 1967). Formerly, precisely the opposite was thought to be true, and it was believed that the major fraction of the total resistance was in the narrower vessels. This belief was in part due to earlier studies (e.g. Rohrer, 1915) which seriously underestimated the calibre of the smaller air passages. This error arose from failure to inflate the excised lung to its normal volume before fixation.

Bronchioles have strong helical muscular bands and a cuboidal epithelium. Contraction of the muscle bands is able to wrinkle the mucosa into longitudinal folds which may cause a very substantial decrease in calibre. In some studies the contraction may have been a post-mortem artefact.

Down to the terminal bronchiole the air passages derive their nutrition from the bronchial circulation and are, therefore, liable to be influenced by changes in systemic arterial blood gas levels. From this point onwards, the small air passages rely upon the pulmonary circulation for their nutrition.

Respiratory bronchioles (seventeenth to nineteenth generations)

Down to the end of the bronchioles, the function of the air passages is solely conduction and humidification. At the next generation (first order respiratory bronchiole) gas exchange occurs to a small extent and this function increases progressively through the three generations of respiratory bronchioles until, in the first order alveolar duct (twentieth generation), the entire surface is devoted to gas exchange (*Plate 3*). The respiratory bronchioles may thus be regarded as a transitional zone between bronchioles and alveolar duct with progressive changes in structure according to the change from conduction to gas exchange. The epithelium is cuboidal between the mouths of the mural alveoli but becomes progressively flatter until it finally gives way entirely to alveolar epithelium in the alveolar ducts. Like the bronchioles, the respiratory bronchioles are embedded in lung parenchyma and rely upon tissue traction for maintenance of their lumen. There is a well marked muscle layer and the muscle forms bands which loop over the opening of the alveolar ducts and the mouths of the mural alveoli. There is no significant change in the calibre of advancing generations of respiratory bronchioles and the total cross-sectional area at this level is of the order of hundreds of square centimetres.

Primary lobule or functional unit.   There is some disagreement about the extent of the primary lobule. Currently the majority view is that the primary lobule is the area supplied by a first order respiratory bronchiole (*Figure 3*). According to this definition, there are about 130 000 primary lobules, each with a diameter of about 3·5 mm and containing about 2 000 alveoli (*Table 2*). They probably correspond to the areas of lung which are seen to pop open at thoracotomy during expansion of collapsed lung by inflation.

Table 2. DISTRIBUTION OF ALVEOLI IN A PRIMARY LOBULE OR ACINUS (SYN. TERMINAL RESPIRATORY UNIT) (AFTER WEIBEL, 1963)

	Generation (as in Table 1)	Number of alveoli per unit (mean)	Number of units per generation (mean)	Number of alveoli per generation (mean)
Respiratory bronchioles				
1st order	17	5	1	5
2nd order	18	8	2	16
3rd order	19	12	4	48
Alveolar ducts				
1st order	20	20	8	160
2nd order	21	20	16	320
3rd order	22	20	32	640
Alveolar sacs	23	17	64	1 088
Total number of alveoli in primary lobule				2 277

Diameter of primary lobule at FRC, 3·5 mm; volume of primary lobule at FRC, 23 μl; number of primary lobules in average lung, 130 000; total number of alveoli in average lung, 300 000 000; diameter of alveolus at FRC, 0·2 mm.

Alveolar ducts (twentieth to twenty-second generations)

Alveolar ducts arise from the terminal respiratory bronchiole from which they differ by having no mucosa at all. The walls are in fact composed entirely of alveoli (about 20 in number) which open widely on to the lumen of the alveolar duct and are separated only by their septa. *Figure 3* shows the alveolar duct system as two successive bifurcations. Miller (1947) presents a somewhat different arrangement with terminal respiratory bronchioles trifurcating into a single generation of alveolar ducts from each of which arise three passages which he terms atria. In fact, Miller's atria are structurally and functionally indistinguishable from alveolar ducts and there seems little point in introducing a separate category. The differences between the model system in *Figure 3* and the reconstructions of Miller are of anatomical interest but need not concern us from the functional standpoint.

The alveolar septa form a series of rings across the length of the alveolar duct. These contain smooth muscle and are capable of contraction causing considerable narrowing of the lumen of the duct. About half of the total number of alveoli arise from ducts and some 35 per cent of the alveolar gas resides in the alveolar ducts and the alveoli which arise directly from them.

Alveolar sacs (twenty-third generation)

The last generation of the air passages are designated alveolar sacs although they are functionally identical to alveolar ducts except for the fact that they are blind. Staub (1963b) does not consider that they merit any distinction from alveolar ducts. About 17 alveoli arise from each alveolar sac, and this accounts for about half the total number of alveoli.

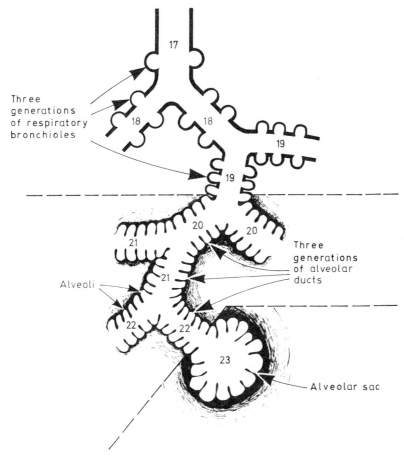

Figure 3. Diagrammatic representation of the terminal air passages of a primary lobule or functional unit. Successive generations are numbered and correspond to Table 1. The strict bifurcation at each generation affords an adequate model for explanation of function, but the actual structure is less regular. Different authors have variously defined the primary lobules as the area of lung supplied by the first, second or third generation of respiratory bronchiole

Alveoli

The mean total number of alveoli is usually stated to be 300 000 000 but ranges from about 200 to 600 million, correlating with the height of the subject (Angus and Thurlbeck, 1972).

The size of the alveoli is proportional to the lung volume and therefore in histological specimens depends critically upon the manner of fixation of the lung. At functional residual capacity the average alveolar diameter in man is 0·2 mm, astonishingly close to the estimate of 1/100 inch made by Stephen Hales in 1731. However, it has now become clear that the size is not uniform throughout the lungs but is largest in the uppermost part of the lung and smallest in the most dependent parts (Glazier et al., 1967). This is a gravitational phenomenon and is increased at high G (during centrifugation, for example). It derives from the fact that the lung is an elastic body with a specific gravity of about 0·3 and its centre of gravity migrates in a downward direction in whatever position the lung is held. This phenomenon has most important implications in the mechanics of breathing, regional distribution of ventilation (page 236), distribution of ventilation/perfusion ratios (page 281), and in the development of pulmonary collapse (page 292).

Alveolar walls which separate two adjacent alveoli consist of two layers of alveolar epithelium on separate basement membranes enclosing the interstitial space. This space contains the pulmonary capillaries, elastin and collagen fibres and nerve endings. The interstitial space is asymmetrically disposed with relation to the capillaries (*Figures 4 and 5*). On one side of the capillary, the space tends to be more than 1–2 μm thick and to contain abundant collagen fibres. This may

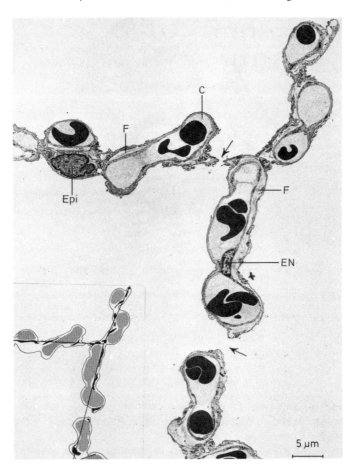

Figure 4. Electron micrograph of the junction of three alveolar septa of inflated lung of dog, showing the form of the continuous network of collagen fibrils, into which the capillary network is interwoven.

C, capillary; EN, endothelial nucleus; Epi, epithelial nucleus (type I); F, collagen fibrils; arrows point to pores of Kohn. (Reproduced from Weibel (1973) by courtesy of the author and the Editors of Physiological Reviews)

be considered as the 'service side' of the capillary and forms the connective tissue framework which maintains the geometry of the alveolus (*Figure 4*). On the other side of the capillary, endothelium and epithelium are closely apposed and the total thickness of the alveolar-capillary membrane is usually less than 0·4 µm (*Figure 6*). This may be considered as the 'active side' of the capillary and the gas exchange function is presumably more efficient on this side. The distinction between active and service sides has considerable pathophysiological significance since the active side tends to be spared in pulmonary oedema

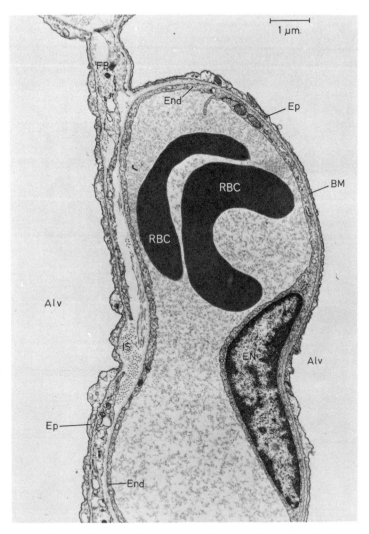

Figure 5. Details of the interstitial space, the capillary endothelium and alveolar epithelium. Note that the thickening of the interstitial space is confined to the left of the capillary (the 'service side') while the total alveolar-capillary membrane remains thin on the right (the 'active side') except where it is thickened by the endothelial nucleus.

Alv, alveolus; BM, basement membrane; EN, endothelial nucleus; End, endothelium; Ep, epithelium; IS, interstitial space; RBC, erythrocyte; FB, fibrolast process.

(Electron micrograph kindly supplied by Professor E. R. Weibel)

(*Figure* 7), as discussed on page 263. This also appears to be the case in fibrosing alveolitis (page 322).

Apart from the mouths of the alveoli, the panels which comprise the walls are approximately flat and in a state of tension due partly to the elastic fibres but more to the surface tension acting at the air/fluid interface. There was formerly considerable doubt as to whether alveolar epithelium existed. This has now been resolved by the electron microscope which reveals a continuous sheet of epithelium containing nuclei which bulge into the lumen of the alveoli (*Figure 4*).

It seems likely that the alveolar septa in man have small fenestrations (pores of Kohn) lying between branches of the capillary network (*Figure 4 and Plate 4*). The pores do not only connect alveoli of the same primary lobule, since communication can be demonstrated between the air spaces supplied by fairly large bronchi (Liebow, 1962). Direct communications have also been found between small bronchioles and neighbouring alveoli (Lambert, 1955).

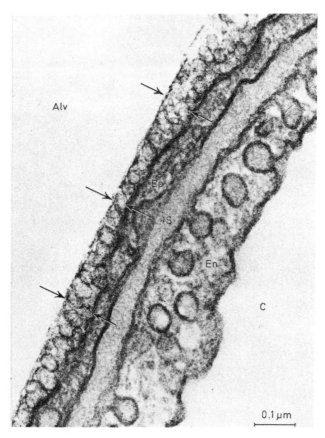

Figure 6. High-powered electron micrograph of the alveolar-capillary membrane of rat, showing the alveolar lining fluid (between arrows) prepared according to the technique described by Weibel and Gil (1968).

Alv, alveolus; C, capillary; En, endothelium; Ep, epithelium; IS, interstitial space.

(Reproduced from Weibel (1973) by courtesy of the author and the editors of Physiological Reviews)

The alveolar epithelium is covered with a very thin film of alveolar lining fluid which forms an interface with the alveolar gas (*Figure 6*). Surface tension at the interface tends to make the alveolar septa contract and this constitutes a major fraction of the lung 'elasticity'. The surface tension is, however, modified in a most important manner by a lipoprotein secreted by the alveolar epithelium, and this is discussed below and in Chapter 3 (page 75).

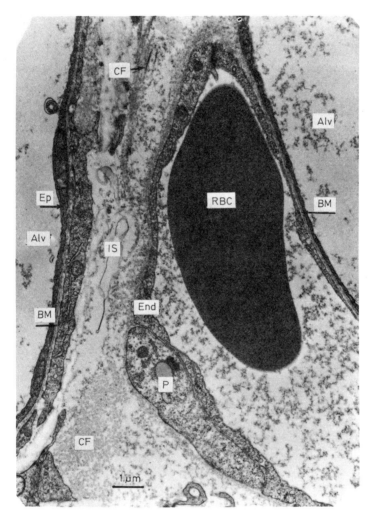

Figure 7. Electron micrograph to show the distribution of interstitial haemodynamic pulmonary oedema. Note that the interstitial space on the 'service side' of the pulmonary capillary has been considerably thickened by oedema fluid while the 'active side' remains unchanged in thickness.

Alv, alveolus; BM, basement membrane; CF, collagen fibres; End, endothelium; Ep, epithelium; IS, interstitial space; RBC, red blood corpuscle.

(Reproduced from Fishman (1972) by courtesy of the author and the Editors of Circulation)

A number of structurally distinct cells may be identified at the alveolar level as follows (see reviews by Weibel, 1973, and Kilburn, 1974).

1. Capillary endothelial cells.   These are continuous with the general circulatory endothelial cells and, in the pulmonary capillary bed, have a thickness of only about 0·1 μm, except where thickened to contain nuclei (*Figures 4 and 5*). It seems likely that pulmonary endothelial cells have many metabolic functions which are described below.

2. Alveolar squamous epithelial cells: Type 1.   These cells constitute the outermost layer of the parenchyma of the lungs and exist as a thin sheet approximately 0·1 μm in thickness except where expanded to contain the nuclei (*Figures 4 and 5*). Type 1 cells have a relatively clear cytoplasm which is devoid of organelles other than pinocytic vesicles.

3. Type II alveolar cells (*syn.* cuboidal or septal cells).   These cells are probably the main site of release of the surfactant which modifies the surface tension of

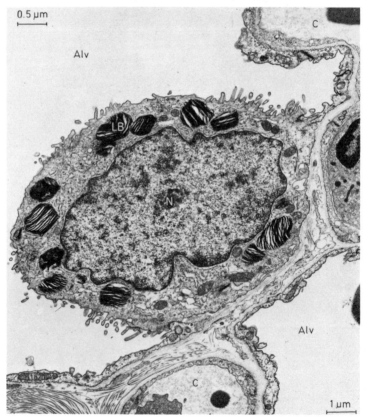

Figure 8. Electron micrograph of an alveolar epithelial cell of type II of dog. Note the large nucleus, the microvilli and the osmiophilic lamellar bodies thought to release the surfactant. Alv, alveolus; C, capillary; LB, lamellar bodies; N, nucleus.
(Reproduced from Weibel (1973) by courtesy of the author and the Editors of Physiological Reviews)

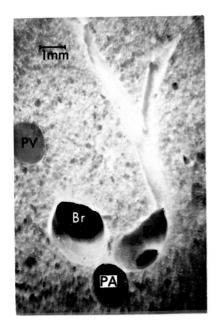

Plate 1

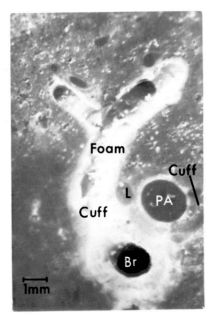

Plate 2

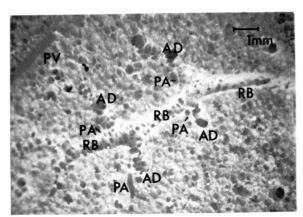

Plate 3

Plate 1. *Branchings of cartilaginous bronchi (BR), together with associated pulmonary artery (PA). The corresponding pulmonary vein (PV) is separate. Rapidly frozen normal cat lung showing natural colours. (Photograph by courtesy of Dr N. A. Staub)*

Plate 2. *Severe pulmonary oedema in freshly frozen dog lung. The bronchi (BR) contain oedema fluid foam and are surrounded by free fluid cuffs. The pulmonary artery and its branches (PA) are also surrounded by cuffs. Note the presence of a distended lymph vessel (L). Lung parenchyma in the background is severely waterlogged. (Reproduced from Staub (1963b) by courtesy of the author and the Editor of* Anesthesiology)

Plate 3. *Branchings of respiratory bronchioles (RB) showing transition to alveolar ducts (AD). Each airway branch is accompanied by its associated branch of the pulmonary artery (PA). The pulmonary vein (PV) lies separate. Fresh frozen cat lung. (Photograph by courtesy of Dr N. A. Staub)*

facing p. 18]

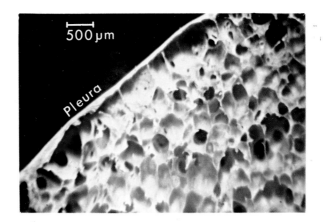

Plate 4

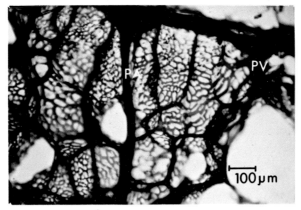

Plate 5

Plate 4. *Fresh frozen human lung showing size and shape of alveoli close to the pleura. Note numerous fenestrations between adjacent alveoli. (Photograph by courtesy of Dr N. A. Staub)*

Plate 5. *Maximally congested pulmonary capillary network in alveolar septum of fresh frozen dog lung. Average length of capillaries from pulmonary artery (PA) to pulmonary vein (PV) is 600–800 µm and crosses several adjacent alveoli. Note capillaries leaving and entering larger blood vessels at right angles. (Photograph by courtesy of Dr N. A. Staub)*

the alveolar lining fluid. They are characteristically sited at the junction of septa and have large nuclei and microvilli on their surfaces (*Figure 8*). They also contain large osmiophilic striated organelles which are probably concerned with storage of the phospholipids. An alternative view is that release takes place in the Clara cells of the terminal and respiratory bronchioles (Smith, Heath and Moosavi, 1974). Both views may be correct.

4. Type III alveolar brush cell. Brush cells are only rarely seen and their function is not yet established. It is possible that they may have a receptor function but neuronal connections have not been demonstrated.

5. Alveolar macrophages. The lung is richly endowed with these phagocytes which are active in combating infection and in scavenging foreign bodies such as dust particles. The alveolar macrophages pass through the alveolar epithelium and lie within the alveolar lining fluid. They contain a variety of destructive enzymes and their death presents a danger of autodigestion of the alveolar septa. This is normally prevented by the protease transport system described below.

6. Mast cells. In common with other organs, the lungs contain numerous mast cells which are located in the subpleural area. They have well developed organelles which secrete heparin, histamine, dopamine and 5-hydroxytryptamine (serotonin).

The pulmonary vasculature

The pulmonary arteries

Although the pulmonary circulation carries roughly the same flow as the systemic circulation, the arterial pressure and the vascular resistance are only one-sixth as great. The media of the pulmonary arteries is about half as thick as in systemic arteries of corresponding size. It consists predominantly of elastic tissue in the larger vessels but in the smaller vessels the media is mainly muscular, the transition being in vessels of about 1 mm diameter. Pulmonary arteries lie close to the corresponding air passages in connective tissue sheaths.

Pulmonary arterioles

The transition to arterioles occurs at a diameter of 100 μm. These vessels differ radically from the corresponding systemic vessels in being devoid of muscular tissue, consisting of merely a thin media of elastic tissue separated from the blood by the endothelium. The structure is, in fact, very similar to that of a pulmonary venule. Branches of the pulmonary arteries lie close to the corresponding branches of the bronchi (*Plate 1*). The general proximity of arterial blood vessels and gas-conducting tubes means that each is subjected to the same pressure changes and they are also conveniently located for the homeostatic mechanisms which provide some compensation for regional inequalities of either ventilation or perfusion.

ARP–2

Pulmonary capillaries

Pulmonary capillaries tend to arise abruptly from much larger vessels, the pulmonary metarterioles (Staub, 1963b). The capillaries form a dense network over the walls of one or more alveoli and the spaces between the capillaries are of the same order as the diameter of the capillaries themselves (*Plate 5*). The actual area of the interalveolar septum occupied by functioning capillaries is about 75 per cent of total but the precise figure varies, particularly in response to the effect of gravity, vascularity being greater in the dependent parts of the lung. This is the basis of the regional scatter of ventilation/perfusion ratios which is of considerable functional importance (page 281). It is generally believed that expansion of the alveoli leads to a reduction of the total cross-sectional area of the capillary bed, and an increased resistance to blood flow. It appears likely that the capillary network may pass continuously from one septum on to a second and possibly a third before draining into a venule. This must clearly have a bearing on the concept of 'capillary transit time' (page 320).

Pulmonary venules and veins

Pulmonary capillary blood is collected into venules which are structurally almost identical to the arterioles. In fact, the pulmonary circulation of the excised lung may be run in reverse, and Duke (1954) has obtained satisfactory gas exchange with an isolated lung of cat perfused from the pulmonary veins. The pulmonary veins do not run alongside the pulmonary arteries but lie some distance away, tending towards the septa separating the segments of the lung (*Plate 1*).

Bronchial circulation

Down to the terminal bronchioles, the air passages and the accompanying blood vessels receive their nutrition from the bronchial vessels which arise from the systemic circulation. Part of the bonchial circulation returns to the systemic venous system but part mingles with the pulmonary venous drainage. This constitutes a shunt and is further discussed on pages 248 and 291.

Bronchopulmonary arterial anastomoses

It is well known that in pulmonary arterial stenosis, blood flows through a pre-capillary anastomosis from the bronchial circulation to reach the pulmonary capillaries. It is less certain whether this occurs in normal lungs (page 249).

Pulmonary arteriovenous anastomoses

There seems little doubt that, when the pulmonary arterial pressure of the dog is raised by massive pulmonary embolization, pulmonary arterial blood is able to reach the pulmonary veins without apparently having traversed a capillary bed. The nature of the communication and whether it occurs in man is discussed in Chapter 9 (page 297), since it offers a possible explanation of some abnormalities of respiratory function which are consistently found during anaesthesia.

Pulmonary lymphatics (see review by Staub, 1974)

The significance of pulmonary lymphatic drainage has long been overlooked. There is in fact a well developed lymphatic system draining the interstitial tissue through a network of channels around the bronchi and pulmonary vessels towards the hilum. When in association with small bronchi (down to generation 11) lymphatics lie in a potential space around air passages and vessels, separating them from the lung parenchyma. This space becomes distended with lymph in pulmonary oedema (*Plate 2*) and accounts for the characteristic butterfly shadow of the chest x-ray. It is uncertain whether lymphatics are present at the alveolar level (Staub, 1974).

In the hilum of the lung the lymphatic drainage passes through the several groups of tracheobronchial lymph glands, where they receive tributaries from the superficial subpleural plexus. Most of the drainage of the left lung usually ends in the thoracic duct and that of the right lung in the right lymphatic duct. However, the pulmonary lymphatics not infrequently cross the midline and may pass independently into the junction of internal jugular and subclavian veins on corresponding sides of the body. Studies in dogs have indicated that approximately 15 per cent of the flow in the thoracic duct derives from the lungs (Meyer and Ottaviano, 1972).

Pulmonary lymphatics are intimately concerned in the pathogenesis of pulmonary oedema (*see* page 263) and in the transport system for inactivated proteases (*see* below).

NON-RESPIRATORY FUNCTIONS OF THE LUNG

The lungs are not solely concerned with gas exchange but also have other important functions. These are important partly because the lungs are favourably placed to process the entire circulation within a single circulation time, and partly because the lungs must inevitably handle toxic material which may be inhaled. Valuable reviews have been written by Heinemann and Fishman (1969) and by Tierney (1974).

Filtration function of the lung

The lungs are uniquely placed to act as a filter between the systemic veins and outflow tract of the left heart. Without this capillary filter there would be a constant risk of particulate matter entering the arterial system where the coronary and cerebral circulations are particularly vulnerable. Throughout life there is probably a continual shower of microthrombi which are arrested at the junction between the pulmonary metarterioles and capillaries. The arrangement of these vessels allows ample bypass circulation so that small particles will not cause any major derangement of the alveolar capillary circulation.

Pulmonary capillaries have a diameter of the order of 8 μm and particles exceeding this size are either delayed in transit or else permanently retained in the lung. Niden and Aviado (1956) have reported that glass beads up to 420 μm in diameter have traversed the pulmonary capillaries through unidentified pathways.

In fulfilling its role as a circulatory filter, the lung would appear to be in danger of circulatory occlusion from accumulation of thromboemboli. In fact, thrombi are cleared more rapidly from the pulmonary circulation than from other organs, and this ability extends to other protein emboli, such as radioactive macroaggregates of albumin used in lung scanning. The lung possesses well developed proteolytic systems not confined to removal of fibrin. Pulmonary endothelium is known to be rich in plasmin activator (Warren, 1963). This converts plasminogen into plasmin which itself converts fibrin into fibrin degradation products. However, it should also be noted that the lung is exceptionally rich in thromboplastin which promotes the conversion of prothrombin to thrombin. Furthermore, the lung is a rich source of heparin and bovine lung is used in its commercial preparation. Heparin is produced in mast cells and we have seen above that the alveoli are particularly rich in mast cells. The lung can thus produce high concentrations of substances necessary to promote or delay clotting and also for fibrinolysis. The interplay of these activities is not fully understood. Apart from the lung's ability to clear itself of thromboemboli, it may play a role in controlling the over-all coagulability of the blood.

Protease transport system

Sputum contains proteases which are released from dead bacteria and the lysozomes of alveolar macrophages. In addition, proteases may be released from sludged polymorphs in the pulmonary capillaries, particularly in the dependent parts of the lungs. The most dangerous enzyme is elastase which destroys elastin fibres, leading to disruption of the alveolar septa.

Two mechanisms protect against this eventuality. Firstly, proteases released into the alveoli are swept up to the larynx with the mucus flow. Secondly, proteases are rendered inactive by conjugation with one of the plasma proteins known as α_1 antitrypsin. Conjugated proteases are then removed by pulmonary blood and lymph and transferred to conjugation with α_2 macroglobulin which is destroyed in the liver.

In 1963, Laurell and Eriksson described patients whose plasma proteins were deficient in α_1 antitrypsin and who had emphysema. The association is now well recognized. The enzyme deficiency is inherited as an autosomal recessive gene and the incidence of homozygous patients is about 1 : 3 000 of the population with, perhaps, a higher incidence in Scandinavia. Homozygotes form a higher proportion of patients with emphysema and estimates range from 3 to 26 per cent. These patients tend to have basal emphysema, onset at a young age and a severe form of the disease (Hutchison et al., 1971). It thus appears that α_1 antitrypsin deficiency is an aetiological factor in a small proportion of patients with emphysema. There may be a family history and heterozygotes may have a slightly increased incidence of the disease.

Alteration of hormone levels

Certain hormones appear to pass through the lungs unchanged, but others may be removed from the circulation; some may be secreted in the lung and others may be chemically changed during transit. Vane (1969) has suggested that substances with local vasomotor effects (e.g. bradykinin and 5-hydroxy-tryptamine) are removed in the pulmonary circulation so that their effects are not broadcast by recirculation, whereas generally active circulating hormones, such as adrenalin, pass unchanged through the pulmonary circulation. Teleo-logical though this argument may be, it contributes to our understanding of what appears to happen. This theme has been developed in the reviews by Gillis (1973) and Bakhle and Vane (1974).

Prostaglandins have various effects on the lung but they are handled in a highly selective manner during transit through the lungs. Approximately 90 per cent of PGE and PGF are removed during a single transit, while PGA passes through the lung untouched (see review by Katz and Katz, 1974). PGE may be released in the lung in response to a variety of mechanical stimuli, including inflation (Berry, Edmonds and Wyllie, 1971). It is possible that this may be a factor in the long-term effects of artificial ventilation.

Angiotensin 1 (a decapeptide formed by the action of the enzyme renin on a plasma α_2 globulin) has a peptide linkage that may be broken to form the octapeptide angiotensin II which has strong vasopressor activity and a half-life of about 2 minutes. The conversion of angiotensin I takes place spontaneously in blood over the course of a few minutes, but at a greatly increased rate during passage through the pulmonary circulation, where about 80 per cent is converted during a single passage (Ng and Vane, 1967). Angiotensin II itself passes through the lung unchanged, as does vasopressin.

There is a striking difference in the effect of passage through the pulmonary circulation of adrenalin and noradrenalin. Each catecholamine has a half-life of about 20 seconds in blood, but as much as 30 per cent of noradrenalin is removed by a single passage through the lungs (Ginn and Vane, 1968). In contrast, adrenalin is unaffected. The removal of noradrenalin by the pulmonary circulation is inhibited by nitrous oxide and halothane in concentrations which are used in clinical anaesthesia (Naito and Gillis, 1973; Bakhle and Block, 1976). It has long been known that acetylcholine is rapidly hydrolysed in blood where it has a half-life of less than 2 seconds. Nevertheless, it is removed even more rapidly during transit through the pulmonary circulation, and it is also removed from solution in saline when passed through the pulmonary circulation (Vane, 1969). It is believed that histamine, dopamine and isoprenaline all pass through the lungs unchanged (Gillis, 1973; Bakhle and Vane, 1974).

5-Hydroxytryptamine (5-HT or serotonin) is very actively removed in the pulmonary circulation, more than 90 per cent being removed during a single passage (Thomas and Vane, 1967). It is thought that 5-HT is taken up into endothelial cells where it may be destroyed by monoamine oxidase activity. 5-Hydroxytryptamine is slowly removed in the systemic circulation and its half-life in blood is 1–2 minutes. However, pulmonary clearance is so rapid that effects due to recirculation are virtually eliminated. Bradykinin is handled in a similar manner, with 80 per cent removal during a single passage through the lungs.

A wide range of drugs are either bound or metabolized in the lungs and the list includes chlorpromazine, imipramine, nortriptyline and propranolol (Gillis, 1973).

Removal of hormones and other substances during passage through the pulmonary circulation has many important implications. Firstly, there will be a substantial difference between arterial and venous levels of angiotensin I, noradrenalin and 5-hydroxytryptamine, so that analyses are only meaningful if the appropriate sampling site is used and specified. Secondly, the route of administration must clearly influence the action of drugs which are substantially cleared by the lungs during a single passage. Thirdly, it seems likely that the lungs have an important role in protecting the body from a wide range of substances which may be liberated in the systemic circulation. Vane (1969) said 'It is intriguing to think that venous blood may be full of noxious, as yet identified, chemicals released from peripheral vascular beds, but removed by the lungs before they can cause effects in the arterial circulation.' Loss of this protective mechanism may be an important effect of prolonged cardio-pulmonary bypass.

Lipid metabolism

The lung is known to be active in the synthesis of fatty acids, esterification of lipids, hydrolysis of lipid–ester bonds and oxidation of fatty acids (Heinemann and Fishman, 1969). Of particular importance is the synthesis of the phospholipids which modify the surface tension of the alveolar lining fluid (page 75). Phospholipids have the general structure shown in *Figure 9*. The fatty acids are hydrophobic while the other end of the molecule is hydrophilic, the whole thus being a detergent. It is believed that in the alveolar lining fluid the fatty acid chains project into the alveolar gas, perpendicular to the interface, while the rest of the molecule is in solution.

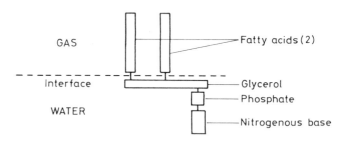

Figure 9. General structure of phospholipids

Lecithins are a series of phospholipids in which the nitrogenous base is choline. Dipalmitoyl lecithin is the most important constituent of the pulmonary surfactant. Palmitic acid is saturated and the fatty acid chains are therefore straight. Harlan and Said (1969) have advanced the attractive theory that straight chain fatty acids will pack together more satisfactorily during lung deflation than would be the case with unsaturated fatty acids (e.g. oleic acid) which are bent at the double bond.

The most important site of release of surfactants is the type II alveolar cell but it is also possible that they may be produced in the Clara cell of the bronchioles (*see* above). The surfactant system has been reviewed by Clements (1970) and King (1974).

Oxygen consumption of the lung

In addition to the functions described above, the lung requires energy for the maintenance of its tissue integrity and repair of damage (ion pumping, protein synthesis, etc.). All of this amounts to a considerable energy requirement which is largely obtained by oxidative phosphorylation (page 376). It has been estimated that the oxygen consumption of the pulmonary tissues is 1–4 per cent of that of the whole body. Its measurement is, of course, technically difficult and its level constitutes a systematic error in the measurement of cardial output by the Fick principle. Adequate oxygenation of pulmonary tissue only becomes a problem when there is failure of ventilation of a large part of the lung (as in lobar pneumonia) when the tissues must depend on the Po_2 of the mixed venous blood.

The above is by no means a comprehensive list of the non-respiratory functions of the lung which must include the elimination of non-respiratory metabolites (e.g. acetone) and drugs (e.g. anaesthetics). The lung also has a role as a store of about 10 per cent of the total blood volume. In addition, it seems likely that the metabolic functions listed above are far from complete and we may confidently expect that the next few years will see a major increase in our understanding of the subject.

This chapter has reviewed the physical behaviour of gases so far as it is relevant to respiratory physiology. It has also described the subdivisions of the lung volume and the micro-anatomy of the air passages and alveoli. In the case of the lungs there are considerable difficulties in explaining function in terms of structure or in explaining the function of every structure which can be seen with the microscope. However, a great deal of progress has been made in recent years and it is evident that a complete understanding of the lung can only come about by a synthesis of studies of structure and function. The subject of non-respiratory functions of the lung has been introduced.

Chapter 2   Control of Breathing

Normal pulmonary ventilation results from rhythmic contraction and relaxation of the voluntary striated muscles concerned with inspiration. Under normal circumstances the subject is not aware of this action, which is continued during sleep or light anaesthesia although it may, within limits, be over-ridden by voluntary cortical control or interrupted by involuntary non-rhythmic acts such as sneezing or coughing. This automatic control of voluntary muscles is an unusual arrangement and its elucidation has proved one of the most formidable problems of physiology.

There is no single mechanism which can be said to control ventilation. Many different mechanisms can be shown to be able to exert an influence on breathing under particular circumstances, although not all are in play at any one time. It appears, for example, that during exercise the mechanisms which control the minute volume are not those which are most important in the resting state. Understanding of such mechanisms is, at present, fragmentary with small islands of knowledge surrounded by seas of uncertainty, and we appear to be far from having an integrated picture of the control of breathing under all circumstances. Of necessity the subject is approached piecemeal with a good deal of detail about individual mechanisms but regrettably little about their relationship to one another.

The plan of this chapter is to commence with a discussion of the origin of the rhythmicity of breathing in the neurones of the hind-brain which appear to subserve respiration ('respiratory centres'). The efferent path is then traced to the muscle of respiration with an account of the important control function of the spindles in these muscles. The next section is concerned with the chemical control of respiration and this is followed by a discussion of the influence of respiratory reflexes and mechanical factors. Finally, some attention is paid to special situations such as breath holding, exercise, altitude and artificial ventilation.

THE ORIGIN OF THE RESPIRATORY RHYTHM

Classical concepts of the respiratory centres

In 1812, Legallois published reports showing that rhythmic inspiratory movements persisted after removal of the cerebellum and all parts of the brain above the medulla, but ceased when the medulla was removed. During the next 150 years a long series of distinguished investigators carried out more detailed localization of the neurones concerned in the control of respiration and studied their interaction. Marckwald and Kronecker (1880) differentiated between inspiratory and expiratory neurones, and Lumsden (1923a-d) described and named the pneumotaxic and apneustic pontine centres. He also advanced the concept of an internal feedback mechanism by which a tonic inspiration was inhibited at the end of inspiration by discharge of the pneumotaxic centre acting through the expiratory centre, the whole loop functioning as an internal pacemaker.

Pitts, Magoun and Ranson (1939a) described the anatomical localization of the overlapping inspiratory and expiratory neurones in the medulla, dispelling any idea of discrete 'centres'. In a later paper (1939b), they advanced the

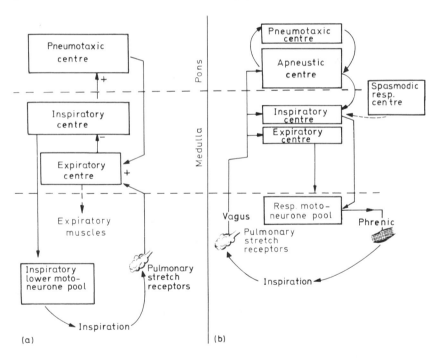

Figure 10. Classical concepts of the organization of the respiratory centres, showing the negative feedback loops believed to maintain the rhythmicity of breathing (see text). Expiratory muscles are not active during quiet breathing in conscious man, and the role of the expiratory neurones is primarily that of inhibition of the inspiratory neurones. However, Freund, Roos and Dodd (1964) have presented convincing evidence that expiratory muscle activity is a normal feature of breathing in the anaesthetized patient. ((a) according to Pitts (1946); (b) from Wang, Ngai and Frumin (1957) courtesy of the authors and the American Physiological Society)

concept of the inhibition of one centre by another, or by vagal afferents from stretch sensors in the lungs. In a third paper Pitts, Magoun and Ranson (1939c) concluded that respiratory rhythmicity is caused by two separate and alternative feedback loops; one based on the pneumotaxic centre, and the other on the vagal reflex sensitive to lung stretch, the two mechanisms being similar and mutually replaceable. When removal of the pneumotaxic areas was combined with bilateral vagotomy, a sustained inspiration, or apneusis, was found to result.

The suggestion of self-limitation of inspiration by vagal impulses arising from inflation of the lung was not new and had first been made in the classical studies of Breuer (1868), previously reported by Hering (1868).* The subject was reviewed in 1946 by Pitts. The next landmark in the long series of studies of the interaction of the various respiratory centres was the paper by Wang, Ngai and Frumin (1957), stressing the pontile apneustic centre as the site of the inspiratory tonicity and also as the site of rhythmic inhibition by both the pneumotaxic centre and the vagus. The general plan of the respiratory centres and the concepts illustrated in diagrams such as *Figure 10* have been widely accepted for a number of years. However, the essential roles of the pneumotaxic centre and the vagus have been strongly challenged on the basis of new experiments and new interpretations of old experiments.

Inherent rhythmicity of the respiratory neurones in the pons and medulla

There is no doubt of the existence of pontile neurones firing in synchrony with different phases of respiration. Bertrand, Hugelin and Vibert (1974) described discrete temporal and spatial distributions of three types of neurones in the pneumotaxic region. According to their firing patterns the three types were defined as inspiratory, expiratory and phase-spanning (inspiratory–expiratory). The spatial relationships and the sequence of firing of the three groups was compatible with the pneumotaxic centre functioning as a rhythm generator by means of a series of feedback loops or, alternatively, as a signal-processing station for a rhythm generated elsewhere. This is not, however, to say that the pneumotaxic centre is essential for the generation of the respiratory rhythm or that it is the normal site of its generation. Eupnoea was demonstrated with an isolated medulla by Wang, Ngai and Frumin (1957):

'In the present study, rhythmic respiration persisted in three medullary animals after section of all cervical dorsal roots and transection of the spinal cord at the level of the sixth cervical segment, in addition to division of all the remaining cervical nerves . . . In conventional medullary preparations, respiration is usually of the gasping type, but occasionally is indistinguishable from eupnea.'

Additional evidence for a medullary origin of the respiratory rhythm was obtained by Hoff and Breckenridge (1949) and Salmoiraghi and Burns (1960). Guz et al. (1964, 1966b) demonstrated that bilateral vagal block had no obvious effect upon the pattern of respiration in man. Reference should also be made to the experiment of St John, Glasser and King (1972) on page 31.

Accounts of how the medullary neurones themselves might generate the respiratory rhythm have been given by Robson (1967) and Salmoiraghi (1963). The concept is advanced that the system is bi-stable with predominant activity

* *See* page 52 for an explanation of the relationship between the papers of Breuer and Hering.

of either the inspiratory or the expiratory neurones. The system thus rests in either inspiration or expiration, normally cycling between the two phases in a rhythmic manner. It may thus be likened to a metronome which has two stable positions but which may be made to oscillate between them. This contrasts with Pitts' concept which is of a uni-stable system with only one resting position, that of inspiration or apneusis, which is rhythmically interrupted by negative feedback from either the pneumotaxic centre or the pulmonary stretch receptors (*Figure 10*).

In the bi-stable system, the inspiratory and expiratory neurones are believed to be separately arranged in two groups of self-re-excitatory chains, capable of raising their activity by internal positive feedback loops. As the burst proceeds, there is a progressive rise in the firing threshold of the group which soon terminates its activity (Salmoiraghi and von Baumgarten, 1961). However, the inspiratory and expiratory groups of neurones are linked by mutually inhibitory pathways which enforce reciprocal activity (*Figure 11*). Therefore, as the activity dies away in one group, it grows in the other, only to be terminated in due course by the development of a raised threshold in that group. Activity then recommences in the original group and so the cycle continues. It should be stressed that cyclical activity in the expiratory neurones does not necessarily imply activity of expiratory muscles and, indeed, under resting conditions, the expiratory neurones are exclusively anti-inspiratory in their action.

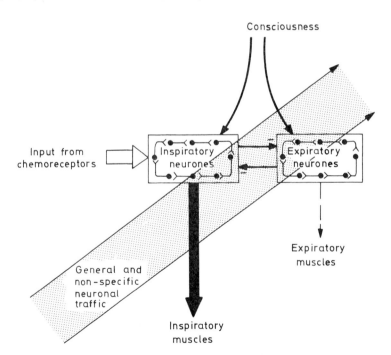

Figure 11. Concept of the generation of the respiratory rhythm within a bi-stable system of medullary neurones. Bursts develop alternately in the inspiratory and expiratory neurones, which are arranged in self-re-excitatory chains and are mutually inhibitory. Bursts in each group are terminated by an elevation of firing threshold within the group. Barbiturates cause respiratory arrest by interference with the pathways of reciprocal inhibition. The system is not self-oscillating in the absence of general neural traffic. (After Robson, 1967)

It is, however, difficult to imagine that the pneumotaxic centre, with its precise spatial and temporal differentiation of neurones according to their time of firing in relation to the respiratory cycle (Bertrand, Hugelin and Vibert, 1974), should play no part in the generation of the respiratory rhythm. Furthermore, Mitchell and Berger (1975) have reviewed the evidence against the possibility that a bi-stable medullary oscillator could generate the respiratory rhythm. They suggest that inhibitory phasing of inspiratory neurones in the dorsal respiratory group of the medulla is responsible for generation of the inspiratory rhythm and that periodic inhibition of tonically active expiratory neurones completes the cycle of the respiratory rhythm. Nevertheless, the actual mechanism and site of origin of the respiratory rhythm remains unknown.

Whatever and wherever may be the origin of the respiratory rhythm, its maintenance appears to depend *inter alia* upon the following factors.

1. *The integrity of the medullary neurones.* They are known to be easily damaged by hypoxia but their intrinsic activity is not apparently depressed by barbiturates (Robson, Houseley and Solis-Quiroga, 1963).
2. *The reciprocal innervation between the inspiratory and expiratory neurones.* Depression of these pathways appears to be the mechanism for the production of apnoea by barbiturates (Robson, Houseley and Solis-Quiroga, 1963). Arrest may be produced with continuous discharge of either inspiratory or expiratory neurones and it is possible to switch activity from one group to the other during arrest by inflation of the lungs, or by peripheral stimulation.
3. *Maintenance of acid–base status between certain limits* (Katz et al., 1963).
4. *The concept of the bi-stable organization of the respiratory neurones in the medulla* does not provide for spontaneous oscillation between inspiration and expiration except in the presence of general neuronal traffic through the brain stem. This may follow non-specific stimulation (such as mechanical stimulation of the larynx or dilation of the anus) or chemoreceptor stimulation by either hypoxia or hypercapnia. However, no less important is what may best be described as the state of wakefulness of the patient. The special significance of this factor for the anaesthetist is considered in the following section.

Influence of wakefulness

Every anaesthetist has noticed the ventilatory depression which accompanies absence of stimulus to the anaesthetized patient and is equally aware of the augmentation of ventilation which follows surgical stimulus even in the presence of deep anaesthesia (Eger et al., 1972). In fact, provided spontaneous respiration is present at all, it is almost impossible to avoid a ventilatory response to a painful stimulus, no matter how deep the anaesthesia. The same phenomenon is observed in sleep, and depression (of the ventilatory response to carbon dioxide) is progressively more marked in the deeper levels of sleep (Ingvar and Bülow, 1963).

The interplay between wakefulness and carbon dioxide is also important in handling the common problem of post-hyperventilation apnoea in the anaesthetized patient. Douglas and Haldane (1909) observed appreciable periods of apnoea following voluntary hyperventilation, in studies which closely followed the classical paper of Haldane and Priestley describing the major role of carbon dioxide in the regulation of breathing (1905). Since ventilation is so easily influenced by voluntary control under experimental conditions, when the subject's attention is focused on his breathing, it seemed worth repeating this study with subjects who had no preconceived ideas on the role of carbon dioxide.

Fink (1961) found that 13 naïve conscious subjects all continued to breathe rhythmically during recovery from reduction of end-expiratory Pco_2 to 3·3 kPa (25 mm Hg) or less, induced by 5–10 minutes of mechanical hyperventilation. It should, however, be noted that Fink's results were not confirmed by Bainton and Mitchell (1965) or Moser, Rhodes and Kwaan (1965), who were able to obtain apnoea after hyperventilation in some, but not all, of their conscious subjects. Whatever the uncertainty which seems to exist in conscious man, there is no doubt of the ease with which apnoea may be produced by moderate hypocapnia in anaesthetized patients (Hanks, Ngai and Fink, 1961), and these studies have a most important practical bearing on the restoration of spontaneous respiration in anaesthetized patients who have been subjected to a period of artificial hyperventilation. If a patient is allowed to regain consciousness rapidly at the end of a period of light anaesthesia, it is common experience that spontaneous respiration will be re-established at a Pco_2 well below the apnoeic threshold (page 47). In contrast, those anaesthetists who favour a more gradual return to consciousness frequently encounter some delay in restoring spontaneous breathing, unless they take steps to raise the Pco_2 to the normal level or higher. After an anaesthetic with artificial ventilation, arterial Pco_2 is very commonly within the range 2·7–4 kPa (20–30 mm Hg). However, Pco_2 may be easily restored to within the range 5·3–6·7 kPa (40–50 mm Hg) by such techniques as the administration of 5 per cent carbon dioxide in the inspired gas for 5 minutes during the continuation of artificial ventilation. It is then usual for spontaneous breathing to be resumed within a few seconds, even if the patient is still deeply unconscious, the additional Pco_2 drive seemingly being able to compensate for the relative absence of neural traffic. Alternatively, neural traffic may be generated by such manoeuvres as moving the endotracheal tube in the larynx, which frequently causes an abrupt resumption of breathing.

It had been the author's hope that a few breaths of electrophrenic respiration might hasten the resumption of spontaneous breathing after a period of artificial ventilation with neuromuscular blockade and opiate-supplemented anaesthesia. It seemed likely that this would, at least, reactivate the feedback loop from the pulmonary stretch receptors. In fact, electrophrenic respiration may very easily be induced with the type of percutaneous nerve stimulator used in anaesthetic practice but the artificially induced inspirations do not usually lead to an earlier resumption of spontaneous breathing.

St John, Glasser and King (1972) have reported an important effect of wakefulness on the breathing of cats with long-term bilateral pneumotaxic lesions and vagotomy. Apneustic breathing was seen during anaesthesia, thus confirming the observations of many investigators working with anaesthetized or decerebrate animals. However, after recovery from methohexitone anaesthesia, eupnoeic respiration returned in all animals except one. Subsequent anaesthesia with diethyl ether or α-chloralose again resulted in the production of apneustic breathing. This study confirms the ability of medullary neurones to generate a respiratory rhythm (*see* above) and also indicates how non-survival experiments in deeply anaesthetized or decerebrate animals may be quite misleading. It suggests that the medullary mechanism for the generation of the respiratory rhythm is particularly sensitive to anaesthesia but that, in the unanaesthetized animal, this may be compensated by an alternative mechanism not operative in cats with pneumotaxic lesions and vagotomy.

Ondine's curse and primary alveolar hypoventilation

This is also perhaps the best place to mention the condition which Severinghaus and Mitchell (1962) have aptly called 'Ondine's curse' from its first description in German legend. The water nymph, Ondine, having been jilted by her mortal husband, took from him all automatic functions, requiring him to remember to breathe. When he finally fell asleep he died. These authors describe three patients who exhibited long periods of apnoea even when awake but who breathed on command. These patients had become apnoeic during surgery involving the high cervical cord or brain stem, but a somewhat similar situation exists in patients with primary alveolar hypoventilation occurring as a feature of many different diseases, including the Pickwickian syndrome and chronic poliomyelitis. Characteristics include a raised P_{CO_2} in the absence of pulmonary pathology, a flat CO_2/ventilation response curve and periods of apnoea. A similar condition is also produced by overdosage with opiates.

MOTOR PATHWAYS CONCERNED IN BREATHING

Three groups of upper motoneurones converge on the anterior horn cells from which arise the lower motoneurones supplying the respiratory muscles. Final integration of respiratory control takes place at the level of the anterior horn cell (Mitchell and Berger, 1975).

The first group of upper motoneurones is mainly concerned with involuntary rhythmic breathing. Efferent fibres from the inspiratory and expiratory medullary neurones cross the midline in the region of the obex and descend in the lateral and ventral columns of the spinal cord respectively. The second group is concerned with voluntary control of breathing (speech, respiratory gymnastics, etc.) and lies in the corticospinal tract of the lateral column but dorsal to the tract from the medullary inspiratory neurones. The third group is concerned with involuntary non-rhythmic respiratory control (cough, hiccup, etc.). This group does not occupy a single compact location in the cord but appears to be separate from the tracts concerned with rhythmic input to the diaphragm (Newsom Davis and Plum, 1972).

The respiratory muscles, in common with other skeletal muscles, have their tension controlled by a servo-mechanism mediated by muscle spindles. They appear to play a more important role in the intercostal muscles than in the diaphragm (Corda, von Euler and Lennerstrand, 1965). Their function is largely inferred from knowledge of their well established role in other skeletal muscles not concerned with respiration (Granit, 1955).

Two types of cell can be distinguished in the motoneurone pool of the anterior horn cell. The α motoneurone has a thick efferent fibre (12–20 μm diameter) and passes by the ventral root directly to the neuromuscular junction

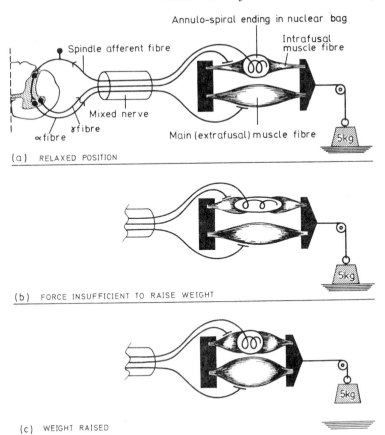

Figure 12. Diagrammatic representation of the servo-mechanism mediated by the muscle spindles. (a) shows the resting state with muscle and intrafusal fibres of spindle relaxed. In (b) the muscle is attempting to lift the weight following discharge of both α and γ systems. The force developed by the muscle is insufficient: the weight is not lifted and the muscle cannot shorten. However, the intrafusal fibres are able to shorten and stretch the annulo-spiral endings in the nuclear bag of the spindle. Afferent discharge causes increased excitation of the motoneurone pool in the anterior horn. α discharge is augmented and the weight is finally lifted by the more powerful contraction of the muscle (c). When the weight is lifted, the tension on the nuclear bag is relieved and the afferent discharge from the spindle ceases. This series of diagrams relates to the lifting of a weight but it is thought that similar action of spindles is brought into play when the inspiratory muscles contract against augmented airway resistance

of the muscle fibre (*Figure 12*). The γ motoneurone has a thin efferent fibre (2–8 μm) which also passes by the ventral root but terminates in the intrafusal fibres of the muscle spindle. Contraction of the intrafusal fibres increases the tension in the central part of the spindle (the nuclear bag) causing stimulation of the annulo-spiral endings. Impulses so generated are then transmitted via fibres which lie in the dorsal root to reach the anterior horn where they have an excitatory effect on the α motoneurones. It will be seen that an efferent impulse transmitted by the γ system may cause reflex contraction of the main muscle mass by means of an arc through the annulo-spiral afferent and the α motoneurone. Thus contraction of the whole muscle may be controlled entirely by efferents travelling in the γ fibres and this has been suggested in relation to breathing (Robson, 1967).

Alternatively, muscle contraction may in the first instance result from discharge of the α and γ motoneurones. If the shortening of the muscle is unopposed, main (extrafusal) and intrafusal fibres will contract together and the tension in the nuclear bag of the spindle will be unchanged (*Figure 12*). If, however, the shortening of the muscle is opposed, the intrafusal fibres will shorten more than the extrafusal fibres, causing the nuclear bag to be stretched. The consequent stimulation of the annulo-spiral endings results in afferents which raise the excitatory state of the motoneurones, causing the main muscle fibres to increase their tension until the resistance is overcome, allowing the muscle to shorten and the tension in the nuclear bag of the spindle to be reduced.

By this mechanism, fine control of muscle contraction is possible. The message from the upper motoneurone is in the form: 'muscles should contract with whatever force may be found necessary to effect such and such a shortening', and not simply: 'muscles should contract with such and such a force'. Clearly the former message is far more satisfactory for such a task as lifting up a suitcase of which the precise weight is not known until an attempt is made to lift it. It is common experience that, provided the weight is not grossly different from the anticipated weight, we can, in fact, raise a suitcase to a predetermined distance from the floor with considerable precision without knowing the exact weight in advance. This feat can only be achieved by means of an efficient servo-system which the spindles appear able to provide. The workings of the system are probably relayed to the cortex and provide information of 'length–tension' relationships which enable us to assess the weight of an object or the elasticity of a piece of rubber.

Campbell and Howell (1962) have presented evidence for believing that a similar mechanism governs the action of the respiratory muscles. According to this belief, the message conveyed by the efferent tract from the inspiratory neurones of the medulla would be in the form: 'inspiratory muscles should contract with whatever force may be necessary to effect such and such a change in length (corresponding to a certain tidal volume)' and not simply: 'inspiratory muscles should contract with such and such a force'.

The use of the servo-loop implies that the action of the respiratory muscles must be dependent upon the integrity of the dorsal roots which contain the efferents from the annulo-spiral endings. This appears to be the case, and dorsal root section at the appropriate level causes temporary paralysis of the respiratory muscles in man (Nathan and Sears, 1960).

The spindle-servo-mechanism provides an excellent mechanism for dealing with sudden changes in airway resistance. The compensation is made at spinal level and operates within the duration of a single inspiration, long before changes in arterial blood gas tensions are able to exert their effect. It is fortunate that this mechanism remains intact during anaesthesia and even withstands moderate curarization which is supposed to act selectively against the γ system. Nunn and Ezi-Ashi (1961) investigated the ability of anaesthetized patients to compensate for added resistance to either inspiration or expiration or both, and found a surprising ability to reinforce the work of the inspiratory muscles before any change in blood gas tensions could influence the picture. In fact the latter effect reinforced (after about 90 seconds' delay) the immediate response of the spindle-servo-mechanism and, in combination, a most reassuring degree of homeostasis of ventilation was achieved. The nature and magnitude of the response to resistance is described in Chapter 4 (page 125). Inspiratory resistance causes an augmentation of tension developed in the inspiratory muscles, while expiratory resistance also causes an augmentation of inspiratory effort resulting in an increase in lung volume, until the increased elastic recoil is sufficient to overcome the expiratory resistance. These changes are explicable in the light of the function of the spindles but cannot be explained in terms of the Hering–Breuer reflexes. Relay to cortical levels is probably the mechanism of detection of external changes in compliance (Campbell et al., 1961) or resistance Bennett et al., 1962).

CHEMICAL CONTROL OF BREATHING

Pflüger in 1868 was the first to demonstrate that breathing could be stimulated either by a reduction of oxygen content or by an increase of carbon dioxide content of the arterial blood. However, the importance of the role of carbon dioxide was not fully established until the classical work of Haldane and Priestley (1905). In one paper they presented their technique for sampling alveolar gas, showed the constancy of the alveolar P_{CO_2} under a wide range of circumstances and also demonstrated the exquisite sensitivity of ventilation to small changes in alveolar P_{CO_2}.

Until 1926 it was thought that changes in the chemical composition of the blood, mainly the P_{CO_2}, influenced ventilation solely by direct action on the respiratory centre, which was presumed to be sensitive to these influences although direct experimental proof was lacking. However, between 1926 and 1930 there occurred a major revision in which the existence of peripheral chemoreceptors was recognized. These receptors were found to be sensitive to hypoxia and the role of the carotid bodies in the control of breathing was clearly established (de Castro, 1926; Heymans and Heymans,* 1927; Heymans,* Bouckaert and Dautrebande, 1930). A similar function for the aortic bodies was reported in 1939 by Comroe.

Division of the afferent nerves from the peripheral chemoreceptors does not greatly diminish the ventilatory response to elevation of the arterial P_{CO_2} and until recently it was generally believed that the respiratory centre itself was sensitive to carbon dioxide. Recent work, however, suggests that the central chemoreceptors, as they have come to be called, may actually be separate from the respiratory neurones of the medulla although located but a short distance away.

The chemical control of breathing is shown schematically in *Figure 13*. The plan of this section of the chapter is first to give a separate account of the peripheral and central chemoreceptors and then to consider the quantitative aspects of their function in combination. The subject has recently been reviewed by Cunningham (1974) and Guz (1975).

The peripheral chemoreceptors

The peripheral chemoreceptors are fast-responding monitors of the arterial blood, responding to a fall in P_{O_2}, a rise in P_{CO_2} or H^+ concentration, or a fall in

* This work resulted in C. Heymans being awarded a Nobel Prize in 1938.

their perfusion rate. Of the peripheral chemoreceptors, the carotid bodies are almost exclusively responsible for the respiratory response.

The carotid bodies contain large sinusoids with a very high rate of perfusion which is about ten times the level which would be proportional to their metabolic rate. Therefore the carotid body arterial/venous Po_2 difference is small. This accords with its role as a sensor of arterial blood gas tensions, and its rapid response which is within the range 1–3 seconds (Ponte and Purves, 1974).

At the cellular level, the main feature is the glomus or type I cell which is in synaptic contact with nerve endings that are probably afferent, with cell bodies in the petrosal ganglion of the glossopharyngeal nerve (McDonald and Mitchell, 1975). Type I cells are partly encircled by type II cells whose function is still obscure. Efferent nerves, which are known to modulate receptor afferent discharge, include post-ganglionic sympathetic fibres from the superior cervical ganglion and centrifugal fibres running in the glossopharyngeal nerve. There is a difference of opinion on whether these efferents supply only the blood vessels of the carotid body or whether they also make synaptic contact with the type I cells.

It is still not clear which structure is the actual chemoreceptor. McDonald and Mitchell (1975) consider the afferent nerve endings themselves as the strongest candidate, with the type I cells functioning as dopaminergic interneurones which modulate the sensitivity of the chemoreceptive nerve endings. However, they do not exclude the possibility that they may act as chemoreceptors in addition to any other functions they may have.

Biscoe reviewed the relationship between structure and function of the peripheral chemoreceptors in 1971 but, since that date, important new evidence has been published, including the paper by McDonald and Mitchell (1975) and others in the proceedings of the workshop edited by Purves (1975).

Discharge in the afferent nerves increases in the following circumstances.

1. *Decrease of arterial* Po_2. Reduced oxygen *content* does not stimulate the bodies, provided that Po_2 remains normal, and there is little stimulation in anaemia, carboxyhaemoglobinaemia or methaemoglobinaemia (Comroe and Schmidt, 1938). The response of ventilation to reduction of arterial Po_2 is non-linear (*Figure 14*) and only becomes prominent below a Po_2 of about 8 kPa (60 mm Hg). Withdrawal of the carotid chemoreceptor response to normal Po_2 by the inhalation of 100 per cent oxygen reduces the ventilatory response of the central chemoreceptors to Pco_2 by about 15 per cent (Cunningham, 1974). This would be represented by interruption of the broken line 'A' in *Figure 13*.

   A small number of otherwise normal subjects lack a measurable ventilatory response to hypoxia when studied at normal Pco_2 (see data of subjects 4 and 5 reported by Cormack, Cunningham and Gee, 1957). This is of little importance under normal circumstances because the Pco_2 drive from the central chemoreceptors will normally ensure a safe level of Po_2. However, in certain therapeutic and abnormal environmental circumstances, it could be dangerous.

2. *Decrease of arterial pH*. Acidaemia of perfusing blood causes stimulation of which the magnitude is the same whether the cause is due to carbonic or to 'non-respiratory' acids such as lactic (Hornbein and Roos, 1963). Quantitatively, the change produced by elevated Pco_2 on the peripheral

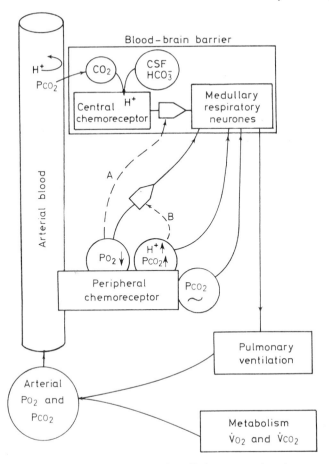

Figure 13. Scheme of chemical control of ventilation. For explanation, see *text*

chemoreceptors is only about one-sixth of that caused by the action on the central chemosensitive areas.

The P_{CO_2} (and consequently the pH) of arterial blood shows small oscillations in phase with respiration (*see Figure 115*), but the oscillations are greatly increased during exercise when the venous/arterial P_{CO_2} difference is increased. The mechanism of the stimulation of the central chemoreceptors is too slow to respond to these changes but the output of the peripheral chemoreceptor in the sinus nerve has been found to vary during the respiratory cycle (Hornbein, Griffo and Roos, 1961). The timing of the nerve discharge suggests that the response is to the rate of rise of P_{CO_2} as well as to its magnitude. A series of square waves of raised P_{CO_2} in the carotid artery of the dog results in a higher level of ventilation than is obtained when the P_{CO_2} is maintained steady at the same mean value (Dutton, Fitzgerald and Gross, 1968), but respiratory oscillations in P_{O_2} do not appear to have this effect.

The effect of oscillations of P_{CO_2} has been demonstrated in the dog, cat and rat but, in man, direct investigation is not possible and recourse has to be made to elaborate experiments involving artificially imposed changes in the composition of the inspired gas (Cunningham and Ward, 1975a, b). Breath-to-breath variations in P_{CO_2} do indeed show a within-breath response with an increased tidal volume when the P_{CO_2} is raised. However, in contrast to animal experiments, there is no evidence that the over-all ventilation is higher than it would be with the same mean P_{CO_2} held at a steady level, and this applies even to hypoxic conditions. However, if the P_{CO_2} is made to rise sharply during inspiration then an augmentation of ventilation occurs (Cunningham, Howson and Pearson, 1973). This mechanism may have relevance to hyperventilation of exercise when the increased mixed venous/arterial P_{CO_2} difference causes a more abrupt rise in arterial P_{CO_2} during expiration. Phase change between the respiratory cycle and the arterial P_{CO_2} cycle may also have an effect on ventilation and play a part in the production of the hyperventilation of exercise (Black and Torrance, 1971).

3. *Hypoperfusion of peripheral chemoreceptors* causes stimulation, possibly by causing a 'stagnant hypoxia' of the chemoreceptor cells. Hypoperfusion may result from hypotension.

4. *Blood temperature elevation* causes stimulation of breathing.

5. *Chemical stimulation* by a wide range of substances is known to cause increased ventilation through the medium of the peripheral chemo-receptors. These substances fall into two groups. The first comprises agents such as nicotine and acetylcholine which stimulate sympathetic ganglia. Action of this group of drugs can be blocked with ganglion-blocking agents (e.g. hexamethonium). The second group of chemical stimulants comprises substances such as cyanide and carbon monoxide* which block the cytochrome system and so prevent oxidative metabolism.

It would be attractive to offer a unified theory which would explain how this wide range of stimuli can excite the chemoreceptors by a common mechanism. For example, thought has been given to the possibility that the chemoreceptor cells might be uniquely sensitive to a fall in intracellular pH. It would then be possible to postulate their stimulation by a rise in P_{CO_2} (which lowers intracellular pH by diffusion of carbon dioxide into the cell), or by reduction of P_{O_2} (which, if sufficiently severe, would cause the cell to utilize anaerobic metabolic pathways). Hypoperfusion and poisoning of cytochrome a_3 would also prevent or diminish aerobic metabolism, and could cause intracellular acidosis from the production of lactic acid. Alternatively, hypoxia might be expected to change electrochemical gradients within the cell, as a result of relatively anaerobic conditions interfering with the sodium pump (Biscoe, 1971). An entirely different mechanism has been proposed by Mills and Jöbsis (1972) who report the presence of a different type of cytochrome a_3 in the carotid body. Unlike the usual cytochrome a_3 (page 377), which is also present in the carotid body, the special type is 50 per cent reduced at the very high level of P_{O_2} of 12 kPa (90 mm Hg) and they suggest that it is the P_{O_2} sensor. It has also been suggested by Neil and Joels (1963) that certain stimuli (e.g. acidosis) may shunt blood past the sinusoids and so cause stagnant hypoxia in the vicinity of the

---

* The apparent paradox between direct stimulation by carbon monoxide and lack of stimulation by the presence of a high level of carboxyhaemoglobin in the arterial blood is explained by Neil and Joels (1963).

chemoreceptor cells, which can then be considered to respond only to hypoxia. At the present time these theories remain conjectural and there is no firm evidence for the mechanism of action.

Apart from the well known increase in depth and rate of breathing, chemoreceptor stimulation causes a number of other effects including brady-cardia, hypertension, increase in bronchiolar tone and adrenal secretion. Stimulation of the carotid bodies has predominantly respiratory effects, while the aortic bodies have a greater influence on circulation.

Bilateral vagal and glossopharyngeal block was studied in two healthy volunteers by Guz et al. (1966b). Apart from the loss of swallowing and phonation, and the development of hypertension, there was no change in the pattern or sensation of breathing. End-tidal Pco_2 and respiratory rate were unchanged but there was a substantial increase in the duration of breath holding. Loss of ventilatory response to hypoxia produced by inhaling 8 per cent oxygen in nitrogen was also reported in another publication by the same team (Guz et al., 1966a). Bilateral vagal block was not found to influence ventilation in five anaesthetized patients (Guz et al., 1964). Interpretation of these studies is complicated by the fact that afferents from pulmonary stretch receptors were unavoidably blocked at the same time as those from the peripheral chemo-receptors.

Studies of patients who have lost their carotid bodies as a result of bilateral carotid endarterectomy (Wade et al., 1970) together with the work of Guz's group, referred to above, clearly show that the carotid bodies are not essential for the maintenance of reasonably normal breathing under conditions of rest and mild exercise. However, patients without peripheral chemoreceptors would be dangerously at risk if exposed to low partial pressures of oxygen in their inspired gas. They would also lose the augmented response to hypoxia in the presence of hypercapnia or exercise, which is considered below in relation to *Figure 14*. There are, in addition, the circulatory responses to chemoreceptor stimulation which generally have the effect of diverting blood flow to vital organs under adverse conditions.

The central chemoreceptors

The ventilatory response to carbon dioxide (i.e. the slope of Pco_2/ventilation curve, as in *Figure 15*) is diminished by denervation of the peripheral chemoreceptors, and some 80 per cent of the respiratory response to inhaled carbon dioxide originates in the central medullary chemoreceptors (Mitchell, 1966). The central response is thus the major factor in the regulation of breathing by carbon dioxide and it has long been thought that the actual neurones of the 'respiratory centre' were themselves sensitive either to Pco_2 (Haldane and Priestley, 1905) or to pH (Winterstein, 1911; Gesell, 1923).

More recently attention has been turned to the role of the cerebrospinal fluid (CSF) in the control of breathing. This followed the important studies of Leusen (1950, 1954) who showed that the ventilation of anaesthetized dogs was stimulated by perfusion of the ventriculo-cisternal system with mock CSF of elevated Pco_2 and reduced pH.

Leusen's work touched off a long series of studies aimed at localizing central chemoreceptors. They were thought to lie in contact with one or other of the reservoirs of CSF, since it seemed unlikely that changes in the composition of the CSF could influence the respiratory neurones within the substance of the medulla in the few minutes required for full development of the ventilatory response to inhaled carbon dioxide.

These studies were carried out mainly in the University of Göttingen (Loeschcke and Keopchen) and the University of California, San Francisco (Mitchell and Severinghaus), although various combinations of many authors appeared in numerous publications which included joint work between members of the two universities. Finally, it appeared likely that the central respiratory response to carbon dioxide was mediated mainly through superficial chemosensitive areas lying within 0·2 mm of the antero-lateral surfaces of the medulla, close to the origins of the glossopharyngeal and vagus nerves, and crossed by the anterior inferior cerebellar arteries (Mitchell et al., 1963).

An elevation of arterial P_{CO_2} causes an equal rise of CSF, cerebral tissue and jugular venous P_{CO_2}, all of which are approximately equal and about 1·3 kPa (10 mm Hg) higher than the arterial P_{CO_2}.* Over the short term and without change in CSF bicarbonate, a rise in CSF P_{CO_2} causes a fall in CSF pH and it was postulated by Mitchell and his colleagues that the reduction in pH stimulated the respiratory neurones indirectly through receptors in the chemosensitive area. The theory was especially attractive because the time course of change in CSF pH accorded with the well known delay in the ventilatory response to a change in arterial P_{CO_2} (Lambertsen, 1963; Loeschcke, 1965). The blood–brain barrier (operative between blood and CSF) is permeable to carbon dioxide but not hydrogen ions. This accords with the old observation that the ventilatory response to a respiratory acidosis is greater than to a metabolic acidosis with the same change in blood pH. Ventilation is, in fact, a single function of CSF pH in both conditions (Fencl, Miller and Pappenheimer, 1966).

Acclimatization to altitude.   Mediation of the central effect of carbon dioxide on respiration through a change in CSF pH also provided a most satisfactory explanation of the delayed ventilatory adaptation to altitude (Severinghaus et al., 1963). The changes which they described are as follows.

1. On acute exposure to an altitude of about 4 000 m the hypoxic drive from the peripheral chemoreceptors stimulates ventilation.
2. As ventilation increases, arterial and CSF P_{CO_2} fall with a concomitant rise in pH. The alkaline shift of CSF reduces the ventilatory drive from the medullary chemoreceptors and this partially offsets the hypoxic drive from the peripheral chemoreceptors. An equilibrium is rapidly attained at which the P_{CO_2} is typically only 0·3–0·7 kPa (2–5 mm Hg) below normal, although the P_{O_2} is about 6 kPa (45 mm Hg). This degree of hypoxaemia is appreciable and, being maximal initially, may explain some of the acute distress of a rapid first ascent.
3. This state of affairs does not persist since the CSF shows a remarkable ability to restore its pH to the normal sea level value of 7·32. When the CSF pH has been raised by hyperventilation, there is an active transport of unknown ions which results in movement of bicarbonate out of the CSF. Thus, within two or three days, the CSF bicarbonate falls by about

---

* Arterial/tissue P_{CO_2} difference is a function of cerebral blood flow, being smaller at high perfusion rates.

5 mmol/l, restoring the pH to within 0·01 units of its original sea level value (Severinghaus et al., 1963). This restores to a normal level the centrally mediated ventilatory drive. The hypoxic drive of the peripheral chemoreceptors is then unopposed and drives ventilation to its full extent. Typically, at 4 000 m, arterial P_{CO_2} settles to about 4 kPa (30 mm Hg) and P_{O_2} to about 7·3 kPa (55 mm Hg), with a substantial improvement in saturation compared with the situation immediately after acute exposure to altitude. Voluntary hyperventilation can further increase P_{O_2} and saturation within the limits imposed by an inspired gas P_{O_2} of about 11·3 kPa (85 mm Hg).

4. On return to sea level, the 'metabolic acidosis' (low bicarbonate) of the CSF persists for a short time and the subject will overbreathe until the CSF bicarbonate has been restored to the normal value by reversal of the active transport mechanism.

The concept of active transport of bicarbonate, restoring the CSF pH to normal, has recently been challenged. Two studies have reported a persistent alkalinity of CSF during acclimatization to altitudes of 3 100 m (Dempsey, Forster and doPico, 1974) and 4 300 m (Forster, Dempsey and Chosy, 1975). It was postulated that some additional drive to ventilation was operative during the early acclimatization period. Furthermore, compensatory changes were found to be similar for blood and CSF. In a separate series of studies, the role of passive distribution of hydrogen and bicarbonate ions between blood and CSF has been evaluated by Pavlin and Hornbein (1975a, b, c) and Hornbein and Pavlin (1975). These workers step-changed arterial P_{CO_2} or blood metabolic acid–base balance in anaesthetized dogs while measuring pH and P_{CO_2} of blood and CSF and also the potential difference between the two liquids. From the Nernst equation, the potential differences due to hydrogen and bicarbonate ion gradients were calculated and, following step-changes of acid–base derangement, were found to return to control values within about 5 hours. The associated changes in CSF hydrogen and bicarbonate ions during this period could thus be explained by passive distribution but the possibility of active ion transfer was not excluded.

Effects of altitude are further considered below (page 58).

Effect of passive hyperventilation. These changes occur during prolonged periods of artificial ventilation with high minute volumes. Semple (1965) pointed out that CSF bicarbonate would be significantly reduced after 1 hour of hyperventilation, and Christensen (1974) reported that CSF pH had returned to normal 30 hours after commencing passive hyperventilation. Hornbein and Pavlin (1975) found substantial resetting of the CSF pH within $4\frac{1}{2}$ hours of a step increase in the ventilation of an anaesthetized paralysed dog. This offers one reason why patients subjected to this treatment may demand high minute volumes, and often continue to hyperventilate after resumption of spontaneous breathing. It is not yet established to what extent there is appreciable loss of CSF bicarbonate during the artificial hyperventilation which is commonly employed during an operation of a few hours' duration.

Response to metabolic acidosis. The stability of the CSF pH is not confined to the circumstances of respiratory alkalosis of altitude but is also found in chronic respiratory acidosis and metabolic acidosis and alkalosis (Mitchell et al., 1965). Mean values of CSF pH in Mitchell's study did not differ by more than 0·011 units from the normal value (7·326) in spite of mean arterial pH values ranging from 7·334 to 7·523. The constancy of CSF pH cannot be explained either by diffusion of bicarbonate between blood and CSF or by renal compensation. Regulation of CSF chemistry in relation to breathing was reviewed by Leusen (1972).

If the bicarbonate of the CSF is altered by pathological factors, the pH is changed and ventilatory disturbances follow. Froman and Crampton-Smith (1966) described three patients who hyperventilated after intracranial haemorrhages. In each case the CSF pH and bicarbonate were persistently below the normal values and it was postulated that this was due to the metabolic breakdown products of blood which contaminated the CSF. In a later communication, Froman (1966) reported correction of hyperventilation by intrathecal administration of 3–5 mmol of bicarbonate.

Location of the central chemoreceptors.   There are considerable difficulties in determining the precise location of the medullary chemoreceptors in relation to the surface of the medulla and also in defining the relative importance of the factors which govern the pH in their vicinity. Although the ionic environment of the receptors is still not known, it appears that the pH is partly influenced by blood pH, Pco_2 and bicarbonate, but primarily by CSF pH, Pco_2 and bicarbonate. Ventilation is increased more when the CSF pH is lowered by reducing its bicarbonate than by raising its Pco_2. This is because attempts to alter the CSF Pco_2 by means of perfusion with mock CSF are frustrated by rapid equilibration of carbon dioxide between perfusate and tissue (Mitchell et al., 1963; Pappenheimer et al., 1965). Abnormal levels of bicarbonate concentration of perfusate are, however, little altered by contact with tissue and the effect of changes in CSF pH may be studied by this means.

In a study of cats with denervated peripheral chemoreceptors, Mitchell et al. (1963) found that, when acid–base variables of arterial blood were held constant, acidifying mock CSF by reduction of bicarbonate resulted in a stimulation of ventilation which was about 60 per cent of the level obtainable by inhalation of the corresponding concentration of carbon dioxide. This result may be compared with the findings of Pappenheimer et al. (1965) who, working with anaesthetized goats, found some 60 per cent of the normal ventilatory response to inhaled carbon dioxide still remained when the pH of the CSF was held constant by perfusion with mock CSF of appropriate bicarbonate concentration. The goats had functioning peripheral chemoreceptors which may explain why less of the total response was found to reside in the CSF receptors than in Mitchell's experiments. There is also the important consideration of species difference since the relative importance of peripheral and central chemoreceptors is known to differ markedly between certain species. The rather small differences between the results of Mitchell and Pappenheimer do not conflict with the general conclusion that the medullary response to carbon dioxide can be expressed as a linear function of the hydrogen ion concentration of the cerebral extracellular fluid (ECF) somewhere close beneath the surface of the ventral aspect of the medulla.

It is not yet clear what is the relative importance of the factors govening pH and bicarbonate concentration of the ECF in this area. Probably the most important factor is the CSF bicarbonate, since it appears that the CSF is able to penetrate into the spaces between the glial cells without crossing any barrier to the free diffusion of ions. Other possible factors are the blood bicarbonate and the extent of active transport of ions across the blood–brain barrier which is interposed between the capillaries and the chemoreceptor areas.

It is probably deceptive to imagine clear-cut models of the receptors and their relationship to blood vessels and bulk CSF. The receptors presumably occupy an area of finite thickness and some of them must be closer to the surface than others. Furthermore, the CSF does not have the same composition in all areas. The brain weeps ECF out into the CSF and, beneath the pia, factors such as blood bicarbonate, intracellular buffers and active transport mechanisms must clearly be important. One cannot expect to control the composition of the CSF in these areas by the experimental perfusion of the cisterna.

It is unlikely that the last word has yet been written on this subject, and in a later paper Fencl, Miller and Pappenheimer (1966) reached the following conclusions.

1. In the resting state, without hypoxic drive, the log of the pulmonary ventilation is directly proportional to the hydrogen ion concentration of the CSF, which they considered equal to the concentration in the interstitial fluid in contact with respiratory neurones.
2. This relationship was unaltered by large changes in bicarbonate concentration of blood or CSF.
3. Respiratory adaptations to chronic acidosis or alkalosis are accounted for quantitatively by observed changes in ion transport between blood and CSF.
4. Concentration gradients of bicarbonate between blood and CSF are maintained by an ion pump at the blood–brain barrier. Brain interstitial fluid and CSF are in diffusion equilibrium with one another and there are no significant bicarbonate, chloride or hydrogen ion concentration gradients between them.

It should also be noted that Cozine and Ngai (1967), working with unanaesthetized (decerebrate) cats with denervated peripheral chemoreceptors, found that apnoea did not follow the application of local anaesthetics to the central chemoreceptor areas on the antero-lateral surface of the medulla, although the minute volume of ventilation was reduced. In anaesthetized cats apnoea was obtained. These studies suggested that the influence of the central chemoreceptors was at least shared with other zones, possibly more deeply placed.

Effect of hypoxia.   Unlike the peripheral chemoreceptors, the central chemoreceptors are not stimulated by hypoxia. In fact, the central respiratory neurones are depressed by hypoxia, and apnoea follows severe medullary hypoxia whether due to ischaemia or hypoxaemia.

Quantitative aspects of the chemical control of breathing

Integration of the chemical factors controlling breathing has been a recurrent and challenging problem of respiratory physiology. It was at one time thought that the various factors interacted so that the resultant ventilation depended on the algebraic sum of the individual factors caused by changes of P_{CO_2}, P_{O_2}, pH, etc. Hypoxia and hypercapnia were, for example, thought to be simply additive in their effect. It is now realized that the interactions between P_{CO_2} and P_{O_2} are far more complex (Lloyd and Cunningham, 1963) and exercise complicates the position further. The P_{O_2}/ventilation response curve will now be considered together with factors which modify it. The P_{CO_2}/ventilation response curve will then receive similar treatment.

The P_{O_2}/ventilation response curve has already been mentioned above. The thick continuous line in *Figure 14* represents a typical normal response, but it must be stressed that there are very wide individual variations, including absence of response at normal P_{O_2} (page 36). The curve may conveniently be considered as a rectangular hyperbola which is asymptotic to the ventilation at high P_{O_2} and to the P_{O_2} at which ventilation theoretically becomes infinite (a parameter usually known as '*C*'). The ventilatory response to P_{O_2} may then be expressed as $W/(P_{O_2} - C)$, where W is a multiplier (i.e. the gain of the system). The ventilatory response would be the difference between the actual ventilation and the ventilation at high P_{O_2}, the P_{CO_2} being unchanged. Others have suggested that the P_{O_2}/ventilation response curve be considered as an exponential function but curve-fitting to available data will not give a clear-cut answer as to which model is the better.

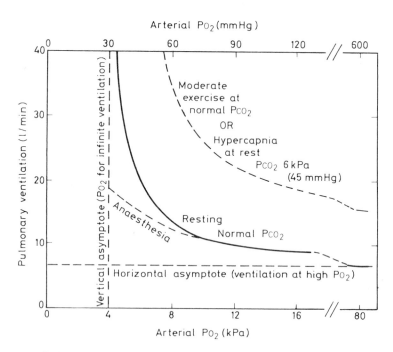

Figure 14. The heavy curve represents the normal P_{O_2}/ventilation response curve at constant (normal) P_{CO_2}. It has the form of a rectangular hyperbola asymptotic to the ventilation at high P_{O_2} and the P_{O_2} at which ventilation becomes infinite. The curve is displaced upwards by both hypercapnia and exercise at normal P_{CO_2}. The curve is depressed by anaesthetics. See text for references

The ventilatory response to hypoxia may be enhanced under either of two circumstances and the upper broken line in *Figure 14* is typical of the enhanced response which may be obtained in man. The first factor causing enhancement is elevated P_{CO_2} (Cormack, Cunningham and Gee, 1957). This effect is well marked and the line in *Figure 14* would correspond to a P_{CO_2} of about 6 kPa (45 mm Hg). This interaction (shown by the broken line 'B' in *Figure 13*) contributes to the ventilatory response in asphyxia being greater than the sum of the response to be expected from the rise in P_{CO_2} and the fall in P_{O_2} considered separately.

The response to hypoxia is also enhanced by exercise even if the P_{CO_2} is not raised (Weil et al., 1972). This may be due to lactacidosis, oscillations of P_{CO_2} or perhaps to catecholamine secretion. The upper broken line in *Figure 14* would also correspond to the response during exercise at an oxygen consumption of about 800 ml/min. Insufficient data exist to define the difference in the form of the curves obtained during hypercapnia and exercise but the general shapes appear roughly similar. It is important to note that the slope of the curve at normal P_{O_2} is considerably increased under both these circumstances and thus there will be an appreciable 'hypoxic' drive to ventilation. Enhanced response to P_{O_2} during exercise appears to be an important component in the over-all ventilatory response to exercise which is considered further below.

Figure 14 also shows the depression of the P_{O_2}/ventilation response curve resulting from halothane anaesthesia in dogs (Weiskopf, Raymond and Severinghaus, 1974). Assuming this also occurs in man, it is clearly of considerable practical importance. Hirshman et al. (1975) have reported substantial loss of hypoxic response in some but not all subjects receiving pentobarbitone (2 mg/kg). It now appears that the earlier belief that the hypoxic ventilatory drive was resistant to anaesthetics was incorrect and the anaesthetist must be prepared to take over the role of the peripheral chemoreceptors which are likely to be depressed by his drugs.

The P_{CO_2}/*ventilation response curve* is linear over the range which is usually studied. It may therefore be defined in terms of the parameters slope and intercept (see Lloyd, Jukes and Cunningham, 1958):

$$\text{ventilation} = S\,(P_{CO_2} - B)$$

where S is the slope (1 min^{-1} kPa^{-1} or 1 min^{-1} mm Hg^{-1}) and B is the intercept at zero ventilation (kPa or mm Hg). The heavy continuous line in *Figure 15* is a typical normal curve with an intercept (B) of about 4·8 kPa (36 mm Hg) and a slope (S) of about 15 l min^{-1} kPa^{-1} (2 l/min/mm Hg). There is in fact a very wide individual variation in P_{CO_2}/ventilation response curves and it may be flattened by disease (page 116) or by drugs (*see* below). Actual values of P_{CO_2} and ventilation depend on the inspired carbon dioxide concentration and the metabolic rate. The broken line in *Figure 15* shows the relationship between arterial P_{CO_2} and ventilation in the resting state when the inspired carbon dioxide concentration is negligible. It is, in fact, the P_{CO_2} in response to changing ventilation (as in *Figure 65a*) and is a section of a rectangular hyperbola. The normal resting P_{CO_2} and ventilation is indicated by the intersection of this curve with the normal P_{CO_2}/ventilation response curve, which is obtained by varying the carbon dioxide concentration in the inspired gas.

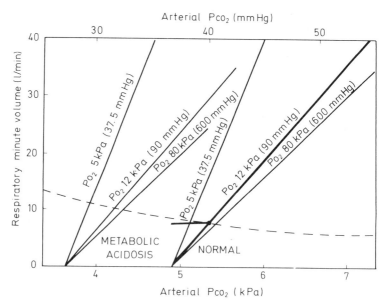

Figure 15. Two fans of PCO_2/*ventilation response curves at different values of* PO_2. *The right-hand fan is at normal metabolic acid–base state (zero base excess). The left-hand fan represents metabolic acidosis. The broken line represents the* PCO_2 *produced by the indicated ventilation for zero inspired* PCO_2, *at basal metabolic rate. The intersection of the broken curve and any response curve indicates the resting* PCO_2 *and ventilation for the relevant metabolic acid–base state and* PO_2. *The heavy curve is the normal curve. For details, see text.*

Slopes and intercepts of PCO_2/*ventilation response curves are subject to very wide individual variation. The curves in this diagram are only intended to indicate general principles and considerable deviations may be found in healthy subjects*

Reference has been made above to the influence of the chemoreceptor drive from PO_2 on the central ventilatory response to PCO_2 (broken line 'A' in *Figure 13*). Typical quantitative relationships are shown in *Figure 15,* with hypoxia at the left of the fan and hyperoxia on the right. The curve marked PO_2 80 kPa represents total abolition of chemoreceptor drive obtained by the inhalation of 100 per cent oxygen. A similar result follows carotid endarterectomy which usually results in destruction of the carotid bodies (Mitchell et al., 1964; Wade et al., 1970). This provides important evidence that the respiratory drive from the peripheral chemoreceptors is almost entirely from the carotid bodies, with the aortic bodies having little respiratory effect.

Metabolic acidosis displaces the whole fan of curves to the left as shown in *Figure 15.* The intercept (B) is reduced but the slope of the curves at each value of PO_2 is virtually unaltered.

The PCO_2/ventilation response curve is the most valuable approach to the study of factors influencing chemical control of breathing because it takes carbon dioxide into full account and PCO_2 is the most important factor of all. The effect of drugs, for example, is best expressed in terms of changes in slope and intercept.

It should, however, be stressed that the PCO_2/ventilation response curve is the response of the entire respiratory system to the challenge of a raised PCO_2. Apart from reduced sensitivity of the central chemoreceptors, the over-all response may be blunted by neuromuscular blockade, obstructive or restrictive lung disease (*see Figure 67*). These factors must be taken into account in drawing conclusions from a reduced response, and diffuse airway obstruction is a most important consideration (Clark, Clarke and Hughes, 1966).

Extensions to the response curves are shown in *Figure 15* below the dotted curve which defines the effect of ventilation on PCO_2. These extensions are of two types. The first is an extrapolation of the curve to intersect the X axis (zero ventilation) at a PCO_2 sometimes known as the apnoeic threshold PCO_2. If PCO_2 is depressed below this point, apnoea may result, particularly in the anaesthetized patient, and the extension of the curve is a graphical representation of Haldane's post-hyperventilation apnoea. The second type of extension is horizontal and to the left, like a golf club, representing the response of the subject who continues to breathe regardless of the fact that his PCO_2 has been reduced. This has been discussed above in relation to wakefulness, but persistent breathing is much more likely to occur in hypoxia.

If PCO_2 is raised above about 10·7 kPa (80 mm Hg), the linear relationship between PCO_2 and ventilation is lost. As PCO_2 is raised a point of maximal ventilatory stimulation is reached (probably within the range 13·3–26·7 kPa or

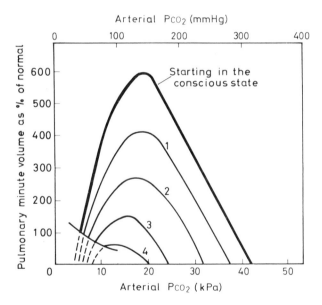

Figure 16. The probable form of complete PCO_2/ventilation response curves carried through to the point of apnoea. Such curves have never been obtained in man and their form is inferred from work on dogs (see text). The heavy curve is the probable form which would be obtained starting in conscious man without additional anaesthesia other than carbon dioxide itself. Curves 1–4 show the likely form which would be obtained in various depths of anaesthesia. Curve 4 is probably similar to that which would be obtained with 2–2·5 per cent halothane (end-expiratory concentration). The broken lines show extrapolation back to apnoeic threshold PCO_2. Rather similar curves have recently been produced for the cat anaesthetized with dial-urethane (Raymond and Standaert, 1967). Apnoea was not obtained and the lowest ventilation was about 50 per cent of control at PCO_2 of about 53 kPa (400 mm Hg)

100–200 mm Hg). Thereafter the ventilatory stimulation is reduced until, at very high P_{CO_2}, the ventilation is actually depressed below control value and finally apnoea results, at least in the dog and almost certainly in man as well. It does not appear to be possible to arrest breathing in the cat by this means in spite of elevation of P_{CO_2} to more than 67 kPa or 500 mm Hg (Hornbein, personal communication; Raymond and Standaert, 1967). The full P_{CO_2}/ventilation curve is thus something like a parabola rising from the apnoeic threshold P_{CO_2} (4·9 kPa or 37 mm Hg), reaching a peak at about 20 kPa (150 mm Hg) and returning to base line at a P_{CO_2} of the order of 40 kPa (300 mm Hg). Few examples of complete P_{CO_2}/ventilation response curves throughout the full range have been published and ethical consideration preclude such studies in man. The general form of the curve is, however, probably not unlike the thick curve in *Figure 16* which is derived from a study of dogs (Graham, Hill and Nunn, 1960). The other curves in *Figure 16* show the progressive modifications occurring with anaesthesia of graded depth (*see* below). The effects of changes in P_{CO_2} on ventilation are also discussed in Chapter 11 (page 366).

The response curves above have been described in relation to arterial P_{CO_2}. It seems likely that internal jugular or CSF P_{CO_2} might be more appropriate and these have been shown to give particularly straight curves. Alternatively, in the clinical environment it may be more convenient to use end-expiratory P_{CO_2} as a substitute for arterial P_{CO_2} although this is not satisfactory in conditions such as chronic bronchitis, which are associated with a marked arterial/end-expiratory P_{CO_2} difference (*see* Chapter 11). Methods of obtaining response curves are summarized at the end of this chapter.

Effect of drugs and anaesthetics. Displacement of the P_{CO_2}/ventilation response curve is probably the best way of defining the 'depressant' or 'stimulant' effect of a drug on ventilation. Determination of the effect of a drug on the response curve is far more informative than simple measurements of ventilation or P_{CO_2}, without regard to the interaction of these two variables. For example, decrease in ventilation may simply reflect a decrease in metabolic rate without any true depression of breathing.

Stimulant drugs have an effect on the P_{CO_2}/ventilation response curve which is similar to hypoxia (*Figure 15*). Mitchell and Herbert (1975) found that, in the cat, graded doses of doxapram produced results which were equal to graded degrees of hypoxia; 3·0 mg/kg, for example, increased integrated phrenic nerve activity to the same extent as a reduction of P_{O_2} to 4·7 kPa (35 mm Hg). Following carotid and aortic body denervation, doxapram had no stimulant effect until a non-specific response was obtained at doses above 6 mg/kg. Aminophylline has a broadly similar effect on the P_{CO_2}/ventilation response curve. It seems likely that doxapram acts by stimulation on the peripheral chemoreceptors. This effect is apparent below the doses which cause general arousal of the central nervous system and, since the response to infusion is sustained, doxapram seems to have a most important role in the pharmacological control of breathing, particularly assistance in difficult cases of weaning from artificial ventilation (page 195).

Inhalational anaesthetics tend to decrease the slope of the P_{CO_2}/ventilation response curve and increase the intercept on the P_{CO_2} axis (*Figure 16*).

The degree of change is a function of the dose of the depressant agent and

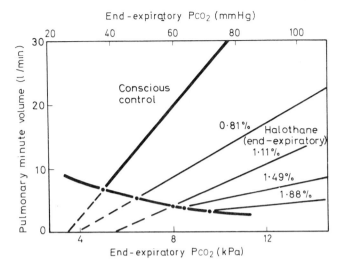

Figure 17. Displacement of PCO_2/*ventilation response curve with different end-expiratory concentrations of halothane. The curve sloping down to the right indicates the pathway of* PCO_2 *and ventilation change resulting from depression without the challenge of exogenous carbon dioxide. The dotted lines indicate extrapolation of apnoeic threshold* PCO_2. *The curves have been constructed from the data of Munson et al. (1966). It will be noted that their curve for the conscious state differs from the normal shown in Figure 15. There is, in fact, wide divergence in the values for slope reported by different workers. A rather similar set of curves has been obtained for methoxyflurane by Dunbar, Ovassapian and Smith (1967) except that these workers did not observe the same degree of displacement to the right of the initial* PCO_2 *at different depths of anaesthesia before the carbon dioxide challenge. Roughly similar changes in slope were reported for equipotent concentrations of the two agents*

itself may be represented on a dose/response curve. Graded effects may be typically produced by halothane, and *Figure 17* has been constructed from the data of Munson et al. (1966). They demonstrated qualitatively similar changes with fluroxene and cyclopropane. Essential points to be noted in *Figure 17* are as follows.

1. Starting points are displaced to the right by deepening anaesthesia along the ventilation/PCO_2 relationship curve. This indicates a rising PCO_2 with a falling ventilation.

2. When challenged with exogenous (or rebreathed endogenous) carbon dioxide, the slope of the PCO_2/ventilation curve is progressively diminished as the anaesthesia is deepened. Finally, the curve becomes flat and there is then no ventilatory response to PCO_2. Beyond this point a negative slope may be found which would mean that an elevation of PCO_2 would depress breathing.

3. The intersection of the extrapolation of the curve on the X axis moves to the right with the curve. The apnoeic threshold PCO_2 is thus raised with deepening anaesthesia.

Full PCO_2/ventilation response curves throughout the range of PCO_2 have very seldom been studied in the anaesthetized state. Data of Graham, Hill and Nunn (1960) and of Merkel, Eger and Severinghaus (quoted in Severinghaus and

Larson, 1965) suggest that curves would have the general form shown in *Figure 16*. Actual values relevant to man are not known and the numbers on the curves simply indicate arbitrary depths of anaesthesia. However, curve 4 is probably similar to that which would be obtained with 2–2·5 per cent halothane (end-expiratory concentration).

In the case of the inhalational anaesthetic agents it is useful to know whether there are significant differences in their respiratory depressant effects, considered in relation to their anaesthetic effects. The most useful approach has been to relate changes in the slope of the P_{CO_2}/ventilation response curve to the concentrations of the different anaesthetics represented on an iso-narcotic scale. This has been done by using multiples of the minimal alveolar concentration required for anaesthesia (MAC—see Saidman and Eger, 1964). The results (*Figure 18*) show halothane and methoxyflurane to be the most depressant agents and cyclopropane and diethyl ether the least (Larson et al., 1969).

Ventilatory effects of inhalational anaesthetic agents are unlikely to be simply a matter of 'central depression of respiratory neurones'. Ether and cyclopropane are known to raise the level of circulating catecholamines, and noradrenalin is known to increase the slope of the P_{CO_2}/ventilation response curve (Cunningham et al., 1963; Dejours, 1966). However, Muallam, Larson and

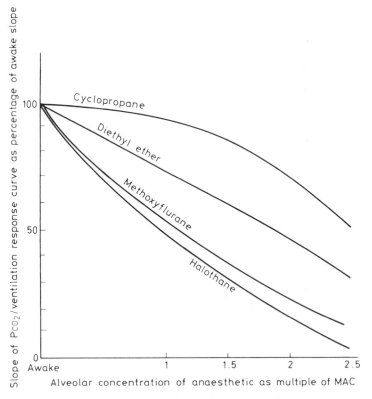

Figure 18. Depression of the slope of the awake P_{CO_2}/ventilation response curve by increasing concentrations of various anaesthetics. The concentrations of the anaesthetics are presented on an equi-narcotic scale as multiples of the minimal alveolar concentration (MAC) required for anaesthesia. (Redrawn from the data of Larson et al. (1969))

Eger (1969) did not find any change in the P_{CO_2} of dogs anaesthetized with ether when they were subjected to vagotomy and high spinal anaesthesia. Ether, furthermore, has a curare-like effect upon neuromuscular transmission in high dosage and may also stimulate ventilation as a result of the development of an arousal state in response to its irritant vapour. Different agents vary greatly in the degree to which they sensitize the pulmonary stretch receptors (*see* page 53), although the relevance of this is not clear. It has now been clearly shown that surgical stimulus will restore a P_{CO_2}/ventilation response curve displaced by a general anaesthetic (Eger et al., 1972). During prolonged anaesthesia without surgical stimulation, there is no progressive change in the response curve up to 3 hours, but some restoration towards the pre-anaesthetic position of the curve has been reported after 6 hours (Fourcade et al., 1972). Impairment of ventilation is greater during anaesthesia of patients with chronic obstructive lung disease (Pietak et al., 1975).

Barbiturates have little effect upon ventilation in sedative or light 'sleep dosage'. However, larger doses which are sufficient to abolish the motor response to skin incisions are probably associated with similar changes to those shown for halothane in *Figure 17* (Bellville and Seed, 1960). Opiates are well known to depress ventilation and, at high dosage, reduction in respiratory frequency is particularly marked. In normal clinical dosage, both tidal volume and frequency are reduced with an increase of resting P_{CO_2} of about 0·4 kPa (3 mm Hg) after 10 mg of morphine and 0·5 kPa (4 mm Hg) after 150 mg of pethidine (Loeschcke et al., 1953). Loeschcke's data may be interpreted as a reduction in slope of P_{CO_2}/ventilation response curve (S) without change in intercept (B), although they did not draw this conclusion in the case of morphine. At higher dosage of morphine, a well marked reduction in slope becomes apparent, with the general effect being again broadly similar to the family of curves shown for halothane in *Figure 17*.

Johnstone et al. (1974) described the ventilatory effect of very large doses of morphine (2 mg/kg) which, when infused over 20 minutes, did not produce respiratory arrest. There was very wide individual variation in the results but the slope of the P_{CO_2}/ventilation response curves were reduced to a mean value of 20 per cent of the control values and the mean intercept on the P_{CO_2} axis was increased to 6·7 kPa (50 mm Hg). Even at this dosage, naloxone resulted in a substantial increase in the slope of the P_{CO_2}/ventilation response curve and a decrease in the P_{CO_2} intercept. Engineer and Jennett (1972) have reported the ventilatory response to pentazocine and pethidine. They also found a reduction in slope of the response curve but reached a point at which further increase in dosage of pentazocine had little further effect on the slope. Taken in conjunction with the study of Johnstone and his colleagues, there is support for the view that there may be a 'ceiling' to the degree of ventilatory depression which can be produced by increasing dosage of opiates. Evans et al. (1974) reported that naloxone produced a well defined reversal of the respiratory depression produced by morphine (0·43 mg/kg) but the action of the morphine outlasted the effect of the naloxone which required repeat doses.

Sleep causes slight reduction in slope of the P_{CO_2}/ventilation response curve, with the degree depending upon the depth of sleep, estimates of P_{CO_2} elevation ranging from zero to 1·2 kPa (9 mm Hg). Response to hypoxia is unimpaired by sleep. This is fortunate since continued hyperventilation is essential for survival at altitude.

ARP–3

REFLEX CONTROL OF BREATHING

Certain reflexes have already been discussed. Firstly, there are the reflex arcs with afferent limbs arising in the peripheral chemoreceptors which have been considered under the heading of chemical control (page 35). Secondly, there is the ventilatory response to pain, which has already been considered in relation to the arousal state which is caused by pain. There remain, however, a number of neural control mechanisms which are more appropriately considered specifically under the heading of reflexes.

Baroreceptor reflexes

The most important groups of arterial baroreceptors are in the carotid sinus and around the aortic arch. These receptors are primarily concerned with regulation of the circulation but a decrease in pressure produces hyperventilation, while a rise in pressure causes respiratory depression and, in the limit, apnoea (Heymans and Neil, 1958). This is the likely cause of apnoea produced by a massive dose of catecholamines. Baroreceptors are sensitized by diethyl ether (Robertson, Swann and Whitteridge, 1956), cyclopropane (Price and Widdicombe, 1962) and halothane (Biscoe and Millar, 1964). This effect has been considered mainly in relation to circulatory control during anaesthesia and the respiratory implications are not yet established.

Pulmonary stretch reflexes

There are a large number of different types of receptors in the lungs (see review by Widdicombe, 1964) sensitive to inflation, deflation, mechanical and chemical stimulation. Afferents from all are conducted by the vagus, although some fibres may be additionally carried in the sympathetic. The stretch receptors of the small air passages and alveoli are of great interest in the control of breathing, and have seldom been far from the centre of the stage since the associated inflation and deflation reflexes were described by Hering (1868) and Breuer (1868).

It is perhaps appropriate at this point to explain the relationship between these two authors who produced two papers of identical title in the same journal from the same department in the same year. Breuer was a clinical assistant and apparently the work was at his own instigation. However, Hering who was a corresponding member of the Vienna Academy of Science published Breuer's work under his own name, in accord with the custom of the time. Breuer's role was clearly stated in Hering's paper but he was not a co-author. Later the same year, Breuer was able to publish a much fuller account of his work under his own name. The extent of the individual contributions of Hering and Breuer has been discussed by Ullmann (1970) who also appended an English translation of the original papers.

The inflation reflex consists of inhibition of inspiration in response to a sustained inflation of the lung. An exactly similar effect may be obtained by obstructing expiration so that an inspiration is retained in the lungs. It has been explained above that, at least in animals, rhythmic breathing may be governed by a negative feedback loop from the pulmonary stretch receptors via the vagus and the expiratory neurones of the medulla (*see Figure 10*).

Generations of medical students have been brought up with the unquestioned belief in the role of the Hering–Breuer reflex in man. This appears to have resulted from an unwarranted extrapolation of animal findings to man without regard for species difference. Widdicombe (1961) compared the strength of the inflation reflex in eight species and found the reflex weakest in man. His method for the human subjects was to weight the bell of a spirometer connected to spontaneously breathing, lightly anaesthetized patients. Inflation to trans-pulmonary pressures of 0·7–1·1 kPa (7–11 cm H$_2$0)* did not produce apnoea lasting longer than 10 seconds, in contrast to the rabbit in which increases of transpulmonary pressure of 0·5–0·7 kPa (5–7 cm H$_2$O) on two occasions killed rabbits by asphyxia during the prolonged apnoea that followed. Widdicombe's traces show some reduction of tidal volume in the human subjects but the movement of a weighted spirometer bell at an increased lung volume is a very indirect measure of inspiratory effort.

The view that the Hering–Breuer inflation reflex is weak if not absent in man is supported by the response of anaesthetized patients to expiratory resistance. This is discussed at some length on pages 126–127, but the essential feature is that the patients respond by an increased inspiratory force until the lung volume is increased to the point at which the increased elastic recoil is sufficient to overcome the expiratory resistance (Campbell, Howell and Peckett, 1957). With high resistance the lung volume increases in a series of steps, with ever-increasing end-inspiratory pressure associated with increasing inspiratory effort (Nunn and Ezi-Ashi, 1961). This remarkable series of changes, which can be confirmed by any anaesthetist, provides clear evidence that lung inflation in the anaesthetized human subject augments the force of contraction of the inspiratory muscles in complete contrast to what might be expected if the effect of the Hering–Breuer inflation reflex were dominant. This provides no proof of the absence of the inflation reflex, but shows that its effect, if present, is overcome by other mechanisms producing an opposite effect. The role of the spindles has been discussed earlier in this chapter (page 33) and on page 127.

It has been shown in cats that the common inhalational anaesthetics, particularly trichloroethylene, sensitize the pulmonary stretch receptors and so would be expected to cause an enhancement of the inflation reflex (Whitteridge and Bülbring, 1944). This is in contrast to Head's conclusion (1889) that ether and chloroform paralysed vagal endings. Whitteridge and Bülbring concluded that the sensitization of the stretch receptors was largely responsible for the shallow breathing seen in trichloroethylene anaesthesia, but observed that trichloroethylene and cyclopropane could have opposite effects on respiratory rate while both agents were causing sensitization of stretch receptors. They further stated that these agents 'must exert another action on a second set of pulmonary endings, or on the respiratory centre, or on extra-pulmonary endings'. Ngai, Katz and Farhie (1965) showed that, in midcollicular decerebrate cats, the marked tachypnoea produced by trichloroethylene was not prevented by bilateral vagotomy and carotid denervation. It would, therefore, seem that there is no solid foundation for the oft repeated view that trichloroethylene causes tachypnoea as a result of sensitization of the pulmonary stretch receptors.

* 1 kilopascal (1 kPa) is approximately equal to 10 centimetres of water (10 cm H$_2$O).

The deflation reflex consists of an augmentation of inspiration in response to deflation of the lung. Guz et al. (1971) studied the effect of sudden unilateral lung deflation in four patients with spontaneous pneumothorax. This was painless, but all patients developed tachypnoea and arterial Po_2 decreased. Breath holding times were decreased and the ventilatory response to carbon dioxide was increased in two patients. Guz concluded that the results were consistent with the hypothesis that lung deflation has a reflex excitatory effect on breathing but that the threshold is higher than for other mammalian species. The deflation reflex in the rabbit is blocked by breathing a local anaesthetic aerosol (Jain et al., 1973)

The inflation and deflation reflexes were the basis of the Selbststeuerung (self-steering) hypothesis advanced by Hering and Breuer in 1868. This concept has played a major role in theories of the control of breathing and, even though its role in man may be questionable, it remains a classical example of a physiological autoregulating mechanism.

Head's paradoxical reflex. Head (1889), working in Professor Hering's laboratory, described a reversal of the inflation reflex, which could be elicited during partial block of the vagus nerves in the course of thawing after cold block. Under these conditions, inflation of the lung of the rabbit causes strong maintained contractions of an isolated diaphragmatic slip (Curve VI, Plate I in Head, 1889). Many authors have reported that, with normal vagal conduction, sudden inflation of the lungs of many species may cause a transient inspiratory effort before the onset of apnoea due to the inflation reflex (Widdicombe, 1961). A similar response may also be elicited in newborn infants (Cross et al., 1960), but it has not been established whether this 'gasp reflex' is analogous to Head's paradoxical reflex. Widdicombe was unable to detect the response in patients anaesthetized with thiopentone but many anaesthetists will know that the response may be elicited in patients who receive opiates (particularly pethidine) in dosage sufficient to reduce the respiratory frequency to less than about five breaths per minute. Transient compression of the reservoir bag often causes an immediate deep gasping type of inspiration and the respiratory frequency may be conveniently raised by manual triggering. This response does not appear to have been studied in detail in anaesthetized man. There is a possible relationship between the reflex and the mechanism of sighing which may be considered a normal feature of breathing (Bendixen, Smith and Mead, 1964).

The cough reflex

The cough reflex may be elicited by mechanical stimuli arising in the larynx, trachea, carina and main bronchi. Chemical stimuli are effective at a lower level (Widdicombe, 1964). The central co-ordination of the motor activity is little understood and the response is complex:

1. an inspiration, which takes into the lungs a volume of air sufficient for the expiratory activity;
2. build-up of pressure in the lungs by contraction of expiratory muscles against a closed glottis;
3. forceful expiration through narrowed airways with high *linear* velocity of gas flow which sweeps irritant material up towards the pharynx.

Irritant receptors have been reviewed by Mills, Sellick and Widdicombe (1970).

The mechanism of the narrowing of the airways is discussed in Chapter 4 (Page 114). Transient changes of pressure up to 40 kPa (300 mm Hg) may occur in the thorax, arterial blood and the CSF during the act of coughing (Sharpey-Schafer, 1953).

Other pulmonary afferents

Pulmonary embolization and pneumothorax may each cause rapid shallow breathing by a reflex arc with afferents carried in the vagi. Changes in blood-gas tensions may also produce secondary changes in ventilation. The pattern of discharge of medullary neurones in these conditions has been reported by Katz and Horres (1972).

J receptors. Paintal (1970) has reviewed his work on the juxtapulmonary capillary receptors (J receptors, for short) which appear to be stimulated by pulmonary capillary distension, and also by inhalational anaesthetics including halothane. Afferent fibres are in the vagi of the same side. These receptors may well be concerned in the dyspnoea of pulmonary vascular congestion and the ventilatory response to exercise and pulmonary embolization. J receptors have been characterized in physiological studies but have never been identified histologically.

Afferents from the musculoskeletal system

Kalia et al. (1972) have shown that a variety of mechanical stumuli applied to the gastrocnemius muscle of the dog can produce a reflex increase in ventilation. This occurred when afferents from the pressure–pain receptors were blocked by antidromic stimulation. The afferents causing stimulation of ventilation were carried by non-medullated fibres. Afferents from the musculoskeletal system probably have an important role in the hyperventilation of exercise (*see* below).

BREATH HOLDING

The understanding of the factors governing the duration of breath holding is a difficult problem which has presented a long-standing challenge to investigators. Induced apnoea is an important feature of practical anaesthesia and its consequences are discussed in various places in this book. This section is restricted to a consideration of the factors influencing the duration of voluntary breath holding.

Blood-gas tensions

When the breath is held after air breathing, the arterial P_{CO_2} is remarkably constant at the breaking point and values are normally close to 6·7 kPa (50 mm Hg). This does not mean that P_{CO_2} is the sole or dominant factor and concomitant hypoxia is probably more important. Oxygen breathing greatly

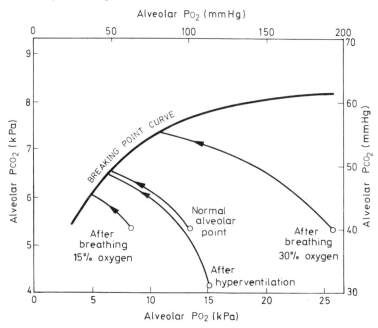

Figure 19. The 'breaking point' curve defines the coexisting values of alveolar PO_2 *and* PCO_2, *at the breaking point of breath holding, starting from various states. The normal alveolar point is shown (*PO_2 *13·3 kPa or 100 mm Hg;* PCO_2, *5·3 kPa or 40 mm Hg) and the curved arrow shows the changes in alveolar gas tensions which occur during breath holding. Starting points are displaced to the right by preliminary breathing of oxygen-enriched gas mixtures, and to the left by breathing mixtures containing less than 21 per cent oxygen. Hyperventilation displaces the point representing the alveolar gas tensions to the right and downwards. The length of the arrows from starting point to the 'breaking point' curve gives an approximate indication of the possible duration of breath holding. This can clearly be prolonged by oxygen breathing or by hyperventilation, maximal prolongation occurring after hyperventilation with 100 per cent oxygen. (Data for construction of the 'breaking point' curve have been taken from Ferris et al. (1946) and Otis, Rahn and Fenn (1948))*

delays the onset of hypoxia during breath holding and times may be considerably extended with consequent elevation of PCO_2 at the breaking point The relationship between PCO_2 and PO_2 at breaking point, after varying degrees of pre-oxygenation, is shown in *Figure 19.* The breaking point curve is displaced upwards and to the left by carotid body resection (Davidson et al., 1974). Guz et al. (1966b) observed marked prolongation of breath holding after vagal and glossopharyngeal block but advanced cogent reasons for believing that this was not due primarily to block of the chemoreceptors. Oxygen breathing would also prevent the chemoreceptor drive but this did not prolong breath holding to the same extent as the nerve block.

Lung volume

Breath-holding time is directly proportional to the lung volume at the onset of breath holding, other factors being constant. In part this is related to the onset of hypoxia, since an appreciable part of the total body oxygen store is in the alveolar gas (page 412). There are, however, other effects of lung volume and its change, which are mediated by afferents arising from both chest wall and the lung itself. Following the experiments of Guz mentioned above, Campbell et al. (1967, 1969) have reported an equally impressive prolongation of breath-holding time following curarization of conscious subjects. Their explanation is that the distress leading to the termination of breath holding is caused by *frustration* of reflex motor response from pulmonary afferents blocked in the experiment of Guz. The motor response consists of involuntary contractions of the respiratory muscles, including the diaphragm, which have been found to increase progressively during breath holding (Agostini, 1963). These contractions *should* produce movement which would be detected by joint and tendon receptors in the chest wall. However, in breath holding, movement is prevented by closure of the glottis and there is an 'inappropriateness' between the muscle activity and the (lack of) movement which results. This accords with the idea of 'inappropriateness' advanced as a general hypothesis to explain the sensation of dyspnoea (Campbell and Howell, 1963). The discomfort of breath holding would then be regarded as an extreme form of inappropriateness, differing only quantitatively from that of mechanically hindered breathing.

According to this hypothesis, the discomfort of breathing could be alleviated at the following points:

1. block of pulmonary afferents causing the involuntary contraction of the respiratory muscles (Guz et al., 1966b);
2. prevention of the involuntary contraction of the respiratory muscles (Campbell et al., 1967, 1969);
3. prevention of the *frustration* of the contractions of the respiratory muscles by permitting chest movement without alleviating the changes in alveolar P_{CO_2} and P_{O_2}.

Eisele et al. (1968) showed that spinal analgesia (affecting intercostal muscles but not the diaphragm) had no effect on breath holding. In contrast, Noble et al. (1971) showed that phrenic nerve block increased breath-holding time. It thus appears that the inappropriateness arises in the diaphragm rather than the intercostals, in spite of the paucity of afferents from the former (Corda, von Euler and Lennerstrand, 1965).

Prolongation of breath-holding time by prevention of frustration of contraction of respiratory muscles may be convincingly demonstrated by Fowler's experiment (1954). After normal air breathing, the breath is held until breaking point, which is usually about 60 seconds. If the expirate is then taken in a bag and immediately re-inhaled, there is a marked sense of relief although it may be shown that the rise of P_{CO_2} and fall of P_{O_2} is quite uninfluenced by the manoeuvre.

Extreme durations of breath holding may be attained after hyperventilation and pre-oxygenation. Times of 14 minutes have been reached and the limiting factor is then reduction of lung volume to residual volume as oxygen is removed from the alveolar gas by the circulating pulmonary blood (Klocke and Rahn, 1959).

EXERCISE

During exercise, ventilation is well matched to the increased oxygen consumption. It has long been clear that the increase in ventilation cannot be explained by changes in the mean level of arterial P_{CO_2} and P_{O_2}, which are the most important factors in the resting state. In fact, during moderate exercise, the P_{CO_2} is usually below and P_{O_2} above the resting level. Nevertheless, the threshold of the central chemoreceptors to P_{CO_2} is reduced by many factors which operate during exercise so that P_{CO_2} drives ventilation more effectively although the actual level of P_{CO_2} is not appreciably raised. In effect the P_{CO_2}/ventilation response curve is moved to the left as in *Figure 15*. The additional factors include raised body temperature and lactacidosis (Bannister, Cunningham and Douglas, 1954). For example, in the post-operative period, Bay, Nunn and Prys-Roberts (1968) showed that pulmonary ventilation was much greater in shivering patients although the mean values for arterial blood gases were almost identical for shivering and non-shivering patients. However, the former group had a lactacidosis which was just about sufficient to explain the difference in ventilation which matched oxygen consumption in both groups.

Even though arterial P_{O_2} is not decreased by moderate exercise at sea level, it seems likely that its effect on ventilation is enhanced by the increased oscillations in arterial P_{CO_2} which are a feature of exercise. This factor might well explain the enhanced ventilatory response to changes in P_{O_2} reported by Weil et al. (1972) to which reference has been made above (page 45).

The modified responses to P_{CO_2} and P_{O_2} together with the effect of noradrenalin are collectively known as the humoral factors and they appear sufficient to account for the greater part of the increased ventilation of exercise. They may be the sole factors during steady state exercise and during repayment of an oxygen debt after exercise (Dejours, 1964). However, there is considerable evidence that neural factors also contribute to the ventilatory drive during exercise. Reference has been made above to the observations of Kalia et al. (1972) which accord with the experiments of Kao (1963). He reported that electrical stimulation of motor nerves produced instant hyperventilation in anaesthetized animals and that there was an abrupt return of ventilation to control levels when the electrically induced exercise was terminated. Chordotomy and crossed circulation experiments showed that only neurogenic stimuli could account for his observations. It should also be noted that hyperventilation usually precedes the start of exercise in man and it seems reasonable that psychological factors should influence ventilation as they do in a wide range of emotional states.

Special considerations apply to very severe exercise, particularly at altitude. Under these conditions, the diffusing capacity of oxygen is probably insufficient for transport of oxygen and arterial hypoxaemia results. A substantial hypoxic drive would then be added to the other factors listed above (West et al., 1962b). Somewhat similar conditions apply to hypoxaemic patients with chronic bronchitis exercising at sea level. Inhalation of 30 per cent oxygen increases the arterial P_{O_2} and reduces ventilation and dyspnoea (King et al., 1973).

HIGH ALTITUDE

With increasing altitude, barometric pressure falls, but the concentration of oxygen in the air and the saturated vapour pressure of water at body temperature remain constant. Therefore the P_{O_2} of the inspired air falls to become zero when the barometric pressure has fallen to a level equal to the saturated water vapour pressure at $37°C$ at an altitude of approximately 20 000 m. Typical values are shown in *Figure 20*.

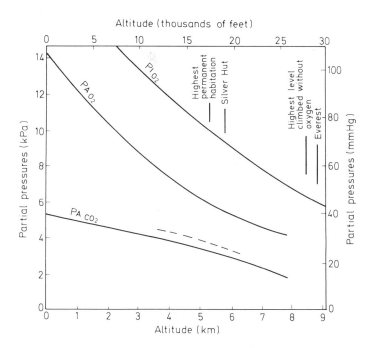

Figure 20. Changes in inspired gas PO_2 (PIO_2), alveolar PO_2 (PAO_2) and alveolar PCO_2 ($PACO_2$) with increasing altitude in acclimatized lowlanders. The broken line above the lowest curve represents observations in highlanders born at an altitude close to the altitude at which measurements were made. Note that observed barometric pressures are usually higher than the International Standard used for aviation. Values are taken from Pugh (1962) and Rahn and Otis (1949)

When a lowlander moves to high altitude, there is an immediate fall in arterial PO_2, and the resultant hypoxic drive tends to increase the ventilation. This, however, lowers the PCO_2 and the ventilatory response to hypoxia is thus diminished. This is clearly disadvantageous and the arterial PO_2 is below the level it would be were it not for this negative feedback. Many years ago, it was recognized that a secondary compensation occurred within the first few days of residence at altitude, during which the pulmonary ventilation gradually improved and the arterial PO_2 rose slightly. These changes were associated with increased tolerance to the altitude.

It had also been observed that the plasma bicarbonate fell during the early stages of residence at altitude as the kidneys compensated for the respiratory alkalosis. For many years it was thought that this metabolic compensation, by restoring the blood pH, was mainly responsible for the increase in ventilation during early acclimatization. Although the induction of a metabolic acidosis certainly increases ventilation by a leftward shift of the fan of PCO_2/ventilation response curves as shown in *Figure 15*, this was not the whole story. Renal

ARP—3*

compensation is too slow to account for the relatively rapid improvement in ventilation, and attention moved to consideration of the possibility of changes in the CSF bicarbonate, which would influence the pH of the central chemo-receptors for a given value of Pco_2. Bradley and Semple (1962) had, in another connection, already obtained evidence that the CSF bicarbonate could be regulated to control CSF pH. Michel and Milledge (1963) suggested that restoration of CSF pH, by means of bicarbonate transport, might explain the acclimatization of ventilation to altitude, a theory which they based on the observations of Merwarth and Sieker (1961). Later in 1963, Severinghaus et al. published the evidence that this was indeed the case (*see* page 40). More recently, data have been produced which show failure of full restoration of CSF pH and there is now evidence that much of the change in CSF bicarbonate levels can be attributed to passive distribution. References for these observations are cited above (page 41).

The homeostatic mechanism for CSF pH continues to function during prolonged residence at altitude (Sørensen and Milledge, 1971). In contrast, the ventilatory response to hypoxia seems to be lost in chronic hypoxaemia whether due to residence at altitude (Severinghaus, Bainton and Carcelen, 1966; Milledge and Lahiri, 1967) or due to such pathological conditions as Fallot's tetralogy. This characteristic seems to be implanted in early life and to persist after highlanders move to sea level. There is thus a tendency for native highlanders to have a higher Pco_2 and a lower Po_2 than acclimatized lowlanders at the same altitude. Nevertheless, their capacity for work is usually superior (Pugh, 1962).

Haemoglobin concentration rises with altitude so that arterial oxygen *content* after acclimatization remains close to normal up to altitudes of at least 6 000 metres. The increased blood viscosity may be responsible for the thrombotic and embolic episodes encountered on the Himalayan Scientific and Mountaineering Expedition (1960–61) at altitudes above 5 700 metres (Pugh, 1962). Haema-tocrits tend to be higher in Andean miners and have been reported to rise from 49 per cent at 3 720 m to 75 per cent at 4 820 m (Severinghaus and Carcelen, 1964). These high levels are not seen in the Himalayas and may be, in part, attributable to chronic bronchitis.

Chronic mountain sickness (Monge's disease) is endemic in the Andes among residents at altitudes in excess of 4 000 m. It is characterized by high haematocrit, cyanosis, finger clubbing, pulmonary hypertension, dyspnoea and lethargy. Such patients tend to have a particularly low or absent ventilatory response to hypoxia.

The highest permanent habitation in the world is at 5 330 m. The Himalayan Scientific Expedition set up temporary residence in the Silver Hut at 5 790 m and concluded that this was too high for satisfactory adjustment by lowlanders. All members of the expedition had loss of appetite and weight and showed general deterioration (Pugh, 1962). Andean miners declined to live in accommodation built for them at 5 790 m, preferring to live at 5 330 m and climb every day to their work.

By careful balance of acclimatization against high altitude deterioration, it has proved possible for man to reach an altitude of about 8 500 m without the use of oxygen. This is only about 350 m below the summit of Everest which, one day, will surely be climbed without the use of oxygen. Nevertheless, it seems a remarkable coincidence that the highest point on earth should be so very close to the highest altitude which it seems possible to reach without artificial aids.

ARTIFICIAL VENTILATION

During artificial ventilation of conscious patients with partial or total respiratory failure, the effector responses are in the hands of the medical attendants while afferent stimuli may still be perceived by the patients. Although patients usually complain if their arterial P_{CO_2} rises above the normal value, they are seldom satisfied by a normal value and frequently demand a ventilation which reduces the P_{CO_2} within the range $3.3-4.7$ kPa ($25-35$ mm Hg). It appears, however, that in most cases what they are seeking is a satisfying movement of the chest wall rather than hypocapnia. Thus, if apparatus dead space is added to the airway or if carbon dioxide is added to the inspired gas, the arterial P_{CO_2} may be elevated without eliciting any complaint until the P_{CO_2} exceeds the normal value (about 5.3 kPa or 40 mm Hg).

Prolonged hyperventilation with hypocapnia partly resets the CSF pH to normal (page 41), requiring the patient to continue hyperventilation during the return to spontaneous breathing. However, it is also possible for a patient to become acclimatized to a high minute volume without hypocapnia. During studies with added apparatus dead space, Smith, Spalding and Watson (1962) showed that, in the transition from artificial ventilation to spontaneous respiration, patients would endeavour to maintain the original high minute volume without regard for the P_{CO_2} which, without added apparatus dead space, would frequently fall substantially below the level maintained during artificial ventilation. In this state the patients appeared to be driven by a volume requirement and did not respond to added carbon dioxide until their P_{CO_2} was raised above the level maintained during artificial ventilation.

OUTLINE OF CLINICAL METHODS OF ASSESSMENT OF FACTORS IN CONTROL OF BREATHING

At the time of writing, it is unusual to make measurements of factors in the control of breathing other than in the course of research. For clinical purposes, ventilatory failure is detected by measurement of P_{CO_2} but, by itself, this measurement does not give any specific information on any factors in the control of breathing. However, if the measurement of P_{CO_2} is combined with simultaneous measurement of ventilation, over a range of values of P_{CO_2} (obtained by increasing the carbon dioxide concentration of the inspired gas), this gives a useful indication of the ability of the ventilatory mechanism to respond to elevation of P_{CO_2}, although the response may be modified by mechanical factors such as resistance to breathing.

The basis of the methods for determination of P_{CO_2}/ventilation response curves consists of measurement of minute volume by any convenient method (*see* Chapter 6, page 207) with various concentrations of carbon dioxide in the inspired gas, usually ranging from 0 to 5 per cent. Ventilation is usually reasonably stable within about five minutes and simultaneous measurements of ventilation and P_{CO_2} are made at that time. P_{CO_2} may be measured in arterial blood or end-expiratory gas and suitable methods are outlined at the end of Chapter 11 (page 371).

Response curves may be determined at different values of P_{O_2} but the study of a fan of curves, as in *Figure 15*, becomes excessively time consuming. Results are obtained more rapidly by keeping ventilation approximately constant while two factors are changed in opposite directions (e.g. P_{CO_2} might be raised while P_{O_2} is also raised: the P_{CO_2} stimulus would thus increase while the hypoxic drive diminished) (Lloyd and Cunningham, 1963).

Determination of the slope of the P_{CO_2}/ventilation curve has now been greatly simplified by introduction of the rebreathing technique of Read (1967). The subject rebreathes for up to four minutes from a 6-litre bag containing 7 per cent carbon dioxide and about 50 per cent oxygen, the remainder being nitrogen. The carbon dioxide concentration rises steadily during rebreathing but the oxygen concentration should remain above 30 per cent. Thus there should be no appreciable hypoxic drive and ventilation is driven by the rising arterial P_{CO_2} which should be very close to the P_{CO_2} of the gas in the bag. Ventilation is measured by any convenient means and plotted against the P_{CO_2} of the gas in the bag. Milledge, Minty and Duncalf (1974) have described an automated technique by which the P_{CO_2}/ventilation response curve is drawn on an $X-Y$ plotter.

The P_{CO_2}/ventilation response curve measured by the rebreathing technique is displaced to the right by about 0·7 kPa (5 mm Hg) compared with the steady state method, but there is good evidence that the slope of normal subjects and patients with obstructive airway disease as measured by the rebreathing technique is the same as the slope measured by the conventional steady state method (Read, 1967; Clark, 1968). However, Linton et al. (1973) have found discrepancies with metabolic acid–base disturbances and Cormack and Milledge (unpublished) have found differences after administration of the benzodiazepine derivative lorazepam.

It has been suggested by Whitelaw, Derenne and Milic-Emili (1975) that a better indication of the output of the respiratory centre may be obtained by measuring the subatmospheric pressure developed in the airways when obstructed for 0·1 seconds at the beginning of inspiration ($P_{0.1}$). This eliminates any effect due to increased airway resistance or reduced compliance and the $P_{CO_2}/P_{0.1}$ response curve is thus a better index of central sensitivity to carbon dioxide.

Chemoreceptor response may be assessed by the inhalation of four vital capacity breaths of 15 per cent carbon dioxide in nitrogen. This should be instantly followed by two or three large breaths before there is time for central chemoreceptor response.

It is fairly simple to measure the ability of an unconscious patient to respond to added external resistance to breathing. A variety of imposed resistors may be used but a simple water bubbler is often convenient (Nunn and Ezi-Ashi, 1961). The immediate response is probably an indication of the integrity of the spindle-servo-mechanism, while the secondary response is probably mediated by change in P_{CO_2}.

Inserted at reprinting of this edition

Effect of anaesthesia on the contribution of the rib cage to breathing

Tusiewicz, Bryan and Froese ((1977) *Anesthesiology*, **47**, 327) have shown that halothane greatly decreases the rib cage contribution to breathing. In conscious man this contribution makes the greater part of the total ventilatory response to raised PCO_2 and this is to a large extent lost during anaesthesia. Thus a major component of the ventilatory depression associated with halothane anaesthesia seems to result from preferential suppression of intercostal muscle function.

Chapter 3   Elastic Resistance to Ventilation

The Functional Residual Capacity (FRC)
Elastic Recoil of the Lungs
Elastic Recoil of the Thoracic Cage
Static Pressure/Volume Relationships of the Lung plus Chest Wall
Principles of Measurement of Compliance

The ventilatory function of the lungs has been extensively analysed as a physical system. This is not to deny that vital processes play an essential role in function and maintenance of structural integrity of the respiratory system, but it is nevertheless true to say that the respiratory movements of the lungs take place largely in accord with the laws of physics. The movements of the lungs themselves are passive and driven mainly by forces external to the lung. The response of the lungs to these forces is largely governed by elasticity and resistance to gas flow which can, in the first instance, best be understood in terms of a mechanophysical system.

Ventilation of the lung normally occurs in response to contraction of the respiratory muscles. Other forces may be used such as the application of intermittent positive pressure to the airways or mechanical deformation of the chest, and these may be almost equally effective. Both natural and artificial forces are employed in overcoming the resistance or hindrance of the lung/chest wall system to movement and the main sources of resistance fall into two main categories:

1. Elastic resistance of tissue and alveolar gas/liquid interface.
2. Frictional resistance to gas flow.

Additional minor sources of resistance are inertia of gas and tissue, and frictional resistance afforded by the viscous flow of tissue during deformation. Work performed on overcoming frictional resistance is dissipated as heat and lost. Work performed in overcoming elastic resistance is stored as potential energy and elastic deformation during inspiration is normally used as the source of energy for expiration.

The present chapter is concerned with the elastic resistance afforded by lungs and chest wall. These structures are arranged concentrically and their elastic resistances are therefore additive.

THE FUNCTIONAL RESIDUAL CAPACITY (FRC)*

It is convenient to start a discussion on the elastic forces by considering the functional residual capacity. This is the relaxed equilibrium volume of the lungs

* Nomenclature of lung volumes is set out in *Figure 1*.

when there is no muscle activity and no pressure difference between alveoli and atmosphere. Equilibrium is attained when the elastic recoil of the lungs is exactly balanced by the elastic recoil of the thoracic cage, which exerts its force in the opposite direction. If the thorax is opened in the paralysed patient, the lung tends to collapse but the chest wall tends to expand to a volume some 500 ml above the FRC. The equlilibrium at the FRC is analogous to two springs joined together at one end, with the other ends anchored separately to fixed points. In equilibrium, the tension in each spring is the same (*Figure 21c*).

Figure 21a shows the static balance at FRC in the upright position when the lung volume is about 3 litres. Anaesthetists and others interested in the unconscious patient are more concerned with the supine position, which is shown in *Figure 21b*. The diaphragm is pressed higher into the thorax by the weight of the viscera, resulting in a reduction of FRC to about 2·2 litres. The reduced lung volume together with the altered direction of the weight of the heart results in important changes of pressure which will be further discussed below.

Failure to recognize the important effects of changes in posture has caused some confusion in the understanding of the respiratory physiology of the anaesthetized patient. Most physiological studies in man are carried out in the upright or sitting posture and it is all too easy to extrapolate the results to anaesthetized man without regard for the effect of the change of posture. Many of the so-called abnormalities of anaesthesia may well prove to be due to nothing more than the prolonged immobility in the supine position.

The intrathoracic pressure

The inward recoil of the lungs is balanced by the outward recoil of the chest wall to produce a subatmospheric pressure in the space between these structures. It might therefore be expected that gas or tissue-fluid would accumulate in the potential space, but fluid is absent because the difference in pressure between the pleural capillaries and the pleural 'space' is normally less than the osmotic pressure of the plasma proteins. Gas is absent because the sum of the partial pressures of gases in venous blood is always less than atmospheric for reasons which are explained in Chapter 12 (page 422). Therefore there will be a pressure gradient between any gas which finds its way into the pleural cavity and the gases carried in systemic venous blood. As a result, gas loculi in the pleural cavity, or elsewhere in the body, must ultimately be absorbed.

The term 'negative intrapleural pressure' is semantically incorrect because there is no intrapleural space to exhibit a pressure and also because a 'negative pressure' is physically impossible. 'Subatmospheric pressure' is the correct term for what is often loosely described as negative pressure. The concept of intrapleural pressure is difficult to understand. If a small bubble of gas is introduced into the pleural cavity, its pressure may be measured but this will be found to vary according to the amount of gas introduced and also according to the location of the bubble (Farhi, Otis and Proctor, 1957; Banchero et al., 1967). The lungs have an over-all specific gravity of about 0·3 so that if two bubbles are introduced into the pleural cavity, one 10 cm below the other, the pressure in the lower bubble will be about 0·3 kPa (3 cm H_2O)* higher than in

---

* 1 kilopascal (1 kPa) is approximately equal to 10 centimetres of water (10 cm H_2O).

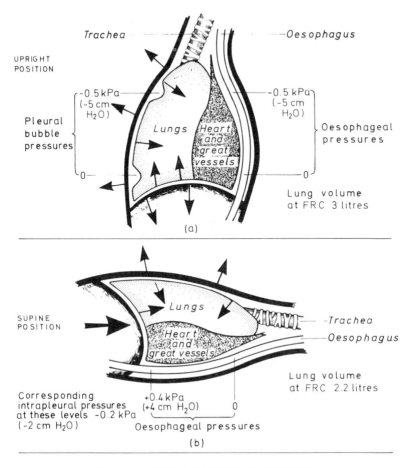

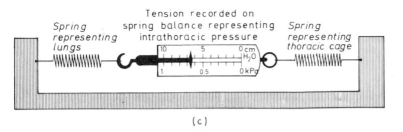

Figure 21. Intrathoracic pressures: static relationships in the resting end-expiratory position. The lung volume corresponds to the functional residual capacity (FRC). The figures in (a) and (b) indicate the pressure relative to ambient (atmospheric). The arrows show the direction of elastic forces. The heavy arrow in (b) indicates displacement of the abdominal viscera. In (c) the tension in the two springs is the same and will be indicated on the spring balance. In the supine position: (1) the FRC is reduced; (2) the intrathoracic pressure is raised; (3) the weight of the heart raises the oesophageal pressure above the intrapleural pressure

the upper bubble. Greater differences may be found in the region of the heart since the mean specific gravity of the thoracic contents approaches unity in the vicinity of the heart and great vessels.

Thus it will be seen that the 'intrapleural pressure' is not an entity with a single value unless there is a large closed pneumothorax. It is nowadays almost invariably measured as the oesophageal pressure, determined with a balloon (about 10 cm in length) passed into the middle third of the oesophagus. Details of technique have been described in two papers by Milic-Emili et al. in 1964.

Oesophageal pressure in the upright subject changes according to the point at which it is measured. The pressure rises as the balloon descends, the change being roughly in accord with the specific gravity of the lung. When the lung volume is 40 per cent of vital capacity, the pressure is about 0·5 kPa (5 cm H_2O) below mouth pressure with the balloon 32–35 cm beyond the nares, the highest point at which the indicated pressure is free from artefacts due to mouth pressure and tracheal and neck movements. When the balloon is advanced, the observed pressure rises, gradually at first, but then more rapidly, to become roughly equal to mouth pressure when the balloon is about 45–50 cm beyond the nares (Milic-Emili, Mean and Turner, 1964).

In the supine position, the lung volume is reduced and this factor alone will bring the oesophageal pressure closer to atmospheric, because the elastic recoil of the lungs is less at lower lung volume. In addition, the heart and great vessels tend to overlie the oesophagus and raise the intra-oesophageal pressure above the level of the true intrathoracic pressure at that level. Further descent of a measuring balloon down the oesophagus increases this effect as the balloon passes behind the heart (*Figure 21*) but there is usually a zone, some 32–40 cm beyond the nares where the oesophageal pressure is close to atmospheric and probably only about 0·2 kPa (2 cm H_2O) above the neighbouring intrathoracic pressure.

The effect of the weight of the mediastinal contents is found only in the supine position and not in the prone or lateral positions (Ferris, Mead and Frank, 1959). With faulty positioning of the oesophageal balloon, the effect may vary during the respiratory cycle, giving fictitiously high swings of intrathoracic pressure (Knowles, Hong and Rahn, 1959).

Factors influencing the FRC

Many studies have reported values for the FRC in normal subjects and the wide scatter of results is due, in part, to the many factors which are known to influence the FRC. The magnitude of the FRC is of considerable practical importance not least because of its relation to the closing volume (*see* below, page 70).

Body size. Most authors relate FRC to height, the relationship being linear throughout the range of normal height. Estimates range from an increase of FRC of 32 ml/cm additional height (Cotes, 1975) to 51 ml/cm (Bates, Macklem and Christie, 1971). Obesity causes a marked reduction in FRC compared with lean subjects of the same height.

Sex.   For the same body height, females have an FRC about 10 per cent less than the corresponding value in males (Bates, Macklem and Christie, 1971).

Age.   There is some difference of opinion on the effect of age. Bates, Macklem and Christie (1971) regard FRC as independent of age in the adult, while others have observed a very slight rise of FRC with increasing age (Needham, Rogan and McDonald, 1954). The nonogram of Cotes (1975) allows for a slight increase with age. Numerous measurements of lung volume in the supine position may be found in the studies of anaesthetized patients cited below. The control observations before anaesthesia may be related to age and the pooled results give no indication of any appreciable change of FRC with age.

Posture   Figure 21 shows the forces which reduce the FRC in the supine position. A very large number of studies have been reported giving a difference between upright and supine within the range 500-1000 ml (*see* Whitfield, Waterhouse and Arnott, 1950; Craig, Wahba and Don, 1971; Craig et al., 1971). Our own observations lie towards the upper part of this range and indicate that the major part of the change takes place between the angles of 0 and 60 degrees to the horizontal (*Figure 22*). Suggested mean values for subjects of 170 cm height are given in *Table 3*.

Anaesthesia.   Bergman (1963b) was the first to suggest that the FRC was reduced during anaesthesia and this has now been amply confirmed by several studies reviewed for spontaneous breathing by Hewlett et al. (1974b) and for artificial ventilation by Hewlett et al. (1974c). A further review has been undertaken by Rehder, Sessler and Marsh (1975). There is reasonable agreement on the magnitude of the change which is indicated in *Table 3*.

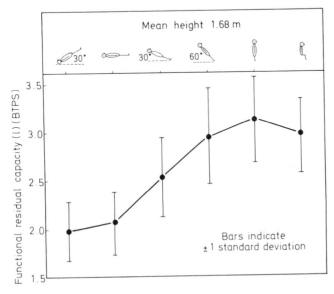

Figure 22. Studies by the author and his co-workers of the functional residual capacity in various body positions

Table 3. VALUES FOR FUNCTIONAL RESIDUAL CAPACITY

Conscious subjects

Seated		3·0 litres	(normalized for body height of 170 cm; mean of normal values from Cotes, 1975, and Bates, Macklem and Christie, 1971).
Supine	mean	2·2 litres	(mean of 125 values in volunteers and patients prior to
	SD	0·64 litres	surgery, reported in studies cited in this chapter.

Anaesthetized patients (supine) mean percentage reductions in FRC following induction of anaesthesia

Spontaneous breathing	31·4%	(Don et al., 1970)
	19·0%	(Don, Wahba and Craig, 1972)
	23·3%*	(Westbrook et al., 1973)
	12·6%	(Hickey et al., 1973)
	16·1%	(Hewlett et al., 1974b)
Mean	20·5%	
Artificial ventilation	9·0%	(Laws, 1968)
	14·0%*	(Rehder et al., 1971)
	25·0%*	(Westbrook et al., 1973)
	15·4%	(Hewlett et al., 1974c)
Mean	15·9%	

* These studies were of healthy volunteers and not patients.

The actual cause of the reduction in FRC has not been elucidated at the time of going to press but the possible explanations include an increase in elastic recoil of the lungs, contraction of alveolar muscle and loss of any pre-existing inspiratory muscle tone which persisted into late expiration. In fact, the existence of such inspiratory muscle tone has not been definitely established in conscious supine man, although the possibility remains.

Although the cause of the reduction in FRC during anaesthesia remains unknown, certain features of the phenomenon have been established.

1. The FRC does not seem to decrease progressively during anaesthesia and appears to have fallen to its final value within the first few minutes of anaesthesia (Don et al., 1970; Don, Wahba and Craig, 1972; Hewlett et al., 1974c).
2. The inhalation of high concentrations of oxygen does not appear to cause an additional reduction of FRC nor does it result in a progressive fall (Don et al., 1970; Hewlett et al., 1974b).
3. The FRC is decreased during anaesthesia, whether or not expiratory muscle activity is present (Don et al., 1970; Hewlett et al., 1974b).
4. The reduction in FRC has a weak but significant correlation with the age of the patient and also with the weight/height ratio, which itself shows a weak correlation with age (Don et al., 1970; Hewlett et al., 1974b).
5. The reduction in FRC is of the same order whether the patient breathes spontaneously or is ventilated artificially. There is only a small reduction in FRC of conscious patients who are ventilated artificially (Hewlett et al., 1974c).

6. The reduction in FRC has been observed in measurements with the technique of helium dilution, nitrogen wash-out and body plethysmography. Studies employing the last technique indicate that the changes observed with the other techniques are not artefacts of measurement nor due to an increase in the volume of trapped gas (Westbrook et al., 1973). This is confirmed by actual measurements of the volume of trapped gas during anaesthesia which increases as would be expected in consequence of the reduction of FRC but not by sufficient to *explain* the reduction in FRC (Don, Wahba and Craig, 1972).

7. There is a difference in observations made during anaesthesia in the sitting position. Rehder, Sittipong and Sessler (1972) used the nitrogen wash-out technique and found no decrease, while Shah et al. (1971) using body plethysmography found substantial and rapid falls of FRC related to the concentration of nitrous oxide inhaled.

8. The reduction of FRC continues into the post-operative period (Alexander et al., 1973).

9. For individual patients, the reduction in FRC correlates well with an increase in the alveolar–arterial P_{O_2} gradient during anaesthesia with spontaneous breathing (Hickey et al., 1973), anaesthesia with artificial ventilation (Hewlett et al., 1974c) and in the post-operative period (Alexander et al., 1973). The likely mechanism for this is discussed below (pages 117 and 292).

10. The reduced FRC may be restored to normal or above normal by the application of positive end-expiratory pressure although this has disappointing effects upon the arterial P_{O_2} (Whyche et al., 1973).

11. The FRC would undoubtedly be reduced by pulmonary collapse but there is at present no evidence that this is the cause of the reduction in FRC observed in uncomplicated anaesthesia.

12. After the induction of anaesthesia, with or without paralysis, the diaphragm moves up into the chest by an amount which roughly accords with the observed reduction in FRC (Froese and Bryan, 1974). These authors concluded that the explanation was loss of inspiratory muscle tone which they believe continues into the expiratory phase in the conscious subject in the supine position. This could result from a reflex mechanism to minimize the reduction in FRC on changing from the upright to the supine position.

Pathological changes in elastic recoil of the respiratory system

The FRC will be reduced by increased elastic recoil of lungs, chest wall or both. Possible causes include diverse conditions such as fibrosing alveolitis (pulmonary fibrosis), organized fibrinous pleurisy, kyphoscoliosis, obesity and scarring of the thorax following burns. Conversely, elastic recoil is diminished in emphysema and asthma, both conditions in which the expiratory airway resistance is predominant (Finucane and Colebatch, 1969).

In emphysema there is an increase of static lung compliance due to destruction of alveolar septa. In asthma, the compliance is only marginally increased but there is an upward displacement of the transmural pressure/lung volume curve (*see Figure 28*).

*The functional residual capacity in relation to closing capacity**

In Chapters 4 and 9 it is explained how reduction in lung volume below a certain level results in absolute or relative underventilation of the dependent parts of the lung, with resultant suboxygenation of the blood perfusing those areas. The lung volume at which this phenomenon first becomes apparent is known as the closing capacity (CC) and rises with increasing age, becoming equal to the FRC in the supine position at a mean age of about 44 years and equal to the FRC in the upright position at a mean age of about 66 years (Leblanc, Ruff and Milic-Emili, 1970). The closing capacity itself appears to be independent of body position and it is the effects of age on CC and posture on FRC which are important in determining whether airway closure exists. Other causes of decreased FRC, such as anaesthesia, will increase the incidence of airway closure and, conversely, an increase of FRC due to positive end-expiratory pressure will tend to decrease airway closure. Hedenstierna and McCarthy (1976) and also Gilmour, Burnham and Craig (1976) reported that the closing capacity is not changed by the induction of anaesthesia.

Shunting of pulmonary blood flow through areas of the lung which are subject to airway closure is an important cause of impaired oxygenation of arterial blood and has resulted in considerable recent interest in the FRC and factors which influence its magnitude.

ELASTIC RECOIL OF THE LUNGS

It is by no means easy to grasp the quantitative aspects of the combined elastic system of lungs plus chest wall. The approach in this chapter is to consider first the elastic recoil of the lungs and then to discuss the chest wall as an elastic system. Finally, the entire system is considered together with an explanation of the rather difficult pressure/volume relationships of the lungs within the intact chest.

The transmural pressure gradient

If the lungs are removed from the thorax and the air passages remain open, the air within the lungs will gradually be expelled. At all lung volumes, the pressure within the alveoli is greater than that surroduing the lungs. The difference (the transmural pressure gradient) is related to the lung volume, and its magnitude at various lung volumes is shown in *Figure 23*. As the lung volume diminishes, three important changes take place.

1. The transmural pressure gradient diminishes.
2. The small air passages become narrower, and one by one become totally obstructed. Airway closure commences at the closing capacity.
3. There is a tendency for alveoli to collapse.

Closure of the smaller air passages tends to prevent total collapse of the alveoli, unless the sequestered gas trapped therein can be removed by the pulmonary blood flow which continues to perfuse the alveoli after the air

* Recommended nomenclature is that closing capacity is the largest lung volume at which airway closure can be detected. Closing capacity = closing volume + residual volume (Cotes, 1975).

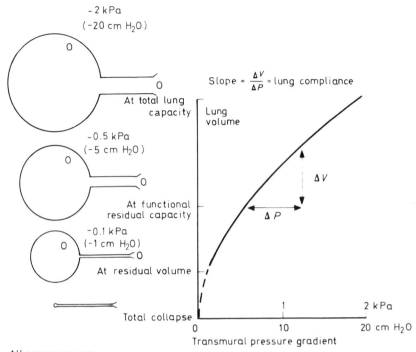

-2 kPa
(-20 cm H₂O)

At total lung capacity

-0.5 kPa
(-5 cm H₂O)

At functional residual capacity

-0.1 kPa
(-1 cm H₂O)

At residual volume

Total collapse

Slope = $\frac{\Delta V}{\Delta P}$ = lung compliance

Lung volume

ΔV

ΔP

All pressures are indicated relative to atmospheric pressure

Transmural pressure gradient

Figure 23. Lung volume bears a curvilinear relationship to the difference in pressure between the alveoli and the intrathoracic space (the transmural pressure gradient). Over the normal tidal range, the relationship approximates to linear and the slope is the lung compliance. The calibre of the air passages falls as the lung volume decreases. At the residual volume (maximal voluntary expiration), some alveoli are isolated by airway closure. Pressure in these alveoli may rise above atmospheric. Once gas is sequestered in an alveolus, collapse can only occur by absorption of contained gases by the pulmonary blood. Values in this diagram relate to the upright position

passages are collapsed. This is most likely to happen if the alveoli contain high concentrations of oxygen or soluble anaesthetic gases such as cyclopropane and nitrous oxide. Absorption is very slow if the trapped alveoli contain air (Webb and Nunn, 1967).

Relationship between lung volume and transmural pressure gradient

The relationship shown in *Figure 23* between lung volume and transmural pressure gradient is typical of an elastic structure. Hooke's law states that stress is proportional to strain. In this case the stress is the change in the transmural pressure gradient, and the strain is the change in the lung volume. The relationship is valid over limited ranges, such as that encountered in normal breathing, and may be stated as follows:

$$\frac{\text{change in lung volume}}{\text{change in transmural pressure gradient}} = \text{a constant}$$

The constant is known as the compliance. The relationship, it should be noted, is independent of the actual pressures and is solely a matter of transmural pressure gradient.

If lung volume is plotted against transmural pressure gradient, the slope ($\Delta V/\Delta P$) of the graph equals the compliance (*Figure 23*). Over a wide range the plot shows a gradual curve with the slope (compliance) falling as the lung volume is increased. However, over the normal range of tidal volumes, the measured compliance is little affected by the magnitude of the tidal volume studied.

Compliance and elastance

It is perhaps unfortunate that two terms are used to define the elasticity of the lung. We have already met the term compliance, which is the volume change per unit change of transmural pressure gradient. Its units of measurement are ml (or litre) per kPa or cm H_2O. Stiff lungs have a *low* compliance.

The other term is *elastance*, which is the reciprocal of compliance:

$$\frac{\text{change in transmural pressure gradient}}{\text{change in lung volume}} = \text{elastance}$$

The units of measurement are kilopascals or centimetres of water per litre. *Stiff* lungs have a *high* elastance.

The nature of the forces causing recoil of the lung

For many years it was believed that the recoil of the lung was due entirely to stretching of the yellow elastin fibres present in the lung parenchyma. However, in 1929, von Neergaard showed that a lung completely filled with and immersed in water, had an elastance which was less than the normal value obtained when the lung was filled with air. He concluded that much of the 'elastic recoil' was due to surface tension acting throughout the vast air/water interface lining the alveoli.

Surface tension at an air/water interface produces forces which tend to reduce the area of the interface. Thus, in a bubble the gas pressure within the bubble will be higher than the surrounding pressure, because the surface of the bubble is in a state of tension. Alveoli resemble bubbles in this respect but differ in their being connected with the exterior through the system of air passages.

The pressure in a bubble is above ambient by an amount depending on the surface tension of the liquid and the radius of curvature of the bubble, according to the Laplace equation:

$$P = \frac{2T}{R}$$

where P is the pressure within the bubble (dyn/cm^2), T is surface tension of the liquid (dyn/cm), and R is radius of the bubble (cm).

In coherent SI units (*see* Appendix A) the appropriate units would be pressure in pascals (Pa), surface tension in newtons per metre (N/m) and radius in metres (m). The millinewton per metre (mN/m) is identical to the old dyne/centimetre, and it follows that:

$$\text{pressure (in pascals)} = \frac{2 \times \text{surface tension (in mN/m)}}{\text{radius (in mm)}}$$

On the left of *Figure 24a and c* is shown a typical alveolus of radius 0·1 mm. Assuming that the alveolar lining fluid has a surface tension of 20 mN/m, the pressure within the bubble will be 0·4 kPa (4 cm H_2O), which is rather less than the transmural pressure gradient at the FRC. It is clear from consideration of the Laplace equation that if the alveolar lining fluid had a surface tension of 72 mN/m (the value for pure water), the lungs would be exceedingly stiff (transmural pressure gradient, 1·44 kPa or 14·4 cm H_2O).

Although it appears inevitable that surface tension must make a contribution to the retractive forces of the lung, two difficulties must be resolved. The first problem is that the pressure in small bubbles is higher than in large bubbles, a conclusion that stems directly from the Laplace equation. From this one might expect that the pressure in a small alveolus would be greater than in a large one. This state of affairs is shown in *Figure 24a,* and would result in a progressive discharge of each alveolus into a larger one, until eventually only one gigantic alveolus would be left. Instability would be inevitable, except in the unlikely event of all the alveoli being exactly the same size. Such a state of affairs would not, of course, be compatible with life, and no such instability exists in the normal lung.

The second problem concerns the relationship between lung volume and the transmural pressure gradient. According to the Laplace equation, one would expect the retractive forces of the lung to increase as the lung volume decreased, a relationship which is certainly true of a bubble. If this were true of the lung, one would expect the lung to decrease in volume according to a viscous cycle, with the tendency to collapse increasing progressively as the lung volume diminished. This, of course, does not happen in the normal lung and the retractive forces decrease as the lung volume is reduced.

The reconciliation of these two problems with the forces which must be produced by the surface tension of the alveolar lining fluid has been one of the most interesting developments in pulmonary physiology. The dilemma was clear to von Neergaard (1929) who concluded that the surface forces in the alveolar lining fluid must be less than would be expected from the properties of simple liquids and, furthermore, that the surface tension must be variable. This has indeed proved to be the case. The original observations of Pattle (1955) on bubbles in lung froth and later studies on alveolar extracts (Brown, Johnson and Clements, 1959) have demonstrated that the surface tension of the alveolar lining fluid is variable and decreases as its surface area is reduced, to attain very low levels which are well below the normal range for body fluids such as plasma.

This effect may be demonstrated by the measurement of surface tension at one end of a trough of alveolar extract. If a floating bar is moved sideways along the trough, the surface film may be concentrated at the end of the trough where the surface tension is being measured. This apparatus is shown diagrammatically in *Figure 24b,* together with a typical result obtained when the area of the surface film is cycled between expansion and contraction.

Alveolar extract with an expanded surface film has a surface tension in the range 30–40 mN/m, a value which is close to that of plasma but, as the surface film is concentrated, the surface tension falls to about 10 mN/m. On expansion, the surface tension rises, but the pathway of change is different during expansion (inspiration) and contraction (expiration).

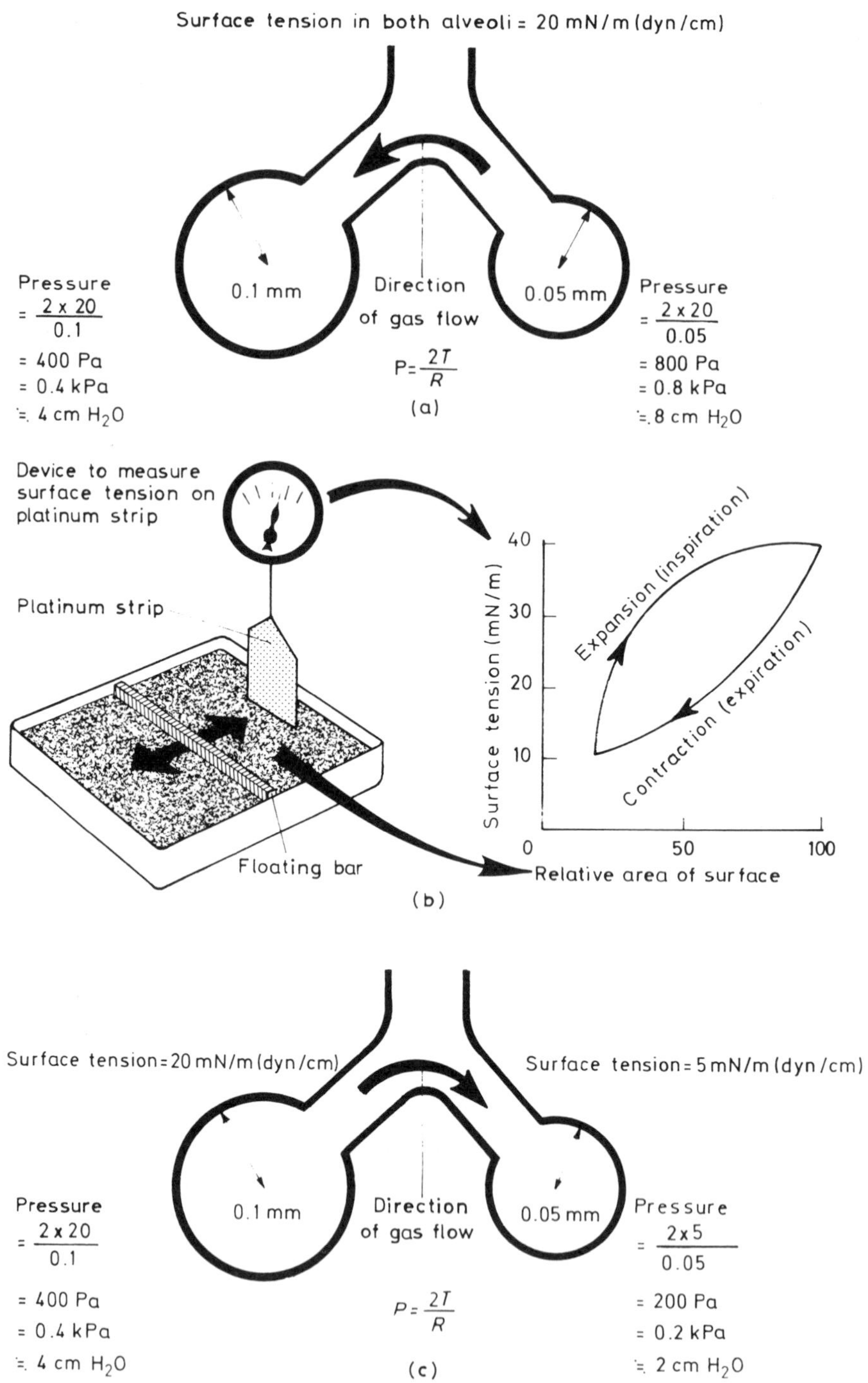

Surface tension in both alveoli = 20 mN/m (dyn/cm)

Pressure
$= \dfrac{2 \times 20}{0.1}$

= 400 Pa
= 0.4 kPa
≃ 4 cm H_2O

0.1 mm

Direction
of gas flow

$P = \dfrac{2T}{R}$

(a)

0.05 mm

Pressure
$= \dfrac{2 \times 20}{0.05}$

= 800 Pa
= 0.8 kPa
≃ 8 cm H_2O

Device to measure
surface tension on
platinum strip

Platinum strip

Floating bar

(b)

Surface tension (mN/m)

Expansion (inspiration)

Contraction (expiration)

Relative area of surface

Surface tension = 20 mN/m (dyn/cm)

Surface tension = 5 mN/m (dyn/cm)

Pressure
$= \dfrac{2 \times 20}{0.1}$

= 400 Pa
= 0.4 kPa
≃ 4 cm H_2O

0.1 mm

Direction
of gas flow

$P = \dfrac{2T}{R}$

(c)

0.05 mm

Pressure
$= \dfrac{2 \times 5}{0.05}$

= 200 Pa
= 0.2 kPa
≃ 2 cm H_2O

Figure 24. Surface tension and alveolar transmural pressure. (a) The pressure relations in two alveoli of different size but with the same surface tension of their lining fluids. (b) The changes in surface tension in relation to the area of the alveolar lining film. (c) The pressure relations of two alveoli of different size when allowance is made for the probable changes in surface tension

When an alveolus decreases in size, the surface tension of the lining fluid falls to a greater extent than the corresponding reduction of radius, so that the transmural pressure gradient (= $2T/R$) diminishes. Therefore the elastic recoil of small alveoli is less than that of large alveoli. This accords with the observed pressure/volume relations shown in *Figure 23*. It also explains why small alveoli do not discharge their contents into large alveoli (*see* lower part of *Figure 24c*).

The alveolar surfactant. The strange features of the surface tension of the alveolar lining fluid are due to the presence of a surface-active material or *surfactant*. In fact, a group of phospholipids are responsible for this activity and the most important is lecithin, but sphingomyelin, phosphatidyl inositol and phosphatidyl dimethylethanolamine are also found (Gluck, 1971). Pulmonary surfactant is highly insoluble and floats on the surface of the alveolar lining fluid, where it offers no appreciable resistance to the diffusion of gases such as oxygen, carbon dioxide and anaesthetics. It is probably secreted mainly by the Type II alveolar lining cells (*see* page 18). Surfactant exerts a surface pressure which counteracts the surface tension of the alveolar lining fluid itself, and this effect is greater when the surface film is reduced in area and the concentration of lecithin at the surface is raised.

It is now well established that surfactant levels are diminished in the respiratory distress syndrome of the newborn, formerly known as hyaline membrane disease (Avery and Mead, 1959; Pattle et al., 1962). The quantity of lecithin in the amniotic fluid rises sharply late in gestation and, if the child is born before this occurs, there is a risk of respiratory distress syndrome (Gluck et al., 1971). In contrast the amount of sphingomyelin remains constant and the lecithin/sphingomyelin (L/S) ratio in the amniotic fluid is a useful measure of the level of lecithin. Chemical differences in the surfactants are considered on page 24). The subject has been reviewed by Clements (1970). It is not clear whether reduction of surfactant activity can explain other pathological conditions but it seems likely that it occurs in the stiff-lung syndrome which sometimes follows cardiac surgery when a pump-oxygenator has been used (Tooley, Finley and Gardner, 1961; Tooley et al., 1961; Nahas et al., 1965a, b).

There has been much speculation whether the increased stiffness of the lungs during anaesthesia (*see* below) is due to an interference with pulmonary surfactant activity. The study of Pattle, Schock and Battensby (1972) suggests that this is not the case, although Forrest (1972) has demonstrated decreased surfactant activity in the lung of the hyperventilated guniea-pig. Woo, Berlin and Hedley-Whyte (1969) showed that ventilation of excised dogs' lungs with air containing clinical concentrations of halothane (1·2 per cent) produced small but significant decreases of compliance. They showed that no such changes occurred when the lungs were filled with liquid and concluded that the anaesthetics might have altered surfactant function. Stanley, Zikria and Sullivan (1972) found that halothane and cyclopropane increased the minimal surface tension of tracheobronchial aspirations from a series of patients. At the time of writing, there is no clear evidence that anaesthetics either decrease surfactant secretion or interfere with its action by physicochemical means, although these possibilities exist.

Pulmonary transudation is also influenced by surfactant activity. Surface tension causes a pressure gradient across the alveolar–capillary membrane (of the order of 0·4 kPa or 4 cm H_2O) which, together with the above-atmospheric pressure in the pulmonary capillaries (about 0·7 kPa or 7 cm H_2O), tends to favour transudation. These pressures are counteracted by the osmotic pressure of the plasma proteins (about 3·5 kPa or 35 cm H_2O) so that transudation does not normally occur. Diminished surfactant activity would elevate the pressure gradient across the alveolar-capillary membrane and, if sufficiently severe, would tip the balance in favour of transudation. This may be the cause of the 'hyaline membrane' in the respiratory distress syndrome of the newborn.

Finally, it is interesting to note that the lung, although it behaves like an elastic body, is not really an elastic body in the usual sense of the term. Its recoil is governed largely by surface tension, but with the surface tension varying with lung volume. Its obedience to Hooke's law appears to be fortuitous.

Time dependence of pulmonary elastic behaviour

For many years it was customary to consider the elastic properties of the lungs as though they behaved as a perfect elastic body obeying Hooke's law. However, it became clear that, in common with other elastic bodies, the stress/strain relationship was greatly influenced by various imperfections in which time was a relevant factor.

If an excised lung is rapidly inflated and then held at the new volume, the inflation pressure rises to its initial value from which it falls exponentially to a lower level which is only attained after several seconds. The same phenomenon can be seen in the intact subject and, following a sustained inflation at constant volume, the pulmonary transmural pressure declines from its initial value to a new value some 20–30 per cent less the original pressure, over the course of about 1 minute (Marshall and Widdicombe, 1961). It is broadly true to say that the volume change divided by the *initial* change in transmural pressure corresponds to the *dynamic compliance* while the volume change divided by the change in transmural pressure, with the second measurement made at the *end* of the period of sustained inflation, corresponds to the *static compliance*, which is clearly larger than the corresponding dynamic compliance. Considerable difficulty attaches to the definition of these terms. Since the secondary decline in transmural pressure is exponential, it can never be said to be complete (*see* Appendix E) and opinions differ on how long the volume change must be sustained to qualify for measurement of static compliance. Similar difficulties apply to the measurement of dynamic compliance which is normally carried out during rhythmic respiration with measurement of pressure at the points of zero air flow (page 91). It will be evident that rate of inflation must influence the transmural pressure gradient at the moment of zero air flow.

The rate of inflation will be altered *inter alia* by the respiratory frequency and it is possible to detect frequency dependence of dynamic pulmonary compliance in the normal subject (Mills, Cumming and Harris, 1963) but it is much more pronounced in the presence of pulmonary disease (Otis et al., 1956; Channin and Tyler, 1962; Woolcock, Vincent and Macklem, 1969).

The effect may be detected during artificial ventilation of patients with respiratory paralysis, and Watson (1962a) found a marked increase in compliance when inspiration was prolonged from 0·5 to 1·7 seconds, with a less marked increase on further extension to 3·0 seconds. Changes in the waveform of inflation pressure, on the other hand, had no detectable effect on compliance.

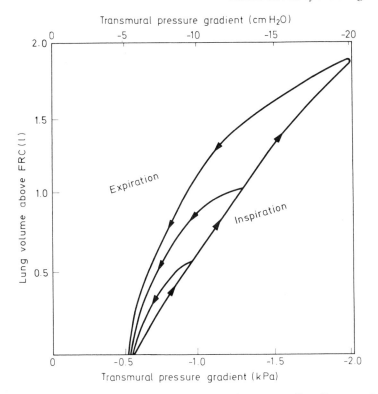

Figure 25. Static plot of lung volume against transmural pressure gradient (intraoesophageal pressure relative to atmosphere at zero air flow). Note that inspiratory and expiratory curves form a loop which gets wider the greater the tidal volume. These loops are typical of elastic hysteresis. For a particular lung volume, the elastic recoil of the lung during expiration is always less than the distending transmural pressure gradient required during inspiration at the same lung volume

Hysteresis.   If the lungs are slowly inflated and then slowly deflated, the pressure/volume curve for static points during inflation differs from that obtained during deflation. The two curves form a loop which becomes progressively broader as the tidal volume is increased (*Figure 25*). (It must be stressed that these loops are not caused by airway resistance although it will be shown in Chapter 4 that airway resistance also causes the production of looped pressure/volume curves during *dynamic* changes in lung volume.) (*See also Figure 31.*)

Expressed in words, the loop in *Figure 25* means that rather more than the expected pressure is required during inflation, and rather less than the expected recoil pressure is available during deflation. This resembles the behaviour of perished rubber which is reluctant to accept deformation under stress and, once deformed, is again reluctant to return to its original shape. This phenomenon is common in elastic bodies, and is given the term 'elastic hysteresis'. Few elastic materials are entirely free of it.

Effect of recent ventilation history.   The compliance of the lung is maintained by recent rhythmic cycling of the lung with the effect being dependent on the tidal volume. Thus a period of hypoventilation without periodic deep breaths may lead to a reduction of compliance, particularly in diseased lungs; compliance can then be restored by one or more large breaths corresponding to sighs. This was first observed during artificial ventilation of patients with respiratory paralysis (Butler and Smith, 1957) and later during anaesthesia with artificial ventilation at rather low tidal volumes (Bendixen, Hedley-Whyte and Laver, 1963). These observations led to the introduction of artificial ventilators which periodically administer 'sighs'. There can be no doubt of the importance of periodic expansion of the lungs during prolonged artificial ventilation of diseased lungs but the case for 'sighs' during anaesthesia is less convincing, since there is no demonstrable effect on arterial Po_2 in an uncomplicated anaesthetic. This is probably because most anaesthetized patients are moderately hyperventilated during artificial ventilation and this is generally sufficient to maintain an acceptable compliance. In Bendixen's study, the beneficial effects of the 'sigh' were most pronounced in patients with the lowest tidal volumes which ranged as low as 250 ml. Watson (1961) reported a 50 per cent reduction in pulmonary compliance within 4 minutes of discontinuing artificial ventilation of a patient with poliomyelitis.

Causes of time dependence of pulmonary elastic behaviour

We have discussed above a variety of phenomena which have in common the influence of recent events on pulmonary compliance. These events include the duration of a sustained inflation, whether the lung is being inflated or deflated and finally the recent history of pulmonary expansion. There are many possible explanations of the time dependence of pulmonary elastic behaviour which may conveniently be considered together although their relative importance varies in different circumstances.

Redistribution of gas.   In a lung consisting of functional units with identical time constants, the distribution of gas will be independent of the rate of inflation, and there will be no redistribution when inflation is held. However, variations in regional time constants will result in distribution being dependent on the rate of inflation. This problem is discussed in greater detail below (page 239) but for the time being we can distinguish 'fast' alveoli and 'slow' alveoli (the term alveoli here referring to a functional unit rather than the anatomical entity). The 'fast' alveolus has a low resistance to inflowing gas and is relatively stiff, while the 'slow' alveolus has a high resistance and a high compliance (*Figure 26b*). These properties give the fast alveolus a shorter time constant (*see* Appendix E) and favour filling during a rapid inspiration. Preferential filling of alveoli with low compliance gives over-all a high pulmonary transmural pressure gradient. A sustained inflation or a slow inflation will permit increased distribution of gas to slow alveoli which have a high compliance and will therefore result in a lower transmural pressure gradient. The extreme difference between fast and slow alveoli shown in *Figure 26b* applies to diseased lungs and no such wide differences exist in the healthy subject. Gas redistribution is therefore unlikely to be a major factor in patients with normal lungs but it can become important in patients with increased airway obstruction as in emphysema, asthma and chronic bronchitis, in whom it is probably the

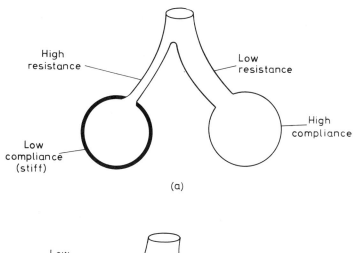

(a)

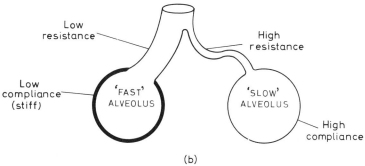

(b)

Figure 26. Schematic diagrams of alveoli to illustrate conditions under which static and dynamic compliances may differ. (a) Represents an idealized state which is probably not realized even in the normal subject. The reciprocal relationship between resistance and compliance results in gas flow being preferentially delivered to the most compliant regions, regardless of the rate of inflation. Static and dynamic compliance are equal. (b) Illustrates a state which is typical of many patients with respiratory disease. The alveoli can conveniently be divided into fast and slow groups. The direct relationship between compliance and resistance results in inspired gas being preferentially delivered to the stiff alveoli if the rate of inflation is rapid. An end-inspiratory pause then permits redistribution from the fast alveoli to the slow alveoli

most important cause of frequency dependence of compliance. Indeed, the demonstration of frequency-dependent compliance is one of the earliest signs of an abnormality of gas distribution (Woolcock, Vincent and Macklem, 1969). The effect of gas redistribution on observed compliance is likely to be completed within a few seconds.

Recruitment of alveoli. Below a certain lung volume, alveoli tend to close and are only reopened at a considerably higher lung volume, in response to a much higher transmural pressure gradient than that at which they closed (Mead, 1961). Reopening of collapsed units (probably primary lobules) may be seen during re-expansion of the lung at the end of a thoracotomy. Recruitment of closed alveoli appears at first sight to be a possible explanation of all the time-dependent phenomena described above but there are two reasons why this is unlikely. Firstly, the pressure required for reopening of a closed unit is very high and unlikely to be realized during normal breathing. Secondly, there is no anatomical evidence for collapsed alveoli in normal lungs at functional residual capacity.

In the presence of pathological pulmonary collapse, a sustained deep inflation may well cause re-expansion with a resultant increased compliance. This is likely to result from 'bagging' patients on prolonged artificial ventilation but opening and closing of alveoli during a respiratory cycle is now considered to be improbable.

Changes in surfactant activity.   It has been explained above that the surface tension of the alveolar lining fluid is greater at higher lung volume and also greater during inspiration than at the same lung volume during expiration (*see Figure 24b*). This is probably the most important cause of the observed hysteresis in the intact lung (*see Figure 25*).

Stress relaxation.   If a spring is pulled out to a fixed increase in its length, the resultant tension is maximal at first and then declines exponentially to a constant value. This is an inherent property of elastic bodies known as stress relaxation: Like hysteresis, it is minimal with metals, detectable with rubber (particularly aged rubber) and very marked with synthetic materials such as polyvinyl chloride. Stress relaxation is also dependent on the form of the material and is, for example, present in woven Nylon though scarcely detectable in mono-filament Nylon thread. The crinkled structure of collagen in the lung is likely to behave similarly and excised strips of human lung show stress relaxation when they are linearly stretched (Sugihara, Hildebrandt and Martin, 1972). The time course is of the same order as the observed changes in pressure when lungs are held inflated at constant volume (*see* above), and Marshall and Widdicombe (1961) concluded that the effect they observed was due to stress relaxation.

Influence of alveolar muscle.   If there are appreciable amounts of muscle in the alveolar walls, it is possible that sustained inflation might be followed by reduction of alveolar muscle tone resulting in changes similar in effect to stress relaxation. Alveolar muscle is present in substantial amounts in some species, particularly the cat, but there is difference of opinion on the presence and importance of alveolar muscle in man.

Displacement of pulmonary blood.   A sustained inflation might be expected to displace blood from the lungs and to increase compliance by reducing the splinting effect of the pulmonary vasculature. The importance of this factor is not known but experiments with excised lungs indicate that all the major time-dependent phenomena of the lung are present when the pulmonary vasculature is empty.

Factors affecting lung compliance

Lung volume.   It is important to remember that compliance is related to lung volume (Marshall, 1957). The same pressure gradient will drive more air into the lungs of an elephant than into the lungs of a mouse, simply because there is more lung in the elephant. Compliance is most conveniently related to the FRC and the actual elasticity of the lung should be expressed by the fraction:

$$\frac{\text{compliance}}{\text{FRC}}$$

This is sometimes known as the specific compliance. The measured compliance of children, and to a less extent women, is less than that of adult men. However, the ratio of compliance to FRC is almost the same for both sexes and all ages down to neonatal. The factor of lung volume is also eliminated when the elastance is recorded as the distension pressure, which is arbitrarily defined as the transmural pressure difference required to increase the lung volume by 10 per cent of total lung capacity (Butler and Smith, 1957).

It has been explained above that the functional residual capacity is significantly reduced during anaesthesia for reasons which remain obscure at the time of writing. This would undoubtedly contribute to the observed decrease of compliance under the same circumstances (*see* below) but, since the fall in compliance is generally greater than the reduction of lung volume, it seems likely that the fall in FRC is secondary to the increased elastic recoil of the lungs rather than the other way about (Rehder, Sessler and Marsh, 1975).

Posture. Attention has already been directed towards the difficult problems associated with the effect of posture on compliance. Not only is the lung volume decreased when posture is changed from upright to supine, but special difficulties are introduced into the measurement of intrathoracic pressure by means of an oesophageal balloon (page 66). When these factors are taken into account, it appears unlikely that changes in posture are associated with appreciable changes of the (specific) compliance.

Pulmonary blood volume. The pulmonary blood vessels probably make a small contribution to the total stiffness of the lungs. Pulmonary vascular congestion is associated with a reduced compliance and this may result from the Müller manoeuvre, left heart disease or septal defects.

Age. One would have expected that age would have influenced the elasticity of the lungs as it appears to influence the elasticity of almost all other tissues of the body. However, Butler, White and Arnott (1957) were unable to detect any correlation between age and compliance, when due allowance had been made for predicted changes in lung volume. This accords with the concept of lung 'elasticity' being determined mainly by surface forces.

Restriction of chest expansion. Elastic strapping of the chest reduces the lung compliance but also causes a roughly proportionate reduction in FRC. The compliance remains reduced if the lung volume is returned to normal, either by a forced inspiration against the restriction or by removal of the restriction. Normal compliance is instantly regained by taking a single deep breath (Caro, Butler and DuBois, 1960).

Recent ventilatory history. This important factor has been considered above (page 77) in relation to the time dependence of pulmonary elastic behaviour.

Anaesthesia.   Ample evidence has been presented above to show that the FRC is reduced during routine anaesthesia with either spontaneous or artificial ventilation (page 67). One possible explanation is that the elastic recoil of the total respiratory system is increased. Indeed, if the inflation pressure of lungs-plus-chest-wall is plotted against *absolute* lung volume, then the reduction of FRC is tantamount to saying that the intercept of the pressure/volume plot at atmospheric pressure will be reduced by the same volume. The displacement of this one point of the pressure/volume curve might be due to a reduction of slope (compliance), an over-all downward shift (without change of compliance) or possibly a combination of reduction of slope with over-all downward displacement. Most studies of the effect of anaesthesia on pulmonary compliance have not considered absolute lung volume and therefore cannot be related directly to change in FRC.

Comparisons of compliance in the same subject awake and anaesthetized are difficult to make. In the first place it is essential to use the same position for both sets of observations to avoid associated changes in FRC, compliance and artefacts of measurement of oesophageal pressure. If total compliance is measured, this is relatively simple in the anaesthetized and paralysed patient, but extremely difficult in the conscious state since voluntary relaxation of respiratory muscles cannot easily be achieved by the untrained patient. If pulmonary compliance is measured, then oesophageal pressure is required and there are considerable difficulties in avoiding posture artefacts or at least in keeping them constant before and after induction of anaesthesia.

Table 4 lists values drawn from the numerous studies of compliance

Table 4. VALUES FOR COMPLIANCE IN HEALTHY SUBJECTS

			l/kPa	ml/cm H_2O
Conscious subjects				
Lungs	upright	static	2·0	200
		dynamic	1·8	180
	supine	static	1·5	150
		dynamic	1·4	140
Chest wall			2·0	200
Total compliance	upright	static	1·5	150
		dynamic	1·0	100
	supine	static	1·2	120
		dynamic	0·9	90
Anaesthetized and paralyzed				
Lungs	(supine)	static	1·5	150
		dynamic	1·0	100
Chest wall			2·0	200
Total compliance		static	0·85	85
		dynamic	0·6	60

These values represent a reasonable mean from a large number of publications. Studies in anaesthetized patients have been reviewed by Rehder, Sessler and Marsh (1975).

undertaken during anaesthesia: there is a considerable measure of agreement and individual studies have not been cited. Bergman (1969) has pointed out that measured values are higher with large tidal volumes and, at 1·5 litres, approach values recorded in conscious subjects.

The relationship of pulmonary pressures to absolute lung volumes is crucial to an understanding of the changes in pulmonary elastic forces which occur during anaesthesia. Such a study has been undertaken by Westbrook et al. (1973) in volunteers who submitted to anaesthesia and paralysis while measurements were continuously made in a body plethysmograph. Elaborate precautions were taken to maintain posture and position of neck constant and also to minimize artefacts in the measurement of oesophageal pressure.

Figure 27 shows the pressure/volume relationships of the total system (lungs and chest wall considered together), the lung and finally the chest wall alone, each considered with the subjects awake, anaesthetized and then anaesthetized and paralysed. For the total system the relevant pressure gradient is airway-to-atmosphere, for the lungs the transmural pulmonary pressure gradient (airway minus oesophageal) and for the chest wall the gradient from oesophagus to atmosphere. All pressure gradients were recorded at zero gas flow maintained for periods of 3–7 seconds. The main features of their findings may be summarized as follows.

1. Following induction of anaesthesia, the pressure/volume curve of the total respiratory system had a reduced slope (lower compliance) and a reduced

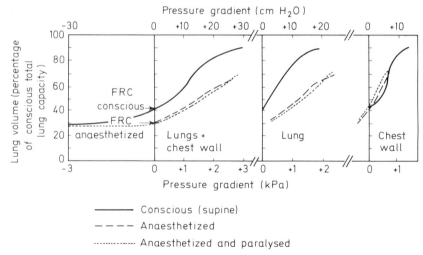

Figure 27. *Pressure/volume relationships in supine volunteers before and after the induction of anaesthesia and paralysis. The first section shows the relationship for lungs plus chest wall where the relevant pressure gradient is alveolar minus ambient. The second section represents lungs alone where the pressure gradient is alveolar minus intrathoracic (transmural). The third section relates to chest wall alone for which the pressure gradient is intrathoracic minus ambient. There are only insignificant differences between observations during anaesthesia with and without paralysis. There are, however, major differences in pressure/volume relationships of the lung and whole system following the induction of anaesthesia. Arrows indicate the FRC conscious and during anaesthesia. The curves meet at a lung volume close to the residual volume. (Redrawn from the data of Westbrook et al. (1973), except that the subatmospheric extensions of the curves for the lungs plus chest wall have been derived from other sources)*

intercept on the volume axis. The elastic recoil of the total system was thus increased for the same lung volume and the changed intercept on the volume axis accorded with the reduction in FRC which was actually observed.

2. The major cause of the change in the pressure/volume relationships of the total system was found to be in the lungs rather than the chest wall. The lungs showed a reduced compliance and a reduced intercept of the pressure/volume curve at the point of resting transmural pressure.

3. There was no major change in the pressure/volume relationships of the chest wall.

4. There were no further changes when paralysis was added to anaesthesia.

5. Changes were not progressive during anaesthesia.

6. After induction of anaesthesia, FRC was reduced to values close to residual volume.

7. Compliance was grossly reduced at lung volumes below FRC during anaesthesia and barely 100 ml of gas could be withdrawn by the application of a pressure of approximately 3 kPa (30 cm H_2O) below atmosphere. (This confirms the observations of Butler and Smith, 1957.)

8. The lung volume attainable by passive inflation to 3 kPa (30 cm H_2O) was barely 70 per cent of the total lung volume measured before anaesthesia.

9. Maximal inflations of the lung did not restore the pressure/volume relationships to control values.

Westbrook's data are in reasonable agreement with the values listed in *Table 4*, and there seems no reason to doubt that the induction of anaesthesia by most of the techniques in current use will result in increased elastic recoil of the lungs and reduced compliance. This is associated with a substantial reduction of FRC.

Although the magnitude of these changes appears to have been established, we remain ignorant of their fundamental cause. It is possible that anaesthesia results in a primary increase in elastic recoil with a secondary reduction in lung volume. Alternatively, the primary change may be in lung volume with a secondary increase in stiffness of the lungs, as suggested by Westbrook et al. (1973).

It is well known that a reduction in lung volume reduces the compliance of the lungs (Caro, Butler and DuBois, 1960). Whatever the primary cause, the observed changes of reduced lung volume and increased stiffness of the lungs may result in pulmonary collapse and it is evident that this sometimes occurs during anaesthesia. Nevertheless, it does not appear to be the primary change and Westbrook's team have added to a considerable body of observation that manual inflation does not restore the pulmonary function to normal during a typical uncomplicated anaesthetic.

Reference has been made above to the elevation of the diaphragm following induction of anaesthesia (page 69) and also to effects of anaesthesia on surfactant activity (page 75).

Disease.   Important changes in lung pressure/volume relationships are found in certain lung diseases (*Figure 28*). Emphysema is unique in that the static pulmonary compliance is increased, as a result of destruction of pulmonary tissue with its elastic recoil and surface retraction. The FRC is increased.

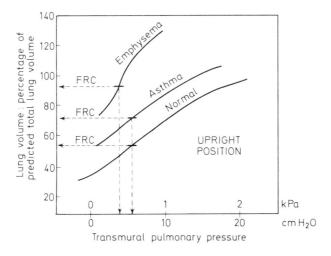

Figure 28. Pulmonary transmural pressure/volume plots for normal subjects, patients with asthma in bronchospasm and patients with emphysema. The broken horizontal lines indicate the FRC in each of the three groups and the corresponding point on the abscissa indicates the resting intrathoracic pressure at FRC. (Redrawn from Finucane and Colebatch, 1969)

However, distribution of inspired gas may be grossly disordered as shown in *Figure 26* and therefore the *dynamic* compliance is commonly reduced. In asthma the pressure/volume curve is displaced upwards without a change in compliance (Finucane and Colebatch, 1969). The elastic recoil is nevertheless reduced at normal transmural pressure and the FRC is therefore increased.

Most other types of pulmonary pathology result in decreased lung compliance. In particular, all forms of pulmonary fibrosis (fibrosing alveolitis), respiratory distress syndrome vascular engorgement, fibrous pleurisy and consolidation will reduce compliance and FRC.

ELASTIC RECOIL OF THE THORACIC CAGE

An excised lung will always tend to contract until all the contained air is expelled, or until all the airways are obstructed. On the other hand the thoracic cage, in the absence of respiratory muscle activity, is tending to expand its volume above the FRC. If air is allowed to enter the pleural cavities freely, the thoracic cage will expand to a volume about a litre greater than the FRC.

It is only in the absence of muscle activity that the thoracic cage can be considered as an elastic structure. During normal inspiration, the pressure difference between the inside and the outside of the thoracic cage reflects the strength of contraction of the muscles rather than the elasticity of the structures. In the conscious subject, the elasticity or compliance of the thoracic cage can only be determined when the respiratory muscles are completely relaxed, and this is difficult to achieve. During anaesthesia with paralysis, the situation is very much easier and the compliance of the thoracic cage is indicated as follows:

$$\frac{\text{compliance of}}{\text{thoracic cage}} = \frac{\text{change in lung volume}}{\text{change in atmospheric-to-intrathoracic}}$$
$$\text{pressure difference}$$

The measurement is actually seldom of much interest in itself. Howell and Peckett (1957), Butler and Smith (1957) and Westbrook et al. (1973) are agreed that thoracic cage compliance is unaltered by anaesthesia. A typical value is of the order of 2 l/kPa (200 ml/cm H_2O).

Effect of posture

When gas enters the lungs, the increase in volume is obtained more by the descent of the diaphragm than by the expansion of the rib cage. Displacement of the viscera is, therefore, an important factor in the measured 'elasticity' of the thoracic cage. Not surprisingly, posture has an important effect, since displacement of the viscera is more difficult in the supine position and this would be shown as a reduction of the observed compliance of the 'thoracic cage'. The study by Ferris et al. (1952) suggests that the thoracic cage compliance is 30 per cent greater when the subject is seated. Lynch, Brand and Levy (1959) have found a reduction of total static compliance of 60 per cent when the anaesthetized patient is turned from the supine to the prone position: much of the difference is likely to be in diminished elasticity of the thoracic cage and diaphragm.

Other factors influencing compliance of thoracic cage

Apart from abdominal muscle tone, there are no physiological factors of importance which influence the compliance of the thoracic cage. External factors of importance are tight clothing and weights resting on the trunk. It is not unusual for surgical assistants to lean on the anaesthetized patient and the effect on respiration of this practice was studied by Nunn and Ezi-Ashi (1961). A weight of 5 kg on the sternum (supine position) caused no appreciable change in minute volume, but when applied to the epigastrium (thus hampering the descent of the diaphragm during inspiration), the minute volume was reduced by 20 per cent per 10 kg applied.

Increased resistance to deformation of the chest wall may occur in obesity, old age or kyphoscoliosis (Lynch, Brand and Levy, 1959). More superficial tissues may offer appreciable resistance in scleroderma and in radiation fibrosis following treatment of carcinoma of the breast.

The restricting effect of the chest wall is lost during thoracotomy when the total compliance rises by 45 per cent (Brownlee and Allbritten, 1956).

STATIC PRESSURE/VOLUME RELATIONSHIPS OF THE LUNG PLUS CHEST WALL

From the clinical standpoint, it is impossible to distinguish between the elasticity of lungs and chest wall. The sensation imparted to the hand during artificial ventilation by manual compression of the reservoir bag is that of a single elastic body, and the simplest measurements of compliance available to the anaesthetist (*see* below) measure the compliance of the lung plus chest wall. This is the value which, together with the airway resistance, governs the practice of artificial ventilation.

The total compliance of lung plus chest wall is related to the individual compliances of lungs and chest wall according to the following expression:

$$\frac{1}{\text{total compliance}} = \frac{1}{\text{lung compliance}} + \frac{1}{\text{thoracic cage compliance}}$$

$$\frac{1}{0 \cdot 85} = \frac{1}{1 \cdot 5} + \frac{1}{2}$$

(static values for the supine anaesthetized subject, l/kPa).

The alternative measure of elasticity, the elastance, may be added directly, and is much more convenient in this respect:

$$\text{total elastance} = \text{lung elastance} + \text{thoracic cage elastance}$$

$$1 \cdot 17 = 0 \cdot 67 + 0 \cdot 5$$

(corresponding values, kPa/l.

Calculation of required inflation pressure

The sustained inflation pressure required for a particular tidal volume is given by the following equation:

$$\text{required sustained inflation pressure} = \frac{\text{required tidal volume}}{\text{total static compliance}}$$

For example, if the total static compliance is 0·85 l/kPa (85 ml/cm H_2O), a tidal volume of 0·85 l will be obtained by a sustained pressure of 1 kPa (10 cm H_2O). This would hardly be a satisfactory method of artificial ventilation as full inspiration would require several seconds. This is because we are considering static values, and have taken no account of the resistance to gas flow which prolongs the time required for entry of gas into the various parts of the lungs. It is common practice to use an inflation pressure at least double the static pressure calculated to produce the required tidal volume. The inspiratory phase may then be cut short before equilibrium is attained, and, by this means, inspiration is reduced to a reasonable duration. In the example quoted above, we might use an inflation pressure of 2 kPa (20 cm H_2O) which, if continued indefinitely, would produce a tidal volume of 1·7 l. We would, however, terminate inspiration before equilibrium and could thus obtain a tidal volume of 0·85 l in a reasonably short time. This approach is fundamental to many aspects of anaesthesia and carries the name 'overpressure'. It is discussed in some detail in Chapter 5 (*see Figure 56*).

Relationship between alveolar, intrathoracic and ambient pressures

Qualitatively, the relationship between these pressures is the same in the upright and supine positions, but the actual values are altered by changes in

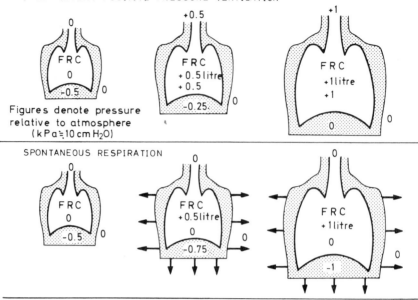

INTERMITTENT POSITIVE PRESSURE VENTILATION

FRC 0
0
-0.5 0

Figures denote pressure
relative to atmosphere
(kPa ≑ 10 cm H₂O)

+0.5
FRC
+0.5 litre
+0.5
-0.25 0

+1
FRC
+1 litre
+1
0 0

SPONTANEOUS RESPIRATION

0
FRC 0
-0.5 0

0
FRC
+0.5 litre
0
-0.75 0

0
FRC
+1 litre
0
-1 0

PRESSURE/VOLUME CURVES FOR THE RELAXED OR PARALYSED SUBJECT

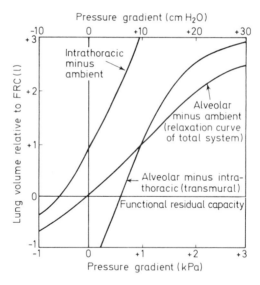

Pressure gradient (cm H₂O)

Intrathoracic minus ambient

Alveolar minus ambient (relaxation curve of total system)

Alveolar minus intra-thoracic (transmural)

Functional residual capacity

Lung volume relative to FRC (l)

Pressure gradient (kPa)

Figure 29. Static pressure/volume relations for the intact thorax for the conscious subject in the upright position. The transmural pressure gradient bears the same relationship to lung volume during both types of ventilation. The intrathoracic-to-ambient pressure difference, however, differs in the two types of ventilation due to muscle action during spontaneous respiration. At all times:

$$\frac{\text{alveolar/ambient}}{\text{pressure difference}} = \frac{\text{alveolar/intrathoracic}}{\text{pressure difference}} + \frac{\text{intrathoracic/ambient}}{\text{pressure difference}}$$

(due attention being paid to the sign of the pressure difference). Lung compliance, 2 l/kPa (200 ml/cm H₂O); thoracic cage compliance, 2 l/kPa (200 ml/cm H₂O); total compliance, 1 l/kPa (100 ml/cm H₂O)

INTERMITTENT POSITIVE PRESSURE VENTILATION

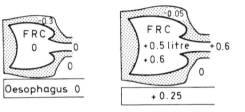

Figures denote pressure
relative to atmosphere (kPa ≈ 10 cm H₂O)

SPONTANEOUS RESPIRATION

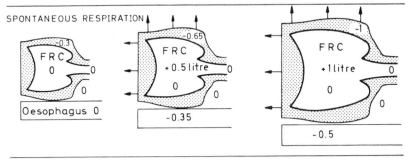

PRESSURE/VOLUME CURVES FOR THE PARALYSED SUBJECT

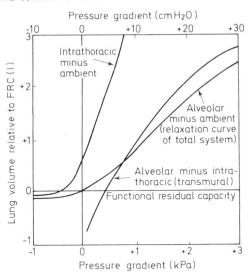

Figure 30. Static pressure/volume relations for the intact thorax for the anaesthetized patient in the supine position. The transmural pressure gradient bears the same relationship to lung volume during both types of ventilation. The intrathoracic-to-ambient pressure difference, however, differs in the two types of respiration due to muscle action during spontaneous respiration. At all times:

$$\frac{alveolar/ambient}{pressure\ difference} = \frac{alveolar/intrathoracic}{pressure\ difference} + \frac{intrathoracic/ambient}{pressure\ difference}$$

(due attention being paid to the sign of the pressure difference). The oesophageal pressure is assumed to be 0·3 kPa (3 cm H₂O) higher than intrathoracic at all times. Lung compliance, 1·5 l/kPa (150 ml/cm H₂O); thoracic cage compliance, 2 l/kPa (200 ml/cm H₂O); total compliance, 0·85 l/kPa (85 ml/cm H₂O)

posture. Two series of diagrams have therefore been prepared to accompany the text. *Figure 29* depicts the upright position and uses typical values drawn from physiological studies in the conscious subject. *Figure 30* depicts the anaesthetized patient in the supine position, and employs values which are culled from a considerable range of published material.

In the paralysed patient, inflation is achieved by raising the alveolar pressure relative to the pressure surrounding the trunk. Either the airway pressure is raised (intermittent positive pressure ventilation) or the pressure surrounding the trunk is lowered (cabinet respirator). In each case, the alveolar/ambient pressure gradient is increased, and the effects are probably identical. At all lung volumes, the intrathoracic pressure is less than the alveolar pressure by an amount equal to the transmural pressure gradient (*see Figure 23*) but, during passive inflation of the lungs, the intrathoracic pressure rises in relation to ambient pressure. Intrathoracic pressure is approximately equal to ambient at a lung volume about a litre greater than the FRC in the upright position, but at a much lower lung volume in the supine position. This is the same volume which would be assumed by the chest wall if air were allowed to enter the pleural cavities freely. If the lungs are then inflated further, the chest wall is stretched beyond its equilibrium position, and consequently the intrathoracic pressure rises above ambient. These changes are shown diagrammatically and are also displayed on static pressure/volume diagrams (*Figures 29 and 30*). At all times, the following relationship holds:

$$\frac{\text{alveolar/ambient}}{\text{pressure difference}} = \frac{\text{alveolar/intrathoracic}}{\text{pressure difference}} + \frac{\text{intrathoracic/ambient}}{\text{pressure difference}}$$

Due attention must be paid to the sign of the pressure differences.

During spontaneous respiration the alveolar pressure equals ambient at the ends of inspiration and expiration when no gas is flowing through the respiratory tract. The alveolar/intrathoracic pressure difference is a function of lung volume and lung compliance exactly as described above for artificial ventilation. As before, the alveolar/ambient pressure difference equals the algebraic sum of its two components, and in this case the two components must always be equal but of opposite sign at the times of zero air flow.

It is not easy to think in terms of intrathoracic pressure during spontaneous or artificial ventilation of anaesthetized patients. However, *Figures 29 and 30* show how it is possible to arrive at a reasonable estimate of its value, which has an important influence on venous return.

PRINCIPLES OF MEASUREMENT OF COMPLIANCE

Compliance of the various structures is defined as follows:

$$\text{total compliance} = \frac{\text{change in lung volume}}{\text{change in alveolar/ambient pressure gradient}}$$

$$\text{lung compliance} = \frac{\text{change in lung volume}}{\text{change in alveolar/intrathoracic pressure gradient}}$$

$$\text{chest wall compliance} = \frac{\text{change in lung volume}}{\text{change in ambient/intrathoracic pressure gradient}}$$

all measurements being made at the time of zero air flow at the end of inspiration or expiration.

Measurements of chest wall compliance (and total compliance, which includes chest wall compliance) are only meaningful if there is no tone in the respiratory muscles. This means that, in practice, such measurements can only be made in paralysed subjects or, so it is said, in trained subjects who are able to relax their muscles completely.

Changes in lung volume are measured with a body plethysmograph, a spirometer or by integration of a pneumotachogram. Points of zero air flow are best detected with a pneumotachograph.

Static pressures can be measured with a simple water manometer, but rapidly changing pressures require the use of transducers which give an electrical output proportional to pressure. Pressure differences can be measured directly by the use of a double-ended manometer (such as a U-tube filled with water) which is connected between the two points concerned. It has been explained above that intrathoracic or intrapleural pressure varies according to the site at which it is measured, and there is now a widespread convention to accept the pressure in the middle third of the oesophagus as representative of the 'intrathoracic pressure'. Details of measurement of oesophageal pressure by an air-filled balloon have been described by Milic-Emili et al. (1964). Alveolar pressure equals mouth pressure when no gas is flowing. It cannot be measured directly.

Static compliance

In the *paralysed subject* this is a simple measurement. The lungs are inflated with a known volume of air by any suitable means (such as the pre-set gas syringe described by Janney (1959)), and the inflation pressure is measured after an interval to allow for equilibration of regional pressure differences, etc. Since this is a static measurement, the simplest form of manometer is adequate and a water-filled U-tube may be used. If only inflation pressure is measured, only total compliance may be determined. If intrathoracic pressure is also measured, it is possible to derive lung and chest wall compliance separately.

Alternatively, the lungs may be inflated by a constant-flow device such as the Pufflator described in the following chapter in relation to *Figure 51* (Don and Robson, 1965) or the measurement may be made during a passive expiration into a spirometer (Nims, Connor and Comroe, 1955) as shown in *Figure 52*.

In the *conscious subject* a known volume of air is inhaled and the subject then relaxes against a closed airway. The various pressure gradients are compared with the resting values (FRC). It is usually very difficult to ensure that the respiratory muscles are relaxed, but the measurement of lung compliance is valid since the static alveolar/intrathoracic pressure difference is unaffected by respiratory muscle activity.

Dynamic compliance

These measurements are made during rhythmic breathing, but compliance is calculated from pressure measurements which are made at the points when no gas is flowing, usually at the end-inspiratory and end-expiratory 'no-flow' turn-round points. When gas is flowing, pressures are dependent in part on the resistance to gas flow and, therefore, compliance cannot be derived directly. Two methods are in general use.

Loops.   The required pressure gradient and the respired volume are displayed simultaneously as X and Y co-ordinates on some device which permits the display of two-dimensional phenomena (e.g. a cathode ray oscilloscope, an X/Y

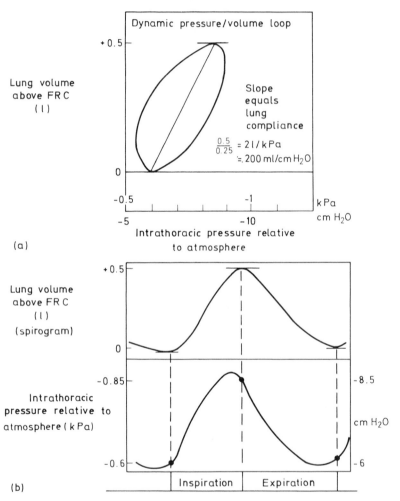

Figure 31. Measurement of dynamic compliance of lung by simultaneous measurement of tidal excursion (lung volume relative to FRC) and intrathoracic pressure (relative to atmosphere). In (a) these parameters are displayed as the Y and X co-ordinates on a two-dimensional plotting device (e.g. cathode ray oscillograph). In (b) they are displayed simultaneously against time on a two-channel oscillograph. In each case, lung compliance is derived as lung volume change divided by transmural pressure gradient change. The transmural pressure gradient is indicated by the intrathoracic pressure (relative to atmosphere) when the lung volume is not changing. At these times the alveolar pressure must equal the atmospheric pressure since no gas is flowing. End-expiratory and end-inspiratory 'no-flow' points are indicated in (b). They correspond to horizontal parts of the loop in (a)

plotter or various photographic devices). The resultant trace forms a loop (*Figure 31a*). The no-flow points, when mouth pressure equals alveolar, are identified as the points when the trace is horizontal. The lung compliance equals the slope of the line joining these points, when mouth/intrathoracic pressure difference is measured. Other parts of the loop reflect the resistance to gas flow, and this is discussed in Chapter 4.

Multi-channel recording of volume, pressure gradient and flow rate. This method differs from the one described above only in the manner of display. The two co-ordinates of the loop (volume and pressure) are plotted simultaneously (against time) on a pen oscillograph (*Figure 31b*). The volume difference is derived from the volume trace and divided by the change in the appropriate pressure gradient measured at the no-flow points. The no-flow points may be identified as the horizontal points of the volume trace (*Figure 31b*) or, more elegantly, by noting the point of phase reversal of a pneumotachogram on a third channel. The pneumotachogram may also be integrated to give volume and, thereby, it is possible to dispense with a spirometer. This method was introduced in 1927 by von Neergaard and Wirz (1927a) and has been used during anaesthesia by Gold and Helrich (1965). Both lung and chest wall compliance may be measured by recording the appropriate pressure differences, and the method is equally suitable for spontaneous and artificial ventilation. Measurement of FRC is described in Chapter 1, on page 6.

Chapter 4   Resistance to Gas Flow

Laminar Flow
Turbulent Flow
Threshold Resistors
Quantification of 'Resistance' when Gas Flow is Partly Laminar and
    Partly Turbulent
Minor Sources of Resistance to Gas Flow
Causes of Increased Airway Resistance
The Effects of Increased Resistance to Breathing
Principles of Measurement of Flow Resistance

Excessive resistance to breathing is the most important cause of ventilatory failure, and total obstruction to breathing constitutes one of the direst emergencies in acute medicine. Particularly in anaesthesia, there is the additional hazard of obstruction to gas flow in apparatus through which the patient is breathing. For these reasons, factors governing resistance to gas flow are of particular relevance to respiratory medicine in general and anaesthesia in particular.

Gas flows from a region of high pressure to one of lower pressure. The rate at which it does so is a function of the pressure difference and the resistance to gas flow of the connecting passage (*Figure 32*). The precise relationship between pressure difference and gas flow rate depends upon the nature of the flow which is usually described as being either *laminar* (streamline) or *turbulent*. This distinction is helpful for gaining an understanding of the problem, but it should not be thought that there is a rigid separation between the two types of flow. In most situations relevant to pulmonary ventilation, the flow pattern is transitional, being neither entirely laminar nor entirely turbulent. Furthermore, the flow pattern may vary between different regions of the respiratory tract. For example, there may be laminar flow in the trachea while there is turbulent flow in the larynx.

Coexistence of laminar and turbulent flow makes the quantification of resistance to gas flow rather untidy and imprecise. The approach in this chapter is to consider laminar and turbulent flow separately and then to consider methods of quantifying resistance in the presence of transitional or mixed flow patterns. Physiological and clinical aspects are discussed later.

LAMINAR FLOW

Characteristics of laminar flow

When gas flows slowly along a straight unbranched tube, the pattern of flow conforms to an infinite series of concentric cylinders of gas which slide, one over

94

the other, with the peripheral cylinder ïtationary, and the central cylinder moving fastest (*Figure 33*). If the composition of the gas entering a region of laminar flow is suddenly changed, the new gas advances down the centre of the tube with a cone front. As a general rule, laminar flow is inaudible.

Flushing effect of laminar flow

The advancing cone front of laminar gas flow means that some gas may reach the end of a connecting tube before the total amount of gas entering the tube equals the volume of the tube (*Figure 33*). In terms of anatomical dead space, laminar flow of inspired gas may result in some gas reaching the alveoli when the inspired tidal volume is less than the actual anatomical dead space (defined as the geometrical volume of the conducting air passages). Although the cone front of laminar flow can reduce the effective volume of conducting tubes, it is for the same reason inefficient for purging an unwanted gas from a tube.

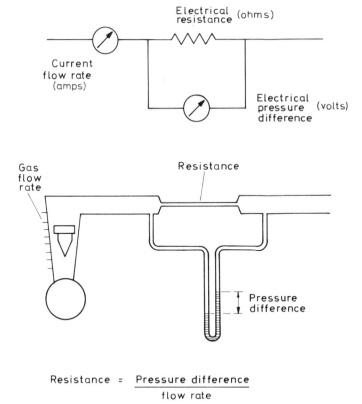

Resistance = Pressure difference / flow rate

Figure 32. Electrical analogy of gas flow. Resistance is pressure difference per unit flow rate. Resistance to gas flow is analogous to electrical resistance (provided that flow is laminar). Gas flow corresponds to electrical current (amps); gas pressure corresponds to potential (volts); gas flow resistance corresponds to electrical resistance (ohms); Poiseuille's law corresponds to Ohm's law

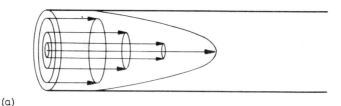

(a)

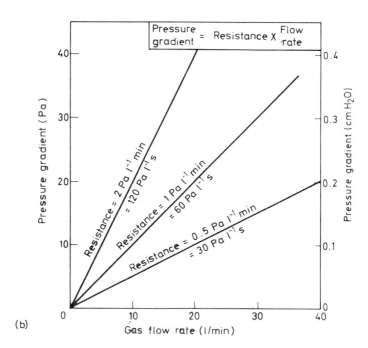

(b)

Figure 33. Laminar flow. (a) shows laminar gas flow down a straight tube as a series of concentric cylinders of gas with the central cylinder moving fastest. This gives rise to a 'cone front' when the composition of the gas is abruptly changed as it enters the tube. (b) shows the linear relationship between gas flow rate and pressure gradient. The slope of the lines indicates the resistance (1 Pa ≒ 0.01 cm H₂O)

Quantitative relationships during laminar flow

Working with long, straight, unbranched tubes, Hagen and Poiseuille independently demonstrated the relationships which are set out in the following expression:

$$\text{gas flow rate} = \text{pressure gradient}\left(\frac{\pi \times (\text{radius of tube})^4}{8 \times \text{length of tube} \times \text{gas viscosity}}\right)$$

Note that gas flow rate is proportional to the fourth power of the radius. Thus, with a constant pressure gradient, a doubling of the tube radius (or diameter) results in a sixteenfold increase in flow. Similarly, a sixteenfold increase in pressure is needed to maintain the same flow rate if the diameter of the tube is halved. This effect is more familiar to the anaesthetist in relation to the selection of cannulas for intravenous infusions, but is also true for endotracheal tubes and their connectors.

It should be stressed that gas viscosity is the only property of the gas which influences resistance during laminar flow. This is in contrast to density, which is the relevant property during turbulent flow. For example, 70 per cent nitrous oxide/30 per cent oxygen is about 10 per cent less viscous than air although it is about 50 per cent more dense. Therefore, under conditions of laminar flow, resistance to 70 per cent nitrous oxide/30 per cent oxygen will be slightly less than to air. The substitution of a gas of low density but high viscosity (such as helium) will do nothing to improve gas flow under these conditions. However, when there is difficulty in breathing due to excessive airway resistance, it is almost axiomatic that gas flow is largely turbulent and, under such conditions, density and not viscosity is important. Therefore, low density is almost always the property to be sought in alleviating the effects of high airway resistance.

Assuming that the gas mixture and the geometric properties of the conducting tubes are constant, the Poiseuille equation indicates that pressure gradient will be directly proportional to gas flow rate. Therefore, for any flow rate, pressure gradient divided by flow rate will be constant.

$$\frac{\text{pressure gradient}}{\text{flow rate}} = \text{a constant}$$

This constant may be called the resistance and is, in fact, equal to:

$$\frac{8 \times \text{length of tube} \times \text{gas viscosity}}{\pi \times (\text{radius of tube})^4}$$

Figure 33 shows a plot of pressure gradient against gas flow rate. For laminar flow the plot is a straight line, of which the slope (pressure gradient/flow rate) equals the resistance. A steep slope means a high resistance, while a shallow slope indicates low resistance.

In the Hagen–Poiseuille equation, the units must all be coherent. CGS units are dyn/sq. cm for pressure, ml/s for flow, cm for length and diameter, which are coherent with the unit of poise for viscosity (dyn sec cm^{-2}). With the introduction of SI units, the position is somewhat complicated by the delay of the biomedical field in the adoption of the kilopascal for measurement of gas pressure. The SI unit for viscosity is newton second $metre^{-2}$ which equals 10 poises (*see* Appendix A).

The concept of a constant value for the resistance is only valid in the presence of laminar flow. It will be seen below that the 'resistance' is not constant when flow is turbulent, and therefore it may be meaningless to give a numerical value for resistance under such circumstances. This is unfortunate as some degree of turbulence is almost always present in the tracheobronchial tree, even in quiet breathing.

One occasionally reads of resistance to gas flow expressed in terms of pressure (strictly a misnomer for pressure gradient). Resistance can only be expressed in terms of pressure gradient if one particular flow rate is stipulated or if the pressure gradient is independent of gas flow rate. This occurs with well designed pressure-relief valves, valves for positive end-expiratory pressure (PEEP), etc. Such devices are known as threshold resistors and are considered below (page 100).

Conductance

It is occasionally convenient to refer to conductance rather than resistance. These two quantities are reciprocally related, and conductance is measured in units such as litres per second per kilopascal or centimetre of water. As with resistance, conductance is only constant during laminar flow, and the term is meaningless when there is an appreciable turbulent component.

TURBULENT FLOW

Characteristics of turbulent flow

High flow rates, particularly through irregular tubes, result in a breakdown of the orderly flow of gas described as laminar. The molecules of gas have an irregular movement superimposed upon their general progression along the tube (*Figure 34*). A cone front does not, therefore, occur and the front of a new gas introduced into the system is square. Turbulent flow will arise in a long, straight, unbranched tube if the flow rate is high enough (*see* below), but turbulence is particularly likely to occur when the diameter or the direction of a tube is changed abruptly, or when branching occurs. It is often possible to hear gas flow when it is largely turbulent.

Effects of turbulent flow

The absence of a cone front means that no new gas can reach the end of a tube until the volume of gas which has entered the tube is close to the geometrical volume of the tube. The effective dead space is thus maximal when flow is turbulent. On the other hand, turbulent flow is the most efficient for purging a tube of the contained gas.

The serious consequences of excessive resistance to gas flow almost always arise under conditions when the gas flow is turbulent. Avoidance of resistance may, therefore, almost always be considered in relation to turbulent gas flow.

Quantitative relationships during turbulent flow

Quantitative relationships differ from those observed with laminar flow in two important respects:

1. The pressure gradient required to produce a given gas flow rate is proportional to the square of the gas flow rate.
2. The pressure gradient required to produce a given gas flow rate through a given passage is proportional to the density of the gas and is independent of its viscosity.

The pressure gradient, in theory, is inversely proportional to the fifth power of the radius (or diameter) of the tube (Fanning equation).

The square law relating pressure gradient and flow is shown in *Figure 34*.

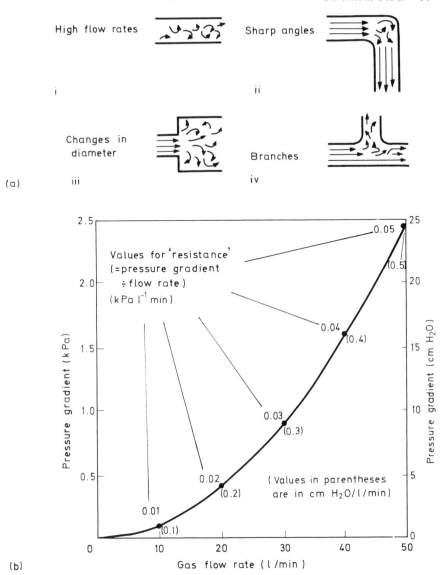

Figure 34. Turbulent flow. (a) shows four circumstances under which gas flow tends to be turbulent. (b) shows the square law relationship between gas flow rate and pressure gradient when flow is turbulent. Note that the value for 'resistance', calculated as for laminar flow, is quite meaningless during turbulent flow

Since resistance is defined as pressure gradient divided by flow rate, it will be seen that the 'resistance' is not constant but rises in proportion to the flow rate. It is thus meaningless to assign a fixed value for the resistance (defined as pressure drop divided by flow rate) when the flow is turbulent. Alternative methods of defining the resistance are discussed below.

Conditions which determine the nature of gas flow

We have seen that irregular and branching tubes tend to result in turbulence which may be confined to the immediate region of the irregularity. Abrupt changes in diameter almost invariably cause turbulence, and the square law relationship between pressure gradient and flow rate may easily be demonstrated for certain types of endotracheal catheter mounts.

In the case of long straight unbranched tubes, the nature of the gas flow may be predicted from the following: (1) the viscosity of the gas; (2) the density of the gas; (3) the diameter of the tube; and (4) the gas flow rate. The prediction is carried out by calculating Reynolds' number. This is a nondimensional quantity derived from the following formula:

$$\frac{\text{mean linear velocity of gas} \times \text{tube radius} \times \text{gas density}}{\text{gas viscosity}}$$

The property of the gas which affects the Reynolds' number is the ratio of the density to the viscosity. This equals the reciprocal of the *kinematic viscosity* which is the ratio of viscosity to density (*Table 5*).

Table 5. PHYSICAL PROPERTIES OF ANAESTHETIC GAS MIXTURES RELATING TO GAS FLOW

	Viscosity relative to air	*Vapour density relative to air*	*Vapour density* / *Viscosity* *relative to air*
Oxygen	1·11	1·11	1·00
70%N_2O/30%O_2	0·89	1·41	1·59
80%He/20%O_2	1·08	0·33	0·31

When Reynolds' number is less than 1000, flow is laminar. Above a value of 1500 flow is entirely turbulent. Between these values both types of flow coexist. The critical values have been determined experimentally, and opinions differ as to the precise values which should be adopted. The figures cited here were chosen by Cooper (1961), in an exhaustive study of the resistance of respiratory apparatus.

An example of the relevance of Reynolds' number to problems of gas flow during anaesthesia is shown in *Figure 35*, which indicates the nature of the gas flow to be expected when air, or a mixture of oxygen with either helium or nitrous oxide, passes at various flow rates through tubes of different diameters.

Viscosities of respirable gases do not differ greatly but densities vary by as much as seventyfold (between hydrogen and sulphur hexafluoride). The use of a less dense gas not only reduces the tendency to turbulence but also reduces the resistance to any turbulent flow which is still present. Different gases make an appreciable difference to resistance and this should be borne in mind when the resistance of anaesthetic apparatus is determined by studying air flow, or when a patient with severe resistance to breathing is anaesthetized with nitrous oxide.

THRESHOLD RESISTORS

Certain resistors are designed to allow no gas to pass until a certain threshold pressure is reached after which gas passes freely without further rise in

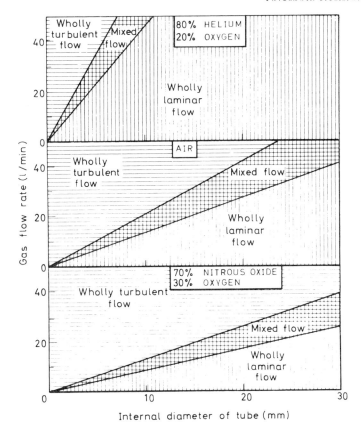

Figure 35. Graphs to show the nature of the gas flow through tubes of various diameters for three different gas mixtures; 25 l/min is a typical peak flow rate during spontaneous respiration. It will be seen that the nature of flow in the trachea and in endotracheal tubes will be markedly dependent on the composition of the gas mixture

pressure. Familiar applications are the safety valves of boilers and pressure cookers. Interest in threshold resistors has recently increased as a result of the discovery of the value of positive end-expiratory pressure (PEEP) in the management of various types of respiratory disorder (*see* page 128). Exhalation through a fixed depth of water provides a rough and ready threshold resistor, but a variety of more sophisticated PEEP valves have now been developed for clinical use. Some anaesthetic relief valves are not true threshold resistors because there is insufficient clearance once the valve is open and the pressure continues to rise with increasing gas flow rate (*see* relief valve in *Figure 37*).

In the field of pulmonary physiology there is a special type of threshold resistor which is best named after Starling who first described it. Fluid flows through a collapsible tube which is exposed on its outside to a particular pressure (*Figure 36*). This outside pressure acts as a threshold pressure below which fluid cannot pass through the tubing. A special characteristic of the Starling resistor is that a reduced pressure on the downward side cannot assist flow by suction since it will merely collapse the walls of the tubing. On the other hand, if both upstream and downstream pressures are raised, then the collapsible

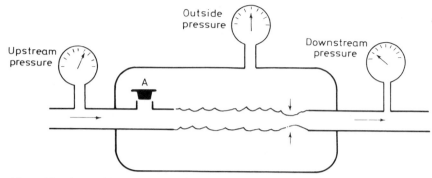

Figure 36. The Starling resistor consists of a length of flaccid collapsible tubing passing through a rigid box. When the pressure outside the collapsible tubing exceeds the upstream pressure, the tubing collapses where shown by the arrows. No gas can flow, whatever the level of the downstream pressure. If the orifice A is opened, the outside pressure rises with the upstream pressure and so limits flow rate to a level which is independent of the magnitude of the upstream pressure. The relevance of this to effort-independent expiratory flow rate is considered on page 114. The relevance of the Starling resistor to the pulmonary capillary circulation is considered on page 260.

tubing is dilated and its resistance is diminished. The resistor in this form is a model of the pulmonary vessels, and its important role in the distribution of the pulmonary circulation is discussed on pages 260 et seq.

The Starling resistor also acts as a model for the behaviour of the air passages during a forced expiration. This situation is complicated by the fact that the upstream driving (alveolar) pressure minus the elastic recoil pressure of the lungs is equal to the (intrathoracic) pressure surrounding the collapsible airways. Thus under static conditions the pressure in the airways is always greater than that which surrounds the airways which should therefore remain patent even in the case of the small airways which have no inherent rigidity. However, with high expiratory flow rates, the pressure gradient down the airways may result in the downstream pressure falling below the surrounding pressure with consequent collapse of the air passages. This mechanism is of great importance and is normally the factor which limits expiratory flow rate (*see* page 114).

QUANTIFICATION OF 'RESISTANCE' WHEN GAS FLOW IS PARTLY LAMINAR AND PARTLY TURBULENT

In a long straight tube, gas flow tends to be laminar at low flow rates, but becomes progressively more turbulent as the flow rate is increased until eventually full turbulence is reached. *Figure 35* shows that the mixed type of flow must occur commonly under the conditions of anaesthesia. There is thus considerable difficulty in ascribing a numerical value to the 'resistance' of either a patient's air passages or a piece of respiratory apparatus. A number of alternative methods are in use and are detailed below, although it is still commonplace to express resistance by a single value (*see Table 6*).

Measurement of pressure difference at a single flow rate

This method has been used as a simple screening test for resistance and it may be useful if the type of flow is similar in every instance. It can, however, be

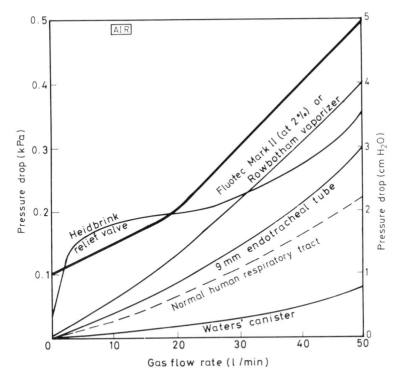

Figure 37. A linear plot of pressure drop against gas flow rate for various pieces of anaesthetic apparatus, compared with the normal human respiratory tract. The heavy line is the author's suggested upper limit of acceptable resistance for an adult patient. With 70 per cent N_2O/30 per cent O_2, the pressure drop is about 40 per cent greater for the same gas flow when the flow is turbulent. There is little difference when the flow is chiefly laminar

grossly misleading if the pattern of flow is different. In the examples shown in *Figure 37*, the Heidbrink relief valve and the vaporizers have the same 'resistance' at a flow rate of 32 litres per minute. However, above and below this flow rate, markedly different pressures are needed to maintain the same flow rate through the two types of resistor. Bergman (1969) has reported respiratory resistance at three different air flow rates and this is an improvement on simple statements of resistance as though it were constant for all flow rates (*see Table 6*).

Determination of two constants for 'resistance'

This approach considers resistance as comprising two components, one for laminar flow and the other for turbulent flow. An equation is then derived which expresses the pressure gradient required to maintain flow as the sum of two terms corresponding to the two types of flow:

$$\text{pressure gradient} = \underbrace{k_1 \text{ (flow)}}_{\substack{\text{laminar} \\ \text{component of} \\ \text{resistance}}} + \underbrace{k_2 \text{ (flow)}^2}_{\substack{\text{turbulent} \\ \text{component of} \\ \text{resistance}}}$$

k_1 contains all the constant factors of the Hagen–Poiseuille equation (gas viscosity, tube radius, etc.), while k_2 includes all the constant factors in the corresponding equation for turbulent flow (gas density, tube radius, etc.). This approach was used by Rohrer in his classical post-mortem study of the human air passages in 1915. He derived the following equation for the flow resistance of the human air passages:

$$\text{pressure gradient} = 0{\cdot}79 \text{ (flow)} + 0{\cdot}81 \text{ (flow)}^2$$

(pressure being measured in cm H_2O and flow rate in 1/sec). More recent studies on living patients (summarized by Mead and Agostoni, 1964) have given the values:

$$\text{pressure gradient} = 0{\cdot}24 \text{ (flow)} + 0{\cdot}03 \text{ (flow)}^2$$
$$\text{(kPa)}$$

$$\text{pressure gradient} = 2{\cdot}4 \text{ (flow)} + 0{\cdot}3 \text{ (flow)}^2$$
$$\text{(cm } H_2O)$$

Both components are increased in emphysema. This type of equation is cumbersome and can only be an approximation of the true relationship, but nevertheless has proved useful.

Determination of constants K and n

Over a surprisingly wide range of flow rates, the equation above may be condensed into the following single term expression:

$$\text{pressure gradient} = K \text{ (flow)}^n$$

In this equation the exponent n has a value of 1 in purely laminar flow and 2 in purely turbulent flow. With mixed flow the value of n varies between 1 and 2. K is an omnibus constant comprising the various constituents of the constants k_1 and k_2 mentioned above. It is clear that this equation cannot apply throughout the whole range of flows since the value of n must change from 1 to 2, as the flow pattern changes from purely laminar to purely turbulent. Nevertheless, it is found in practice that the values of both K and the exponent n are often reasonably constant throughout the range of flows encountered in clinical practice. This method of statement of resistance has the advantage that the nature of the flow is indicated by the value of n. However, it must be remembered that the expression is at best an approximation and, furthermore, is only applicable between limits which should be stated. The expression has been used by Cooper (1961) for assessment of the resistance of breathing apparatus.

Using this convention, resistance of the normal human respiratory tract may be expressed as follows:

$$\text{pressure gradient} = 0{\cdot}24 \text{ (flow)}^{1{\cdot}3}$$
$$\text{(kPa)}$$

$$\text{pressure gradient} = 2{\cdot}4 \text{ (flow)}^{1{\cdot}3}$$
$$\text{(cm } H_2O)$$

This does not differ by more than 10 per cent from the two-term expression over the range of flow $0{\cdot}2$–$3{\cdot}0$ l/s.

Table 6. PULMONARY RESISTANCE STUDIES IN HEALTHY
ANAESTHETIZED PATIENTS (VALUES EXCLUDE APPARATUS
RESISTANCE) (*see page 119*)

	$kPa\ l^{-1}\ s$	$cm\ H_2O\ l^{-1}\ sec$
Newman, Campbell and Dinnick (1959)	0·05–0·3	0·5–3·0
Bodman (1963) *	0·12–0·32	1·2–3·2
Bergman (1966)	0·55–0·60	5·5–6·0
Bergman (1969)* at 1·5 l/s	0·50–0·57	5·0–5·7
at 1·0 l/s	0·44–0·49	4·4–4·9
at 0·5 l/s	0·36–0·39	3·6–3·9
Hedenstierna and McCarthy (1975)	0·4 –0·6	4·0–6·0
Bergman and Waltemath (1974)	0·4 –0·6	4·0–6·0

* These series also report patients with physical and radiographic evidence of pulmonary disease, who showed much greater levels of resistance.

Flow rate/pressure gradient plot (linear)

Probably the best all-round method of describing resistance to gas flow is by constructing a plot of pressure gradient against flow rate on linear graph paper. This, of course, will relate only to a particular air passage and a particular gas or gas mixture. *Figure 37* shows a typical plot for a variety of anaesthetic components compared with the normal human air passages. This method of presentation is particularly valuable for describing the performance of threshold resistors. Once these are beyond their opening pressure, gas flow often tends to be turbulent and so they commonly present S-shaped flow rate/pressure gradient characteristics which cannot be conveniently expressed in mathematical form.

Cathode ray tubes or $X–Y$ recorders may be used to make direct plots of pressure gradients against flow rates during respiration. This is a particularly elegant method for displaying the resistance of the nose or external breathing apparatus. One deep breath is sufficient for displaying the characteristics of flow in both directions.

Flow rate/pressure gradient plot (logarithmic)

Logarithmic plots have two great virtues. Firstly, they enable a wide range of values to be displayed. Secondly, many curves become straight lines when values are plotted as their logarithms. Both considerations apply to the problems of display of resistance to gas flow. When log pressure is plotted against log flow, the curve will be a straight line for both linear and turbulent flow, with a slope of 1 in the former case and 2 in the latter. The slope equals the value for the exponent n in the expression:

$$\text{pressure gradient} = K\ (\text{flow})^n$$

Figure 38 shows the data from *Figure 37* replotted on logarithmic co-ordinates. The following advantages of the logarithmic plot may be claimed.

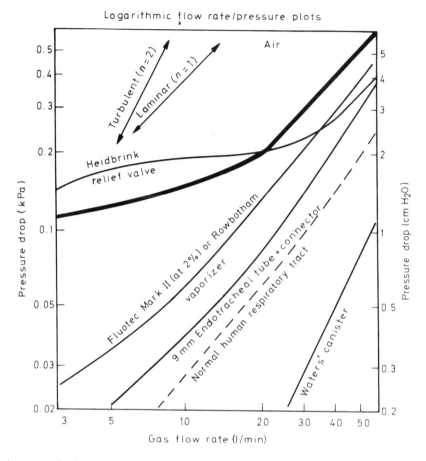

Figure 38. The data of Figure 37 replotted on logarithmic co-ordinates. Note that many of the curves become straight lines. A slope of 2 indicates wholly turbulent flow; a slope of 1 indicates wholly laminar flow; a slope of zero indicates a threshold resistor

1. Low flow rates may be distinguished on the same plot as very high flow rates.
2. Laminar flow is distinguished by a slope of 1·0. Turbulent flow is distinguished by a slope of 2·0. The degree of turbulence may thus easily be derived from the slope.
3. The slope is often fairly constant throughout a wide range of flows. Under these circumstances, the flow rate/pressure gradient characteristics can be plotted from only two experimental observations.

MINOR SOURCES OF RESISTANCE TO GAS FLOW

The major component of the total resistance to breathing is afforded by the resistance to gas flow discussed above. However, certain techniques of measurement of resistance include other minor sources of resistance to breathing which are listed below. The total resistance to breathing is generally known as the *pulmonary resistance* to distinguish it from the frictional resistance to gas flow itself which is known as *airway resistance.*

1. The frictional resistance of lung tissue to deformation offers a resistance to gas flow which is probably less than one-fifth of the resistance to gas flow through the air passages. Pulmonary tissue resistance is increased in pulmonary oedema, hyaline membrane disease and in the diseases grouped together as pulmonary fibrosis.
2. The thoracic cage, diaphragm and abdominal contents offer a small resistance to the flow of gas, but this component is difficult to measure.
3. Respired gases, moving parts of breathing apparatus, lung and chest wall have appreciable inertia and, therefore, offer resistance to changes in direction of gas flow. This component is usually negligible.

In addition to the sources of resistance listed above, it is important to remember that external breathing apparatus, endotracheal tubes, etc. usually offer an appreciable amount of resistance to breathing. In a typical anaesthetized patient this *apparatus resistance* is equal to about half of the patient's *pulmonary resistance* and it is important to specify whether it has or has not been included in a measurement or a figure used in calculations providing a specification for a ventilator. For purposes of calculation it is usually assumed that the effect of two resistances in series is additive.

CAUSES OF INCREASED AIRWAY RESISTANCE

It is unusual to measure airway resistance in clinical practice, and the degree of resistance is commonly assessed in terms of the response of the patient. Four grades may be recognized.

Grade 1. Slight resistance, against which the patient is able to sustain indefinitely an increased respiratory effort sufficient for the maintenance of alveolar ventilation. Arterial blood gas levels remain within normal limits (arterial Pco_2, 4·8–5·9 kPa or 36–44 mm Hg).

Grade 2. Moderate resistance, against which a considerable respiratory effort is required to avert a deterioration in blood gas levels. In some patients increased effort is well sustained and the arterial Pco_2 does not rise appreciably in spite of substantial resistance. In cases of obstructive airway disease, such patients have been referred to as 'pink puffers', in contrast to 'blue bloaters' who allow their ventilation to decrease in the face of a similar degree of resistance.

Grade 3. Severe resistance, against which no patient is able to sustain an increased respiratory effort sufficient to prevent a deterioration in blood gas levels which threatens the life of the patient. This means a rise in Pco_2 in the range 10–12 kPa (75–90 mm Hg). The corresponding fall of Po_2 is often influenced by abnormalities of distribution which are usually present. Thus, in patients with obstructive airway disease, the fall in Po_2 is usually greater than the rise in Pco_2 and the latter is a better indication of the ventilatory state.

Grade 4. Respiratory obstruction may be defined as an increase of airway resistance against which neither the patient himself, nor artificial ventilation, can achieve a ventilation sufficient to maintain life. The limiting factor is usually hypoxia.

It is not possible to define the actual levels of resistance which separate these grades, since much will depend on the duration of the obstruction and the ability of the patient to increase his respiratory effort. The disturbance of ventilation and blood gas levels are the most practicable methods of assessment.

Sites of increased airway resistance

External apparatus

Respiratory apparatus often causes resistance which is considerably higher than that afforded by the normal human respiratory tract (*Figure 37*). It is difficult to say what level of resistance is unacceptable and when design must be considered faulty. It should be remembered how very high the airway resistance of a 'normal' patient may be during anaesthesia (Bodman, 1963), and how very powerful are the compensatory powers of the anaesthetized patient (page 125). As a general guide, the heavy line in *Figure 37* indicates a level of resistance which may be considered excessive. A somewhat higher limit has been proposed for patients in labour and this is relevant to inhalational apparatus for obstetric analgesia (Hogg et al., 1974).

When a number of resistors are joined in series to form an anaesthetic gas circuit, they may interact upon one another in a very complex manner. In general, they summate after the manner of electrical resistors in series, but detailed studies show that they may alter the pattern of air flow through one another so that the combined resistance cannot be predicted (Smith, 1961). It is even possible that the total resistance may be *less* than that of individual components.

The most important sources of external resistance are narrow tubes, and generators of turbulence such as sharp bends and sudden changes in diameters. It is well known that a reduction in diameter of a tube will increase the pressure gradient between its ends by a factor equal to at least the fourth power of the reduction in diameter. *Figure 39* shows this effect illustrated by various sizes of endotracheal tubes.

Vaporizers are classified fairly sharply into those which are suitable for draw-over use and those which require an external source of energy to drive gas through them. The Rowbotham and Fluotec (Mark II) vaporizers are normally regarded as falling within the latter category but, in fact, offer less resistance than a catheter mount with an 8 mm Magill tube (provided the setting of the Fluotec does not exceed 2 per cent; Nunn, 1961b). The Fluotec Mark III vaporizer has a resistance about 100 times greater than that of the Mark II and is entirely unsuitable for draw-over use (Paterson, Hulands and Nunn, 1969).

Countless published articles describe the resistance of anaesthetic apparatus. Very simple methods of measurement of resistance are available, and it is valuable for anaesthetists to spend a little time on the measurement of the

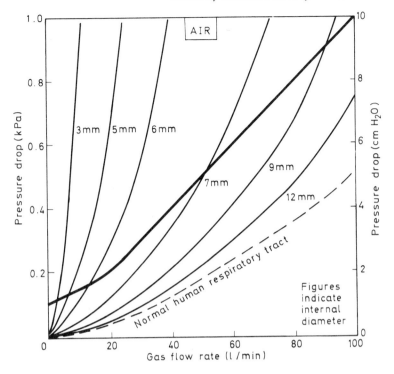

Figure 39. Flow rate/pressure drop plots of a range of endotracheal tubes, with their connectors and catheter mounts. The heavy line is the author's suggested upper limit of acceptable resistance for an adult. Pressure drop does not quite increase according to the fourth power of the diameter (inverse) because the catheter mount offered the same resistance throughout the range of tubes. With 70 per cent N_2O/30 per cent O_2, the pressure drop is about 40 per cent greater for the same gas flow rate when flow is turbulent, but little different when the flow is chiefly laminar

resistance of the apparatus which they customarily use. Not only will they derive valid figures for their own apparatus, but they will also learn a great deal about the concept of 'resistance' which cannot easily be gleaned from a textbook.

No aspect of apparatus resistance approaches the clinical importance of obstruction. This is prone to occur at certain well known sites and is always potentially lethal.

1. Closure of taps fitted to the Y-piece of some makes of circle apparatus. Such taps should be removed.
2. Closure of taps to reservoir bags during use with low flows of fresh gases.
3. Kinking of endotracheal tubes, and clenching of teeth on them.
4. Obstruction of endotracheal tubes and their connectors by foreign bodies, herniated cuffs, dilatations of their walls, etc.

The danger is greatest when using unfamilar apparatus, but it is always incumbent on the anaesthetist to carry out a functional test of the apparatus before commencing an anaesthetic.

The upper air passages

As in the case of external apparatus, the effects of moderate changes in resistance are of small importance compared with obstruction. The causes of upper respiratory tract obstruction may be conveniently classified in the customary manner:

1. Obstruction due to foreign material within the lumen.
2. Obstruction due to thickening or contraction of the walls of the air passages.
3. Obstruction due to displacement of the walls of the air passages, by forces acting from outside.

Obstruction due to foreign material within the lumen.   Gastric contents, blood and forgotten packs are the most important foreign bodies which may obstruct the upper air passages.

Obstruction due to contraction of muscles occurs in laryngeal spasm, inspiratory stridor and coughing, but *thickening of the mucosa* is the dominant factor in nasal resistance and in laryngeal and cricoid oedema. The larynx may also be obstructed by neoplasm and by membranous diphtheria.

Obstruction due to outside forces may occur with retropharyngeal abscess, Ludwig's angina and thyroid enlargement. A special problem of the unconscious patient is relaxation of the muscles of the tongue which then falls back against the posterior pharyngeal wall. Practical aspects of this are considered below (page 119) in relation to anaesthesia and resuscitation. Three studies have correlated lateral radiographs with the degree of pharyngeal obstruction occurring in the unconscious patient (Safar, Escarraga and Chang, 1959; Morikawa, Safar and DeCarlo, 1961; Ruben et al., 1961). In the conscious subject, the anteroposterior distance from the back of the tongue to the posterior pharyngeal wall is about 10 mm. Relaxation of the muscles between the tongue, larynx and chin causes marked reduction of this clearance in the unconscious subject, changes being similar for prone and supine positions provided the position of the head is unchanged relative to the trunk. Clearance is, however, markedly dependent upon the angle of the head at the atlanto-occipital joint. Flexion usually results in total obstruction, while extension usually increases the clearance to a value comparable with that in the conscious subject. Further improvement is obtained by closing the mouth, which puts further tension on the soft parts. Finally, the mandible may be protruded (*see Figure 45*).

Clearing of the airway by these means inevitably increases the anatomical dead space of the pharynx. A study by Nunn, Campbell and Peckett (1959) showed that, between the positions of neck flexion and neck extension with jaw protrusion, the anatomical dead space is increased by 70 ml. A patient with hypoventilation might thus pass over the narrow margin into respiratory failure as a result of over-enthusiastic attempts to minimize resistance in the pharyngeal airway. Therefore, if for some reason artificial ventilation is not practicable, it is preferable to secure the airway with an endotracheal tube or at least an oropharyngeal artificial airway. The significance of upper airway obstruction during use of the manual methods of artificial ventilation (e.g. Holger Nielsen technique) is outlined on page 174.

Carcinoma of the larynx, diptheria, cricoid and subcricoid oedema can all give rise to a severe narrowing of the air passages which may remain undetected in the hospital patient who is at rest. Provided he remains calm, he can withstand suprisingly high resistance. However, once he is alarmed and starts to struggle, he enters a vicious cycle of raised oxygen consumption, increased ventilatory demand, increased pressure gradients, panic and struggle, leading to further increase in oxygen consumption.

The lower air passages

In the healthy subject, airways of less than 2 mm diameter make only a small contribution to total airway resistance. However, they are the main site of obstruction in most diseases characterized by airway obstruction, including chronic bronchitis, emphysema, bronchiectasis, cystic fibrosis, asthma and bronchiolitis (Macklem, 1971). The smaller airways have been termed the 'quiet zone' because pathological increase in their resistance must be extensive before it can be detected by tests of over-all airway resistance which is dominated by the resistance of the larger airways in the healthy subject. The calibre of all air passages is influenced by lung volume which therefore has a major effect on airway resistance (*see Figure 43*).

Obstruction of the lower air passages is especially serious since it cannot be relieved by intubation or tracheostomy. Increased resistance is a most important feature of many respiratory diseases.

Obstruction due to foreign material within the lumen may result from inhaled gastric contents, blood, ruptured lung abscess, excessive secretions, drowning, pulmonary oedema or displacement of tumours fungating into the bronchi. Inflatable blockers and packing may be deliberately introduced during thoracic surgery. In the absence of effective coughing, obstruction by foreign material can only be cleared by suction or by postural drainage if the material is sufficiently liquid.

Mucus and other secretions lining the air passages do more than simply diminish the effective diameter, with resistance rising inversely to the fourth power of the radius. When the air flow rate increases beyond a critical level, the secretions are thrown up into a series of waves travelling in the direction of air flow, and flow becomes turbulent (Clarke, Jones and Oliver, 1970). Although this is an essential preliminary to clearance of secretions by the cough mechanism, it results in a gross increase in resistance before the secretions are actually cleared. If the peak air flow rate is sufficient to raise the waves but insufficient to clear the secretions, then there may be a serious increase in airway resistance. This commonly arises when secretions are thick and tenacious. Airway resistance may, in these circumstances, be reduced by tracheobronchial toilet especially after bronchial lavage with 50–100 ml of isotonic saline.

Thickening of the mucosa or constriction of the bronchiolar musculature is a common response to a wide variety of allergens and irritants such as sulphur dioxide, including bronchial instrumentation with inadequate anaesthesia. Of particular importance to the anaesthetist is the development of these forms of resistance after inhalation of gastric contents. In the rabbit at least, it appears to be the acid of the gastric contents which is primarily responsible (Mendelson, 1946), and a solution of sodium bicarbonate may be used for bronchial lavage when acid contamination is suspected. In many forms of respiratory disease, particularly asthma, swelling of the mucosa and bronchoconstriction are important features. Bronchoconstriction may be induced by histamine, para-sympathomimetic drugs, β-adrenergic receptor blockers or anticholinesterases, particularly some of the nerve gases. Certain anaesthetic agents including thiopentone and althesin are believed to render the patient more liable to bronchoconstriction. *d*-Tubocurarine, with its reputation for histamine release, has been suspected as a potential bronchoconstrictor, but Gerbershagen and Bergman (1967) found no significant change of airway resistance when large doses of *d*-tubocurarine were administered to a series of anaesthetized patients. The subject of bronchomotor tone has been reviewed by Aviado (1975).

A number of agents will dilate the bronchioles. Atropine in dosage of 1·0 mg increases the anatomical dead space by about 20 ml (Nunn and Bergman, 1964). Aminophylline (200 mg) is a popular therapeutic agent but probably not as effective as a β-sympathomimetic agent such as isoprenaline, or, preferably, salbutamol. Since these agents may also cause cardiac arrhythmias, they are usually given by droplet inhalation, although intravenous administration may be used in emergencies (isoprenaline 1–2 μg, salbutamol 100–300 μg).

Obstruction by pressure from outside the lumen is of great practical importance and not least because it is seldom amenable to treatment. The subject is best approached by consideration of the mechanisms which hold the airways open. These are as follows.

1. *Structural rigidity* is only present in those air passages which have cartilage in their walls (*see Table 1*).
2. *Elastic recoil of alveolar septa* is important for the small air passages which are embedded directly in the lung parenchyma (*see Table 1*). This force may be reduced when there is destruction of alveolar tissue as in emphysema.
3. *Transmural pressure gradient* has an important influence on all air passages with the normally subatmospheric intrathoracic pressure holding open the air passages which usually have an intraluminal pressure close to atmosphere.

The large intrathoracic air passages are held open by a combination of factors (1) and (3), while small air passages are held open by a combination of factors (2) and (3). The effect of transmural pressure gradient is common to both and, if it is reversed, may lead to closure of both small and large air passages.

Collapse of large air passages by a reversed transmural pressure gradient is the normal mechanism limiting maximal expiratory flow rate and the phenomenon is best considered in terms of the flow/volume plot. *Figure 40* shows such a plot in which the lung volume is on the abscissa and the instantaneous respiratory flow rate on the ordinate. Time is not directly indicated. In the upper part of the figure, the small loop shows the normal tidal excursion above the FRC and with air flow rate ranging on either side of zero air flow. Arrows show the direction of the trace during normal breathing. At residual volume the black square indicates the patient at the end of a maximal expiration with zero air flow rate. The lower part of the curve then shows the course of a maximal inspiration taken in the patient's own time and reaching total lung capacity at the point shown by the black circle, again at zero air flow rate. The four expiratory curves starting from total lung capacity show four levels of expiratory effort, each with its own peak expiratory flow rate. Within limits, the greater the effort, the greater is the resulting peak flow rate. The striking feature of the experiment is that all the

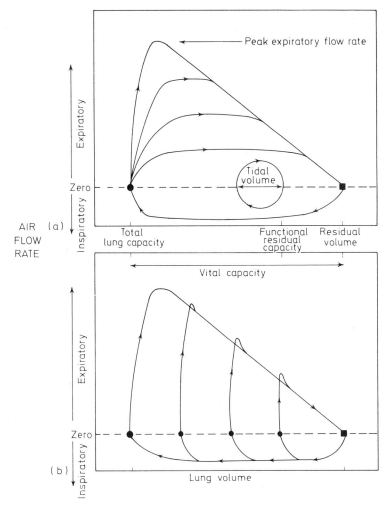

Figure 40. Normal flow/volume curves. Instantaneous air flow rate (ordinate) is plotted against lung volume (abscissa). (a) shows the normal tidal excursion as the small loop. In addition, it shows expirations from total lung capacity at four levels of expiratory effort. Within limits, peak expiratory flow rate is dependent on effort but, during the latter part of expiration, all curves converge on an effort-independent section where flow rate is limited by airway collapse. (b) shows the effect of forced expirations from different lung volumes. The pips above the effort-independent section probably represent air expelled from collapsed airways

expiratory curves terminate in a final common pathway which is therefore called the effort-independent part of the curve. This is the part where flow rate is limited by airway collapse and maximal air flow rate is directly related to the lung volume. The greater the effort, the greater is the degree of airway collapse and the resultant air flow rate for a particular lung volume is the same. Maximal expiratory effort from total lung capacity should produce a brassy noise, and radiographic studies with tantalum dust lining the air passages have shown that the major site of obstruction is in the trachea and large bronchi (Jones, Fraser and Nadel, 1975).

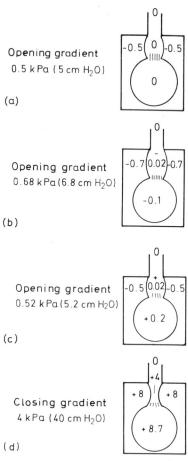

Opening gradient
0.5 kPa (5 cm H$_2$O)

(a)

Opening gradient
0.68 kPa (6.8 cm H$_2$O)

(b)

Opening gradient
0.52 kPa (5.2 cm H$_2$O)

(c)

Closing gradient
4 kPa (40 cm H$_2$O)

(d)

Figure 41. Typical transmural pressure gradients of the intrathoracic air passages under various conditions of ventilation. Note the pressure drop occurring in the smallest air passages, leading to a pressure difference between the alveoli and the larger air passages. (a) Static pressures at the end of expiration (upright, conscious subject). (b) Pressures at the middle of a normal inspiration. Note the increased favourable transmural pressure gradient of the intrathoracic airway. (c) Pressures at the middle of a normal expiration. Note the decreased (but still favourable) transmural pressure gradient of the intrathoracic airway. (d) Typical pressures during a forced expiration. Note the unfavourable transmural pressure gradient of the intrathoracic airway—leading to collapse

The lower part of *Figure 40* shows a series of maximal expiratory efforts, each starting from a different lung volume. This also shows the phenomenon of the final common pathway of the effort-independent part of the curve and also illustrates the importance of a maximal inspiration in measurement of the peak flow rate. The overshoots are not fully explained but are, in part, due to the collapse of the air passages with expulsion of the air in the anatomical dead space.

The mechanism by which this collapse occurs is shown in *Figure 41*. During expiration, the resistance to gas flow in the smaller air passages results in a pressure gradient between the alveoli and the larger air passages. However, during normal breathing the pressure in the lumen of the air passages should remain well above the (subatmospheric) pressure in the thorax and there will be no tendency towards airway collapse. *Figure 41d* shows the situation during a maximal forced expiration where the intrathoracic pressure rises far above atmospheric. This pressure is communicated to the alveoli which have a pressure higher still, due to the elastic recoil of the alveolar septa. However, at high gas flow rates, the pressure drop down the air passage is increased and there will be a point where it equals the intrathoracic pressure. At that point (the equal pressure point) the air passages are held open by elastic recoil of lung parenchyma (in the small air passages) and by cartilage (in the large air passages). Downstream of this point, the transmural pressure gradient is reversed and at some point will overcome these forces and result in airway closure. As lung volume decreases, the point of collapse moves progressively from the larger to the smaller air passages. As collapse becomes imminent, an additional factor is the Bernoulli or Venturi effect by which gas flowing over a convex surface creates a low pressure which would tend to accentuate collapse in the situation shown in *Figure 41d*.

Airway closure during a forced expiration, otherwise known as trapping, occurs at lower gas flow rates in emphysema and in asthma. In the former case this is mainly due to destruction of lung parenchyma, resulting in loss of elastic recoil which is required to hold open the small air passages embedded in the lung parenchyma. Elastin may be lost in patients with α_1-antitrypsin deficiency (*see* page 22). There may also be some weakness of the cartilaginous air passages with increased tendency to collapse by invagination of the posterior wall of intrathoracic trachea and large bronchi. Increased small airway resistance may exaggerate the pressure gradients along the airways shown in *Figure 41*.

In asthma, there is a high bronchomotor tone and mucosal oedema which augments forces tending to collapse the air passages, and small airway resistance will enhance the reversed transmural pressure gradient in the large air passages. The adverse effect of increased secretions has already been described above. When bronchospasm is a major factor, relief should be obtained from bronchodilators but this is absent in uncomplicated emphysema.

The effect of pathological closure of small airways on a forced expiration is shown in the upper part of *Figure 42*. Residual volume is commonly increased and vital capacity diminished. Inspiration is relatively normal but a maximal forced expiration is characterized by a peak flow rate which is diminished in both rate and duration. Expiratory flow rate then falls markedly to give a long drawn-out expiration with a characteristically concave flow/volume plot. There will also be a reduced forced expiratory volume (page 137) and expiration will be prolonged. Various bedside tests have been devised to give a clinical indication of the condition. Large airway obstruction (as, for example, due to carcinoma of the larynx) produces the type of flow/volume curve shown in the lower part of *Figure 42*. There is a flat cut-off to the expiratory curve (and also the inspiratory curve) and the level of the cut-off is highly effort-dependent. This may be reflected in the peak flow rate being reduced more than the forced expiratory volume.

An impairment of maximal expiratory flow rate of the type shown in the upper part of *Figure 42* has an obviously deleterious effect on the ability of the patient to clear his secretions. A stage is reached in which he is unable to generate an air flow rate sufficiently high to raise the secretions into waves prior to ejection as described on page 111. Ultimately the impairment becomes so grave that the patient is unable to maintain an adequate alveolar ventilation. He then passes into ventilatory failure with a progressive rise of arterial Pco_2. There is no fixed relationship between ventilatory capacity (commonly assessed as the forced expiratory volume) and the Pco_2. Most patients with emphysema fall into the class of *pink puffers* and maintain a normal arterial Pco_2 by a greatly increased work of breathing even in the face of grave reduction of forced expiratory volume (FEV) and it is not uncommon to find the FEV (1 second) as low as 0·5 litres with a normal arterial Pco_2. This is also true of patients with asthma. In contrast, most patients with chronic bronchitis fall into the class of

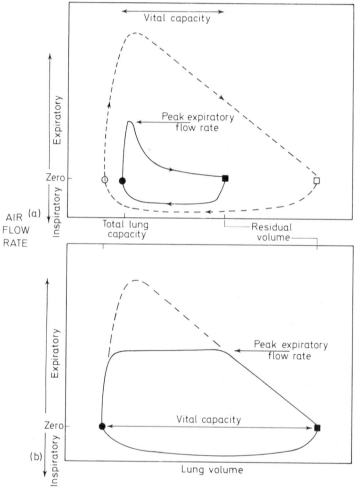

Figure 42. (a) Shows a flow/volume curve which is typical of a patient with obstructive airway disease of the smaller air passages. Note the diminished vital capacity and flattening of the effort-independent sector of the curve (compared with the broken curve which shows the normal). The expiratory curve is characteristically concave upwards. (b) shows the cut-off of high flow rates which is characteristic of upper airway obstruction (e.g. due to carcinoma of the larynx). The plateau is highly effort-dependent

blue bloaters and allow their Pco_2 to rise while they still have a reasonable ventilatory capacity. They may be shown to have a reduced ventilatory response to carbon dioxide (page 45).

It will be clear from *Figure 40* that airway collapse occurs at higher flow rates at higher lung volumes. This is the basis of pursed lip breathing, a device which emphysematous patients use to raise their end-expiratory lung volume. A similar effect may be obtained by the use of a positive end-expiratory pressure (PEEP) in patients who are being ventilated artificially, and by continuous positive airway pressure (CPAP) in patients breathing spontaneously. These techniques are, however, more commonly used for their beneficial effect on arterial Po_2 in various pathological conditions of the lungs such as are encountered in intensive therapy units (page 128 et seq.).

Volume-dependent but effort-independent limitation of expiratory air flow rate by airway collapse is a dynamic phenomenon which occurs only at maximal air flow rates. It must be clearly distinguished from the static phenomenon of airway closure which is simply a function of lung volume and is not appreciably affected by air flow rate or by expiratory effort.

The effect of lung volume—the closing capacity

When the lung volume is reduced, there is a reduction in the size of all air-containing parts. Thus the alveoli and their ducts diminish in size and the air

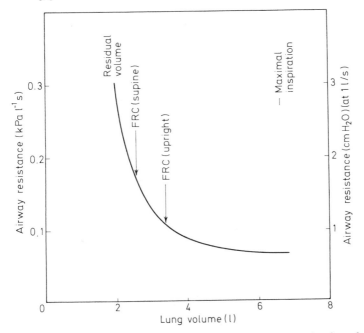

Figure 43. Airway resistance is a function of lung volume. This curve is a hyperbola and conductance (reciprocal of resistance) is linearly related to lung volume. Note that a reduction of FRC of about 0·4 l, which is known to occur during anaesthesia, would itself increase the airway resistance sufficiently to account for most of the actual increase in resistance which has been reported under these circumstances. (This curve is compounded of curves reported by Mead and Agostoni (1964) and Zamel et al. (1974))

passages show an over-all reduction of calibre. It follows that airway resistance must be a function of the lung volume at which the measurement is made (*Figure 43*).

In addition to the over-all change of airway resistance with reduction of lung volume, there are most important effects on regional resistance. This is because the airways and alveoli in the dependent parts of the lungs are smaller than those at the top of the lung, except at inspiratory capacity. Thus, when the lung volume is reduced, the airways in the dependent parts are always those which are most likely to close (*Figure 44*). In fact, it seems very likely that total or almost total obstruction of dependent airways does occur in normal subjects when they exhale down to what is known as their closing capacity, measurement of which is outlined at the end of this chapter.

Closing capacity was considered on page 70 in relation to FRC. It tends to rise during life, becoming equal to the FRC in the supine position at a mean age of about 44 years and to the FRC in the upright position at a mean age of about 66 years (Leblanc, Ruff and Milic-Emili, 1970). If the tidal range is below the closing capacity, a part of the pulmonary blood flow will be distributed to underventilated areas, producing in effect a shunt and tending to cause a reduction in arterial Po_2.

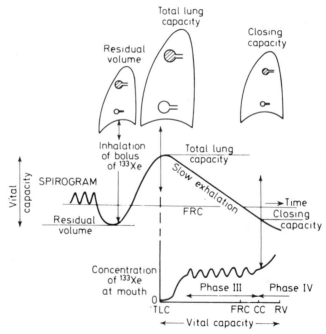

Figure 44. Measurement of closing capacity by the use of a tracer gas such as ^{133}xenon. The bolus of tracer gas is inhaled near residual volume and, due to airway closure, is distributed only to those alveoli whose air passages are still open (shown shaded in the diagram). During expiration, the concentration of the tracer gas becomes constant after the dead space is washed out. This plateau (phase III) gives way to a rising concentration of tracer gas (phase IV) when there is closure of airways leading to alveoli which did not receive the tracer gas

Resistance to breathing during anaesthesia

There seems to be general agreement that total respiratory resistance is approximately doubled when a healthy patient is anaesthetized, and typical values are of the order of $0.3–0.6$ kPa l^{-1} s (3–6 cm H_2O l^{-1} sec). Results obtained in a number of studies are listed in *Table 6* (page 105). In older patients, particularly those with respiratory disease, considerably higher values are obtained, and in the series of Bodman (1963) and Bergman (1969) were as high as 1.6 kPa l^{-1} s (16 cm H_2O l^{-1} sec) excluding the resistance of endotracheal tube and connector. It is important to remember that this apparatus resistance is commonly in the range $0.4–0.6$ kPa l^{-1} s (4–6 cm H_2O l^{-1} sec) and total respiratory resistance of a healthy anaesthetized patient together with his endotracheal tube and connector is likely to be of the order of 1 kPa l^{-1} s (10 cm H_2O l^{-1} sec) and double this in many patients with lung disease.

Until recently there was no obvious explanation for the increase in respiratory resistance when a healthy patient is anaesthetized. It now seems likely that this is due to the decreased FRC which seems to be a normal feature of an uncomplicated anaesthetic (*see* page 67). The over-all reduction in all components of the lung volume results in a reduced calibre of airway which not only increases resistance but also increases any tendency towards airway collapse. The relationship between airway resistance and lung volume is well established (*Figure 43*) and the observed reductions in FRC, firstly on assuming the supine position (about 0.8 l) and secondly following the induction of anaesthesia (about 0.4 l), are sufficient to explain the increased airway resistance seen in the healthy anaesthetized patient.

In addition to this 'normal' increased airway resistance in the anaesthetized patient, there are a number of pathological causes, some of which result in a life-threatening interference with ventilation. Most of these have been mentioned above in connection with the relevant part of the respiratory tract. Of the greatest practical importance is pharyngeal obstruction, which can be considered to be a normal feature of unconsciousness (*see* page 110). Maintenance of a clear airway by correct positioning of the head and jaw is an essential skill which must be learned by all those responsible for the care of unconscious patients. A minor degree of this type of obstruction occurs in snoring and the degree of obstruction from this cause can be alarming to a trained anaesthetist.

In 1959, Safar published a most important paper in which he showed that pharyngeal obstruction was almost always present during resuscitation and was not relieved by the methods which were currently being taught to first-aid workers. In particular, manual methods of artificial ventilation, in which both hands were required for compression of the chest had little hope of success. Even placing the patient in the prone position, or the use of a pharyngeal airway, does not guarantee that the obstruction will be relieved. In a subsequent paper, Safar, Escarraga and Chang (1959) showed that the most effective manoeuvres are extension of the atlanto-occipital joint (*Figure 45*) and protrusion of the mandible. Much of the success of mouth-to-mouth resuscitation depends on the fact that the rescuer's hands are already placed where they can clear the airway by these manoeuvres as well as steady the head (*see* page 174).

Laryngeal spasm is a dreaded complication in situations where effective methods of treatment are lacking. It usually results from stimulation, particularly when the depth of anaesthesia is insufficient to suppress the laryngeal reflex. Once obstruction is complete, the alveolar P_{O_2} falls, the P_{CO_2} rises and the alveolar partial pressure of anaesthetics is reduced (at least during the early part of an anaesthetic). Various courses of action may be followed. One school

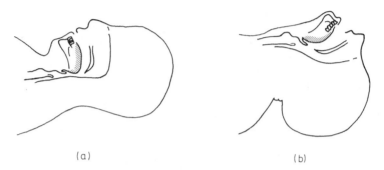

(a)   (b)

Figure 45. Clearance of airway by extension of the atlanto-occipital joint. (a) The outline of the pharynx in the unconscious patient. Turning into the prone position does little to improve the obstruction between the base of the tongue and the posterior pharyngeal wall. This may be cleared by maximal extension of the atlanto-occipital joint (b). The airway may also be cleared by protrusion of the mandible in the manoeuvre familiar to all anaesthetists

of thought advocates masterly inactivity on the grounds that the larynx will always open before the patient's life is threatened. Alternatively, a rapidly acting relaxant will open the glottis more quickly and perhaps before the P_{O_2} is seriously reduced. In appropriate situations, it may be possible to slide an endotracheal tube through the larynx but force must never be used under these circumstances. Much depends upon the alveolar P_{O_2} before obstruction supervenes. If the patient has been breathing oxygen, the alvolar gas will contain sufficient oxygen to maintain a safe P_{O_2} for several minutes and the situation is far less urgent than in cases when the patient has been breathing a 20 per cent oxygen mixture.

THE EFFECTS OF INCREASED RESISTANCE TO BREATHING

The effects of increased resistance to breathing are of profound importance in chest medicine, anaesthesia and intensive therapy. On the one hand, there are therapeutic endeavours designed to overcome pathological resistance in the patient's respiratory system and now, more recently, there is the question of deliberate imposition of various forms of resistance to breathing for the purpose of improving gas exchange in the lungs. This form of therapy, however, has important circulatory implications largely in relation to resultant changes in the intrathoracic pressure.

The plan of this section is to deal first with the relationship between peak flow rate, mean flow rate and minute volume of respiration and then with the effect of resistance on mean intrathoracic pressure. After that, the respiratory response to increased resistance will be considered. After these preliminaries we are then able to consider the reaction of the patient as a whole to increased resistance to breathing: firstly, flow-dependent resistance, and secondly, flow-independent resistance which includes PEEP.

The relationship between peak flow rate, mean flow rate and minute volume

Some of the more important effects of increased resistance to breathing are due to the abnormal pressure gradients resulting from the tidal flow of gas past the elevated resistance. It is, therefore, important to appreciate the relationship

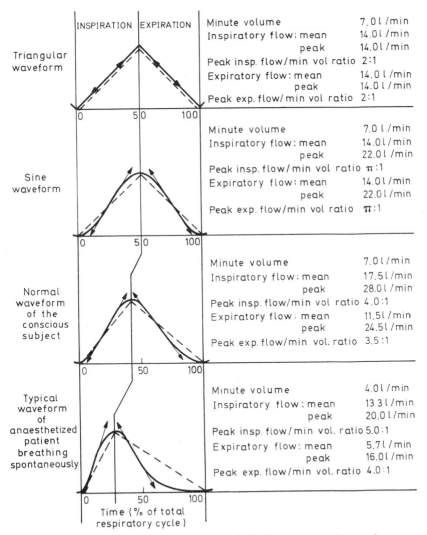

Figure 46. Respiratory waveforms showing the relationship between minute volume, mean flow rates (broken lines) and peak flow rates (indicated by arrows). The normal waveform of the conscious subject is taken from Cain and Otis (1949). The waveform of the anaesthetized patient is derived from 44 spirograms of patients during surgery

between the instantaneous rate of gas flow and the minute volume. In the examples below, the minute volume is assumed to be 7 l/min.

Triangular waveform.   If inspiration and expiration have equal duration and constant gas flow rates without any pauses, it follows that the peak flow rates will equal the mean inspiratory and expiratory flow rates which must be twice the minute volume or 14 l/min (*Figure 46*). This peak flow/minute volume ratio of two is the lowest which can be attained and would be appropriate for breathing through a very high resistance.

Sine wave.   The triangular waveform is seldom found in respiration but a sine waveform is closely approximated during spontaneous hyperventilation. Like the triangular pattern, there are no pauses and the durations of inspiration and expiration are equal (*Figure 46*). Therefore, the *mean* inspiratory and expiratory flow rates again equal twice the minute volume. However, the peak flow in each direction will exceed the mean flow rate when the flow rate reaches a maximum at the middle of inspiration and expiration. It may be shown that the peak flow is in fact equal to π times the minute volume. Thus, if the minute volume is 7 l/min, the peak flow rate will be about 22 l/min.

The normal respiratory waveform does not conform to a sine wave. The inspiratory phase is usually less than half the duration of the total respiratory cycle, and the peak inspiratory flow rate usually has a value of about four times the minute volume. Expiration lasts about half the cycle, but reaches its peak flow early, thereafter declining exponentially into the post-expiratory pause (*Figure 46*).

Anaesthesia.   Nunn and Ezi-Ashi (1962) studied the respiratory waveforms of 44 anaesthetized patients breathing spontaneously and found that post-expiratory pauses tended to be longer with lower minute volumes.

Thus as minute volume fell, the peak flow/minute volume ratio tended to rise and the peak flow rates remained roughly constant within the range 15–30 l/min (*Table 7*). These values were derived from a spirometer trace which tends to

Table 7. RELATIONSHIP BETWEEN PEAK FLOWS AND MINUTE VOLUME OF ANAESTHETIZED PATIENTS BREATHING SPONTANEOUSLY WITH VARIOUS POST-EXPIRATORY PAUSES

Mean minute volume (l/min)	Duration of post-expiratory pause(s)	Peak flow/minute vol. ratio	Peak flow rate (l/min)
6·2	Less than 0·5	4–5 (insp.) 2–3 (exp.)	25–31 (insp.) 12–19 (exp.)
4·0	0·5–2·0	4·5–6	18–24
2·9	2·0–4·0	5·5–7	16–20

overlook some of the more transient peaks of high flow rate; nevertheless, 15–30 l/min seems a reasonable range of peak flow rates as a basis for consideration of the effects of resistance to breathing during anaesthesia with spontaneous respiration.

During artificial ventilation, the anaesthetist may impose any peak flow rate he chooses up to a limit of about 120 l/min. In practice, the highest level usually encountered is about 75 l/min associated with a minute volume of the order of 20 l/min.

The effects of resistance on intrathoracic pressure

Expiratory resistance alone will always result in an increased intrathoracic pressure during expiration. In the case of an expiratory threshold resistor (e.g. a 'PEEP' valve), the end-expiratory lung volume will be increased according to the static pressure/volume curve of lung and chest wall (alveolar/ambient pressure difference line in *Figure 30*). From the new end-expiratory lung volume, the intrathoracic pressure may be read from the intrathoracic/ambient pressure difference line on the same graph. Using the data of *Figure 30*, a PEEP of 0·5 kPa (5 cm H_2O) will increase the end-expiratory lung volume by about 300 ml above the original FRC and this will cause the end-expiratory intrathoracic pressure to change from 0·3 to about 0·1 kPa (3 to 1 cm H_2O) below atmospheric.

During inspiration, the effect of an expiratory resistance will depend upon the manner of breathing. If the patient is breathing spontaneously with his end-expiratory lung volume elevated by an expiratory resistor, he will normally compensate by a more forceful inspiration (*see* page 126) even if he is deeply anaesthetized. This will require a greater than normal reduction in intrathoracic pressure (*see Figure 30*) which will partly offset the elevated intrathoracic pressure during expiration and in the post-expiratory pause. If the patient is being ventilated artificially, additional inflation pressure is required when PEEP is used. Therefore the intrathoracic pressure will be higher during inspiration than when PEEP is not used, to maintain the same ventilation.

It is important to appreciate that the intrathoracic pressure is usually much lower than the inflation pressure used on an artificial ventilator. Firstly, while gas is flowing, there will be a pressure drop between the ventilator and the alveoli: this is a function of instantaneous gas flow rate and airway resistance. Secondly, there is a further pressure drop between alveoli and the intrathoracic space: this is a function of the actual lung volume and the lung compliance.

Inspiratory resistance alone will result in a decrease of both intra-alveolar and intrathoracic pressures during inspiration. Mean pressure will also fall since expiratory pressures are unchanged. The fall of pressure during inspiration can only be produced by the inspiratory muscles or by a cabinet respirator. No reduction can occur during artificial ventilation by intermittent positive pressure.

A combination of inspiratory and expiratory resistances will result in a change of intrathoracic pressure, the direction of which will depend upon the relative magnitude of inspiratory and expiratory resistance and peak flow rates. It is possible that alveolar and intrathoracic mean pressures may be unchanged if the swings in each direction are of equal duration and magnitude.

The effects of changes in the intrathoracic pressure are usually considered in relation to the *mean* pressure with respect to time. The mean pressure may be determined graphically from a record of the instantaneous pressure, by

ARP–5*

construction of a rectangle of area equal to that under the curve and length equal to a respiratory cycle. The height of the rectangle will then indicate the mean pressure (*Figure 47*). This technique is the same as that used for determination of the mean arterial blood pressure. Alternatively, the mean pressure can be measured directly by using a manometer, which is so damped that it cannot respond to the rapid changes in pressure (*Figure 47*). Electronic damping of a transduced signal is generally used in practice. Consideration of these methods of measurement will make it clear that the mean pressure depends upon the duration as much as the actual level of the pressure transients.

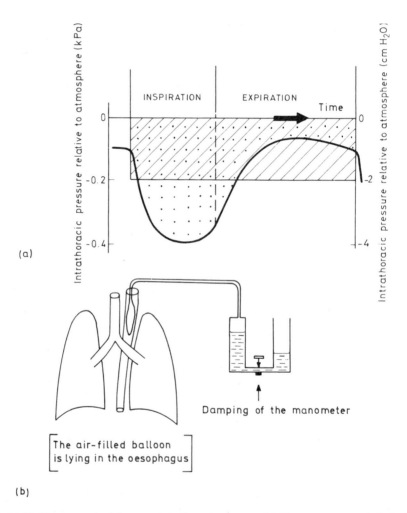

Figure 47. *Measurement of the mean intrathoracic pressure. (a) The mean pressure is derived from the instantaneous pressure by construction of a rectangle (shaded) equal in area to that (dotted) above the instantaneous pressure curve. The height of the rectangle then indicates the mean intrathoracic pressure (0·2 kPa = 2 cm H_2O below atmospheric). (b) A simple manometer is used which cannot follow individual breaths. If suitably damped, it will indicate the mean intrathoracic pressure*

The respiratory response to increased resistance to breathing

The normal response to *inspiratory resistance* is an increased inspiratory effort with little change in the FRC (Fink, Ngai and Holaday, 1958). Accessory muscles are brought into play according to the degree of resistance. There is considerable individual variation in the ability of subjects to compensate for the added resistance, and ventilation is diminished or even abolished if the resistance is sufficiently high. Maximal voluntary inspiratory effort at the FRC will attain an alveolar pressure about 9 kPa (90 cm H_2O) below atmospheric (Rahn et al., 1946b). Campbell (1958, p. 79) has pointed out that the inspiratory muscles are not contracting maximally at this level, and appear to be subject to reflex inhibition. He added that pressures of 9 kPa (90 cm H_2O) below atmospheric would result in a tendency for gases to be drawn out of solution in the tissues.

The respiratory response of the anaesthetized patient to inspiratory resistance was studied by Nunn and Ezi-Ashi (1961), who found a remarkable ability of patients to compensate for an inspiratory threshold resistor (*Figure 48*). Patients

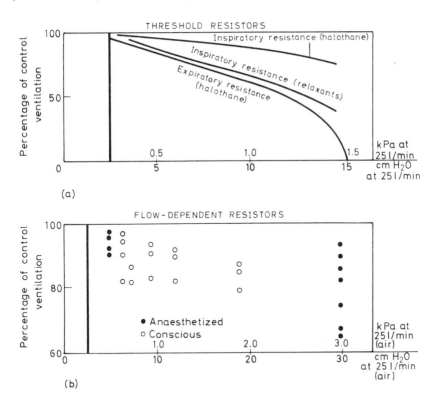

(a)

(b)

Figure 48. Ventilatory response to added resistance to breathing. (a) The response of anaesthetized patients to threshold resistors (Nunn and Ezi-Ashi, 1961). (b) The response to anaesthetized patients is compared with the published results in conscious subjects (McIlroy et al., 1956; Zechman, Hall and Hull, 1957). The conscious subjects breathed air through resistors with laminar flow. The anaesthetized patients breathed 70 per cent N_2O/30 per cent O_2 through tubular resistors with predominantly turbulent flow. In both diagrams the heavy vertical line indicates the author's suggested upper limit of acceptable resistance for an anaesthetized patient

who had received relaxants responded rather less favourably than those anaesthetized with halothane, who suffered only a 15 per cent reduction of ventilation against an inspiratory threshold resistor of 1 kPa (10 cm H_2O)—a level which is distinctly unpleasant to the conscious subject.

Asthmatic patients also show a remarkable capacity to compensate for increased airway resistance. Twenty patients in status asthmaticus studied by Palmer and Diament (1967) were found to have a mean Pco_2 in the lower reaches of the normal range. Isoprenaline aerosols give symptomatic relief from dyspnoea but may cause little change in Pco_2. Hypercapnia in the asthmatic patient is a sign of serious deterioration.

Mechanism of compensation.   There is a twofold mechanism for the augmentation of inspiratory effort in the face of resistance. The first mechanism operates immediately and even during the first breath in which the resistance is applied. It seems probable that the muscle spindles indicate that the inspiratory muscles have failed to shorten by the intended amount, and their afferents augment the activity of the motoneurone pool. The resemblance of the inspiratory muscle control to a servo-mechanism has already been described in Chapter 2 (page 32). It is of interest that the conscious subject is able to detect very small increments in external resistance, and it is clear that the afferent pathway of the reflex is in existence (Campbell et al., 1961). A second compensatory mechanism develops over about 90 seconds and overacts for a similar period when the resistance is removed (Nunn and Ezi-Ashi, 1961). It is probable that this delayed response depends upon elevation of the arterial Pco_2 which is an inevitable consequence of underventilation. After the resistance is removed, hyperventilation continues until the Pco_2 returns to normal.

A similar two-phase response to inspiratory obstruction was demonstrated in dogs (Bendixen and Bunker, 1962). The first breath after obstruction developed a subatmospheric pressure of about 1·5 kPa (15 cm H_2O), which corresponds to a much greater tension in the inspiratory muscles than would be present during normal unobstructed respiration. Thereafter the dogs further augmented their inspiratory tension during the 50 seconds of the observation period.

Expiration against pressures of 1 kPa (10 cm H_2O) results in no contraction of the abdominal muscles or rise of intragastric pressure. Above this pressure, expiratory muscles are brought increasingly into play, up to pressures of 1·7 kPa (17·5 cm H_2O) at which level their use is invariable.

At expiratory pressures below 1 kPa (10 cm H_2O), the additional work of expiration is performed entirely during inspiration by a most remarkable mechanism, in which *inspiration* is augmented until the lung volume is increased to a point at which the elastic recoil is sufficient to overcome the expiratory resistance (Campbell, 1957). The increase in lung volume, divided by the expiratory pressure to be overcome, is, in fact, a measure of the total static compliance of the subject. The same mechanism is found in anaesthetized patients (Campbell, Howell and Peckett, 1957; Nunn and Ezi-Ashi, 1961). The latter workers found that expiratory resistance tended to diminish the pulmonary ventilation rather more than did the same level of inspiratory resistance. There was, furthermore, a rather sharp cut-off of ventilation with expiratory pressures in excess of 1·5 kPa = 15 cm H_2O (*Figure 48*).

It will be noticed that the response to expiratory resistance runs counter to what might be expected from demonstration of the Hering–Breuer inflation reflex in animals. In Chapter 2 it has been explained that in man this reflex is extremely weak in response to pressures of less than about $1\cdot2$ kPa = 12 cm H_2O (page 53).

The actual mechanism of the increased inspiratory effort is rather complicated and seems likely to depend on the ability of the intrafusal fibres of the inspiratory muscle spindles to accommodate themselves to the altered FRC brought about by the impairment of expiration. This resets the developed inspiratory tension in accord with the increased FRC (Nunn and Ezi-Ashi, 1961).

Perhaps of greater importance is the response of the patient to the *combination of inspiratory and expiratory resistance.* Nunn and Ezi-Ashi (1961) found that a combined inspiratory and expiratory threshold resistor produced much the same decrease of minute volume as was obtained with the same expiratory threshold resistor alone. They also studied the effect of two tubular resistors through which the flow was largely turbulent. The resistance of the larger was equivalent to a 6 mm endotracheal tube, and the smaller to a $3\cdot5$ mm endotracheal tube (*see Figure 39*), both being well above the external resistance considered acceptable for an anaesthetized patient. These resistors caused no measurable change in FRC, and less decrease of ventilation than was caused by comparable pressure gradients produced by the threshold resistors. The larger tubular resistor reduced the mean ventilation by 7 per cent, and the smaller by 21 per cent (*Figure 48*). It is unlikely that a 7 per cent reduction would be of clinical significance.

Studies of the response of the conscious subject to external resistance to breathing have been reported by Davies, Haldane and Priestley (1919), Killick (1935), Cain and Otis (1949), McIlroy et al. (1956), and by Zechman, Hall and Hull (1957). In *Figure 48b,* some of their results are shown (open circles) for comparison with results obtained during anaesthesia with tubular resistors (solid circles). It is surprising that anaesthetized patients seem able to compensate for the added load just as well as conscious subjects, although their control minute volumes (without resistance) were substantially less than those of the conscious subjects. On a cautionary note, it should be mentioned that these experiments have all been acute and there are no data on the ability of an anaesthetized patient to tolerate long-standing resistance to breathing.

The good ventilatory response of the anaesthetized patient to resistance joins an interesting list of previously unsuspected factors which help anaesthetized patients to survive some of the insults to which they are, at times, subjected. Many other factors appear in this book.

General physiological response to flow-dependent resistance

Whether the resistance be in external apparatus or in the respiratory tract, the effect on minute volume of ventilation depends upon the severity of the resistance and the ability of the patient to compensate by the mechanisms described above. When there is a reduction in ventilation, it is important to consider separately the effect on carbon dioxide, oxygen and other gases such as anaesthetics. Detailed consideration is postponed to page 186 but the essential features are as follows. P_{CO_2} must rise but will do so comparatively slowly since this is dependent upon the rate of carbon dioxide production and its considerable storage capacity in the body. With total failure of carbon dioxide elimination, arterial P_{CO_2} should rise by 0·4–0·8 kPa/minute (3–6 mm Hg/min). However, with partial obstruction the rate of rise should be less. The equilibrium level of P_{CO} attained may be inferred from *Figure 118*. Arterial P_{O_2} falls with reduced minute volume and the change is much more rapid than the change in P_{CO_2} (*see Figure 141*) because of the very small storage capacity of the body for oxygen. Much depends upon lung volume and alveolar P_{O_2} before the start of obstruction but, under the worst conditions, P_{O_2} may fall to dangerous levels within as little as 1 minute. It is often forgotten that the levels of other gases, such as anaesthetics, also change during obstruction. During induction of anaesthesia, the level of anaesthetic in the alveoli will fall as the agent is distributed through the body and the level of narcosis will lighten. If the obstruction is due to reflex laryngospasm or bronchospasm, this may temporarily exacerbate the condition. During recovery from anaesthesia, the reverse happens and the alveolar level rises. Since the tension of anaesthetic in the brain follows that in the alveoli, it will be seen that changes are unfavourable during both induction and recovery.

If the patient is breathing a high concentration of oxygen, the danger of hypoxaemia is postponed but, as an alternative hazard, obstruction imposes the possibility of absorption collapse. It is all a matter of the ventilation/perfusion ratio. In round figures, 1 ml of pulmonary arterial blood can remove 0·05 ml of oxygen. Therefore, if a lung or part of a lung containing 100 per cent oxygen has a ventilation/perfusion ratio of less than 0·05 it must inevitably collapse within 5–10 minutes. If nitrogen is present, this will delay collapse (*see Figure 105*) but the P_{O_2} will fall more rapidly and the consequences are generally more serious.

We have discussed above the rather complex factors governing change in intrathoracic pressure due to flow-dependent resistance to breathing. In general, changes in intrathoracic pressure are of secondary importance compared with the effect on ventilation.

General physiological response to flow in dependent threshold resistance

This subject has assumed great practical importance because of the demonstration of the beneficial effect of an expiratory threshold resistance on the arterial P_{O_2} of a wide range of patients undergoing intensive therapy. In current nomenclature, an expiratory threshold resistor during artificial ventilation is known as PEEP (positive end-expiratory pressure) and during spontaneous breathing as CPAP (continuous positive airway pressure).

Respiratory effects.   We have already seen that, during spontaneous respiration, most patients are able to maintain a well compensated minute volume in the face of an expiratory threshold resistor of about 0·5 kPa (5 cm H_2O) even if anaesthetized. During artificial ventilation, there should be no problems in adjusting the ventilator to give an adequate minute volume, even with considerably higher expiratory pressure. The respiratory benefits of an expiratory threshold resistor are as follows.

1. FRC is increased and over-all airway resistance should be reduced (*see Figure 43*).

2. The increased FRC may lift the tidal volume above the closing capacity, and thereby avoid the underventilation of dependent parts of the lung.
3. There should be a tendency towards re-expansion of areas of collapse.
4. There tends to be removal of lung water (*see* page 267).

The over-all result is that the percentage of pulmonary blood flow through non- or underventilated areas should be reduced, and in many conditions it has been shown that shunt or pulmonary venous admixture is markedly reduced. The benefits will clearly be minimal if there is pathological reduction in blood flow to the dependent parts of the lungs as in cases of long-standing mitral stenosis (Trichet et al., 1975).

Circulatory effects.   The respiratory advantages outlined above may, in some situations, be offset by circulatory disadvantages due to the inevitable rise in intrathoracic pressure which accompanies the use of PEEP or CPAP. This pressure is communicated to the right atrium and impedes the return of venous blood from the periphery. If the patient has a normal relationship between ventricular filling pressure and myocardial contractility (i.e. the normal Frank–Starling curve), the impaired diastolic filling will reduce the strength of myocardial contraction, resulting in a reduced cardiac output which will in turn lower the blood pressure unless systemic vascular resistance is increased. In the healthy subject there is a rise in peripheral venous pressure, which provides some measure of compensation. This can be studied in the response to the Valsalva manoeuvre which is blocked by deep anaesthesia and by β-adrenergic blockers or head-up tilt in the lightly anaesthetized patient (Blackburn et al., 1973).

In the case of healthy anaesthetized dogs, there is no doubt that PEEP causes a substantial reduction in cardiac output (Braunwald, Binion and Morgan, 1957; Sykes et al., 1970; Qvist et al., 1975). The last group showed that the reduction was maintained for as long as 8 hours with no evidence of adaptation. Braunwald's group demonstrated that cardiac output could be restored to control levels with an α-adrenergic stimulator (metaraminol), and both Sykes' and Qvist's groups showed that overtransfusion was equally effective.

In clinical practice the situation is much more complicated because disease and drugs have profound effects upon the circulatory response to PEEP or CPAP. It is interesting that certain conditions aggravate the depression of cardiac output but others actually oppose the reduction in cardiac output, and it is in these situations that PEEP is of particular clinical value. Firstly, there is the ability of the patient to raise his peripheral venous pressure to match the increased intrathoracic pressure. There are obvious dangers in patients with vasomotor paralysis and hypovolaemia but, on the other hand, venous pressure can be supported with transfusion and vasopressor drugs. Secondly, there is the question of the pulmonary compliance of the patient. If the lungs are excessively stiff (e.g. respiratory distress syndrome of both infants and adults, fibrosing alveolitis, etc.) much of the applied end-expiratory pressure will be opposed by the excessive pulmonary transmural pressure, thus minimizing the rise in intrathoracic pressure. Therefore, the stiffer the lungs, the safer it is to apply PEEP, other things being equal. Thirdly, it is necessary to consider the ventricular response to raised filling pressure. If the patient has a flat Frank–Starling curve or, due to congestive failure, is already on the flat part of a normal curve, then a further reduction in filling pressure (reduced transmural end-diastolic ventricular pressure) will not necessarily reduce the strength of ventricular contraction and may even effect some improvement. Thus in many clinical situations, the worse the cardiac state, the less likely it is to be further embarrassed by PEEP. There are, of course, important exceptions to this rule. Finally, we should note that pulmonary vascular disease in the dependent parts of the lung (e.g. long-standing mitral valve disease) may also protect the circulation from the adverse effects of PEEP (Trichet et al., 1975).

Clinical response to PEEP or CPAP.   It will be seen that, in essence, PEEP is likely to confer respiratory benefits and circulatory disadvantages. These interact in a most complicated way and the question of benefit to the patient can only be settled by direct measurements of the relevant physiological variables. Patients with different conditions may respond quite differently and there are also differences between individual patients with a particular condition.

Initially, there was great reluctance to use PEEP because of the circulatory hazard of intermittent positive pressure breathing with sustained expiratory pressure, which had been stressed in the classic paper by Cournand et al. (1948). Not many papers in this field count two Nobel prize winners amongst their authors. Earliest reports of the value of PEEP were in relation to postoperative cardiac surgical patients (Hill et al., 1965), acute respiratory distress in adults (Ashbaugh et al., 1967), inhalation of gastric contents (Adams et al., 1969) and pulmonary oedema (Uzawa and Ashbaugh, 1969). This was followed by a report of its use in 108 patients with a wide range of respiratory pathology (Kumar et al., 1970) and the use of CPAP for the respiratory distress syndrome of infants (Gregory et al., 1971).

In a second generation of studies, Downs, Klein and Modell (1973) described the use of incremental PEEP to obtain the optimal improvement in arterial P_{O_2}, and Suter, Fairley and Isenberg (1975) extended this concept to optimize the oxygen flux which occurred at what they called 'best PEEP'. The latter study thus defined the level of PEEP at which the most favourable combinations of respiratory and circulatory changes occurred. They also reported that compliance was optimal at this level of PEEP. The use of very high levels of PEEP has been presented by Kirby, Downs and Civetta (1975). CPAP and PEEP have been briefly reviewed by Downes (1976).

During routine anaesthesia, the results of PEEP are disappointing. In 1965, Nunn, Bergman and Coleman reported that 0·5 kPa (5 cm H_2O) PEEP did not improve arterial P_{O_2}. Similar results have been obtained by subsequent workers. Whyche et al. (1973) showed that PEEP during anaesthesia raised FRC as might be expected but that arterial P_{O_2} was only significantly improved in those patients with a particularly low arterial P_{O_2} before the application of PEEP. Such patients might have had some pulmonary collapse. A study in anaesthetized dogs by Colgan, Barrow and Fanning (1971) showed that PEEP increased FRC and reduced pulmonary venous admixture but also reduced cardiac output and mixed venous saturation. The net result was no change in alveolar–arterial P_{O_2} gradient. At the present, this seems to be a plausible explanation of what happens in the anaesthetized patient. One may summarize by saying that, in the routine anaesthetized patient, PEEP is unlikely to raise arterial P_{O_2} but will probably reduce cardiac output and therefore the oxygen flux. There would seem to be no indication for using PEEP under these circumstances.

PRINCIPLES OF MEASUREMENT OF FLOW RESISTANCE

Resistance to respiratory gas flow is determined by the simultaneous measurement of gas flow rate and the appropriate pressure gradient, as outlined in *Figure 32*. Measurement of gas flow rate usually presents no insuperable problem, and the difficulties centre around the measurement of the pressure gradient. Methods of presentation of results are described earlier in this chapter.

Apparatus resistance

Continuous flow of gas offers the simplest method of measurement of airway resistance. The pressure difference is then static and may be measured by simple methods such as liquid U-tube manometers.

Reciprocating flow has the advantage of testing the apparatus under the actual conditions of use, but requires manometers with rapid response. Cooper (1961) has shown that it is generally possible to use data derived from continuous flow studies to deduce the resistance offered to reciprocating flow.

Nasal resistance

The resistance of the nose can easily be determined by measuring the mouth-to-atmosphere pressure difference, while the subject breathes through his nose, with the mouth closed around the tube leading to the manometer. Either continuous or reciprocating flow can be used, powered either by the patient's respiratory muscles or by some external device (Seebohm and Hamilton, 1958; Butler, 1960).

Airway and pulmonary resistance

Simultaneous measurement of air flow rate and mouth-to-intrathoracic pressure gradient. In Chapter 3, it was shown how simultaneous measurement of tidal volume and intrathoracic pressure yielded the dynamic compliance of the lung (*Figure 31*). For this purpose pressures were selected at the moments of zero air flow when pressures were uninfluenced by air flow resistance. The same experimental arrangement may be used for the determination of flow resistance, but for this purpose, steps are taken to eliminate the component of pressure which is produced by the elastic forces. *Figure 49* shows a suitable experimental arrangement in which a pneumotachograph is used to measure the instantaneous flow rate which may then be integrated to give respired volumes. A second differential manometer measures the difference between mouth and intrathoracic pressure.

From the flow trace it is easy to select the points of zero flow at which the pressure gradient is opposed only by elastic forces. It is then possible to construct the dotted line in the pressure trace (*Figure 49*), which shows the pressure changes which would be seen in a hypothetical patient with zero resistance to gas flow, and in whom pressure gradients would relate only to elastic forces. The difference between this and the observed pressure gradient (shaded zone) is the component due to flow resistance. It is then a simple matter to read off the flow resistance component of the pressure gradient for different flow rates as given by the pneumotachogram above it. A flow rate/pressure gradient plot may then be derived, or else the resistance may be expressed according to any of the mathematical conventions discussed earlier in this chapter.

Alternatively, the mouth-to-intrathoracic pressure gradient and respired

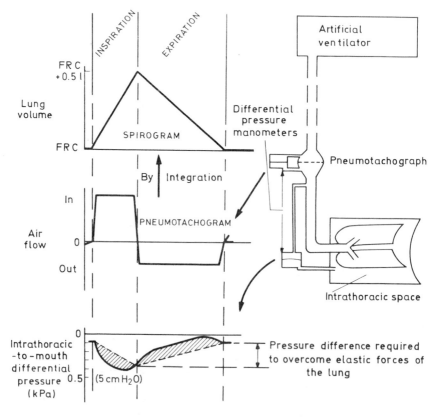

Figure 49. The measurement of pulmonary resistance and dynamic compliance by simultaneous measurement of air flow and intrathoracic-to-mouth differential pressure (Neergaard and Wirz, 1927b). The spirogram is conveniently obtained by integration of the pneumotachogram. In the pressure trace, the dotted line shows the pressure changes which would be expected in a hypothetical patient with no pulmonary resistance. Compliance is derived as shown in Figure 31. Pulmonary resistance is derived as the difference between the measured pressure differential and that which is required for elastic forces (shaded area) compared with the flow rate shown in the pneumotachogram. Note that the pneumotachogram is a much more sensitive indication of the no-flow points than the spirogram

volume may be plotted as X and Y co-ordinates to give a loop. *Figure 31* showed how dynamic compliance could be derived from the no-flow points of such a loop. In our hypothetical patient with zero resistance to gas flow, the 'loop' would consist of a straight line (*Figure 50a*). The greater the resistance, the

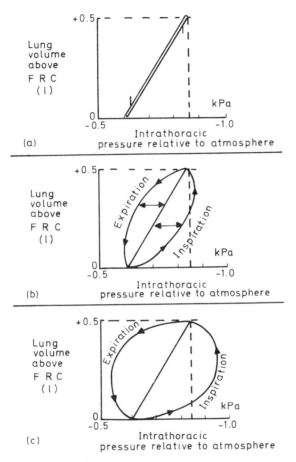

Figure 50. *Dynamic pressure/volume loops obtained in conscious upright subjects with varying degrees of pulmonary resistance. It is not possible to determine the actual resistance from a loop, but the area of the loop indicates the amount of work done in overcoming pulmonary resistance. The diagonals joining the no-flow points of the loop correspond very closely with the transmural pressure curve in Figure 29. (a) A hypothetical subject with zero pulmonary resistance; pressure changes solely in accord with elastic forces:*

$$compliance = \frac{volume\ change}{pressure\ change}$$

$$= \frac{0 \cdot 5}{0 \cdot 25}$$

$$= 2\ l/kPa\ (200\ ml/cm\ H_2O)$$

(b) Subject with normal pulmonary resistance; horizontal displacement of points from the diagonal (shown by arrows) indicates pressure required to overcome pulmonary resistance. (c) Subject with excessive pulmonary resistance; the higher the resistance, the fatter the loop becomes.

fatter the loop becomes, with the horizontal deflections of the points from the 'no resistance' line indicating the pressure gradient required for gas flow at that particular flow rate. Elegant though this method of display may be, it is not possible to derive the actual instantaneous gas flow rate from the loop and, therefore, the resistance cannot be quantified according to the methods described above. Nevertheless, we shall see in Chapter 6 that the work required to overcome the flow resistance corresponds to the area of the loop.

The interrupter technique.   A single manometer may be used to measure both the mouth and the alveolar pressure if the air passages distal to the manometer are momentarily interrupted with a shutter. The method is based on the assumption that, while the airway is interrupted, the mouth pressure comes to equal the alveolar pressure, a concept open to some doubt. Flow resistance may thus be derived from the difference between the alveolar pressure (measured during interruption) and the mouth pressure (measured immediately before and after interruption). Both this and the preceding methods were first described in the classic paper of Neergaard and Wirz in 1927b.

The pufflator.   This simple device for the measurement of inspiratory resistance of the paralysed patient was described by Don and Robson (1965). A constant-flow generator is used to inflate the lungs of a patient for a known period of time, after which the flow abruptly ceases, the mouth or tracheal pressure being measured throughout this process. The static pressure after flow ceases is the elastic component for that particular tidal volume, and the appropriate fraction of this elastic pressure may then be subtracted from the dynamic pressure during inflation to indicate the pressure required to overcome flow resistance (*Figure 51*). The technique thus yields compliance (lungs and chest wall) and pulmonary resistance.

The body plethysmograph.   If the hypothetical patient with zero resistance to gas flow were to sit in a sealed box and inhale, there would clearly be no change in the pressure within the box. However, if he had appreciable airway resistance, the pressure of the alveolar gas would fall below ambient during inspiration and the thorax would expand in accord with Boyle's law. The increased displacement of the thorax would then increase the pressure in the box in accord with the airway resistance (DuBois, Botelho and Comroe, 1956). It is possible to obtain a direct plot of pressure gradient against respiratory flow rate on a cathode ray oscilloscope or $X-Y$ plotter. A patient may be studied without instrumentation in a few minutes and functional residual capacity may be measured at the same time. The body plethysmograph measures only the *airway resistance*.

Analysis of the passive spirogram.   Perhaps the simplest method of assessment of resistance is the study of the slope of a passive spirogram—either a passive expiration into an ordinary spirometer (Comroe, Nisell and Nims, 1954), or the discharge of a weighted spirometer into a relaxed patient (Newman, Campbell and Dinnick, 1959). Both methods are suitable only for paralysed patients. The first stage in the analysis of the result is to determine the static compliance, which is given by the volume change divided by the pressure change. The resistance to flow may then be derived by a number of different methods.

1. Spirograms obtained by this method appear to approximate closely to simple exponential functions and, therefore, a time constant may be derived (*Figure 52*). Assuming that resistance remains constant throughout the breath, the resistance may be derived from the equation:

$$\text{resistance} \times \text{compliance} = \text{time constant}$$

The concept of the time constant is discussed more fully in the following chapter and in Appendix E. During expiration it seems feasible that the resistance (in the sense of pressure divided by flow) may remain constant. Initially the flow rate is high but increased tendency to turbulence is probably offset by the wider calibre of the air passages.

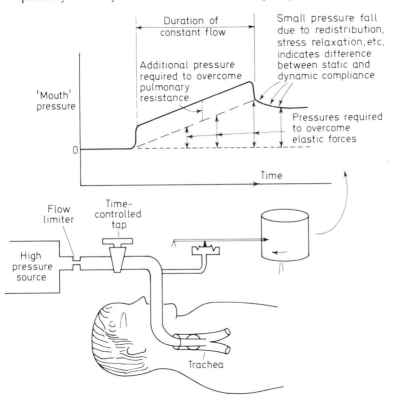

Figure 51. Measurement of compliance and resistance with the Pufflator. With this simple device a constant flow rate of gas is passed into the patient for a pre-set time interval. The broken line on the pressure trace indicates the pressure which would be required for a hypothetical patient with no pulmonary resistance. The difference between this and the actual pressure is the pressure required to overcome pulmonary resistance. In this example it is constant throughout the inflation.

$$\textit{Tidal volume} = \underset{\textit{(pre-set)}}{\textit{constant flow rate}} \times \underset{\textit{(pre set)}}{\textit{duration of flow}}$$

$$\textit{Static compliance} = \frac{\textit{tidal volume}}{\textit{static end-inflation pressure}}$$

$$\textit{Pulmonary resistance} = \frac{\textit{additional pressure required to overcome pulmonary resistance}}{\textit{constant flow rate (pre-set)}}$$

2. The initial pressure gradient is known and the tangent to the first part of the curve will indicate the flow rate at that point (*Figure 52*).

3. At any point of the curve, the flow rate may be derived as the tangent to the curve. The mouth pressure is known (assumed equal to the pressure within the spirometer), and the alveolar pressure may be derived from its initial pressure and final pressure (assumed equal to the pressure within the spirometer) assuming that the alveolar pressure changes in proportion to the volume change (indicated by the spirometer).

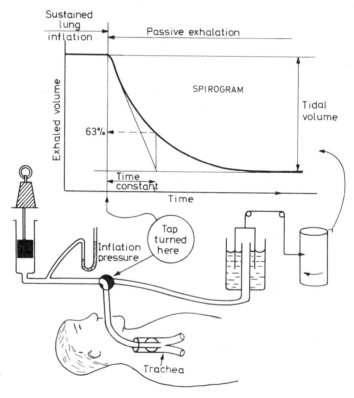

Figure 52. Measurement of resistance and compliance by analysis of the passive spirogram. This method is only applicable to the paralysed patient. Only a water manometer and a spirometer are required

$$Static\ compliance = \frac{tidal\ volume}{inflation\ pressure}$$

$$Compliance \times resistance = time\ constant$$

$$Initial\ resistance = \frac{initial\ pressure\ gradient}{initial\ flow\ rate} = \frac{inflation\ pressure}{tidal\ vol/time\ constant}$$

Clinical tests of ventilatory capacity

It is rather unusual to carry out a formal measurement of airway resistance in the clinical investigation of a patient. The more usual procedure is to measure the ventilatory (or more specifically the expiratory) capacity of the patient. In most cases this approach is satisfactory as it is usually obvious when ventilatory capacity is impaired by increased resistance to breathing. However, there are many other possible causes of reduction of ventilatory capacity (*Figure 67* and page 190) and it is important to distinguish increased resistance from such conditions as restriction of lung volume, diminished force of contraction of respiratory muscles and lesions of the lower motoneurone.

Formerly the standard test of ventilatory function was to measure the maximal breathing capacity (MBC). This test consisted of urging the patient to breathe maximally in and out of a lightweight spirometer for a period of 15 seconds. The ventilation over this period was then multiplied by four to give the value which would be obtained if ventilation had been sustained for a full minute. About 50 per cent of MBC is required for heavy work loads (80 per cent of capacity) and 75 per cent of MBC can be maintained with difficulty for 15 minutes by fit young subjects (Shephard, 1967). Normal values depend upon body size, age and sex, the range being 47–253 l/min for men and 55–139 l/min for women (Cotes, 1975). The average young adult male should have a value of about 170 l/min. It is difficult to obtain repeatable results with this test, which may be quite exhausing for the patient. It has therefore become more usual to assess the ventilatory capacity of a patient indirectly by study of a forced expiration. This carries the assumption that the major component of the resistance is operative during expiration, and this is true in most patients with obstructive airway disease of the type which typically occurs in emphysema.

The forced expiration may be quantified in many ways but the commonest are measurement of the peak flow rate or the forced expiratory volume (one second). The former may be measured by three methods: as the slope of a spirometer trace, with a peak flowmeter (Wright and McKerrow, 1959), or by observation of the pneumotachogram. Normal values will depend upon the method since the spirometer method overlooks transients of very high flow rate while the pneumotachogram method is particularly sensitive to these transients. The peak flowmeter is intermediate (for details of calibration, *see* page 207). The peak flow measured by the Wright peak flowmeter tends to be about four times the MBC.

Forced expiratory volume (FEV) is measured by instructing the patient to take a maximal inflation and then to exhale maximally into a spirometer of low inertia. The volume expired in the first second is measured and designated the $FEV_{1.0}$. Some prefer to measure over three-quarters or half a second. The $FEV_{1.0}$ is a valid measurement of expiratory capacity, but some find it easier to derive the indirect MBC which equals:

$$35 \times FEV_{1.0}$$

Water spirometers are inconvenient and lack portability. Much ingenuity has been devoted to the design of suitable dry spirometers such as the Vitalograph.

A reduction of MBC or $FEV_{1.0}$ below the predicted value for the patient may provide valuable information about the ventilatory capacity of the patient but does not indicate the cause of the impairment. Further light may be shed by taking the following steps.

1. The investigator should satisfy himself that the patient's ability to exhale is not being curtailed by failure to develop the appropriate tension in the

expiratory muscles. This maý be due to a wide range of conditions including malingering, poliomyelitis, muscular dystrophies and abdominal pain. Without appreciation of this point, a reduced FEV could be erroneously interpreted as indicating increased airway resistance although the FEV is not unduly sensitive to effort (Kemm and Kamburoff, 1970). Failure to take a full inspiration before a forced expiration will also give a low value for FEV and peak flow rate (*Figure 40*).

2. Restrictive disease of the chest (e.g. kyphoscoliosis) will also give a reduction of the FEV which might be confused with increased airway resistance. The distinction may be made by comparison with the vital capacity which is reduced more in restrictive disease than in obstructive disease. $FEV_{1.0}$ may with advantage be expressed as a percentage of the vital capacity, with values below about 85 per cent indicating an abnormal airway resistance.

3. Bronchoconstriction may be distinguished from stuctural causes of increased airway resistance by repeating measurement of the $FEV_{1.0}$ or peak flow after the use of a bronchodilator aerosol spray (e.g. salbutamol). No change of a reduced FEV which is less than 75 per cent of vital capacity is usually indicative of increased airway resistance caused by structural changes leading to trapping but the lower limit of normal decreases with advancing age.

The flow/volume plot has been illustrated in *Figures 40 and 42*. It has considerable diagnostic value in distinguishing different types of increased airway resistance and is particularly useful for detecting malingerers. It may be generated by a variety of methods, but the commonest is a wedge (dry) spirometer which gives the volume signal from a linear potentiometer. This signal is then differentiated to give flow rate. Display is either on an $X-Y$ plotter or on a storage oscilloscope.

Closing volume

This is perhaps the most convenient place to describe the measurement of closing volume (*see* page 117 and *Figure 44*). The technique measures the lung volume at which airways begin to close in the dependent part of the lung. This is done by arranging for there to be different concentrations of a tracer gas in the upper and lower parts of the lung by inspiration of a bolus of the tracer gas at residual volume when airways are closed in the dependent parts of the lung. Then, after a maximal inspiration, the patient exhales slowly while the concentration of the tracer gas is continuously analysed at the mouth. When airways again begin to close in the dependent parts of the lungs, the tracer concentration begins to rise (phase IV) above the alveolar plateau level (phase III). Suitable tracers are ^{133}xenon (Dollfuss, Milic-Emili and Bates, 1967), 100 per cent oxygen measured as fall in nitrogen (Anthonisen et al., 1969) or sulphur hexafluoride enhancement of the nitrogen method (Newberg and Jones, 1974).

For further information on these tests and data for prediction of normal values, the reader is referred to Cotes (1975). Techniques for measurement of gas volumes and flow rates are described in Chapter 6 (pages 204 et seq.).

Chapter 5 Mechanisms of Pulmonary Ventilation

I. TIDAL EXCHANGE PRODUCED BY THE DEVELOPMENT OF A PRESSURE GRADIENT BETWEEN THE MOUTH AND THE AIR SURROUNDING THE TRUNK

Phases of the Respiratory Cycle
Ventilation by Intermittent Step Increases in Mouth Pressure (Constant Pressure Generators)
Variable or Flow-limited Pressure Generators
Requirements of Artificial Ventilation by Intermittent Positive Pressure

II. TIDAL EXCHANGE PRODUCED BY FORCES ACTING DIRECTLY ON THE BOUNDARIES OF THE THORACIC CAVITY

Spontaneous Respiration
Artificial Ventilation Produced by Forces Acting Directly on the Thorax

•

The previous chapters have described the various structures, factors and mechanisms which play a part in pulmonary ventilation. This chapter is concerned with the tidal exchange resulting from the interaction of the factors already considered.

The flow of respiratory gases may always be considered as secondary to the development of a pressure gradient between the mouth* and the alveoli. Inspiration may result either from raising the mouth pressure (e.g. artificial ventilation by intermittent positive pressure—IPP), or from lowering the alveolar pressure (e.g. spontaneous breathing). In either case, the pressure gradient is developed in the same direction and the resultant gas flow is roughly similar.

Apart from normal breathing, there are many alternative methods of achieving adequate tidal ventilation of the lungs. This chapter considers the various methods in two groups. The first part of the chapter discusses methods of ventilation in which gas flow results from a change in gas pressure induced by external means (e.g. artificial ventilation by IPP). The second part of the chapter

---

* Throughout this chapter, 'mouth' should be taken to read 'tracheal' when the mouth is bypassed by a tracheostomy or endotracheal tube.

139

considers methods of ventilation in which the driving pressure gradient is secondary to forces acting directly on the boundaries of the thoracic cavity. Although this group includes normal spontaneous respiration, it is considered later as the fundamental principles of ventilation are easier to understand when ventilation results directly from changes in mouth pressure.

Part I   Tidal Exchange Produced by the Development of a Pressure Gradient Between the Mouth and the Air Surrounding the Trunk

The cumbersome title of the first part of this chapter represents an attempt to consider together techniques which are similar from the physiological point of view. Artificial ventilation by IPP is, from the clinical standpoint, quite different from artificial ventilation by means of a whole-body cabinet respirator. However, the two methods are almost identical in terms of pressure gradients and the resultant gas flow. Furthermore, the similarity extends to the effects upon the venous return.

PHASES OF THE RESPIRATORY CYCLE

Inspiration

During artificial ventilation by IPP, the mouth pressure is intermittently raised above ambient. When a cabinet respirator is used (with subatmospheric pressures only), the ambient pressure around the trunk is rhythmically lowered below the mouth pressure. In each case, a mouth-to-ambient pressure gradient is developed during inspiration, and then allowed to decay at the start of expiration. From the point of view of ventilation, the two techniques seem to be identical. They are compared in *Figure 53*, and it will be seen that the various pressure gradients are the same although actual pressures, particularly intrathoracic, differ between the two methods.

If inspiration is slow, inspired air will be distributed according to the compliance of the different parts of the lungs and chest wall, the most compliant parts receiving the largest quantity of inspired air. If, however, there are regional variations in airway resistance and inspiration is completed fairly quickly, distribution will be influenced by the tendency of gas to take the paths of least airway resistance. This problem has already been mentioned in Chapter 3 in connection with the distinction between static and dynamic compliance (page 78). It will be discussed in greater detail in Chapter 7 which is devoted to problems of distribution of inspired gas.

Expiration

During IPP ventilation, it is usual to allow a passive expiration by letting the mouth pressure fall to atmospheric. With the cabinet respirator the equivalent procedure is to allow cabinet pressure to rise to atmospheric. In terms of pressure differentials, the two are identical.

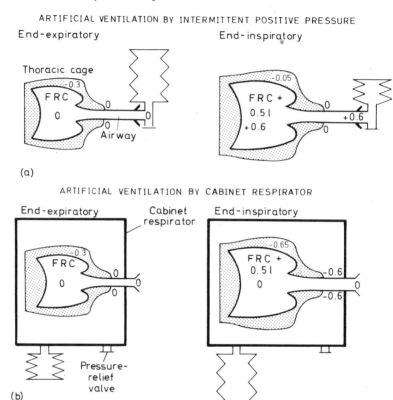

Figure 53. Comparison of artificial ventilation by (a) intermittent positive pressure (IPP) and (b) cabinet respirator (subatmospheric pressures only). The actual pressures differ in the two techniques, but the following pressure gradients are the same in both cases: mouth-to-ambient; alveolar-to-intrathoracic (transmural); intrathoracic-to-ambient. Ambient pressure refers to the pressure surrounding the trunk and is therefore cabinet pressure in the latter case. Static values for supine anaesthetized patient: lung compliance, 1·5 l/kPa (150 ml/cm H$_2$O); thoracic cage compliance, 2 l/kPa (200 ml/cm H$_2$O); total compliance, 0·85 l/kPa (85 ml/cm H$_2$O). (Intrathoracic space is shown stippled.) Figures indicate pressures relative to atmosphere in kilopascals

With either technique, expiration may be assisted in a manner analogous to the use of expiratory muscles during spontaneous respiration. During IPP ventilation, the mouth pressure may be reduced below atmospheric—the so-called 'negative phase' or negative end-expiratory pressure (NEEP). With the cabinet respiratory, the equivalent technique is the raising of the cabinet pressure above atmospheric during expiration. Formerly, this was common practice and pressure swings as much as 1·5 kPa (15 cm H$_2$O)* on either side of atmospheric were usual.

The use of subatmospheric pressure with IPP or the use of raised pressure in the cabinet will both tend to reduce the lung volume below the FRC. We have seen in Chapter 4 that this may increase airway resistance and cause pulmonary collapse, although the systemic venous return may be improved. When the lung

---

* 1 kilopascal (1 kPa) is approximately equal to 10 centimetres of water (10 cm H$_2$O).

volume falls below the FRC in this manner, pressure volume relationships follow the extrapolation of the curves in *Figures 29 and 30* downwards and to the left. The picture is, however, complicated by alveolar collapse and airway trapping.

Nowadays, rather than assisting expiration with a subatmospheric airway pressure, it is more usual to impede expiration by applying a positive end-expiratory pressure (PEEP). This increases the functional residual capacity (pages 128 et seq.) and improves arterial oxygenation under certain conditions. It should also be noted that, at high respiratory frequencies, the duration of expiration may be too short for the lung volume to return to functional residual capacity and this will have a similar effect to the application of PEEP. Bergman (1972) found that approximately three time constants were required for expiration to proceed to within 100 ml of FRC.

VENTILATION BY INTERMITTENT STEP INCREASES IN MOUTH PRESSURE (CONSTANT PRESSURE GENERATORS)

The subject of time relations is best approached by considering the type of IPP ventilation in which the mouth pressure is suddenly raised to a level which is maintained throughout inspiration. At the end of inspiration, the pressure is allowed to fall immediately to atmospheric, where it remains until the start of the next inspiration. This type of pressure profile is known as 'square wave' (*Figure 54*), and may be produced by many commercially available ventilators such as the Manley, the Bird (with air entrainment) or the Barnet, and is approached by many others including the Radcliffe. If the inflating pressure is maintained for several seconds, the tidal volume will be indicated by the following relationship:

tidal volume = sustained inflation pressure x total compliance

When the mouth pressure is raised during inspiration, it is opposed by the two forms of resistance which have already been considered; the elastic resistance of lungs and chest wall, and the frictional (non-elastic) pulmonary resistance.* At any instant, the inflation pressure equals the sum of the pressures required to overcome these two forms of resistance:

$$\frac{\text{inflation}}{\text{pressure}} = \frac{\text{pressure required to overcome}}{\text{elastic resistance}} + \frac{\text{pressure required to overcome}}{\text{pulmonary resistance}}$$

The pressure required to overcome elastic resistance equals the lung volume above FRC divided by the total compliance, while the pressure required to overcome the pulmonary resistance equals the pulmonary resistance multiplied by the instantaneous air flow rate (assuming for the moment that the air flow is entirely laminar).

The equation may now be rewritten:

$$\frac{\text{inflation}}{\text{pressure}} = \left(\frac{\text{lung volume above FRC}}{\text{compliance}}\right) + \left(\frac{\text{instantaneous}}{\text{air flow rate}} \times \frac{\text{pulmonary}}{\text{resistance}}\right)$$

The equation can be elaborated to allow for dynamic (as opposed to static)

* Pulmonary resistance = airway resistance + pulmonary tissue resistance (page 107).

compliance, and for the turbulent component of gas flow, but this simplified form is sufficient for the present.

The right-hand side of the equation has two terms, one of which is directly related to lung volume and the other to rate of gas flow. When the lung volume

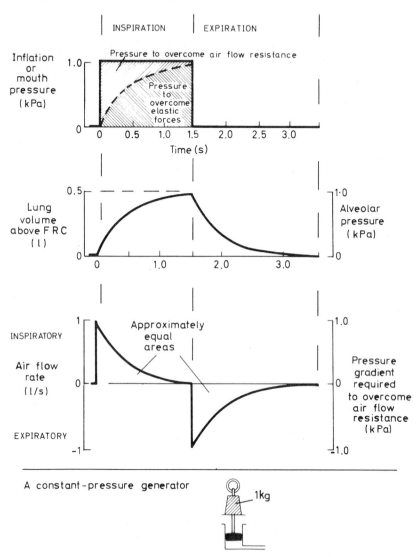

Figure 54. Artifical ventilation by intermittent application of a constant pressure (square wave). Passive expiration. Inspiratory and expiratory flow rates are both exponential. Assuming that air flow resistance is constant, it follows that flow rate and pressure gradient required to overcome resistance may be shown on the same graph. Lung volume and alveolar pressure may be shown on the same graph if compliance is constant. Values are typical for an anaesthetized supine paralysed patient: total dynamic compliance, 0·5 l/kPa (50 ml/cm H_2O); pulmonary resistance, 0·3 kPa l^{-1} s (3 cm H_2O/l/sec); apparatus resistance, 0·7 kPa l^{-1} s (7 cm H_2O/l/sec); total resistance, 1 kPa l^{-1} s (10 cm H_2O/l/sec); time constant, 0·5 s

is equal to the FRC (e.g. at the start of inspiration) the first term is zero, and inflation pressure is acting solely against the pulmonary resistance to gas flow. When gas flow ceases (at the end of inspiration) the second term is zero and inflation pressure is acting solely against elastic recoil. At the end of a normal expiration when the lung volume equals the FRC and gas flow ceases, both terms are zero.

During inspiration both terms have finite values. *Figure 54* shows how the two components of the inflation pressure vary during inspiration while their sum remains constant. The component opposed by elastic forces (which equals the alveolar pressure) increases in proportion to the˝ lung volume, while the component opposed by air flow resistance is proportional to the instantaneous air flow rate (which equals the slope of the plot of the lung volume against time). With a square pressure wave, flow is maximal at first and then declines exponentially. Therefore, the component of the inflation pressure opposed by airway resistance is maximal at first and also declines exponentially.

If expiration is passive and mouth pressure remains at ambient, the driving force is the elevation of the alveolar pressure above atmosphere, caused by elastic recoil of the lungs and chest wall. This pressure is dissipated in overcoming the airway resistance during expiration. In *Figure 54*, it will be seen that during expiration, the alveolar pressure (proportional to lung volume above FRC) is directly proportional to the expiratory flow rate.

Time relations

In the example shown in *Figure 54*, typical values for the anaesthetized patient were chosen as follows: total compliance 0·5 l/kPa (50 ml/cm H_2O); pulmonary plus apparatus resistance, 1 kPa l^{-1} s (10 cm H_2O/l/sec) (flow assumed laminar). These two quantities alone determine the rate of inflation and deflation for any particular inflation pressure. Assuming that compliance and resistance remain constant, all the curves shown in *Figure 54* are *exponential*. Changes of this type are of great importance in anaesthesia, and Appendix E describes some of the practical aspects of exponential functions as they concern anaesthetists.

During inflation with a constant mouth pressure, the lung volume follows a typical exponential 'wash-in' curve (shown in *Figure 153* of Appendix E). The expiratory curve approximates to a 'wash-out' curve and also features in Appendix E (*Figure 152*).

Exponential changes may be relatively fast or slow and their rate may be quantified by the *half-life* or the *time constant*. The former is preferred for measuring the rate of radioactive decay but the latter is more convenient for biological systems. Factors determining the time constant are considered in Appendix E, and for the example shown in *Figure 54* the relationship is as follows:

$$\frac{time}{constant} = \frac{total}{compliance} \times \frac{pulmonary}{resistance}$$

$$= 0{\cdot}5 \text{ l kPa}^{-1} \times 1 \text{ kPa l}^{-1}\text{s} = 0{\cdot}5 \text{ s}$$

(or, in non-SI units) = 0·05 l/cm H_2O × 10 cm H_2O/l/sec = 0·5 sec

Table 42 (Appendix E) provides the necessary information for calculating the changes in lung volume for any time during inspiration or expiration. Only two quantities need be known. The first is the time constant (0·5 s in this example) and the second is the equilibrium tidal volume, which would be attained if inspiration were maintained for several seconds. The latter equals inflation pressure multiplied by compliance (1 x 500 = 500 ml in this example). We may now tabulate the changes occurring during inspiration (wash-in) as in *Table 8*.

Table 8.

Duration of inflation		Lung volume increase	
s	time constants	percentage of final value	ml
0·35	0·69 (half-life)	50	250
0·5	1	63	315
1·0	2	86·5	433
1·5	3	95	475
2·0	4	98	490
2·5	5	99	495
Infinity		100	500

Once we know the change in lung volume for any duration of inspiration, we also know the alveolar pressure (equal to volume above FRC divided by compliance). This is the pressure opposing elastic recoil forces, and the balance of the inflation pressure opposes resistance to air flow (*see Table 9*).

Table 9.

Time	Pressure* opposed by elastic recoil	+	Pressure* opposed by air flow resistance	=	Total inflation pressure*
At start of inspiration	0	+	1·0	=	1·0
After 0·35 s	0·5	+	0·5	=	1·0
After 0·5 s	0·63	+	0·37	=	1·0
After 1·0 s	0·87	+	0·13	=	1·0
After 1·5 s	0·95	+	0·05	=	1·0
Infinite duration	1·0	+	0	=	1·0

* Pressures in kPa.

Pressure opposed by air flow resistance is directly proportional to air flow rate in our example, for which laminar flow was specified. Note that, at the beginning of inspiration, the whole inflation pressure is available to overcome air flow resistance. In this example, the inflation pressure of 1 kPa (10 cm H_2O) is sufficient to produce a flow rate of 1000 ml/s. If this rate were maintained, a tidal volume of 500 ml would be attained in 0·5 s—one time constant.

Time relations during expiration may be derived in a similar fashion using the values for rate of decay in a wash-out exponential curve (*Table 42*, Appendix E), as in *Table 10*.

The flow rate of gas falls exponentially during expiration in proportion to the alveolar pressure.

Table 10.

Duration of expiration		Lung volume remaining above FRC		Alveolar pressure remaining to overcome flow resistance	
s	*time constants*	*percentage of tidal volume*	*ml*	*kPa*	*cm H₂O*
0	0	100	500	1·0	10
0·35	0·69 (half-life)	50	250	0·5	5·0
0·5	1	37	185	0·37	3·7
1·0	2	13·5	67	0·13	1·3
1·5	3	5	25	0·05	0·5
2·0	4	2	10	0·02	0·2
2·5	5	1	5	0·01	0·1
Infinity		0	0	0	0

The effect of changes in inflation pressure, resistance and compliance

Changes in *inflation pressure* do not alter the time constant but directly influence the amount of air introduced into the lungs in a given number of time constants. In our example, an inflation pressure of 1 kPa (10 cm H$_2$O) introduced 433 ml gas into the lungs in 1 second (2 time constants). A pressure of 2 kPa (20 cm H$_2$O) would have introduced 866 ml.

Changes in *compliance* directly influence the tidal volume obtained if the same inflation pressure is maintained indefinitely. Compliance also directly affects the time constant.

Changes in flow *resistance* cannot by themselves alter the tidal volume obtained if inflation is maintained indefinitely (unless the resistance becomes total). However, the time constant increases in proportion to the resistance. Proportional increases in either compliance or resistance cause identical increases in time constant. These effects are illustrated in *Figure 55*.

Overpressure

If the duration of inflation is limited, the inflation pressure required for a particular tidal volume cannot be derived simply from the equation:

$$\text{inflation pressure} = \frac{\text{required tidal volume}}{\text{compliance}}$$

This relationship takes no account of time and is only true after the passage of infinite time. It is true that 98 per cent of inspiration is complete in 4 time constants. However, with a time constant of 0·5 second, this corresponds to an inspiration of 2 seconds which may be too long. To minimize mean intrathoracic pressure, expiration should last about one and a half times as long as inspiration, and therefore we would be faced with a total of 5 seconds per breath and a maximum respiratory rate of 12 breaths per minute. Means must therefore be found of inflating the lungs more quickly.

The solution to the problem requires no knowledge of mathematics, and is soon discovered by all who are responsible for ventilating paralysed patients. The

ARP–6

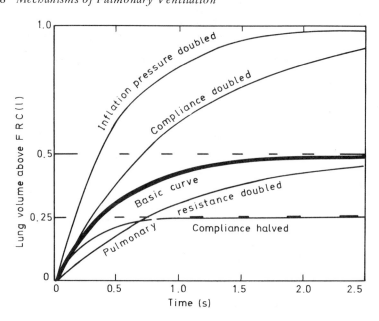

Figure 55. Effect of changes in various factors on inflation of the lungs. Fixed relationships: ultimate tidal volume = inflation pressure x compliance; time constant = compliance x resistance. (See also Table 11).

63% of inflation completed in 1 time constant
86·5% of inflation completed in 2 time constants
95% of inflation completed in 3 time constants
98% of inflation completed in 4 time constants
99% of inflation completed in 5 time constants

Table 11.

	Basic curve	Pulmonary resistance doubled	Inflation pressure doubled	Compliance doubled	Compliance halved
Inflation pressure					
(kPa)	1	1	2	1	1
(cm H₂O)	10	10	20	10	10
Compliance					
(l/kPa)	0·5	0·5	0·5	1	0·25
(ml/cm H₂O)	50	50	50	100	25
Ultimate tidal					
volume (l)	0·5	0·5	1	1	0·25
Pulmonary resistance					
(kPa l⁻¹ s)	1	2	1	1	1
(cm H₂O/l/sec)	10	20	10	10	10
Time constant					
(s or sec)	0·5	1	0·5	1	0·25

principle is called *overpressure,* and is especially important to the anaesthetist as it is analogous to speeding the induction of inhalational anaesthesia by the use of higher concentrations of the agent at the start of induction.

If resistance and compliance are fixed, there is nothing which can be done to alter the time constant. However, the introduction of a certain volume of gas into the lungs can be hastened by employment of a higher pressure and a shorter duration of inflation. In effect one *aims* at a higher tidal volume but cuts short the inflationary phase while gas is still entering the chest at a fast rate. In this

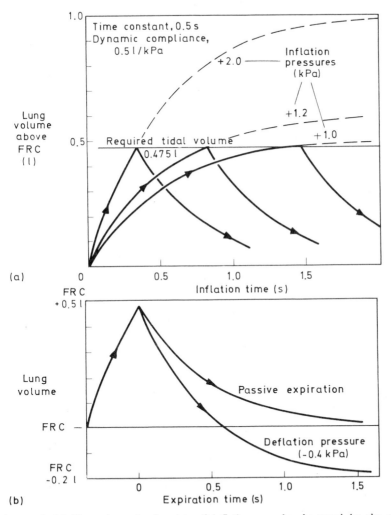

Figure 56. (a) Shows how the duration of inflation may be shortened by the use of overpressure. Inflation curves are shown for +2 kPa (+20 cm H₂O) (equilibrium 1 l), +1·2 kPa (+12 cm H₂O) (equilibrium 0·6 l) and +1 kPa (+ 10 cm H₂O) (equilibrium 0·5 1). With a required tidal volume of 0·475 l note the big reduction in duration of inflation needed when the inflation pressure is increased from 1 to 1·2 kPa (10 to 12 cm H₂O). (b) shows how expiration is influenced by the use of a subatmospheric pressure or 'negative phase'. Expiration may be terminated at the FRC after 0·6 s, or may be prolonged, in which case the lung volume will fall to 0·2 l below the FRC

way one avoids the tedious creep up to equilibrium between 2 and 5 time constants and only the first part of the exponential wash-in is used, over the first 1 or 2 time constants. This process is shown in *Figure 56*. It will be seen that quite a small increase in inflation pressure results in a considerable reduction of duration of inspiration. The effects of various increases in inflation pressure can be calculated from the data in *Table 42* (Appendix E).

It is important to remember that, if overpressure is inadvertently sustained, the lung volume and alveolar pressure will be increased more than was intended. The greater the degree of overpressure employed, the greater will be the danger of lung distension in the event of failure of the mechanism which terminates the inflation phase. The risk of rupture of the lung is real in infants. Unfortunately, a safety valve cannot be effectively used as the development of the high pressure is essential for the shortening of inspiration. Unless the resistance to air flow is pathologically high, it is probably wise to restrict the inflation pressure to no more than double the inflation pressure given by the equation:

$$\text{inflation pressure} = \frac{\text{required tidal volume}}{\text{compliance}}$$

Possible failure of the mechanism to terminate inflation (e.g. sticking of a valve) will then only result in double the intended tidal volume. In most cases this would be harmless.

The use of a subatmospheric pressure during expiration (the 'negative phase') speeds up expiration in exactly the same way as overpressure speeds inflation (*Figure 56*). This may be useful if the patient is exhaling through narrow-bore tubes. As in the case of inflation, much depends on how long the subatmospheric pressure is maintained. If it is cut short, then expiration is hastened, the lung volume does not necessarily fall below the FRC, and the intrathoracic pressure does not fall below the normal end-expiratory value. If, however, the subatmospheric pressure is maintained for several seconds, the lung volume must fall below the FRC and the intrathoracic pressure will fall below its normal end-expiratory value.

Deviations from true exponential character of the passive exhalation

Our understanding of the flow of air during artificial ventilation is greatly assisted by the assumption that inflow at constant inflation pressure and passive exhalation are both exponential in character. As a rough approximation, observations fit the theory, but a detailed analysis of the passive exhalations of anaesthetized patients has shown consistent deviations from the single exponential described above and in Appendix E. In a series of healthy patients, Bergman (1969) showed that respiratory resistance consistently decreased as air flow fell from 1·5 to 0·5 l/s, presumably due to reduction in the turbulent component of the flow pattern (*see Table 6*). Therefore the final part of the exhalation was completed more quickly than would be expected from extrapolation of a semi-logarithmic plot. In sharp contrast were observations in four patients with physical and radiological evidence of pulmonary disease. They showed a sharp *increase* in respiratory resistance at lower air flow rates which occurred at lower lung volumes. The likely explanation is that the lung volume had fallen below the closing capacity and airway closure was taking place. In these cases, a semi-logarithmic plot (of the type shown in *Figure 152*, of Appendix E) has an inflexion with a tail of reduced slope. A similar two-phase exponential is found in the nitrogen wash-out curve of patients with defective gas distribution and mixing (*see* page 241).

VARIABLE OR FLOW-LIMITED PRESSURE GENERATORS

The application of a constant or 'square' pressure wave has been considered first because it is easier to consider the relationship between pressure and flow when the first variable is held constant. We must now consider artificial ventilation by IPP when the flow of gas from the apparatus to the patient is regulated in such a way that the mouth pressure is not constant throughout inspiration. Such devices have been classified as 'flow generators' (Mapleson, 1962) which implies that the intended flow is produced under all circumstances. However, a reduced compliance or a raised airway resistance may reduce the flow below the intended rate and it is probably better to consider the inspiratory flow rate as governed by the mouth pressure which itself is dependent on the flow generated by the apparatus.

The simplest pattern of flow generation is a constant flow rate throughout the inspiratory phase. This has already been considered in *Figure 51*, for the measurement of air flow resistance and compliance with the Pufflator. When constant flow is used for artificial ventilation it is usual to commence the expiratory phase as soon as inflation is complete and, therefore, the pressure and volume changes are cut short compared with those obtained during measurement of compliance and resistance with the Pufflator. *Figure 57* shows the changes which may be expected with constant-flow generators such as the Blease Pulmoflator or Bird respirators (the latter used without air entrainment).

The other common pattern of flow is sine wave. This is the flow pattern which is developed by a cylinder and piston, driven from a rotating crank with a long connecting rod. It may also be obtained by the use of an eccentric or a Yorkshire coupling (*Figure 58*). The first type of linkage is used in the Starling 'Ideal' pump (intended for laboratory animals), and the Mörch III Piston ventilator. An eccentric drive is used in the Beaver ventilator, while the Smith–Clark ventilator uses a Yorkshire coupling. The Engström ventilator is fundamentally a sine-wave generator with a piston and connecting rod, but the beginning and end of the inspiratory piston stroke are cut off, leaving only the middle of the stroke which approximates to constant flow. The volume and pressure changes with sine-wave flow are difficult to analyse, and vary in a complex manner with changes in the characteristics of the patient (*Figure 58*). Cabinet respirators usually have sine-waveform.

Between the extremes of constant flow and sine-wave flow lie an infinite variety of devices for artificial ventilation. Consideration of their individual characteristics must lie outside the scope of this book, and the reader is referred to *Automatic Ventilation of the Lungs* by Mushin et al. (1969). Manual ventilation still remains the commonest method of artificial ventilation during anaesthesia, and may be regarded as flow generation. The pattern of flow is usually intermediate between constant flow and sine wave, depending mainly on the habits of the individual anaesthetist.

Expired air resuscitation

This is a special form of IPP ventilation with flow limitation in which the donor exhales into the respiratory tract of the patient. The recipient is then allowed to exhale to atmosphere while the donor inhales ready for the next

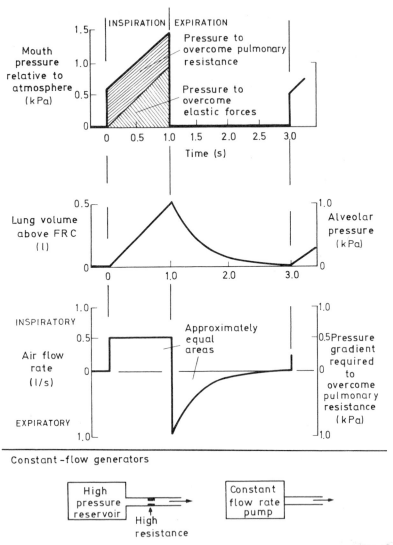

Figure 57. *Artificial ventilation by intermittent application of a constant-flow generator with passive expiration. Note that inspiratory flow rate is constant. Assuming that pulmonary resistance is constant, it follows that a constant amount of the inflation pressure is required to overcome flow resistance. Lung volume and alveolar pressure may be shown on the same graph if compliance is constant. Values are typical of an anaesthetized supine paralysed patient: total dynamic compliance, 0·5 l/kPa (50 ml/cm H_2O); pulmonary resistance, 0·3 kPa l^{-1} s (3 cm H_2O/l/sec; apparatus resistance, 0·7 kPa l^{-1} s (7 cm H_2O/l/sec); total resistance, 1 kPa l^{-1} s (10 cm H_2O/l/sec); time constant, 0·5 s*

breath. The technique is suggested in a number of passages in the Bible and, without doubt, its origin is lost in the distant past. The first clear account of expired air resuscitation is in a manual for the rescue of people, apparently drowned, published in Holland in the eighteenth century (Herholdt and Rafn, 1796).

At first sight, it might appear that expired air, being 'vitiated', would not constitute a suitable inspired air for the recipient. However, if the donor doubles his ventilation, he is able to 'breathe for two'. If neither party had any

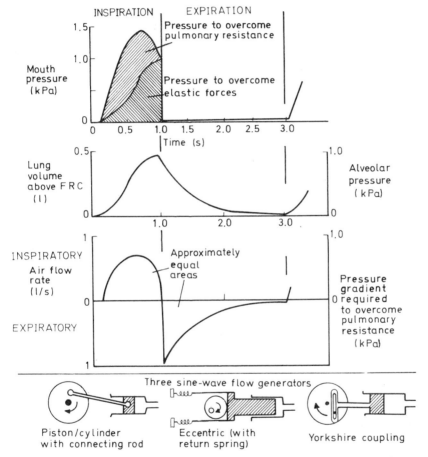

Figure 58. Artificial ventilation with inspiratory gas flow conforming to a sine wave. Passive expiration. Note that inspiratory gas flow rate is out of phase with the change in lung volume. (The latter conforms to a sine wave and the former to the differential of the sine which is the cosine.) Assuming that air flow resistance is constant, it follows that flow rate and pressure gradient required to overcome resistance may be shown on the same graph. Lung volume and alveolar pressure may be shown on the same graph if compliance is constant. Peak inspiratory flow rate equals π times the minute volume times 1·5. (The factor 1·5 is inserted because in this example inspiration does not last half the respiratory cycle.) Values are typical of an anaesthetized supine paralysed patient: total dynamic compliance, 0·5 l/kPa (50 ml/cm H₂O); pulmonary resistance, 0·3 kPa l⁻¹ s (3 cm H₂O/l/sec); apparatus resistance, 0·7 kPa l⁻¹ s (7 cm H₂O)/l/sec); total resistance, 1 kPa l⁻¹ s (10 cm H₂O/l/sec); time constant, 0·5 s

respiratory dead space, the simple relationship shown in *Table 12* would apply. In fact the existence of the donor's respiratory dead space makes the situation more favourable. The donor's dead space is filled with fresh air at the end of his inspiration, and this is the first gas to be delivered to the recipient. An increased dead space will, therefore, improve the freshness of the gas the patient receives and also helps to prevent hypocapnia in the donor. The beneficial effect of dead space is exploited in certain instrumental aids to the technique which add an external apparatus dead space to the donor (Elam, 1962).

Table 12.

	Normal spontaneous respiration	Expired air resuscitation with doubled ventilation	
		donor	recipient
Alveolar CO_2	6%	3%	6%
Alveolar O_2	15%	18%	15%

(Doubling the donor's ventilation increases his alveolar O_2 concentration to a value midway between the normal alveolar oxygen concentration and that of room air.)

Within the last few years, expired air resuscitation has been widely accepted as superior to the manual methods of artificial respiration which are discussed below. The success of the technique rests upon the following considerations.

1. Safar (1959) has demonstrated that airway obstruction is usual in unconscious patients, and cannot easily be cleared without the continuous use of the hands of the rescuer. In contrast to the manual methods of artificial respiration, expired air resuscitation leaves the rescuer's hands free to control the victim's airway.
2. During expired air resuscitation, information is fed back to the rescuer who can see the chest expansion, hear any airway obstruction and sense the tidal exchange by means of his proprioceptive receptors.
3. The donor is usually able to ventilate the victim adequately with only 20 per cent of his total ventilatory capacity (Elam and Greene, 1962). There is thus seldom difficulty in obtaining adequate ventilation, which may be maintained for long periods without fatigue (Greene et al., 1957; Cox, Woolmer and Thomas, 1960).
4. The method is extremely adaptable. It may, for example, be used before drowning persons have been removed from the water, and by linesmen electrocuted whilst working on pylons (Elam and Greene, 1962).
5. The method appears to be 'natural', and many rescuers have achieved success after the minimum of instruction.

Expired air resuscitation has been extensively reviewed by Elam and Greene (1962), and by Elam (1962). Essential features of the technique are as follows.

1. The airway must be cleared, firstly by removal of foreign matter and, secondly, by opening the pharynx either by extension of the atlanto-occipital junction or by protrusion of the mandible (page 110).
2. The rescuer should employ a tidal volume about double normal. Most rescuers appear to do so intuitively.

3. The first few breaths should be delivered at the fastest possible rate; thereafter a normal respiratory rate should be employed.
4. Alternative variants of the technique should be learned as no one method can be applicable to all situations. For example mouth-to-nose may be required when trismus precludes the use of mouth-to-mouth.
5. No potential rescuer should be led to believe that success is dependent on the use of ancillary apparatus (discussed by Elam, 1962). A rescue is such a rare event in the life of all except professional rescuers, that there is little chance of having apparatus to hand.

Use of the Venturi principle for ventilation during bronchoscopy

Maintenance of adequate pulmonary ventilation during bronchoscopy has been a perennial problem of the anaesthetist. Sanders (1967) described the use of an oxygen injector which intermittently entrained air to inflate the lungs without obscuring vision through the bronchoscope. All that is necessary is to arrange for an intermittent supply of oxygen at pipe-line pressure (400 kPa or 60 p.s.i. gauge) to be applied to a 16 s.w.g. needle or cannula (internal diameter 0·7 mm) lying to one side of the lumen of the bronchoscope, near the open end and pointing towards the patient's feet. Suitable ventilation may be obtained by allowing inspiratory periods of 1–2 seconds at a frequency of 15–20 breaths per minute. Air is entrained from the open end of the bronchoscope to give inflation pressures of the order of 2–3 kPa (20–30 cm H_2O) and an inspired oxygen concentration of 40–70 per cent oxygen (Ball, Dundee and Stevenson, 1973). These workers reported values for arterial Pco_2 within or below the normal range, but, using a similar system, Komesaroff and McKie (1972) reported generally satisfactory results although with some cases of moderate elevation of Pco_2. Giesecke et al. (1973) have compared injection systems with ventilating bronchoscopes and their own results, together with other studies which they have reviewed, leave one with little doubt of the superiority of the Venturi system both for convenience of the bronchoscopist and for maintaining satisfactory blood gas levels. The system may be regarded as one providing intermittent constant inflating pressure.

Glossopharyngeal respiration (frog breathing)

This remarkable technique is suitable for patients who have paresis of the respiratory muscles but retain the use of the muscles used in swallowing. Gulps of air are taken into the mouth and passed into the lungs, which are thus inflated stepwise. After a number of swallows, a passive expiration takes place and the cycle starts again (Dail, Affeldt and Collier, 1955). Not everyone can master the technique, but it is often useful for supplementing weakened breathing, and for taking an extra large breath before a cough.

REQUIREMENTS OF ARTIFICIAL VENTILATION BY INTERMITTENT POSITIVE PRESSURE

This topic has been discussed endlessly but few clear guidelines have emerged. A remarkably large number of automatic ventilators are available (*see* Mushin et

ARP–6*

al., 1969) and there is no universal consensus of opinion on what constitutes the ideal ventilator. In some situations, such as anaesthesia, there is not even agreement on whether automatic is preferable to manual ventilation. The plan of this section is to consider the various requirements of a system of ventilation together with a discussion of the types of apparatus which are available to meet the requirement.

Attainment of adequate pulmonary ventilation

The first essential of a ventilator is to attain an adequate minute volume of pulmonary ventilation, which may be defined as that which will maintain the arterial P_{CO_2} at or preferably below the normal range. Maintenance of a satisfactory P_{O_2} is a more complicated problem and depends on other factors.

Chapter 6 deals with this problem in greater detail, but for the present we may note that the requirement ranges from about 0·5 l/min in a small neonate to about 20 l/min in a large adult with the largest physiological dead space likely to be compatible with life. The problem for the ventilator is to attain any minute volume within these limits in the face of pathological levels of impedance to gas flow.

It appears that manual ventilation by compression of a reservoir bag can meet any requirement likely to be met. The performance of a mechanical ventilator in the face of altered impedance depends partly upon whether it is a *pressure generator* or a *flow generator*. The first type generates a constant pre-set mouth pressure during inspiration while the second generates a particular gas flow pattern with the resultant mouth pressure secondary to the flow rate and impedance to its flow. However, the manner of operation, particularly in the face of changed characteristics of the patient, is mainly dependent on the manner of cycling of the ventilator, which may be:

time-cycled (inspiration terminated after a pre-set time);
volume-cycled (inspiration terminated after passage of a pre-set volume);
pressure-cycled (inspiration terminated after a pre-set pressure is attained at the mouth or elsewhere in the apparatus).

Tables of classification of ventilators tend to be unhelpful, because the manner of operation often combines features of different types. For example, a time-cycled pressure generator may have an inspiratory flow rate limiter and thus behave partly as a flow generator. The most profitable approach is the detailed study of those ventilators which one uses.

If inspiration is limited to a pre-set time (*time-cycled*), a pressure generator will deliver a smaller volume in the face of increased resistance. A true flow generator will deliver almost the correct volume provided the raised mouth pressure does not exceed the setting of the safety valve. If compliance is diminished the flow generator should again deliver almost the correct volume, while the pressure generator would deliver a reduced tidal volume in proportion to the reduction in compliance.

If inspiration is terminated by the passage of the intended volume (*volume-cycled*), a flow generator should deliver the correct tidal volume in the normal time (unless the developed mouth pressure exceeds the setting of the safety valve). The minute volume should thus be independent of moderate changes in compliance or resistance. The response of a constant-pressure generator is a little more complicated. If air flow resistance is increased, the time constant will be increased proportionately and more time will be needed for inflation (*see Figure 55*). Even if tidal volume remains normal, respiratory frequency will fall, and so the minute volume will be diminished. If the compliance is decreased, the time constant of inflation will be decreased. However, the tidal volume produced by the inflation pressure will also fall, and it is then possible that the volume required for cycling would never be attained and the ventilator would stop cycling.

The third group of ventilators terminate the inflation phase after the development of a pre-set mouth pressure (*pressure-cycled*). Only flow generators can be pressure-cycled and a constant-pressure generator must be cycled either by time or volume, the latter being unusual but possible. Cycling by pressure carries the disadvantage that, should resistance increase or compliance decrease, the mouth pressure will reach the critical level at a smaller tidal volume than with normal respiratory function. The apparatus may thus appear to be functioning normally although an unsuspected change of lung characteristics has occurred and tidal volume is substantially reduced. It is, however, possible that the duration of inspiration will be sufficiently reduced to increase the respiratory frequency enough to maintain a normal minute volume.

The danger of a ventilator clicking rhythmically with no one aware of a reduction of ventilation is much reduced if there is one moving part which bears a relation to the volume of gas passed into the lung. The Blease Pulmoflator, for example, cycles when a predetermined pressure has been reached. However, the movements of the gas reservoir give some indication of the tidal exchange.

This account of ventilator performance in the face of changed parameters in the patient is necessarily very condensed and largely theoretical. In practice, the subject is extremely complex, largely because a precise definition of a ventilator's function is seldom possible, and Mushin et al. (1969) repeatedly refer to 'hybrid types' and to 'qualifications and reservations' about the mode of operation of individual ventilators. Frequently more than one method of cycling is included in one apparatus. Mapleson (1962) has presented a more detailed account of the effect of changes in the pulmonary characteristics of the patient.

Servo-operation. Protagonists of manual ventilation proclaim that the 'educated hand' detects changes in compliance and resistance and adjusts the inflation pressure accordingly to maintain a satisfactory ventilation. Experiment has cast doubt on the discrimination of the 'educated hand' (Egbert and Bisno, 1967; Robinson, 1968) but the concept of a feedback system is in accord with sound engineering principles. Ventilators such as the Pneumotron (British Oxygen Co.) have transducers for monitoring inspiratory and expiratory tidal volumes and, by a special-purpose analogue computer, vary the inspiratory flow rate of the ventilator to maintain a pre-set minute volume. The system can be further elaborated, for example, to detect a leak at the cuff as a difference between inspired and expired tidal volumes. At the time of writing it is too early to say whether servo-operated ventilators are likely to gain general acceptance in intensive therapy.

Optimizing gas exchange at a given minute volume

There are two separate problems. The first is to minimize the physiological dead space/tidal volume (V_D/V_T) ratio to maximize carbon dioxide elimination (pages 213 et seq.). The second is to minimize the alveolar/arterial (A–a) Po_2 difference to maximize the arterial Po_2 (pages 388 et seq.). These aspects of lung function are considered in greater detail elsewhere but we may now consider how the function of a ventilator may influence these two parameters.

Duration of inspiration and expiration. For a given minute volume of ventilation, it is possible to vary between wide limits the duration of inspiration and expiration and the ratio between the two. The commonest pattern is probably 1 second of inspiration followed by 2–4 seconds of expiration, giving a respiratory frequency of 12–20 breaths per minute. The problem is whether changes from this pattern have any appreciable effect on gas exchange.

In theory, one would expect that a moderately prolonged inspiration would tend to equalize the distribution of the tidal volume between the fast alveoli (short time constant) and slow alveoli (long time constant) as shown in *Figure 26.* One would further expect that this would reduce the V_D/V_T ratio and (A–a) Po_2 difference, so improving both indices of gas exchange as ventilation tended towards greater uniformity. The difficulty has been in demonstrating that the theoretical advantages are borne out in practice. There is no guarantee that a study of dogs or fit anaesthetized human subjects will give any guide as to what happens in patients with bad lungs and few studies have been carried out on such patients.

Bergman (1963a) found in anaesthetized, paralysed and artificially ventilated dogs, that longer inspirations (with higher mean airway pressures) resulted in the lowest values for (A–a) Po_2 difference and (a–E') Pco_2 difference, the latter being related to the V_D/V_T ratio. However, Finlay et al. (1970) found only small and statistically insignificant reductions of V_D/V_T ratio and (A–a) Po_2 difference with longer inspirations in a somewhat similar study of normo-, hypo- and hypervolaemic greyhounds. Evidence from patients is scarce. Watson (1962b) demonstrated a substantial increase in V_D/V_T ratio of patients in an intensive therapy unit when the duration of inspiration was reduced below 1 second (*see Figure 82*). A similar but less marked change was found in anaesthetized patients with healthy lungs by Bergman (1967) and Fairley and Blenkarn (1966). Sykes and Lumley (1969) reported the same effect during cardiac surgery. However, the changes have mostly been too small to be of much clinical significance except in the study of Watson. It seems reasonable to conclude that 1 second is a reasonable minimum for the duration of inspiration and that, above that figure, changes have little effect on the V_D/V_T ratio. Spalding and Smith (1963) have suggested 1·3 seconds.

There appears to be no convincing evidence in any of the studies cited above that the duration of inspiration (within the range 0·5–3 s) has any effect on the (A–a) Po_2 difference. Sykes and Lumley (1969) have suggested that this may be because the patients were breathing at least 30 per cent oxygen which would minimize the effect of ventilation/perfusion inequalities (*see page 284*).

Other things being equal, a longer duration of inspiration will increase the effective compliance since this parameter is well known to be frequency-dependent (page 76).

Waveform. Mouth pressure may be built up as a square wave (*Figure 54*), a ramp (*Figure 57*), sine wave (*Figure 58*) or in any other waveform which may take the fancy of the investigator. Much effort has been devoted to seeing whether any one waveform is preferable to another but the only significant changes are those related to duration of inspiration outlined above. With constant duration of inspiration, Adams et al. (1970) found no significant changes of V_D/V_T ratio or (A–a) P_{O_2} difference when four different waveforms were used in normo-, hypo- and hypervolaemic greyhounds. However, de Almeida (1975) has reported a study in which he found lower values for alveolar/arterial P_{O_2} difference and physiological dead space when anaesthetized patients were ventilated artificially with a falling waveform of inspiratory flow rate than when they were ventilated with a steady or rising waveform, other respiratory parameters being held constant. The falling waveform can be considered as prolonging the effective duration of inspiration.

Positive end-expiratory pressure (PEEP).   Unquestionably the most important development in the optimization of gas exchange for given values of minute volume and inspired oxygen concentration has been the introduction of PEEP. Various aspects of this technique are considered on pages 69, 128 and 267. The circulatory effects are discussed below.

Negative end-expiratory pressure (NEEP).   This has no beneficial effect on gas exchange and increases V_D/V_T (*see Figure 82*) and usually (A–a) P_{O_2} difference as well. Sykes et al. (1970) showed very large rises in (A–a) P_{O_2} difference with NEEP in artificially ventilated dogs when normo- or hypervolaemic. They did not, however, confirm the increased V_D/V_T ratio observed by Watson (1962b).

Minimizing circulatory embarrassment

The classic paper of Cournand et al. (1948) stressed the circulatory hazard of a mean airway pressure which was higher than necessary due to faulty selection of the airway pressure waveform during artificial ventilation with IPP. They recommended a gradual increase of pressure during inspiration, a rapid drop in pressure after cycling, a mean mask pressure during expiration as near atmospheric as possible and an expiratory time equal to or exceeding the inspiratory time.

From these observations, it was reasonable to conclude that IPPV, with its inevitable rise in mean intrathoracic pressure, must be worse than spontaneous breathing in its effect on the circulation and that PEEP would make matters worse still. NEEP, on the other hand, should diminish the adverse effect of IPPV. Once again the problem has been to establish whether a theoretical hazard is a significant hazard in the practical clinical situation and the results are rather conflicting and difficult to interpret.

Maloney et al. (1953) were early in the field and reported that IPPV did not greatly reduce the cardiac output of healthy anaesthetized patients but that there was an adverse effect in three patients with 'circulatory inadequacy'. In these patients, cardiac output was increased by 42 per cent following the use of NEEP. This paper was widely accepted and the use of NEEP became widespread.

More recent studies have had the benefit of improved methodology and have tended to control more of the variables, particularly P_{CO_2} (*see* below). The effect of P_{CO_2} on the circulation is discussed on page 366.

Duration of inspiration and expiration.   Evidence from artificial ventilation of dogs is conflicting. Morgan and her co-workers (Morgan et al., 1966; Morgan, Crawford and Guntheroth, 1969) found that cardiac output and stroke volume were both decreased by relative prolongation of inspiration, and increased inflation pressure at constant P_{CO_2}. This was not confirmed by Finlay et al. (1970), who investigated the effect of variations of duration of inspiration between 0·5 and 2·0 seconds in normo-, hypo- and hypervolaemic greyhounds. They found no significant change in cardiac output but a small increase in arterial pressure when the hypovalaemic dogs were given the shortest inspiration.

Waveform.   Adams et al. (1970) found that changes in respiratory wave forms, with constant duration of inspiration, had no effect on arterial pressure or cardiac output of normo-, hypo- or hypervolaemic greyhounds.

Positive end-expiratory pressure (PEEP).   The circulatory effects of PEEP have been discussed on pages 129 et seq., where references have been cited. There is little doubt that, in the subject with healthy lungs, there is a progressive reduction of cardiac output as PEEP is applied and it has been explained how this nullifies the benefit of PEEP in routine anaesthesia. However, in patients with diminished pulmonary compliance, congested lungs or right heart failure, there is much less impairment of circulatory function. In such patients the respiratory benefit of PEEP tends not to be counteracted by adverse circulatory effects, and a marked reduction of the $(A-a)$ P_{O_2} difference is commonly seen.

Negative end-expiratory pressure (NEEP).   The value of NEEP was anticipated by the study of Cournand et al. (1948) and later demonstrated by Maloney et al. (1953). However, there has been little recent evidence to support the value of NEEP in man. Scott, Stephen and Davie (1972), using NEEP of 0·5–0·7 kPa (5–7 cm H_2O), found no significant improvement in either cardiac output or arterial blood pressure of six patients undergoing artificial ventilation in an intensive therapy unit. Similar results have been reported during anaesthesia: Prys-Roberts et al. (1967a) found that the introduction of NEEP during IPPV did not increase either cardiac output or arterial blood pressure in spite of a substantial reduction of mean intrathoracic pressure.

Weaning from artificial ventilation

After an extended period of artificial ventilation, great difficulty may be encountered in re-establishing spontaneous respiration in a patient with marginal lung function. The commonest technique of weaning is the abrupt cessation of artificial ventilation for periods of 2–3 minutes with gradual prolongation of these periods depending upon the performance of the patient during the last period. Whereas this technique is satisfactory for an uncomplicated case and for patients recovering from curarization, it is unsatisfactory for patients in whom ventilatory capacity and gas exchange function are barely adequate for unassisted respiration. There is usually a grossly unsteady state during short trial periods of spontaneous respiration and there are obvious problems in monitoring. In particular, the arterial P_{CO_2} may rise progressively and initial values may be misleading. It is usual to rely upon measurements of minute volume but there is no guarantee that a minute volume adequate to maintain a normal P_{CO_2} during artificial ventilation will be sufficient when the patient is breathing for himself. *Figure 59* shows the pattern of change of certain respiratory variables during a trial period of spontaneous breathing in a patient with considerable impairment of all parameters of respiratory function and emphasizes the difficulties of monitoring. It should be stressed that the transition from artificial to spontaneous ventilation may result in an increase in metabolic rate, V_D/V_T ratio and $(A-a)$ P_{O_2} difference. There are many patients in whom it may be quite fallacious to be satisfied with what appears to be an adequate minute volume without evidence that this is, in fact, achieving satisfactory levels of arterial P_{CO_2} and P_{O_2}.

Triggering and assisted breathing. A valuable aid to weaning is the provision of a device which triggers a passive inflation when the patient lowers his airway pressure by a spontaneous attempted inspiration (*Figure 60a*). The sensitivity of

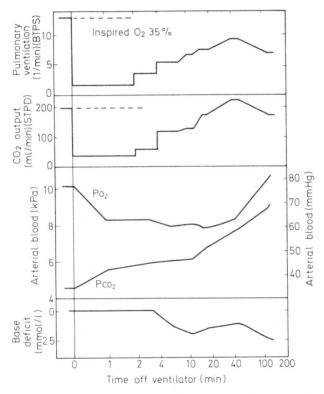

Figure 59. Typical progress of respiratory variables during an abrupt wean from artificial ventilation. Pulmonary ventilation fell from the pre-wean level of 12 l/min to 1·5 l/min but increased during the first few minutes. Carbon dioxide output fell from the steady state level of 200 ml/min as carbon dioxide production was diverted to body stores during the period of acute hypoventilation. Output did not match the steady state level (presumably the value for carbon dioxide production*) for half an hour. P*CO_2 *rose progressively for 2 hours and the attempted wean was abandoned. The base deficit probably reflects hypoxia. Not shown is the oxygen consumption which undoubtedly rose during the period of the attempted wean. (Note that the time scale is logarithmic)*

the trigger may be progressively reduced so that the patient has to make a progressively greater effort to initiate the passive inflation. To safeguard the patient in the event of failure of spontaneous efforts, it is usual to provide for a mandatory inflation at a pre-set interval after the previous inspiration. The system is generally used with a time-cycled pressure generator and effectively prevents a patient wasting energy in 'fighting' the ventilator. The disadvantage of the system is that the patient does not actually accomplish the inspiration with

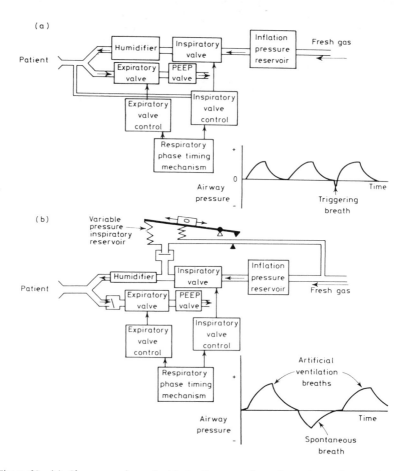

Figure 60. (a) Shows a schematic block diagram of a triggered ventilator. The basic ventilator is a time-cycled pressure generator. A respiratory phase timing mechanism operates inspiratory and expiratory valves by controls. The inspiratory valve control may be over-ridden by a subatmospheric pressure generated by the patient attempting to inspire. This immediately initiates a forced inspiration as shown in the graph of airway pressure plotted against time. (b) shows the same basic ventilator without the trigger but equipped to enable the patient to breathe spontaneously between artificial breaths, the whole arrangement being described as intermittent mandatory ventilation. A suitable reservoir of fresh gas is separated from the inspiratory circuit by a unidirectional valve, and a second unidirectional valve is placed in the expiratory circuit. If PEEP is used, it is necessary to raise the pressure in the reservoir to a level slightly below the end-expiratory pressure. Otherwise, the inspiratory effort required may be excessive. The trace of airway pressure shows a spontaneous breath between two artificial breaths

his own efforts and has still to make the transition to wholly spontaneous respiration.

A form of manual triggering may be undertaken by manual compression of the reservoir bag of a circle system when a spontaneous inspiration is felt. This is widely practised in the United States during routine anaesthesia of patients who are not fully curarized but is not a usual feature of anaesthetic practice in Great Britain.

Intermittent mandatory ventilation.   An important new development in the problem of weaning has been the provision of a double circuit whereby a patient can breathe spontaneously from a separate circuit which is independent of a ventilator providing the 'mandatory' passive inflations at predetermined intervals. Although the concept seems obvious in retrospect, it was not formally introduced until 1973 by Downs et al. The secondary circuit provides a source of gas of appropriate oxygen concentration which should be humidified before it reaches the patient. Gas is drawn from the secondary circuit through a non-return valve whenever the patient makes an inspiratory effort. This usually requires the addition of a second non-return valve in the expiratory line to prevent the patient inspiring expired gas (*Figure 60b*).

Weaning is accomplished by progressively reducing the frequency of the mandatory inflations while maintaining the tidal volume constant. During the intervals between inflations, the patient is able to breathe as shown in *Figure 60b*. The system avoids the abrupt transitions between the two modes of breathing, and the progressive reduction of frequency of mandatory inflations may be extended over several days if necessary in difficult cases. The avoidance of sudden transitions simplifies monitoring and there is no difficulty in reversing the weaning procedure if it appears that arterial Pco_2 and Po_2 are not being satisfactorily maintained. At any time there is a guaranteed minimum mandatory ventilation but it is important that ventilation should be continually monitored during weaning. At Northwick Park Hospital it is our practice to record separately spontaneous and mandatory ventilation with periodic blood-gas estimations. It is convenient to measure the total ventilation with an electronic recording Wright Respirometer (British Oxygen Co.) and subtract the mandatory ventilation to indicate the spontaneous breathing.

Mandatory minute volume (MMV) ventilation

A further logical development to the problem of weaning has recently been proposed by Hewlett (unpublished). His circuit provides for a pre-set minute volume of which the patient takes as much as he is able by spontaneous breathing. That which he is unable to take is passed to an automatic ventilator such as the Brompton Manley which is a minute volume divider (*Figure 61*). At the time of writing it is too early to report on the efficacy of this system in clinical practice.

'Pharmacological' weaning

Weaning of patients with reduced sensitivity to carbon dioxide may be simplified by the use of sustained respiratory stimulation. No very satisfactory

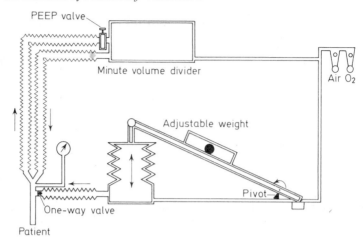

Figure 61. Hewlett's circuit for mandatory minute volume ventilation. Fresh gas, metered to the required minute volume, is passed to the variable-pressure inspiratory reservoir, from which the patient breathes as much as he is able, through a unidirectional valve circuit. If he is unable to breathe the pre-set flow rate of gas, the surplus is diverted, when the reservoir is full, into a gas-powered minute volume divider artificial ventilator (such as the Manley). PEEP and CPAP may be applied by means of the PEEP valve, but the inspiratory reservoir pressure must then be adjusted to rather less than the PEEP

drug was available for this purpose until the introduction of doxapram. Preliminary experience in the author's hospital has given very promising results with continuous intravenous administration in the dose range 1–8 mg/min, started just before disconnecting the ventilator and tapering off in the course of the next day or two.

General considerations

In addition to provision of the facilities described above, there are a number of extremely important considerations which affect the choice of a ventilator.

Environment.   Different considerations apply to the choice of a ventilator for use in the operating theatre, intensive therapy unit and special care baby unit. For use in the operating theatre, manual ventilation is considered preferable by some although others, including the author, believe it is important for the single-handed anaesthetist to have his hands free for attending to other duties. For general use the ventilator should be small and convenient in use. Elaborate facilities for varying the waveform do not seem to be important. A minute volume divider such as the Manley ventilator has the advantage that the minute volume and the composition of the inspired gas can be read directly from the rotameters. The cost of gases and vapours is trivial in the United Kingdom (Barton and Nunn, 1975) but economy can be achieved with a closed or partially closed circuit, in which case some form of 'bag squeezer' is required which may operate through a bag-in-box system.

For the intensive therapy unit, there is at least a two-level requirement. There are many patients in whom ventilation and weaning present no great difficulty and for whom a simple ventilator is adequate. Other patients, however, present formidable problems of low compliance, high airway resistance, bronchopleural fistulas, difficult weaning and so on. It is therefore essential to have some ventilators which meet the more advanced requirements. Ventilation of infants is really a separate subject and the reader is referred to reviews by Inkster and Pearson (1967), Mattila (1974) and Downes and Raphaely (1975).

Ease of teaching.   It is often overlooked that the majority of time patients spend on ventilators in intensive therapy units is without direct medical supervision. It is therefore important that nursing and technical staff should be thoroughly conversant with the operation of the ventilator, its response to altered parameters of impedance of the patient and to detection of malfunction. This depends on the calibre of the staff and the complexity of the ventilator. Recruitment difficulties are widespread and there is an obvious advantage in a ventilator which is easy to understand and has a high reliability.

Sterilization.   There is now general recognition of the problem of sterilization of a ventilator between cases. In earlier models it was often necessary to undertake gas sterilization with ethylene oxide, which was extremely inconvenient and time consuming. The modern tendency is to make the part of the circuit with which the patient comes in contact detachable and suitable for autoclaving. Alternatively, the ventilator may be isolated with bacterial filters (Holdcroft, Lumley and Gaya, 1973).

Cost and size.   Although certain sectors of the market are attracted primarily by high cost, for most of us there is a limit to the amount which can be spent on hospital equipment. Considerations of cost cannot therefore be excluded in the choice of a ventilator, neither can versatility which affects the total number of ventilators required. The size of a ventilator may be a factor if treatment and storage rooms are small. Ideally, 15 square metres of floor area are required for treatment of a patient on a ventilator.

Prolonged extracorporeal membrane oxygenation (ECMO) (see review by Zapol, 1977)

It is technically possible to maintain oxygenation of arterial blood for as long as three weeks by the use of venoarterial bypass through an extracorporeal membrane oxygenator. Blood is drawn from the central venous pool by a femoral venous catheter and passed, via a roller pump, through an oxygenator and returned by a long femoral arterial catheter to a point as near the aortic valve as possible. It is essential to maintain some lung perfusion (approximately 2 l/min) and to continue ventilation of the lung (preferably with 30 per cent oxygen in nitrogen). The pulmonary venous blood is generally of very low Po_2 in patients deemed to require ECMO and the blood in the ascending arch of the aorta will have a Po_2 intermediate between that of the pulmonary venous blood and that of the blood returned from the ECMO. Blood from the right radial artery should give the lowest value of Po_2 of blood perfusing any of the major vessels of head, neck and upper extremity, but coronary perfusion is likely to have a lower Po_2.

The clinical value of ECMO is currently under investigation in a multi-centre randomized trial in the United States. The indications for treatment are that the arterial P_{O_2} should be less than 6·7 kPa (50 mm Hg) for 2 hours while breathing 100 per cent oxygen, or for 12 hours while breathing 60 per cent oxygen with a shunt greater than 30 per cent. Measurements should be made after tracheo-bronchial suction and three lung hyperinflations together with an appropriate level of PEEP. It is well known that patients who fulfil these criteria have an extremely poor prognosis.

There is no doubt that ECMO is technically feasible although the cost in labour and resources is very high. The crucial question is whether it improves the chances of survival. ECMO is in no way curative and only buys time for spontaneous resolution of the underlying pulmonary pathology. When the disease is progressive or irreversible, the use of ECMO merely postpones death and its eventual withdrawal introduces yet another agonizing decision into the practice of intensive therapy. At the time of writing the multi-centre trial has not yet shown any evidence of improved survival of treated patients compared with the control group.

Part II   Tidal Exchange Produced by Forces Acting Directly on the Boundaries of the Thoracic Cavity

The first part of this chapter has considered artificial ventilation produced by the development of a pressure gradient between the mouth and the air surrounding the chest. The second part considers tidal exchange produced by forces acting directly on the boundaries of the thoracic cavity. These boundaries may be moved by contraction of the subject's own muscles or by external forces applied by a second person (e.g. in the manual methods of artificial ventilation) or by a machine (e.g. cuirass respirator). It is a common feature of all these forms of ventilation that the geometric pattern of expansion of the thorax is partly dependent upon the action of local forces, and does not depend solely on the response of the regional elasticity to the development of a pressure gradient as in the forms of ventilation discussed in the first part of the chapter.

SPONTANEOUS RESPIRATION

The muscular pattern of contraction during normal breathing has been the subject of controversy for many years. Elucidation has been hampered by the difficulty in detecting contraction of many of the muscle groups concerned. It is difficult to detect active contraction of the diaphragm and also to distinguish active movement from passive movement secondary to displacement of the abdominal viscera by the abdominal muscles. Even greater difficulty is encountered in demonstrating the localization of contraction within the intercostal group of muscles. The most effective methods of study have proved to be electromyography, measurement of pressures within the thorax and abdomen, and studies (particularly radiographic) of the change in shape of the thorax. These methods are usually correlated with spirometric demonstration of the respiratory phase.

Electromyography is the only method of demonstrating contraction in muscles such as pectoralis minor and the internal intercostals, which are covered by other muscles and which produce no skeletal movement that could not be attributed to other muscles. Nevertheless, the technique is difficult to apply in these circumstances and it is not easy to separate the actions of different layers of the intercostals by accurate placing of the electrodes. Recordings from the abdominal muscles may easily be made. Electromyography of the diaphragm is difficult but may be accomplished with a bipolar oesophageal lead (Agostoni, Sant'Ambrogio and Carrasco, 1960; Agostoni, 1962). This lead records from the crura but recordings from other parts of the diaphragm are almost impossible in man.

The measurement of pressures within the thorax and abdomen is particularly valuable as evidence of contraction of expiratory muscles. Effective contraction of the abdominal muscles cannot take place without the appearance of characteristic peaks of oesophageal and intragastric pressure.

Radiographic and stethographic methods will show changes in shape of the confines of the thorax but will not necessarily indicate the muscle groups responsible. Ribs may be elevated, for example, either by contraction of the intercostals or by contraction of the diaphragm. For a detailed account of the muscles of breathing the reader is referred to *The Respiratory Muscles* by Campbell (1958). This monograph contains an extensive bibliography of the classical and more recent work in the field.

The diaphragm is the most important inspiratory muscle. During contraction, the origin and insertion are approximated, resulting both in descent of the domes and in elevation and rotation of the lower ribs (*Figure 62*). The normal

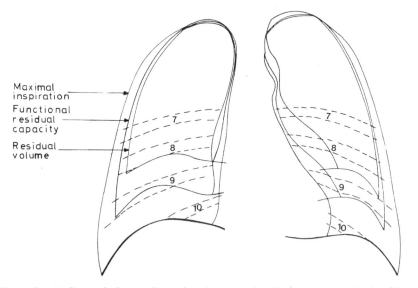

Maximal
inspiration
Functional
residual
capacity
Residual
volume

Figure 62. Outlines of chest radiographs of a normal subject at various levels of lung inflation. The numbers refer to ribs as seen in the position of maximal inspiration. (I am indebted to Dr R. L. Marks who was the subject)

excursion of the domes is 1·5 cm, increasing to 6–7 cm during deep breathing (Wade and Gibson, 1951). Although the diaphragm plays the major part in inspiration, there is a large reserve of function in the other inspiratory muscles. Thus unilateral paralysis of the diaphragm causes little reduction of ventilatory capacity, while even bilateral phrenic interruption is compatible with reasonably good ventilatory function (Dowman, 1927; Eisele et al., 1972).

The intercostal muscles acting alone are able to maintain a high level of ventilation (Otis, Fenn and Rahn, 1950), and contract during inspiration in most, but not all, subjects (Campbell, 1955). Inspiratory activity is less in the higher than in the lower intercostal spaces. Campbell (1955) was unable to demonstrate in man the expiratory activity which has been reported in animals. Other muscles, particularly the scaleni, may occasionally be found to contract during normal quiet breathing.

Expiration is passive in the normal resting subject but active when making expulsive efforts, talking, breathing against high expiratory resistance or when the minute volume is greater than about 40 l/min. There is normally no myographic or manometric evidence of contraction of abdominal or intercostal muscles during quiet breathing provided that these muscles are not in sustained contraction for the maintenance of posture. However, the contraction of the inspiratory muscles is not suddenly terminated at the start of expiration. Instead, there appears to be a gradual 'let-down' of tone so that expiration starts slowly. Only after the expiration of about a quarter of the tidal volume does inspiratory tone finally disappear, and expiration of the remaining part of the tidal volume proceeds according to a wash-out exponential function (*see Figure 54*). In this respect expiration differs between spontaneous respiration and artificial ventilation by IPP. In the latter, the whole of expiration usually proceeds according to the simple exponential process shown in *Figure 54*, while in the former, the expiratory spirogram follows the rather complex S-shaped curve shown in *Figure 46*. Modifications of the pattern of spontaneous respiration occurring during anaesthesia are described on page 170.

Active hyperventilation

As ventilation is increased, the inspiratory muscles contract more vigorously and accessory muscles are recruited. The first group to be recruited is usually the scaleni, and considerable hyperventilation (about 50 l/min) is attained before the sternomastoids and extensors of the vertebral column are brought into use (Campbell, 1958). Extreme hyperventilation (as during the measurement of the maximum breathing capacity) requires the use of a great many different muscle groups. The pectorals, for example, reverse their usual origin/insertion and help to expand the chest when the arms are fixed by grasping a suitable support. During voluntary hyperventilation, expiratory muscle activity remains absent until a minute volume of about 40 l/min is attained (Campbell, 1952). Thereafter, it plays an increasingly important role as respiration progressively assumes the quasi sine-wave push-pull pattern of extreme hyperventilation (Cooper, 1961).

Effect of posture

Throughout this book, the effect of posture is stressed, since so many studies of normal human physiology relate to standing or seated subjects. The anaesthetist, on the other hand, is concerned almost exclusively with supine patients, and must constantly be mindful of the differences consequent on change of posture. In fact, the simplified account above of the action of the respiratory muscles refers primarily to supine subjects. An important difference in the upright position is the tonic contraction of the postural (anti-gravity) muscles. Many of these, including the abdominal muscles, show a variation in tone according to the respiratory phase.

In the supine position the diaphragm is some 40 mm (4 cm) higher in the chest (Wade and Gibson, 1951) and this accords with the reduction of FRC (*see Figure 21*). The dimensions of the rib cage are probably little altered. Although the reduction of FRC is undesirable from the point of view of airway and alveolar closure, the diaphragm is able to contract more effectively the higher it is forced into the chest.

In the lateral position (*Figure 63*), the lower dome of the diaphragm is pushed higher into the chest while the upper dome is flattened. It follows that

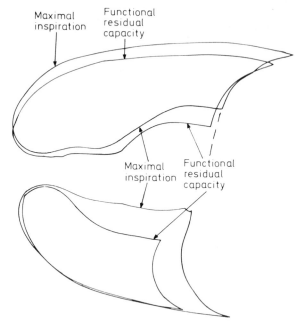

Figure 63. Radiographic outlines of the lungs at two levels of lung volume in a conscious subject during spontaneous breathing in the lateral position (right side down). This is the same subject as in Figure 62: comparison will show that, in the lateral position at FRC, the lower lung is close to residual volume while the upper lung is close to inspiratory capacity. The diaphragm therefore lies much higher in the lower half of the chest. Both these factors contribute to the greater volume changes which occur in the lower lung during inspiration. The mediastinum seems to rest on a pneumatic cushion at FRC and rises during inspiration.

the lower dome can contract more effectively than the upper, and the ventilation of the lower lung is found to be about twice that of the upper lung. This is fortunate since gravity causes a somewhat similar discrepancy between the blood flow of the two lungs. Thus the ventilation/perfusion ratio of each lung remains approximately constant, regardless of position (Svanberg, 1957). This subject is discussed more fully in Chapters 7 and 9.

Effect of anaesthesia

Jones, Faithfull and Minty (1976) have extended the classical observation of Miller (1938) that there is a consistent reduction in the contribution of the chest wall to breathing during anaesthesia with spontaneous respiration. The decline in chest movement was related to the depth of anaesthesia and was accompanied by a phase shift. When the alveolar halothane concentration reached 1·5 per cent, there was a complete phase reversal in some patients, with decrease in chest volume during inspiration. This was associated with an increased alveolar/arterial Po_2 difference, suggesting maldistribution of inspired gas.

The spirogram is also different during anaesthesia (*see Figure 46*). Instead of the gradual onset of expiration with progressive release of inspiratory muscle tone, there tends to be an abrupt start to expiration consistent with a sudden cessation of inspiratory muscle tone and expiration is roughly exponential in form. Inspiration lasts only 30 per cent of the respiratory cycle compared with 40 per cent in the conscious subject.

Froese and Bryan (1974) have made the most important observation that the diaphragm rises into the chest during anaesthesia with or without muscle paralysis. This accords with the observed reduction in FRC (page 67), and appearances suggested that the diaphragm was fully relaxed at the end of expiration during anaesthesia but only partially relaxed at the same phase of breathing when the patient was conscious. These authors suggest that, contrary to accepted beliefs, the diaphragm is not fully relaxed at the end of an expiration in the conscious supine subject. During anaesthesia, on the other hand, the diaphragm is fully relaxed throughout expiration which is therefore passive. This hypothesis is difficult to confirm by direct observation but it would seem to explain the change in pattern of breathing, the radiographic appearances and the difference in FRC following the induction of anaesthesia. Observations in animals do not necessarily indicate what happens in man and electromyographic recordings from the crura are not necessarily representative of the whole of the diaphragm.

Certain special patterns of inspiration may be seen during anaesthesia. Sighing appears to be more common under ether anaesthesia and during the administration of nitrous oxide supplemented with pethidine than under halothane. It has been suggested that the sigh is useful to re-expand collapsed areas. A most curious pattern occasionally seen is the double inspiration, producing a spirogram like the outline of a Bactrian camel. The significance of the double inspiration is not known, but it is unlikely to be a particularly effective method of ventilation. Reversed rhythm has been described as a feature of profound anaesthesia; the pause is said to occur at the end of inspiration instead of at the end of expiration. It is certainly rare and has never been observed by the author.

It has long been thought that expiratory muscle activity occurs during anaesthesia. An electromyographic study by Freund, Roos and Dodd (1964) showed that expiratory activity in the abdominal muscles is, in fact, an invariable feature of anaesthesia and is not related to any particular technique. This phenomenon has been further investigated by Freund (1973) and by Kaul, Heath and Nunn (1973). The latter group found expiratory muscle activity absent (in the supine position) in all of 22 subjects before induction but it developed within about half an hour in all but 2 patients. Deepening halothane anaesthesia reduced the activity but only abolished it in 1 case. Topical anaesthesia to the larynx, endotracheal intubation and the passage of a pharyngeal airway had no effect other than initial stimulation. On the other hand, surgical stimulation and respiratory obstruction both caused marked increases in expiratory muscle activity. Hewlett et al. (1974b) showed that expiratory muscle was unrelated to the reduction of FRC which followed induction.

Every surgeon knows that expiratory muscle tone diminishes as anaesthesia deepens. When anaesthesia lightens, contraction of the expiratory muscles becomes apparent in one of the following ways.

1. Detection by the surgeon during abdominal surgery.
2. Observation of the abdomen by the anaesthetist.
3. Detection of an 'expiratory push' visible in the reservoir bag.

The expiratory push is one of the most sensitive indices of lightening anaesthesia and is noticed instinctively by the experienced anaesthetist. An excellent demonstration of the return of expiratory muscle activity may be made by connection of a simple manometer to a balloon in the oesophagus. Pronounced peaks of pressure may be seen at the same time as the appearance of the expiratory push. The reason for the enhanced expiratory muscle activity of the anaesthetized patient is unknown.

Deep anaesthesia and carbon dioxide retention are sometimes associated with a characteristic phenomenon known as tracheal tug. During inspiration, the larynx and lower jaw are jerked downwards and this movement is usually attributed to traction from the diaphragm transmitted through the mediastinum to the trachea. Mitchinson and Yoffey (1947) suggested that downward movement of the larynx was normally prevented by a stabilizing contraction of the elevators of the larynx; it is postulated that tracheal tug develops when the stabilizing muscles are paralysed while the diaphragm is still contracting vigorously. Observations in hypercapnic dogs (unpublished) have led the author to believe that contraction of the infrahyoid and hyomandibular muscles may make some contribution to the development of tracheal tug.

We shall see in later chapters that there is ample evidence to suggest that the distribution of inspired air relative to pulmonary blood flow is defective during anaesthesia. This *could* be explained by a spatial maldistribution of inspired gas due to abnormal functioning of the ventilatory mechanism as a result of anaesthesia. This view is supported by the studies of Jones et al., cited above.

Dysco-ordinated breathing

All clinicians working in the field of intensive therapy are familiar with the type of breathing in which there is lack of co-ordination between thoracic and diaphragmatic components. In its extreme form, there is failure to synchronize and the chest wall moves inwards during inspiration, as has been described above in relation to deep anaesthesia. Pontoppidan, Geffin and Lowenstein (1972) have discussed this problem in their review of acute respiratory failure, pointing out that it is relatively common and may exist between the two sides of the diaphragm, which is difficult to diagnose by bedside observation. Respiratory muscle dysco-ordination increases the work of breathing and reduces the effective tidal volume. It may delay successful weaning from artificial ventilation.

Comparison between spontaneous respiration and IPP ventilation

IPP ventilation results in a spatial pattern of distribution of inspired gas which is determined solely by the regional variations in compliance, except in so far as regional variations in airway resistance may influence distribution if inflation is fairly rapid. It is still not clear to what extent similar considerations apply to the distribution of inspired gas during spontaneous respiration. It used to be taught that the diaphragm descended in inspiration, creating a 'vacuum' in the pleural cavities, and that gas then entered the lungs because 'nature abhors a vacuum'. This facile explanation overlooks the fact that the pleural space does not exist and the lungs cannot, therefore, freely expand into the space after the manner of the familiar bag-in-a-bottle 'model' of the respiratory system. In fact, the lungs remain firmly in contact with the parietal pleura, although the two layers slide over one another to a certain extent. Thus the lungs must follow the changes in the shape of the confines of the thorax and the spatial pattern of distribution of inspired gas must be influenced by the pattern of change of shape of the confines of the thorax. It may then be argued that it could only be coincidental if this pattern were identical to the pattern obtained with IPP ventilation. Froese and Bryan (1974) produced clear radiological evidence of a difference in the pattern of movement of the diapragm. In the supine awake and anaesthetized patient, breathing spontaneously, respiratory excursion was predominantly in the posterior part of the diaphragm. However, with paralysis and artificial ventilation, movement was predominantly in the anterior part.

Although the *geometrical outline of the lungs as a whole* must follow the movements of the chest wall, it does not follow that the entry of air into specific lobes and lobules is so influenced. The boundaries between the lobes and lobules have considerable freedom of movement so that the fraction of the tidal air admitted to a particular lobule may well be largely independent of the spatial pattern of expansion of the confines of the thorax. If, for example, the left dome of the diaphragm were paralysed and respiratory movement on that side were confined to expansion of the upper ribs, the radiological appearance would show distribution of inspired gas in favour of the upper parts of the lungs. However, inspiration would be associated with ascent of the interlobar fissure, so that the lower lobe would be better ventilated than radiological appearances might suggest. Nevertheless, the observations of Froese and Bryan (1974) suggest that regional ventilation is greater near that part of the diaphragm which shows the greatest excursion.

Reference has already been made to the differences in expiratory waveforms. Artificial ventilation by IPP is usually associated with a passive expiration conforming to a simple exponential wash-out. During spontaneous respiration, this is modified by the initial slow let-down of inspiratory muscle tone while, during anaesthesia, there usually is active expiratory muscle activity.

ARTIFICIAL VENTILATION PRODUCED BY FORCES ACTING DIRECTLY ON THE THORAX

This section is concerned largely with manual methods of artificial ventilation of the type used in first aid. Their importance is now greatly reduced following the recognition of the superiority of expired air resuscitation (page 152).

Shortly after World War II, the advent of nerve gases stimulated interest in simple methods of artificial ventilation. Attention was first directed to the manual methods, and the December 1951 issue of the *Journal of Applied Physiology* (vol. 4, no. 6) was devoted to comparative studies of the various methods. Unfortunately, these studies employed either conscious non-apnoeic subjects or else anaesthetized volunteers who had been paralysed and intubated. In neither case was there airway obstruction and this vitally important factor was overlooked.

It was not until 1959 that the iconoclastic paper of Safar showed that airway obstruction was almost always present in the unconscious subject and could not be satisfactorily cleared by the use of an oropharyngeal airway or by placing the patient in the prone position. Effective ventilation by the manual methods was shown to be ineffective unless the trachea was intubated. A subsequent paper by Safar, Escarraga and Chang (1959) demonstrated the nature of the pharyngeal obstruction and showed that the pharyngeal airway was most effectively cleared either by extension of the atlanto-occipital joint or by protrusion of the mandible (*see Figure 45*). These manoeuvres are now regarded as essential adjuncts to the manual methods of artificial respiration (Karpovich, 1962) but, unfortunately, either two rescuers are required, or else a single rescuer uses his legs to maintain the victim's head in a favourable position. In either event the procedure is complicated, tiring and difficult to teach.

Nevertheless, it should be remembered that the manual methods have saved lives in the past. Although normal ventilatory exchange is desirable, life may be sustained on an alveolar ventilation which is only half the normal value.

Some manual methods of artificial ventilation employ an active expiratory phase with passive inspiration. This is the exact opposite of spontaneous respiration or artificial ventilation by IPP. Other methods employ an active inspiratory phase which is intended to stimulate spontaneous respiration. A third group has both active inspiration and active expiration. These methods are known as 'push-pull' and are analogous to spontaneous respiration with expiratory muscle activity, or to IPP ventilation with a subatmospheric pressure phase during expiration.

Group I—Active expiratory phase only

Generally speaking these techniques are unsatisfactory. They operate within the patient's expiratory reserve (*see Table 13*), which is appreciably reduced in the supine or prone position. (The figures in *Table 13* are taken from Whitfield, Waterhouse and Arnott (1950).)

Table 13.

Number of subjects		Expiratory reserve volume (l) (ATPS)	
		mean	*range*
Male:	64 sitting	1·269	0·27–2·540
	41 lying	1·005	0·20–2·600
Female:	32 sitting	0·884	0·30–1·580
	16 lying	0·663	0·17–1·120

The normal airway resistance rises very sharply as the residual volume is approached and, in practice, it is doubtful if effective use can be made of more than half of the expiratory reserve volume. Therefore, an active expiratory phase alone is unlikely to produce effective tidal exchange. The following are the more important methods employing an active expiratory phase alone.

Belt respirator (Paul Bragg Pneumobelt). This device consists of an inter- mittently inflated belt which surrounds the lower chest and abdomen. It cannot be relied upon to produce an effective tidal exchange in the totally paralysed patient, but finds some use for assisting breathing in the *partly* paralysed patient.

Back pressure (Schafer's method, 1904). Intermittent pressure is applied to the lower ribs with the patient in the prone position. Even with a clear airway, the tidal exchange seldom approaches normal. Gordon et al. (1951b) reported a mean tidal volume of 238 ml in apnoeic intubated subjects but this was increased to 469 ml by 'spring-off' at the end of the patient's expiratory phase. Karpovich, Hale and Bailey (1951) obtained a mean exchange of 451 ml in conscious volunteers simulating apnoeic victims. It is, however, unlikely that conscious volunteers are able to relax completely and they probably tend to supplement their ventilation; such studies almost always indicate higher tidal volumes than are found with paralysed patients.

External cardiac massage. All concerned with resuscitation should understand clearly that external cardiac massage by itself is most unlikely to achieve an effective tidal exchange. In healthy, intubated curarized patients, Safar et al. (1961) recorded a mean tidal volume of 156 ml resulting directly from external cardiac massage. However, in 12 victims of cardiac arrest, they were unable to detect any tidal exchange in spite of tracheal intubation. Cardiac massage must be supplemented by artificial ventilation and, when single handed, the rescuer should alternate 15 strokes of cardiac massage with 2 breaths of expired air, repeated as rapidly as possible.

Group II—Active inspiratory phase only

These methods operate within the inspiratory capacity, which is approxi- mately three times the expiratory reserve when the patient is lying down (Whitfield, Waterhouse and Arnott, 1950). However, this advantage is largely offset by the mechanical difficulty of expanding the thorax by manual means. The more important inspiratory methods are as follows.

Rocking bed. This technique closely simulates the normal movements of the diaphragm. Active contraction is replaced by varying the gravitational load of the abdominal viscera on its lower surface. However, the pattern of thoracic expansion differs from normal since passive descent of the diaphragm does not expand the rib cage, which therefore tends to move paradoxically. When the feet are lowered from the horizontal, the lung volume increases in proportion to the sine of the angle of tilt (Colville, Shugg and Ferris, 1956). There is little change when the feet are elevated, and the most effective range of rocking is between horizontal and 20 degrees, feet down (Radford and Whittenberger, 1962). The method is most effective in tall adults in whom it is generally possible to obtain adequate ventilation (*see Figure 22*).

Hip lift and hip roll (Gordon et al., 1951a).   The victim lies prone while the rescuer lifts the hips with or without rolling them to one side over his thigh. This manoeuvre extends the spine and allows the abdominal viscera to fall. This produces inspiration and tidal exchange occurs above the FRC. In conscious volunteers, Karpovich, Hale and Bailey (1951) obtained a mean tidal volume of 888 ml, but less satisfactory results would be expected when airway obstruction complicated the picture.

Cuirass respirators.   Cuirass respirators exert an intermittent subatmospheric pressure over the lower part of the chest. The area of application varies from the epigastrium (shell cuirasses) to the greater part of the trunk (Tunnicliffe jacket). The greater the area of application the more efficient is the ventilation although at the cost of convenience of application. With a large area of application the efficiency and general effects approach those of a cabinet respirator. The smaller cuirasses, however, tend to hamper movement of the chest and are, therefore, chiefly suitable for the reinforcement of ventilation in patients with partial respiratory paralysis.

Group III—Both active inspiratory and expiratory phases (push-pull)

These techniques are now accepted as the most efficient of the manual methods of artificial respiration. Tidal exchange occurs above and below the FRC. The following methods are in use.

Rocking stretcher (Eve, 1932).   This method differs from the rocking bed in the range of tilt, which is much greater. The patient must be secured to the stretcher which is commonly tilted about 40 degrees on either side of horizontal. Tidal exchange occurs above and below the FRC measured in the horizontal position. Comroe and Dripps (1946) found the method greatly superior to Schafer's method.

Arm lift, back pressure (Holger Nielsen method, 1932). The victim lies prone. The rescuer kneels at the head of the victim and produces inspiration by drawing the elbows towards the head. Expiration is produced by back pressure as in Schafer's method. Both phases are active, and tidal exchange takes place above and below the FRC. In curarized intubated subjects, Gordon et al. (1951b) obtained a mean tidal volume of 957 ml, most of the exchange occurring below the FRC (i.e. in the expiratory reserve). Safar (1959) reported an exchange of only 619 ml under similar circumstances. Karpovich, Hale and Bailey (1951) obtained a mean tidal volume of 938 ml in conscious volunteers.

Arm lift, chest pressure (Silvester's method, 1857).   The victim lies supine. The rescuer kneels at the head of the victim and produces inspiration by raising the victim's arms above his head. Expiration is produced by laying the victim's arms on his chest and exerting pressure. Both phases are active and tidal exchange takes place above and below the FRC. Karpovich, Hale and Bailey (1951) obtained a mean tidal volume of 1068 ml in conscious volunteers, but Safar (1959) obtained an exchange of only 503 ml in intubated curarized subjects.

Hip roll, back pressure.   Studies of this combination have given results broadly similar to those of Silvester's method and the Holger Nielsen technique. Gordon et al. (1951b) reported mean tidal exchanges of 1057 ml (hip lift) and 903 ml (hip roll). Karpovich, Hale and Bailey (1951) obtained a mean tidal exchange of 1015 ml.

All the push-pull manual methods of Group III are capable of producing an adequate tidal exchange if the airway is perfectly clear. Unfortunately, this is seldom the case and the data of Safar (1959) given in *Table 14* clearly demonstrate the significance of this factor.

Table 14. CURARIZED ANAESTHETIZED PATIENTS–ARTIFICIAL VENTILATION BY BACK PRESSURE, ARM LIFT METHOD (HOLGER NIELSEN METHOD, 1932)

Airway	Mean tidal volume (ml)	Percentage of patients with tidal volume less than dead space
Natural (head in flexion)	126	75
Oropharyngeal airway (head in flexion)	178	71
Natural (head in extension)	328	31
Oropharyngeal airway (head in extension)	351	20
Endotracheal tube	619	0

Finally, it must be stressed that the production of a normal tidal volume does not necessarily guarantee normal arterial blood gas levels. Gordon et al. (1951c) found a marked degree of desaturation during artificial respiration with Schafer's method, which could not be entirely explained by hypoventilation. It is likely that reduction of the lung volume below the FRC resulted in sufficient airway closure to cause appreciable shunting, and this accords with the study of Nunn et al. (1965b) in which shunting was caused by normal subjects breathing within their expiratory reserve. There is no doubt that shunting might be considerably aggravated by inhalation of foreign material in many situations confronting the first aid worker.

Chapter 6 The Minute Volume of Pulmonary Ventilation

Definition of Adequacy of Ventilation
The Effect of Different Levels of Ventilation on Alveolar Gas
Tensions
Causes of Failure of Ventilation
Treatment of Ventilatory Failure
The Work of Breathing
Measurement of Ventilation

So far, most of this book has been concerned with mechanisms and factors related to the tidal flow of gas into and out of the lungs. The present chapter considers what ventilatory exchange may be regarded as adequate and classifies the causes of failure of ventilation. The work and energy cost of breathing are discussed and finally, the principles of measurement of ventilation are presented.

DEFINITION OF ADEQUACY OF VENTILATION

It is the function of the respiratory system to ensure normal levels of oxygen and carbon dioxide in the arterial blood. It is then the function of the circulatory system to transport the arterial blood to the tissues. An adequate minute volume of ventilation may be defined as follows.

The respiratory minute volume which will ensure satisfactory levels of both oxygen and carbon dioxide in the arterial blood, under prevailing conditions of barometric pressure, composition of the inspired gas, dead space, distribution, shunting, diffusing capacity and metabolic activity of the patient.

A minute volume which is adequate for a healthy resting subject at sea level will not be adequate if the subject is on the top of Mount Everest, is exercising, is breathing 9 per cent oxygen or if he has developed diseases such as emphysema which impair pulmonary function.

Our definition hinges on what is considered a satisfactory level of oxygen and carbon dioxide in the arterial blood. The P_{CO_2} is the more important consideration in defining the adequacy of ventilation under hospital conditions, since the P_{O_2} can easily be altered by changes in the concentration of oxygen in the inspired gas and is, therefore, less dependent on the minute volume. For example, a patient with a grossly inadequate minute volume (as regards P_{CO_2}) may have a normal or elevated P_{O_2} if the concentration of oxygen in the inspired gas is increased by the appropriate amount.

Optimal value for Pco$_2$

The normal range of arterial Pco$_2$ is 4·8–5·9 kPa (36–44 mm Hg), and should not rise appreciably during moderately heavy exercise. Low values may occur in patients who hyperventilate, particularly in response to hypoxaemia as, for example, in cases of Fallot's tetralogy or lobar pneumonia. High values occur in patients with ventilatory failure, the causes of which are discussed below (page 190). When patients are ventilated artificially, it is usually sound policy to aim for a Pco$_2$ slightly below the normal range. However, in patients with chronic hypercapnia it may be preferable to allow the Pco$_2$ to rise towards their usual value, particularly before attempting to wean from the ventilator.

There is no consensus of opinion on the optimum Pco$_2$ during anaesthesia. Whereas it might appear reasonable to keep the Pco$_2$ within the normal range, many anaesthetists feel it is preferable to hyperventilate the patient and so reduce the Pco$_2$ to levels within the range 2·7–4 kPa (20–30 mm Hg) (Gray and Rees, 1952; Geddes and Gray, 1959). The following advantages have been claimed.

1. In cases of doubt, it is better to err on the side of overventilation rather than underventilation.
2. The chances of pulmonary collapse are minimized by a large tidal volume.
3. Apnoea is considered by many to be a desirable feature of an anaesthetic and this may be maintained by the reduction of Pco$_2$ (page 47). It is now thought to be unlikely that stimulation of the Hering–Breuer reflex plays a part in causing apnoea (page 52).
4. Hypocapnia with alkalosis causes changes in distribution and duration of action of certain drugs, and such changes have been considered desirable (Dundee, 1952; Utting, 1963).
5. There are a number of situations in which cardiac arrhythmias are less likely to arise if the Pco$_2$ is reduced (page 367).
6. Carbon dioxide has an arousal effect on the brain and some believe that suppression of this effect by hyperventilation can make a useful contribution towards the maintenance of anaesthesia.

There seems little doubt that patients remain quiet and relaxed on the operating table with smaller doses of relaxants and anaesthetics if they are passively hyperventilated. Whatever their motives, most anaesthetists employ hyperventilation with hypocapnia during the conduct of an anaesthetic with paralysing doses of relaxants (Nunn, 1958a). Opposition to this practice is based principally on the reduction of cardiac output and cerebral blood flow which results from hypocapnia. (The effects of abnormal levels of Pco$_2$ are considered in Chapter 11.)

During operations in which patients are allowed to breathe spontaneously, there is usually a rise in Pco$_2$ (Nunn, 1958a). Anaesthetists vary in the extent to which they will permit this to occur. Elevation as far as about 10 kPa (75 mm Hg) seems to be commonplace even during operations not requiring much relaxation. However, during laparotomy with spontaneous respiration, levels as high as 20 kPa (150 mm Hg) have been reported (Birt and Cole, 1965).

Against this wide spectrum of Pco$_2$ values, it may be argued that the exact level is unlikely to be very important. For the healthy patient this may well be true, but the skill of the anaesthetist is also measured by his ability to carry bad risk patients through extensive surgical procedures with the minimum mortality. Under such conditions, the maintenance of PCO_2 at the optimum level may be critically important, and the next section of this chapter considers how this may be accomplished. This is linked to a consideration of the influence of ventilation on PO_2 in those situations where the anaesthetist cannot or does not wish to adjust the concentration of oxygen in the inspired gas. If, for example, he is relying upon nitrous oxide to keep the patient unconscious, it is not possible to raise the inspired oxygen concentration much above 30 per cent.

Optimal PO_2

Normal arterial PO_2 varies widely within the range 9·3–14·7 kPa (70–110 mm Hg) and is markedly dependent on age (*see* page 411). It is generally sound policy to aim for the upper part of the normal range but, in patients with severe respiratory disease, it may not be feasible to achieve the normal value without exposure to the dangers of oxygen toxicity (*see* page 424). Under these conditions it may be necessary to accept a level as low as 8 kPa (60 mm Hg) or sometimes 7 kPa (52·5 mm Hg). The lowest safe level depends upon many factors, which are considered in detail in Chapter 12. Higher than normal levels of arterial PO_2 may be required in exceptional circumstances such as severe anaemia, hypoperfusion or in anticipation of a period of respiratory arrest (e.g. extubation).

In practice, the PO_2 is seldom a factor in determining the adequacy of pulmonary ventilation. This is because oxygenation depends upon a number of factors which do not apply to carbon dioxide homeostasis. In particular, arterial PO_2 can usually be adjusted by altering the oxygen concentration of the inspired gas. Therefore, during artificial ventilation, it is the usual practice to control the PCO_2 by adjusting the pulmonary ventilation, and then to control the PO_2 by adjusting the inspired oxygen concentration.

The relationship between ventilation and arterial gas tensions during artificial ventilation

During prolonged artificial ventilation, continuous monitoring of arterial PO_2 and PCO_2 is at present inpracticable for the control of minute volume and inspired oxygen concentration. It is therefore necessary to be able to make a reasonable prediction of the blood-gas tensions which will result from a particular setting of these variables. Blood-gas tensions may then be checked from time to time and adjustments made.

Under the conditions of routine clinical anaesthesia, monitoring of blood-gas tensions is seldom practised and it is usual to rely almost entirely on prediction of the likely values for arterial PO_2 and PCO_2 which result from the selected minute volume and inspired oxygen concentration.

Calculation of ventilation required for CO_2 homeostasis during anaesthesia

Certain simplifying assumptions are usually made, based on typical conditions during uncomplicated anaesthesia. Appropriate corrections can be applied later if they are required.

1. Barometric pressure is 101·3 kPa (760 mm Hg). Water vapour pressure at 37°C is 6·3 kPa (47 mm Hg), and so the dry barometric pressure of alveolar gas is 101·3 − 6·3 = 95 kPa (713 mm Hg).
2. The inspired gas is free of carbon dioxide.
3. The patient's metabolic activity is basal on the English Standard (Robertson and Reid, 1952), or about 15 per cent below basal on the American Standard (Aub and DuBois, 1917; Boothby and Sandiford, 1924) (*see Table 15*).

Table 15. PREDICTED VALUES FOR OXYGEN CONSUMPTION AND CARBON DIOXIDE OUTPUT DURING UNCOMPLICATED ANAESTHESIA (ml/min) (STPD)

Age	Oxygen consumption			Carbon dioxide output		
	small patient	*average patient*	*large patient*	*small patient*	*average patient*	*large patient*
Male						
14–15		190			152	
16–17		200			160	
18–19	168	210	252	134	168	202
20–29	162	203	243	130	162	194
30–39	162	203	243	130	162	194
40–49	158	198	237	126	158	190
50–59	155	194	233	124	155	186
60–69	150	187	224	120	150	179
Female						
14–15		174			139	
16–17		188			150	
18–19	156	194	233	125	155	186
20–29	152	190	228	122	152	182
30–39	150	187	224	120	150	179
40–49	148	184	221	118	147	177
50–59	144	180	216	115	144	173
60–69	140	175	210	112	140	168

Values for CO_2 output will only apply in a steady respiratory state.
Values are probably about 6 per cent lower during artificial ventilation.
Figures are based on 85 per cent of basal according to data of Aub and Dubois (1917) and Boothby and Sandiford (1924).

4. The respiratory exchange ratio (RQ) is 0·8.
5. The physiological dead space and distribution have the values known to apply to healthy anaesthetized patients. General considerations commonly exclude apparatus dead space, allowance for which is postponed until consideration of an individual patient and his gas circuit.

Charts and nomograms for prediction of correct ventilation are all based on the following axiomatic relationship:

$$\frac{\text{volume of } CO_2 \text{ eliminated}}{\text{in one minute}} = \frac{\text{alveolar}}{\text{ventilation}} \times \frac{\text{concentration of } CO_2}{\text{in alveolar gas}}$$

Therefore:

$$\frac{\text{alveolar}}{\text{ventilation}} = \frac{\text{volume of } CO_2 \text{ eliminated per minute}}{\text{concentration of } CO_2 \text{ in alveolar gas}}$$

$$= \frac{\text{volume of } CO_2 \text{ eliminated per minute}}{\text{* alveolar } P_{CO_2} \div 95}$$

For all practical purposes,

$$\text{arterial } P_{CO_2} = \text{alveolar } P_{CO_2}$$

Therefore:

$$\frac{\text{alveolar}}{\text{ventilation}} = \frac{\text{volumes of } CO_2 \text{ eliminated per minute}}{\text{arterial } P_{CO_2} \div 95}$$

So far these equations make no assumptions which are likely to be invalid. Unfortunately, they are of little practical use until alveolar ventilation (which cannot be measured) is related to minute volume of respiration (which can be measured). This relationship depends upon the physiological dead space which, excluding apparatus dead space, approximates to one-third of the tidal volume in healthy, anaesthetized intubated patients (Nunn and Hill, 1960). Therefore the alveolar ventilation will approximate to two-thirds of the minute volume.

However, it is important to remember that the dead space is increased under certain circumstances, and that the alveolar ventilation will then be less than two-thirds of the minute volume. The most important causes of an increase of dead space are certain respiratory diseases, pulmonary embolus and conditions associated with a reduction of pulmonary blood flow (pages 220 et seq.). The *total* dead space includes apparatus dead space which will vary widely with different gas circuits and is often an important factor. For example, a value of 100 ml, at a respiratory frequency of 20 breaths per minute, will cause a reduction in alveolar ventilation of 2 litres per minute. Not without significance is the difference in total dead space between intubated and non-intubated patients. Kain, Panday and Nunn (1969) found the total dead space to be about 85 ml greater in unintubated patients breathing from a facemask.

If we confine our attention to healthy intubated patients and ignore, for the moment, apparatus dead space, the following relationship applies:

$$\text{required minute volume} = \frac{\text{predicted oxygen consumption x RQ}}{\text{required arterial } P_{CO_2} \div 95} \times 1.5$$

where the factor 1·5 represents the ratio of minute volume to alveolar ventilation.

However, minute volume is normally expressed under conditions of body temperature (BTPS), while oxygen consumption is expressed under conditions of standard temperature and pressure, dry (STPD). To convert gas volumes at STPD to BTPS the factor is approximately 1·2 (*see* Appendix B). Also, oxygen consumption is usually expressed in millilitres per minute and a factor of 0·001 is required to convert this to litres per minute, which is the customary unit for expression of minute volume.

---

* P_{CO_2} in kPa.

Allowing a value of 0·8 for the RQ, the equation may now be written as follows:

$$\text{*required minute volume (l/min)} = \frac{\text{predicted oxygen consumption (ml/min)}}{\text{required arterial } P_{CO_2} \text{ (kPa)}} \times 0·14$$

(If P_{CO_2} is expressed in mm Hg, the value of the constant is very close to unity.) This equation forms the basis of the charts of Nunn (1960a), subsequently presented in the form of a slide rule (Nunn, 1962a). Radford's nomogram (1955) employs the same basic equation but assumes a fixed dead space related to the weight of the patient (*Figure 64*). Both methods give reasonable results

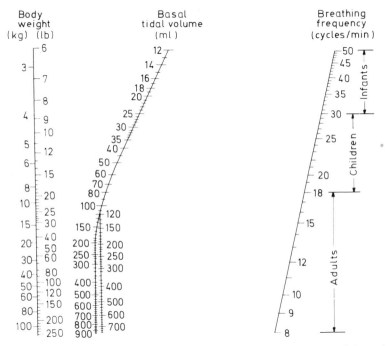

Figure 64. Radford's (1955) ventilation nomogram. (Reproduced by courtesy of the author and the Editor of the Journal of Applied Physiology)

during steady artificial ventilation, when the calculated minute volume usually gives an arterial P_{CO_2} within the range 4·5–6·1 kPa (34–46 mm Hg) (Scurr, 1956). However, predicted relationships are far less accurate during anaesthesia with spontaneous respiration, when ventilation tends to fluctuate from minute to minute, in response to surgical stimulus (Nunn, 1960a).

Although these methods give satisfactory results during routine anaesthesia of patients without cardiorespiratory disease, the problem is much more complicated when patients with severe respiratory disease are ventilated, during either anaesthesia or intensive therapy. It is not unusual to underestimate the minute volume required for CO_2 homeostasis, particularly during the return to

* The apparent inconsistency of the dimensions in this equation is explained by the constant 0·14 which has the dimensions of pressure.

spontaneous respiration. Arterial P_{CO_2} is proportional to the ratio of CO_2 output to alveolar ventilation and estimates of both these variables may be in error. The output of CO_2 may be raised in febrile or agitated patients and in those who are struggling to breathe out of phase with the ventilator. Values of double the basal output are common. This factor may easily be checked by collecting expired air during a period of two or three minutes. The product of the expired minute volume and the mixed expired CO_2 concentration equals the CO_2 output and, since a steady state is usual during prolonged ventilation, CO_2 production will be close to output.

The estimate of the alveolar ventilation from the imposed minute volume will also be in error if the physiological dead space is increased. This problem is discussed in Chapter 7 but we may note at this stage that values for the physiological dead space (including apparatus dead space) are often as high as 75 per cent of tidal volume in patients being ventilated in the intensive therapy unit. Thus a patient with twice his basal CO_2 output and twice the expected physiological dead space will require four times the minute volume indicated by Radford's nomogram or derived from basic considerations. The requirement for a high minute volume will normally be indicated by routine blood-gas analysis, but during weaning from artificial ventilation it is most important to be satisfied that the patient's spontaneous minute volume is appropriate to his own conditions (particularly CO_2 output and dead space) and not to accept some arbitrary value for minute volume or tidal volume as good enough. Not infrequently the highest ventilatory requirements occur in just those patients whose ventilatory capacity is inadequate to meet the requirement.

Adequacy of oxygenation when ventilation has been adjusted to maintain CO_2 homeostasis

When efforts are made to calculate the 'correct' ventilation for a patient, they are usually based on an attempt to attain an arterial P_{CO_2} of the desired level. For a patient breathing air, the attainment of a normal P_{CO_2} ensures that the *alveolar* P_{O_2} will also be normal. However, in many clinical situations it does not follow that a normal *alveolar* P_{O_2} results in a normal *arterial* P_{O_2}. The level of oxygen in the arterial blood is influenced by two important factors which do not significantly affect the level of carbon dioxide. The first is the concentration of oxygen in the inspired gas; the second is the degree of admixture of venous blood with arterial blood, a condition which seems to be almost always present to some degree in patients requiring intensive therapy and also during anaesthesia. Oxygen enrichment of the inspired gas will compensate for a considerable degree of venous admixture, and it is important to grasp the quantitative aspects of this difficult and markedly non-linear relationship. So far as intensive therapy is concerned, one can never assume that a ventilation adequate for CO_2 homeostasis will ensure adequate arterial oxygenation if the inspired gas is air. It is usually necessary to measure the arterial P_{O_2} at intervals and adjust the inspired oxygen concentration to give an acceptable value for P_{O_2}. Factors governing the relationship between inspired oxygen concentration and arterial P_{O_2} in this situation are complex and are discussed elsewhere (*see* pages 290 and 387).

During routine anaesthesia for patients without cardiorespiratory disease, the arterial oxygenation is more predictable. Numerous studies have shown that there is an increased alveolar/arterial P_{O_2} difference during anaesthesia with spontaneous respiration, and it cannot be assumed that the arterial Po_2 will be normal in a patient breathing 21 per cent oxygen, even if the ventilation is adequate to ensure a normal Pco_2. During anaesthesia with artificial ventilation, most authors have also found the alveolar/arterial Po_2 difference to be increased so that arterial Po_2 values of 13·3 kPa (100 mm Hg) cannot be guaranteed with an inspired oxygen concentration of 21 per cent even if the patient is hyperventilated (*see* page 434). There may be an exception in the case of patients who are passively hyperventilated with air-ether mixtures, and satisfactory values for arterial Po_2 have been reported with this technique (Roberts et al., 1974). In contrast, Bodman and Latimer (1975) report many unacceptably low values for arterial Po_2 (less than 6 kPa (45 mm Hg)) during ether-air anaesthesia with spontaneous respiration when the anaesthetic was administered by experienced nurse anaesthetists under supervision of physician anaesthetists. Many very low values of Po_2 were observed at a time when the minute volume was over 7 l/min. It should, however, be remembered that the normal arterial Po_2 falls with age (page 411) and 10 kPa (75 mm Hg) is to be expected in a healthy man aged 70.

During anaesthesia, the defect in arterial oxygenation is due mainly to shunting, although it may be due in some part to maldistribution. The malfunction during the inhalation of 21 per cent oxygen may be expressed conveniently as a difference between ideal alveolar and arterial Po_2 of the order of 4·7 kPa (35 mm Hg)* (compared with a normal value of less than 1·3 kPa or 10 mm Hg):

mean alveolar Po_2 with standard ventilation	14 kPa	105 mm Hg
mean arterial Po_2 (observed)	9·3 kPa	70 mm Hg
alveolar/arterial Po_2 difference	4·7 kPa	35 mm Hg

Table 16. INSPIRED OXYGEN CONCENTRATIONS REQUIRED FOR MAINTENANCE OF NORMAL ARTERIAL Po_2 IN THE MAJORITY OF INTUBATED, ANAESTHETIZED PATIENTS AT SEA LEVEL

Minute volume of respiration (l/min) (BTPS)	*Inspired oxygen concentration (%)*
Infinity	28
20	29·5
10	31·5
7	32·5
6	33·5
5	34·5
4	36·5
3	39
2	44·5
1	61

Values for minute volume below about 5 l/min will usually be associated with carbon dioxide retention which will be severe when the minute volume is less than 3 l/min. Enrichment of the inspired gas mixture with oxygen will not prevent carbon dioxide retention.

* The alveolar arterial Po_2 difference in a particular patient varies with the actual Po_2 (*see* page 391). The difference noted here only applies to an alveolar Po_2 close to 13·3 kPa (100 mm Hg).

Arterial P_{O_2} may be restored to the normal value of 13·3 kPa (100 mm Hg) by increasing the alveolar P_{O_2} to approximately 20 kPa (150 mm Hg). This may be achieved by increasing the concentration of oxygen in the inspired gas mixture, and an increase to 30 per cent is sufficient in the average patient. A greater increase will be needed in certain patients with larger shunts and, of course, if the ventilation is less than standard. *Table 16* gives an approximate indication of the concentration of oxygen in the inspired gas which is required to ensure a normal arterial P_{O_2} at different levels of ventilation in the healthy intubated, anaesthetized patient.

THE EFFECT OF DIFFERENT LEVELS OF VENTILATION ON ALVEOLAR GAS TENSIONS*

As ventilation increases, the composition of the alveolar gas tends to approach that of the inspired gas. The difference between inspired and alveolar concentrations of a gas is equal to the ratio of the output (or uptake) of the gas, to the alveolar ventilation.

$$\begin{array}{c} \text{alveolar} \\ \text{concentration} \\ \text{of gas } X \end{array} = \begin{array}{c} \text{inspired} \\ \text{concentration} \\ \text{of gas } X \end{array} + (\text{or}-) \left(\frac{\text{output (or uptake) of gas } X}{\text{alveolar ventilation}} \right)$$

Note:

1. Concentrations are here expressed as fractions and must be multiplied by 100 to give percentages.
2. The equation does not correct for any difference in the inspired and expired minute volumes and, in the case of oxygen, is usually subject to a slight error which may be avoided by the use of a small correction factor which may be ignored for general clinical purposes.
3. The sign on the right-hand side is + for output and − for uptake.
4. Tension of a gas X may be obtained by multiplying both sides of the equation by the dry barometric pressure (barometric pressure *minus* water vapour pressure at body temperature).
5. The figures of gas exchange and alveolar ventilation must both be expressed under the same conditions of temperature and pressure. BTPS is used for the examples given below.

In the case of carbon dioxide:

$$\text{alveolar } P_{CO_2} = \text{dry barometric pressure} \left(\begin{array}{c} \text{inspired } CO_2 \\ \text{concentration} \end{array} + \frac{CO_2 \text{ output}}{\text{alveolar ventilation}} \right)$$

$$\text{e.g.} \quad 5{\cdot}3 \quad = \quad 95 \quad \left(0 \quad + \quad \frac{0{\cdot}18}{3{\cdot}2} \right)$$

$$\text{kPa} \qquad\qquad \text{kPa} \qquad\qquad\qquad \text{l/min} \div \text{l/min}$$

$$\text{or:} \quad 40 \quad = \quad 713 \quad \left(0 \quad + \quad \frac{180}{3200} \right)$$

$$\text{mm Hg} \qquad\qquad \text{mm Hg} \qquad\qquad\qquad \text{ml/min} \div \text{ml/min}$$

* This subject receives extended treatment for the case of oxygen in Chapter 12 (pages 384 et seq.).

And in the case of oxygen:

$$\text{alveolar } P_{O_2} = \text{dry barometric pressure} \left(\frac{\text{inspired } O_2}{\text{concentration}} - \frac{O_2 \text{ uptake}}{\text{alveolar ventilation}} \right)$$

$$\text{e.g.} \quad 13 \cdot 3 \quad = \quad 95 \quad \left(\frac{21}{100} - \frac{0 \cdot 225}{3 \cdot 2} \right)$$

$$\text{kPa} \qquad\qquad \text{kPa} \qquad\qquad \text{l/min} \div \text{l/min}$$

$$\text{or:} \quad 100 \quad = \quad 713 \quad \left(\frac{21}{100} - \frac{225}{3200} \right)$$

$$\text{mm Hg} \qquad\qquad \text{mm Hg} \qquad\qquad \text{ml/min} \div \text{ml/min}$$

The relationship between alveolar ventilation and alveolar gas tensions is non-linear and rather difficult to visualize. It is best displayed on a graph, and *Figure 65* shows the relationships based on conditions which are typical of anaesthesia. The diagram will repay careful study and the following points should be noted.

1. The relationship between alveolar gas tensions and alveolar ventilation is hyperbolic. When the ventilation is increased above the normal range, the alveolar gas tensions approach the inspired tensions asymptotically but dramatic changes do not occur on the flat part of the curves. Thus the hyperventilation does not raise the alveolar P_{O_2} markedly, unless the alveolar ventilation was previously reduced. On the other hand, reductions of alveolar ventilation may cause severe deterioration in alveolar gas tensions. Alveolar P_{O_2} falls steeply after reduction of ventilation below a critical level. The critical level is reduced by oxygen enrichment of the inspired gas, but the transitional zone then becomes narrower—often alarmingly so. For example, when the subject in *Figure 65* breathed 30 per cent oxygen, an alveolar ventilation of 1·2 l/min would result in an alveolar P_{O_2} of 10·7 kPa (80 mm Hg), a level which is not dangerous in an otherwise healthy patient. If the alveolar ventilation were then reduced by only 400 ml/min, the alveolar P_{O_2} would fall to 1·9 kPa (14 mm Hg), a level which is not compatible with life.

2. A change in the inspired P_{O_2} produces an equal change in the alveolar P_{O_2} if other factors remain the same (pages 387 et seq.). Consider an alveolar ventilation of 1·2 l/min during air breathing. In the example shown in *Figure 65* this would result in an alveolar P_{O_2} of 2·1 kPa (16 mm Hg), which would not be compatible with life. If, however, the inspired air were enriched with oxygen to 30 per cent that would increase the P_{O_2} of the inspired gas by 8·5 kPa (64 mm Hg). If other factors remained the same, the alveolar P_{O_2} would also rise by 8·5 kPa (64 mm Hg) to 10·6 kPa (80 mm Hg), a level which is not much below the normal range. As a general rule, it may be said that, if hypoxaemia due to hypoventilation is to be treated with oxygen-enrichment of inspired gas, then a modest level of enrichment will be sufficient. If more than 30 per cent oxygen is required, it follows that the hypoventilation should be treated by methods which increase the ventilation. There are some cases in which this is not possible and greater increases in the inspired oxygen concentration will then be required, but it must be appreciated that this will do nothing to

reduce the concomitant elevation of P_{CO_2}. The addition of carbon dioxide to the inspired gas raises the alveolar P_{CO_2} in the same way as addition of oxygen raises the alveolar P_{O_2}.

3. *Figure 65* shows clearly the dangers of decreasing the inspired oxygen concentration below 21 per cent as was formerly common practice in dental anaesthesia and obstetric 'gas-air' analgesia. The maintenance of a high ventilation rate is essential during oxygen curtailment and the patient is exposed to grave risk if ventilation is reduced as, for example, by airway obstruction.

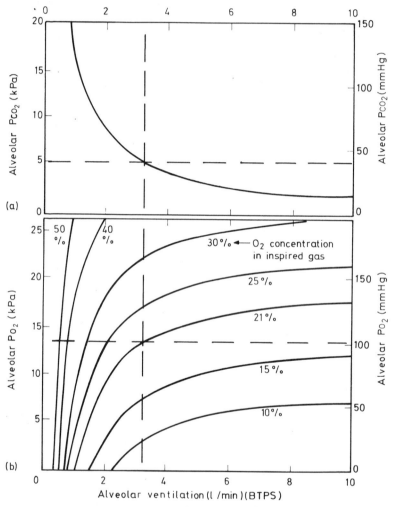

Figure 65. Alveolar gas tensions produced by different levels of alveolar ventilation. (a) The hyperbolic relationship between alveolar P_{CO_2} and alveolar ventilation. (b) The relationship between alveolar P_{O_2} and alveolar ventilation for different levels of oxygen concentration in the inspired gas. The broken vertical line indicates an alveolar ventilation of 3·2 l/min. Dry barometric pressure, 95 kPa = 713 mm Hg; carbon dioxide output, 150 ml/min (STPD) = 180 ml/min (BTPS); oxygen uptake, 190 ml/min (STPD) = 225 ml/min (BTPS). No allowance has been made for the difference between inspired and expired minute volumes

It must be stressed that the discussion of *Figure 65* relates to the alveolar P_{O_2} and not the arterial P_{O_2}. It will be seen in Chapters 9 and 12 that the arterial P_{O_2} may be much less than the alveolar P_{O_2}, and the difference constitutes a major cause of hypoxaemia associated with pulmonary disease and anaesthesia. *Figure 66* shows, on a P_{O_2}/P_{CO_2} diagram, the typical pattern of deterioration of arterial blood gases in respiratory failure due to chronic obstructive airway disease compared with the values which would result from pure ventilatory failure. The diagram also shows the pattern of changes in arterial blood gases

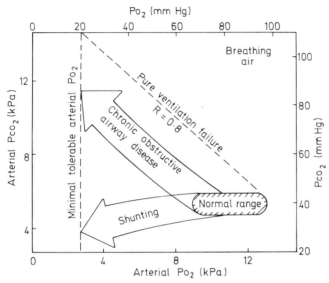

Figure 66. Pattern of deterioration of arterial blood gases in chronic obstructive airway disease and pulmonary shunting. The shaded area indicates the normal range of arterial blood-gas tensions in which P_{O_2} decreases with age. The oblique broken line shows the theoretical changes in alveolar P_{CO_2} and P_{O_2} resulting from pure ventilatory failure. In chronic obstructive airway disease, the arterial P_{O_2} is always less than the value which would be expected in pure ventilatory failure at the same P_{CO_2} value. Discussion of shunting is postponed to Chapter 9.

with progressive shunting of pulmonary blood flow past ventilated alveoli. If oxygen saturation is considered instead of P_{O_2}, the non-linearity of the dissociation curve is added to the non-linearity of the rectangular hyperbolas in *Figure 65*. When ventilation is reduced, arterial saturation falls even more abruptly than the P_{O_2}.

It is also important to bear in mind the time course of changes in P_{CO_2} and P_{O_2} resulting from changes in ventilation (page 357). The values indicated in *Figure 65* relate to the steady state which is attained some time after a change in ventilation. Oxygen levels change quickly but, in the case of carbon dioxide, the changes are slow due to the large stores of carbon dioxide present in the body. The problem is considered in some detail in Chapters 11 and 12, but for the present it should be noted that, after a step change in ventilation, there is an exponential approach towards the equilibrium values shown in *Figure 65*. (Exponential changes are discussed in Appendix E.) Changes in P_{O_2} are rapid and have a half-life of 30 seconds. Changes in P_{CO_2} are much slower, with a half-life of 4 minutes for a falling P_{CO_2} (Farhi and Rahn, 1955a; Nunn and Matthews, 1959). When P_{CO_2} is rising (following a reduction in ventilation) changes are even slower, with half-lives ranging from 4 to 15 minutes (Ivanov and Nunn, 1968).

CAUSES OF FAILURE OF VENTILATION

So far, most of this book has been devoted to factors influencing ventilation and most causes of ventilatory failure have already been described. This section is intended to classify the causes of ventilatory failure and present them as a unified scheme (*Figure 67*).

The 'Respiratory Centre' (see Chapter 2)

The rhythmicity of respiration in man appears to have its origin in the neurones of the medulla (A in *Figure 67*). These neurones are very susceptible to oxygen lack, and central respiratory failure is an early effect of anoxia. Temporary apnoea often follows a severe anoxic episode, but fortunately spontaneous respiration usually returns after restoration of normal oxygenation. Hypoxia may be due to arterial desaturation, circulatory failure or raised intracranial pressure.

The respiratory neurones may also be depressed by very high levels of arterial P_{CO_2}, probably of the order of 40 kPa (300 mm Hg) in the unanaesthetized subject, but at a lower P_{CO_2} in the presence of narcotic drugs (page 48). Reduction of P_{CO_2} below the apnoeic threshold level causes apnoea in the

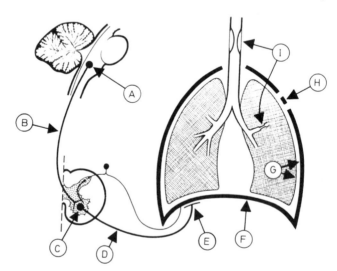

Figure 67. Summary of sites at which lesions, drug action or malfunction may result in ventilatory failure. (A) The 'respiratory centre'. (B) Upper motoneurone. (C) Anterior horn cell. (D) Lower motoneurone. (E) The neuromuscular junction. (F) The respiratory muscles. (G) Altered elasticity of lungs or chest wall. (H) Loss of structural integrity of chest wall and pleural cavity. (I) Increased airway resistance

unconscious but usually not in the conscious patient (page 30). Loss of respiratory sensitivity to carbon dioxide in patients with chronic bronchitis is a potent cause of ventilatory failure. It may also occur in patients with chronic ventilatory failure due to other causes.

A wide variety of drugs will produce central apnoea; these include the opiates and all anaesthetic agents, provided the dosage is sufficiently high. Respiration may be reflexly arrested by a variety of noxious stimuli applied to the respiratory tract and other areas. However, the Herring–Breuer inflation reflex is weak in man and inflation to moderate pressures does not normally inhibit inspiration in an anaesthetized man (page 52).

The commonest form of central apnoea encountered by the anaesthetist is failure of a patient to breathe at the end of an anaesthetic which has been conducted with paralysis and artificial hyperventilation. The condition is not serious although often troublesome and time wasting. It appears that the apnoea is due to the absence of general neuronal traffic when the P_{CO_2} is below the apnoeic threshold. Breathing can usually be restarted either by waking the patient or by elevation of P_{CO_2} above the threshold level (Ivanov and Nunn, 1969).

Finally, it should be noted that the respiratory neurones may be affected by pressure, trauma, infection, neoplasm or vascular catastrophe.

Upper motoneurone

The upper motoneurones serving the respiratory muscles are liable to interruption in the neck. Those connecting with the phrenic nerves (cervical 3, 4 and 5) are seldom interrupted since the upper cervical cord is relatively well protected against trauma although fracture-dislocation of the cervical vertebrae may occur at the level of cervical 1–2. The upper motoneurones connecting with the inspiratory muscles are interrupted by the more usual type of cervical dislocation (cervical 5–6). Upper motoneurones may be involved in various disease processes including tumour and demyelination, although seldom in syringomyelia.

Anterior horn cell

The anterior horn cells concerned with respiration may be affected by various disease processes, of which the most important is anterior poliomyelitis. All degrees of involvement occur including total paralysis of all respiratory muscles. The anterior horn cells are reversibly depressed by the drug mephenesin (Myanesin) which was formerly used as a relaxant in anaesthesia.

Lower motoneurone

The motor nerves of the respiratory muscles are prone to the normal traumatic risks and the phrenic nerves may be surgically interrupted. However, apnoea due to traumatic damage of the nerves supplying the respiratory muscles is improbable. Polyneuritis (e.g. Guillain–Barré syndrome) and motoneurone disease are the principal conditions which may cause apnoea from disruption of conduction by these nerves. Interference with the γ fibres (page 32) would cause severe dysfunction but there is no clear evidence of the occurrence of specific lesions of these fibres.

The neuromuscular junction

The most important disease processes acting at this site are myasthenia gravis and botulism. Drugs acting on this site include all the relaxants used in clinical anaesthesia, neostigmine and certain organophosphorus compounds. Procaine acts by preventing the synthesis of acetylcholine.

The respiratory muscles

Disease of the respiratory muscles may rarely cause respiratory failure, but discussion of the muscular dystrophies also lies outside the scope of this book. The efficacy of the inspiratory muscles may be impaired by deformity, injury and 'splinting' of the diaphragm by abdominal distension. A flattened diaphragm (as may be seen in tension pneumothorax) may contract forcefully but have little effect upon tidal ventilation.

Elasticity of lungs and chest wall

Ventilatory failure may result from increased elastic resistance to breathing. This may arise in the lungs (e.g. respiratory distress syndrome or pulmonary fibrosis), in the pleura (e.g. chronic empyma with fibrinous deposit), in the chest wall (e.g. kyphoscoliosis or contracted burn scars) or external to the chest (e.g. traumatic asphyxia due to burial under sand or bodies). A sustained pressure on the chest wall of no more than about 6 kPa (45 mm Hg) is sufficient to prevent breathing. This is equivalent to immersion in water to a depth of about 60 cm, when airway pressure is close to atmospheric.

Loss of structural integrity of chest wall and pleural cavity

The introduction of air into the pleural cavity (closed pneumothorax) reduces the volume, the ventilation and probably the perfusion of the lung on that side. If the pressure of gas in the pleural cavity rises appreciably above atmospheric (tension pneumothorax), the ipsilateral lung is totally collapsed, the mediastinum is displaced and the contralateral lung partially collapsed; the convexity of the diaphragm is lost and ventilation may be critically impaired. The correction of this condition is a matter of urgency and the possibility of its occurrence must always be borne in mind. Deviation of trachea and apex beat, combined with hyper-resonance, usually make the diagnosis simple provided the possibility is considered. When the pleural cavity communicates with the atmosphere (open pneumothorax) there is danger of the contralateral lung inhaling gas from the ipsilateral lung, which is not subjected to the normal reduction of intrathoracic pressure during inspiration. The degree of dysfunction depends on the size of the opening in the chest, but is also influenced by the degree of airway obstruction produced, for example, by approximation of the vocal cords. Pendulum movement of gas between the two lungs may be prevented by collapsing the exposed lung, a manoeuvre familiar to a former generation of surgeons who used local analgesia for thoracotomy.

Loss of rigidity of the rib cage may result in regional or general ventilatory failure. This may be therapeutic (thoracoplasty) or traumatic (crushed chest).

Various local devices may improve ventilation when failure results from impairment of structural integrity of the chest wall but artificial ventilation, by intermittent positive pressure, is almost always effective and was the long-awaited solution to the problem posed by thoracic surgery and crushed chest.

Airway resistance

Chapter 4 has been devoted to the problems of airway resistance. It is much the most important cause of ventilatory failure, whether due to overt massive obstruction of the upper air passages or to diffuse, progressive disease of the small air passages.

Diagnosis of cause of ventilatory failure

In cases of ventilatory failure, it is usually obvious whether respiratory efforts are being made or not. This distinction is of prime importance and divides the causes of failure into two groups of approximately equal importance.

Absent or diminished respiratory effort implies defective function in the central nervous system, peripheral motor nerves, neuromuscular junction or respiratory muscles (A–F in *Figure 67*). Ventilatory failure from dysfunction at any of these sites may present a broadly similar clinical picture. However, the history of events leading to ventilatory failure is usually sufficient to indicate the actual site and nature of the dysfunction. Nevertheless, after anaesthesia with induced neuromuscular block, it may be difficult to distinguish between ventilatory failure due to central causes and persistent neuromuscular block. Under these circumstances, it is useful to note the muscular contraction when a peripheral nerve (e.g. ulnar) is stimulated. Alternatively, the demonstration of action potentials in the phrenic nerve would also distinguish between the two conditions, although this is technically difficult. In practice, the distinction is often made by means of a variety of therapeutic tests which afford the anaesthetist an opportunity to display his acumen.

Forceful respiratory efforts in the presence of ventilatory failure mean reduced compliance, increased airway resistance or loss of structural integrity of the thoracic cage. Usually the latter is immediately apparent although it may be overlooked in cases of severe multiple injuries. The distinction between loss of compliance and increased resistance may be difficult. Attempts by the patient to ventilate with minimum work usually dictate an increased respiratory frequency with shallow breathing when compliance is reduced. Increased resistance, on the other hand, is usually associated with slow breathing, Expiratory resistance, particularly due to trapping, leads to an increased lung volume and often the patient deliberately checks expiratory air flow at the mouth to dilate his air passages (pursed-lip breathing). Inspiratory resistance shows characteristic in-drawing of soft tissues around the bony thorax during inspiration. Auscultation is helpful and may define the presence and the phasing of obstruction. It should also help to distinguish between obstruction due to liquid material in the air passages and that due to narrowing of the air passages. Spasm of the air passages is most convincingly demonstrated by study of the response to bronchodilators, while absence of response in a chronic case is often evidence of structural causes of obstruction (e.g. trapping). Oedema of the mucosa may be confused with spasm and both may respond to salbutamol, isoprenaline or adrenaline.

TREATMENT OF VENTILATORY FAILURE

It is self-evident that the first line of treatment is to remove the cause of the ventilatory failure. Neuromuscular blockade should be reversed, airway obstruc-tion should be relieved, an open pneumothorax should be closed, and so on. However, there remain for consideration many patients in whom it is not possible to treat the cause of the ventilatory failure. Such patients cover a wide range of conditions including chronic bronchitis (with airway obstruction and diminished ventilatory response to carbon dioxide), motoneurone disease, chronic poliomyelitis (with respiratory involvement) and fibrosing alveolitis. Crushed chest, drug overdose and severe chest infections are examples of causes of ventilatory failure which can be expected to be of limited duration. Nevertheless, during the short term, it may not be possible to restore normal spontaneous ventilation.

Symptomatic treatment of ventilatory failure depends upon the cause and the degree of failure. In its mildest form it may be permissible to allow the arterial Pco_2 to rise and the Po_2 to fall. In the case of patients with chronic bronchitis, they may live an independent though relatively inactive existence with a Pco_2 as high as 8 kPa (60 mm Hg) and a Po_2 as low as 5·5 kPa (41 mm Hg). Po_2 falls more than Pco_2 rises because there are usually disordered ventilation/perfusion relationships in these patients. Such levels of arterial blood gases may be tolerated in a patient with progressive pulmonary disease in the interest of maintaining his independence of cumbersome therapeutic devices but, in hospital practice, it would be usual to treat hypoxia before the arterial Po_2 had fallen to 5·5 kPa. Even in domiciliary practice, the use of oxygen would be considered at this level of hypoxia.

The most dangerous feature of ventilatory failure is hypoxia, and it is possible to restore a normal arterial Po_2 by appropriate augmentation of the inspired oxygen concentration even in very severe degrees of ventilatory failure. However, it is of the utmost importance that all concerned in the treatment of patients with ventilatory failure should understand that oxygen therapy cannot reduce the Pco_2 and will often raise it through withdrawal of the hypoxic drive to breathing. In practice, the role of oxygen therapy in the treatment of ventilatory failure is confined to patients with only slight to moderate rise of Pco_2 and oxygen should be used with great caution when the Pco_2 is above 10 kPa (75 mm Hg). It is also important that the correct level of inspired oxygen should be employed. *Figure 65* shows that only modest oxygen enrichment is required. For example, a reduction in alveolar ventilation which results in an alveolar P_{CO_2} of 10 kPa (75 mm Hg) will give an alveolar P_{O_2} of about 7 kPa (53 mm Hg) when the patient is breathing air. If this level of alveolar ventilation is maintained, 25 per cent inspired oxygen will be sufficient to raise the alveolar P_{O_2} to 11 kPa (83 mm Hg). Use of excessively high concentrations of oxygen carries the danger of precipitating severe ventilatory failure from withdrawal of the hypoxic drive to respiration on which so many patients in chronic ventilatory failure depend. *Figure 65* also shows that if more than 30 per cent oxygen is required to restore a normal alveolar P_{O_2}, then the P_{CO_2} will be over 12 kPa (90 mm Hg) and steps must be taken to increase the alveolar ventilation as the patient is in danger of carbon dioxide narcosis. Fortunately, inspired oxygen concentrations in the range 24–35 per cent can be easily and economically provided in the form of air-oxygen mixtures using such devices as the Venturi Mask and walking oxygen sets.

Depending upon the circumstances, there is a degree of ventilatory failure when oxygen therapy alone is insufficient and steps must be taken to increase the alveolar ventilation. Firm guidelines cannot be given since much depends upon the cause of the ventilatory failure, the prognosis and many other factors. There are, in general, three methods of increasing the alveolar ventilation.

1. *Respiratory stimulants.* When the best available stimulant was nikethamide, this line of treatment was unreliable. Initial stimulation tended to be followed by depression and results were poor. With the advent of doxapram, the situation was changed and continuous intravenous infusion at the rate of 1–8 mg/min is worth considering if there is reasonable hope of spontaneous improvement within a day or two. It may therefore be useful for treating an intercurrent infection in a chronic bronchitic or temporary failure to ventilate after weaning from artificial ventilation.

2. *Endotracheal intubation* alone may be sufficient to reduce the P_{CO_2} to a safe level. Anatomical dead space is reduced, upper airway obstruction is relieved and tracheobronchial secretions may be aspirated.

3. *Artificial ventilation* will restore a normal alveolar ventilation in almost all patients with ventilatory failure. It is now very widely used but it requires a high level of medical and nursing cover, preferably in an intensive therapy unit. Perhaps the major reason for withholding this form of therapy is a hopeless prognosis as, for example, in patients with severe brain injury.

Finally, it should be stressed that control of tracheobronchial secretions is paramount in the management of ventilatory failure. This factor alone may indicate endotracheal intubation.

THE WORK OF BREATHING

During spontaneous respiration, the work of breathing is accomplished by the respiratory muscles of the patient. During artificial ventilation, the work of breathing is performed by the machine or person who has taken over responsibility for tidal exchange. In spite of the obvious difference in the source of energy, there are many similar features in the two types of breathing. In each case, the work is normally performed during inspiration; expiration is powered by the potential energy stored in the tissues which have been distorted from their resting position during inspiration. All the work is eventually used to overcome air flow resistance which results in its dissipation as heat. Approximately half the inspiratory work is so dissipated during inspiration, while the

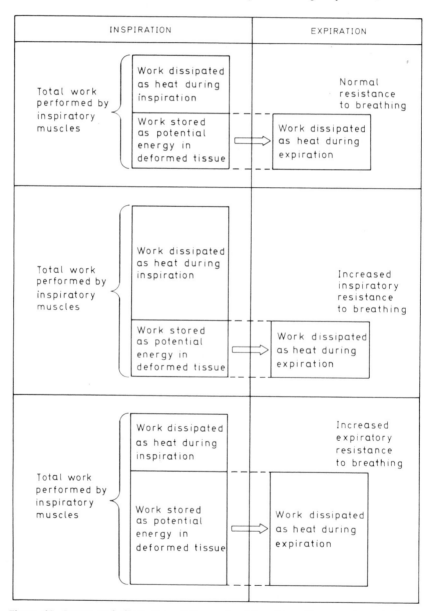

Figure 68. Source and dissipation of the work of breathing. The areas in each diagram correspond to the work of breathing. The total area on the left indicates the work done by the inspiratory muscles during inspiration

remainder is stored temporarily and then dissipated during expiration. Elasticity thus enables the work of *expiration* to be performed by the *inspiratory* muscles (*Figure 68*).

During both spontaneous and artificial respiration, there may be occasions when additional work is performed during expiration to hasten the expulsion of gas from the lungs. Typical examples are the use of expiratory muscles in coughing and the use of a subatmospheric pressure phase during IPP ventilation of the lungs (NEEP).

The actual rate of work performed by the respiratory muscles is quite remarkably small in the healthy resting subject. Under these circumstances the oxygen consumption of the respiratory muscles is only about 3 ml/min, or less than 2 per cent of the metabolic rate. Furthermore, of this tiny amount of energy, about 90 per cent is lost as heat within the respiratory muscles, so that only 10 per cent is available for moving gas. The efficiency is further reduced in many forms of respiratory disease, certain deformities, pregnancy and when the minute volume is increased (*Figure 69*). When approaching maximal ventilation, the efficiency falls to such a low level that additional oxygen made available by further increase of ventilation will be entirely consumed by the respiratory muscles (Otis, 1954). It is clear that under these circumstances a further increase in ventilation would result in net oxygen loss. This effectively limits the changes in the alveolar gas which can be brought about by *active,* though not *passive,* hyperventilation. This 'ceiling' of ventilation is only reached at very high levels of ventilation in the healthy patient. However, in diffuse obstructive respiratory

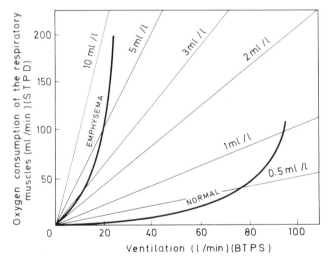

Figure 69. Oxygen consumption of the respiratory muscles plotted against minute volume of respiration. The isopleths indicate the oxygen cost of breathing in millilitres of oxygen consumed per litre of minute volume. The curve obtained from the normal subject shows the low oxygen cost of breathing up to a minute volume of 70 l/min. Thereafter the oxygen cost rises steeply. In the emphysematous patient, the oxygen cost of breathing is not only much higher at the resting minute volume, but it rises steeply as ventilation is increased. At a minute volume of 20 l/min, the respiratory muscles are consuming 200 ml oxygen per minute, and a further increase of ventilation would consume more oxygen than it would make available to the rest of the body. (Reproduced after Campbell, Westlake and Cherniak (1957) by courtesy of the Editor of the Journal of Applied Physiology*)*

disease, the 'ceiling' may be sufficiently low to impose a severe limit on exercise tolerance.

Units of measurement

There is a good deal of confusion over the terminology and units of measurement of work.

Work is done when a force moves its point of application, and the amount of work is equal to the product of force and distance moved. The force may be applied to the plunger of a syringe raising the pressure of a gas contained therein. In this case, the work done is equal to the product of the mean pressure and the change in volume, or alternatively to the product of the mean volume and the change in pressure. The units of work are identical whether the product is *force x distance* or *pressure x volume*. The various units which may be used are listed in Appendix A.

Power is a measure of the rate at which work is being (or can be) performed. The 'work of breathing', when expressed in watts, is thus a misnomer, since we are referring to the rate at which work is being done. Power is the correct term and work is appropriate to a single event such as one breath.

Dissipation of work of breathing

The work of breathing overcomes two different sources of resistance. The first is the elastic recoil of the tissues (Chapter 3). The second is the frictional resistance to gas flow afforded by the air passages and, to a much smaller extent, the frictional resistance of the movements of the tissues during ventilation (page 107). It is usual to ignore the very low resistance afforded by the inertia (or momentum) of static (or moving) gases and tissues.

Work against elastic resistance

When a perfectly elastic body is deformed, none of the work is dissipated as heat and all is stored as potential energy. No body is perfectly elastic, but satisfactory conversion to potential energy is obtained in such devices as the clockwork motor.

In the case of respiration, it is easiest to consider inflation of the lungs by positive pressure. *Figure 70a* shows a section of the pressure/volume diagram taken from *Figure 30*. As the lungs are inflated from the expiratory position to the inspiratory position, the alveolar pressure/volume line forms the hypotenuse of a triangle whose area will represent the work done against elastic resistance during inspiration. The area of a triangle (half the base times the height) will thus equal half the tidal volume times the pressure change (or the mean pressure times the volume change). This indicates the potential energy available for expiration. In *Figure 70b* the pressure/volume curve is flatter, indicating stiffer or less compliant lungs. For the same tidal volume, the area of the triangle is increased. This represents a greater amount of work performed against elastic resistance and greater potential energy available for expiration.

Work against resistance to gas flow

Figure 70 describes conditions under which air flow resistance has been ignored by measuring alveolar pressure. In practice, of course, additional inflation pressure is required to overcome the resistance to gas flow afforded by the respiratory tract. At any instant, during inspiration, the mouth (or inflation) pressure will always be above the alveolar pressure, and simultaneous plots of volume and *mouth* pressure will describe a curve bowed to the right as in

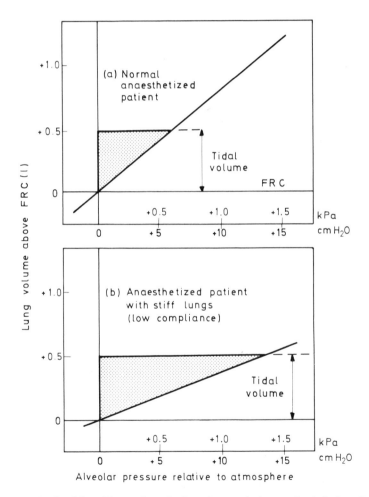

Figure 70. Work of breathing against elastic resistance during passive inflation. Pressure/volume plots of the lungs of anaesthetized patients (see Figure 30). The length of the pressure/volume curve covered during inspiration forms the hypotenuse of a right-angled triangle whose area equals the work performed against elastic resistance. Note the area is greater when the pressure/volume curve is flatter (indicating stiffer or less compliant lungs)

Figure 71. Figure 71b represents a patient with normal compliance but with particularly high airway resistance. In each case the area between the curve OAC, and the alveolar pressure/volume line OYC represents the work expended in overcoming the frictional resistance to gas flow during inspiration. When the gas drawn into the lungs is represented by the vertical distance OX (on the volume axis), the horizontal distance XY indicates the alveolar pressure (overcoming elastic resistance), YA indicates the mouth-to-alveolar pressure difference (overcoming flow resistance) while XA indicates the mouth pressure (overcoming both sources of resistance). The division of the inflation pressure into two components overcoming two sources of respiration is shown in *Figures 54,*

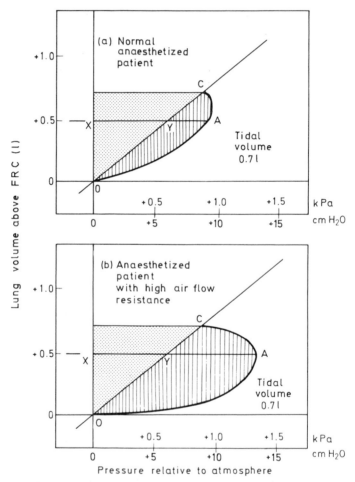

Figure 71. Work of breathing against air flow resistance during passive inflation. The sloping line (OYC) is the alveolar pressure/volume curve. The curve (OAC) is the mouth pressure/volume curve during inflation of the lungs. The area shaded with vertical stripes indicates the work of inspiration performed against air flow resistance. This work is increased in the patient with high resistance (b). At the point when 500 ml gas has entered the patient, XY represents the pressure distending the lungs, while YA represents the pressure overcoming air flow resistance. XA is the inflation pressure at that moment. The stippled areas represent work done against elastic resistance (see Figure 70)

57 and 58 which indicate the changes in lung volume, mouth and alveolar pressures when the lungs are inflated by an increase in mouth pressure. Methods are available for recording the changes shown in *Figures 71 and 73*. Such recordings are suitable for the direct calculation of the work of breathing from the various areas enclosed.

In the last few pages, we have considered the elastic recoil of the expiratory system as though it were a single entity, exerted by a single structure. This, of course, is not the case. It is true that the lungs exert an active elastic resistance opposing the inflation of the lungs, and store potential energy for powering expiration. However, it will be remembered that the equilibrium position of the chest wall is at a volume greater than the functional residual capacity. Therefore the elasticity of the chest wall is actually assisting the inflation of the lungs and it will similarly oppose expiration. The separation of the two sources of elastic resistance is far from simple. Those who are interested in this problem are referred to Chapter 15 of the monograph by Campbell (1958).

There is an interesting dichotomy in studies of elastic recoil made by respiratory physiologists on the one hand, and anaesthetists on the other. Broadly speaking, the physiologist studies conscious subjects who are seldom, if ever, able to relax completely their respiratory muscles. Now it is impossible to measure the elasticity of a structure which has a variable amount of muscular tone and, therefore, the physiologist cannot easily study thoracic wall compliance or, indeed, total compliance which includes that of the thoracic wall. He therefore tends to concentrate on lung compliance studies with the aid of an oesophageal balloon for measurement of intrathoracic pressure. The anaesthetist, on the other hand, is frequently concerned with paralysis of the respiratory muscles and so avoids the difficulty of an indefinite thoracic compliance. However, he does have difficulties in measuring the intrathoracic pressure in a supine subject (page 66) and, therefore, in separating lung and thoracic wall compliance. Consequently, he tends to concentrate his studies on total compliance which is, after all, of considerable practical importance in artificial ventilation.

The active expiratory phase

Passive expiration is normally adequate, not only for resting respiration, but also for respiration under moderately difficult conditions. Thus minute volumes as high as 20 l/min are normally obtained without the use of expiratory muscles, and we have seen in Chapter 4 that expiration against pressures up to about 1·2 kPa (12 cm H_2O) is normally accomplished by augmentation of *inspiratory* effort without participation of expiratory muscles. This results in hyperinflation of the lung with increased elastic recoil available to overcome expiratory resistance. Nevertheless, for very high minute volumes and for expiration against very high pressures, the expiratory muscles are brought into play and their work must be included in the total work of breathing.

The minimum work of breathing

For a constant minute volume, the work done against elastic resistance is increased when breathing is deep and slow. On the other hand, the work done against flow resistance is increased when breathing is rapid and shallow. If the two components are summated, and the total work plotted against the respiratory frequency, it will be found that there is an optimal respiratory frequency at which the total work of breathing is minimal (*Figure 72*). It is

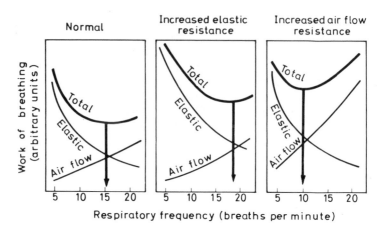

Figure 72. *The diagrams show the work done against elastic and air flow resistance separately and summated to indicate the total work of breathing at different respiratory frequencies. The total work of breathing has a minimum value at about 15 breaths per minute under normal circumstances. For the same minute volume, minimum work is performed at higher frequencies with stiff (less compliant) lungs and at lower frequencies when the air flow resistance is increased*

interesting to find that human subjects and animals tend to select a respiratory frequency which corresponds very closely to the frequency which may be calculated to require the minimum work (McIlroy et al., 1956). This applies to different species, different age groups in the same species and to patients with diseased lungs. When elastic resistance is high (pulmonary fibrosis, small animals, infants, etc.), the optimum frequency is high and rapid shallow breaths are favoured. When airway resistance is high, the optimum frequency is low and slow deep breaths are favoured. When supervising artificial ventilation, it would appear reasonable to form some estimate of the respiratory frequency likely to be associated with minimal work and to use a frequency of that order for artificial ventilation. It is, however, also necessary to bear in mind that frequency affects the dynamic compliance (page 76) and also to consider the effect of different frequencies on distribution (Chapter 7).

Work of breathing through apparatus

It has already been pointed out that there are difficulties in expressing the resistance to breathing offered by a piece of breathing apparatus (pages 102 et seq.). For this reason, it may be preferable to measure the actual work done by the patient in breathing through the apparatus, and this figure may be readily compared with the patient's own work of breathing. It is clearly advantageous to measure the work of breathing through apparatus using the patient's respiratory waveform and with the gas mixture which the patient is actually breathing. The technique is not particularly difficult and may be used with little modification for measurement of work done in breathing against nasal resistance (Butler, 1960). A plot is prepared of gas volume passed against the pressure drop across the apparatus (*Figure 73*). With the two variables plotted simultaneously, this yields a loop of which the area represents the work done in breathing through the apparatus for a single breath. This method was used extensively by Cooper (1961) in the evaluation of the resistance afforded by breathing apparatus used in mines rescue work.

It is often sufficient to assess the work of breathing through apparatus more simply by multiplying the gas volume passed by the pressure drop across the apparatus at the 'effective mean flow rate' of gas. The latter quantity is not easy to define but may be taken as somewhat less than the peak gas flow rate (about 25 l/min during anaesthesia with spontaneous respiration). The pressure drop at this flow rate may then be read off a graph of pressure drop plotted against flow rate (e.g. *Figure 37*), and multiplied by tidal volume to indicate work, during a single phase of the respiratory cycle. Multiplied by the respiratory frequency, this will indicate the work expended in one minute in overcoming apparatus resistance in one direction of flow. As an example 1 litre moved against a pressure gradient of 1 kPa requires the expenditure of 1 joule of energy. This will need the consumption of about 0·5 ml oxygen or one-sixth of the normal oxygen cost of breathing.

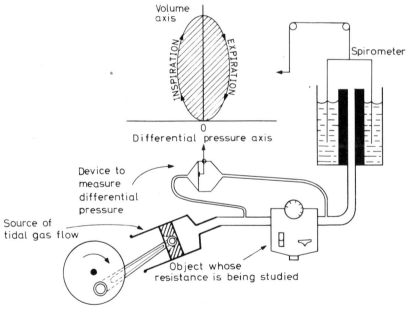

Figure 73. Experimental arrangement for studying the work of breathing through apparatus. Gas is made to pass to and fro through the apparatus, with the volume exchange recorded from a spirometer. A differential pressure manometer records the pressure drop across the apparatus. Various devices may be employed to arrange for volume to be plotted on one axis while pressure is simultaneously recorded on the other axis. A loop is then traced out, whose area is equal to the work of breathing through the apparatus. This apparatus is particularly suitable for studying the effect of different gas mixtures and different respiratory waveforms

MEASUREMENT OF VENTILATION

In the measurement of ventilation we are concerned with gas flow rates and gas volumes, the former having the dimensions of volume/time ($L^3 T^{-1}$) and the latter the dimensions of volume (L^3) (*see* Appendix A). There is some doubt as to whether the term 'minute volume' refers to a flow rate (litres/minute) or a volume (litres). Semantically the latter may be correct but it is clear that a flow rate is implied.

If volume is plotted against time (as on a spirometer trace) the slope of the line will indicate gas flow rate. When the flow rate is rapidly changing, the slope of a tangent to the curve will indicate the instantaneous flow rate (*Figure 74*).

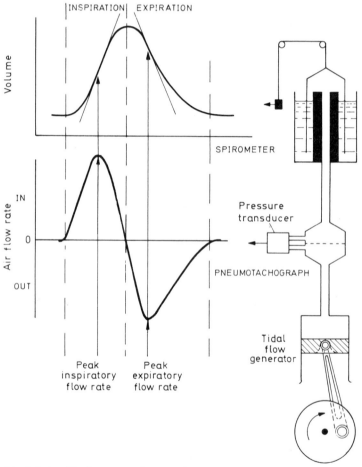

Figure 74. Relationship between volume and flow rate. The upper graph shows volume plotted against time; this type of tracing may be obtained with a spirometer. The lower graph shows instantaneous air flow rate plotted against time; this type of tracing may be obtained with a pneumotachograph. At any instant, the flow-rate trace indicates the slope of the volume trace, while the volume trace indicates the cumulative area under the flow-rate trace. Flow is the differential of volume; volume is the integral of flow rate. Differentiation of the spirometer trace gives a 'pneumotachogram'. Integration of the pneumotachogram gives a 'spirometer trace'

The slope of the tangent is the differential of volume with respect to time (dV/dt). Alternatively, when flow rate is plotted against time (as in a pneumotachogram), the area under the curve between two points indicates the volume change between these points. The integral of the flow rate equals the volume change.

It is important to distinguish between two entirely different flow rates. The *minute volume* is defined as the tidal volume multiplied by the respiratory frequency. The *instantaneous flow rate* is the actual rate at which gas flows into or out of the respiratory system at any instant (dV/dt). Peak flow rates are the maximum flow rates occurring during breathing and are usually about four or five times greater than the minute volume (*Figure 46*). It is appropriate to consider peak flow rates when assessing the effects of resistance to breathing.

Sometimes it is necessary to distinguish between the inspiratory and expiratory minute volumes (or tidal volumes). Under normal circumstances, the inspiratory minute volume is about 50 ml larger than the expiratory minute volume, this being the amount by which the oxygen uptake exceeds the carbon dioxide output. However, during anaesthesia, exchange of nitrous oxide can result in very large differences between inspired and expired minute volume. As a rough approximation, the uptake of nitrous oxide (in ml/min) equals:

$$\frac{1000}{\sqrt{\text{duration of anaesthetic (minutes)}}}$$

(Severinghaus, 1954)

For example, after 16 minutes the uptake of nitrous oxide approximates to 1000 divided by the square root of 16, which is 250 ml/min. Separate measurement of inspired and expired minute volume presents considerable difficulty and the problems have been discussed by Nunn and Pouliot (1962) and by Smith (1964a).

The minute volume of ventilation may vary from as little as 3 l/min in a deeply anaesthetized patient allowed to breathe spontaneously, to over 100 l/min in an exercising subject and, for short periods of time, over 200 l/min during the measurement of the maximum breathing capacity (MBC). Techniques of measurement of pulmonary ventilation must satisfy the following requirements.

1. The resistance to breathing must not be excessive at the ventilation rate which is to be measured.
2. The apparatus must not impose a significant addition to the dead space through which the patient must breathe.*
3. The response of the apparatus should be as flat as possible and must be appropriate to the ventilation rate which is being measured.
4. The response must not be unduly influenced by the respiratory waveform or the nature of the respired gas.

Most clinical methods of measurement of ventilation afford negligible resistance at minute volumes up to 40 l/min. However, above this figure, and particularly during the measurement of MBC, a very low level of resistance is essential. Resistance to gas flow may be minimized by increasing the calibre of

* This consideration is not relevant during the measurement of maximum breathing capacity (MBC).

the tubes through which the patient breathes: inertia may be minimized by reduction of weight of moving parts, and resonant frequency may be kept high by suitable design.

In connection with accuracy, we shall make reference to the 'response' of an apparatus. This is defined as the indicated volume divided by the actual volume passed, and is often expressed as a percentage. The reciprocal of the response is the correction factor which must be applied. Response presents an important problem since, with most techniques, the response of the apparatus is not constant but tends to increase with increasing minute volume.

Measurement of gas flow rate

Rotameters and ball-in-tapered-tube flowmeters afford a most convenient method of measuring steady gas flow and are used widely for the measurement of fresh gas flow rate on anaesthetic apparatus. They can only be used for one specified gas since their calibration is influenced by the viscosity and specific gravity of the gas. (These properties are similar for air and oxygen so that rotameters for these two gases are interchangeable.) Rotameters are available in a wide variety of ranges, for each of which the maximum flow rate is usually ten times the minimum but the range may be extended by the use of double-taper tubes.

The pneumotachograph is the most versatile method of measurement of gas flow rates, being particularly well suited to rapidly changing flow rates and the direction of transients, which are smoothed out in the record of any mechanical device such as a spirometer. The pneumotachograph is based on the measurement of the pressure gradient across a resistor through which the gas flow is laminar. In accordance with the Hagen–Poiseuille relationship (page 96), the pressure gradient will be directly proportional to the flow rate. A variety of resistors are in use and many different types of pressure transducers are available, all of which convert displacement of a metal diaphragm into an electrical signal (*Figure 74*). The pressure gradient need not exceed a few millimetres of water and the resistance offered to the patient is therefore negligible. The volume constitutes only a small increase in apparatus dead space, and the patient may breathe to and fro through the pneumotachograph head.

When the highest levels of accuracy are required, pneumotachography presents very severe problems arising from the composition of the gases and their actual temperature as they pass through the laminar resistor. Both factors influence the viscosity of the gas on which the calibration depends (page 97). Smith (1964a) has considered these problems in detail and suggested means by which they may be overcome.

The slope of a spirometer trace (*Figure 74*) will give an idea of mean flow rates but is not well suited to detecting transients. Irregularities of flow rate are faithfully recorded on a pneumotachogram, but they tend to be smoothed out in the differential of a spirometer trace due to the inertia of moving parts.

Wright's peak flowmeter is a useful method for the measurement of maximum peak expiratory flow which is a valuable index of expiratory airway resistance (page 137). In this instrument the expiratory gas stream displaces a baffle whose peak displacement is indicated on a dial. The peak flowmeter is calibrated to indicate the peak flow sustained for 10 ms, as recorded by a pneumotachograph (Wright and McKerrow, 1959). Thus it usually reads lower than the highest transient recorded by a pneumotachograph but higher than the value derived from the slope of a spirometer trace. The apparatus is highly convenient and portable, being particularly suitable for pre-operative assessment of patients scattered through different wards (Bodman, 1963). Normal values for adults are in the range 400–700 l/min but this is markedly dependent upon age, body size and sex (Cotes, 1975).

Measurement of ventilatory volumes

Spirometry

The water-sealed spirometer is the most accurate clinical method of measurement of minute volume and is the method against which the accuracy of other techniques is assessed. Unfortunately, spirometers are cumbersome, difficult to transport and cannot easily be incorporated in gas circuits without entailing rebreathing. At low respiratory frequencies, their calibration (linear displacement per litre) is constant and is the reciprocal of the cross-sectional area. As the frequency increases, spirometers over-read until they reach their resonant frequency at which the whole system oscillates and the reading is grossly in error. About the resonant frequency, damping occurs until finally the spirometer ceases to respond at all. The presence of soluble gases does not cause the error which might be expected and it is difficult to detect any loss of nitrous oxide into the water of a spirometer bath (Nunn, 1958b).

Tissot spirometers usually have a capacity of over 100 litres and are not used for measurement of tidal exchange. They are employed either as reservoirs for inspired gas or else for collection of expired gas. Minute volume is usually read direct from the total movement of the bell occurring over a period of several minutes.

General purpose spirometers are now of a pattern which was originally designed for measuring the MBC. Although the MBC is seldom measured nowadays, the general design has been found satisfactory for general respiratory purposes such as measurement of FEV, lung volume and minute volume. In contrast to the old Benedict–Roth type of spirometer, the currently favoured design has low inertia and a high resonant frequency. This minimizes errors due to the response changing with respiratory frequency (Bernstein and Mendel, 1951; Bernstein, D'Silva and Mendel, 1952).

Bronchospirometers have a small diameter to magnify the small unilateral tidal volume. Similar dimensions are suitable for recording low levels of ventilation and the specification in *Table 17* is satisfactory up to frequencies of 35 breaths per minute, with an error of less than 2 per cent when used in conjunction with anaesthetic gas circuits (Nunn, 1956).

Table 17. SPECIFICATIONS FOR A WET SPIROMETER SUITABLE FOR RECORDING
THE VENTILATION OF ANAESTHETIZED PATIENTS BREATHING
SPONTANEOUSLY

Capacity of bell	2 litres
Diameter of bell (internal)	9·2 cm
Length of bell	30 cm
Weight of bell	89·5 g
Thickness of bell	0·314 mm
Material of bell	Anodized aluminium
Diameter of core (external)	7·9 cm
Distance from core to sides of tank	6·8 cm
Weight of counterweight (including pen)	75·5 g
Suspension	Thin cord
Pulleys	Two in number, 37 mm diameter, aluminium, mounted on ball races.
Sensitivity	1 cm per 67 ml (ATPS)

The resonant frequency of the system is 96 breaths per minute (BPM). The response is less than 105 per cent of static response up to 50 BPM. Its use in association with the continuous-flow spirometer causes some damping up to frequencies of 35 BPM, resulting in an error of less than ±2 per cent within this range of respiratory frequency. The sensitivity is sufficient for recording the depressed ventilation of deep anaesthesia.

The box–bag spirometer is a system which permits spirometric measurements of minute volume without rebreathing (Donald and Christie, 1949). The system has been adapted to the circumstances of anaesthesia by Nunn and Pouliot (1962), and may be converted for use during artificial ventilation (Nunn, Bergman and Coleman, 1965). It probably affords the most accurate method for the separate measurement of inspired and expired minute volumes (*Figure 75*).

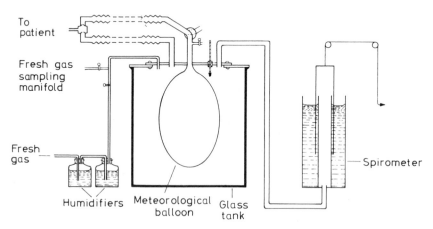

Figure 75. In the box–bag spirometer system, the patient inhales from the box and exhales into the bag. The tidal volume and the difference between the inspiratory and expiratory respiratory volumes are read directly from the spirometer. Inspiratory and expiratory gas may be samples and analysis permits measurement of exchange of all gaseous components. The system may be reversed (i.e. inspiration from the bag) for studying the response to different inhaled gas mixtures. (Reproduced from Nunn and Pouliot (1962) by courtesy of the Editor of the British Journal of Anaesthesia)

The continuous-flow spirometer (Nunn, 1956) is a derivative of the box–bag spirometer which permits continuous spirometric measurement of minute volume during anaesthesia using any of the gas circuits in clinical use (*Figure 76*).

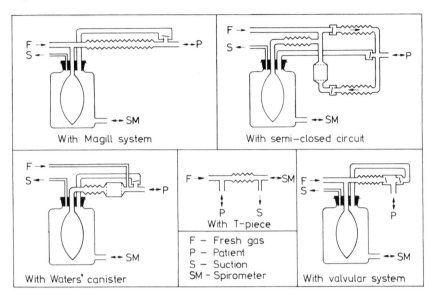

With Magill system

With semi–closed circuit

With Waters' canister

With T-piece

F – Fresh gas
P – Patient
S – Suction
SM – Spirometer

With valvular system

Figure 76. The continuous-flow spirometer enables spirometric records to be made when patients are breathing spontaneously with any anaesthetic gas circuit. Gas is aspirated from the tube marked 'S' until the spirometer trace is level, the amount aspirated being approximately equal to the fresh gas flow rate. When the trace is level, the tidal exchange is indicated with an accuracy of ±2 per cent. (From Nunn (1956) by courtesy of the Editor of British Journal of Anaesthesia)

Wedge spirometers are entirely dry and resemble bellows with two plates hinged together. The frequency response is good and they tend to be more portable and convenient than water-sealed spirometers. Simple instruments such as the Vitalograph have a mechanical recording system and are widely used for the routine measurement of vital capacity and FEV. More elaborate wedge spirometers have electrical outputs for volume and flow rate and are particularly suitable for recording flow/volume curves (*see Figure 40*).

Display for spirometers is traditionally by ink registration on a rotating kymograph. However, the pulley over which the cord passes may be made to rotate the wiper of a potentiometer from which an electrical read-out can easily be obtained. A differentiating circuit can then be used to indicate gas flow rate.

Gas meters

Apart from a spirometer, the most accurate method of measuring gas volumes is by the use of a wet gas meter. This device records the volume of gas which flows past a type of paddle wheel in which a water-seal is used to contain the gas within each successive compartment. The apparatus is fairly expensive and requires careful handling since displacement of the water level influences the calibration. It is most suitable for continuous low flow rates of gas and it is therefore customary to collect expired air in a Douglas bag before passing the contents through a wet gas meter. Gas volumes to be measured must be at pressures close to atmospheric.

Dry gas meters are more robust and cheaper than wet meters, but less accurate. The mechanism is analogous to a two-cylinder double-acting steam engine. The stream of gas is diverted by a system of valves to act alternately on either side of a pair of leather bellows which are linked to a shaft out of phase by 90 degrees. The system has undergone many decades of refinement and is used widely for the metering of domestic gas. Potentially it is extremely repeatable and it may therefore be calibrated to indicate gas flow with a very high level of accuracy, but unfortunately errors can arise from failure of the valves to seat correctly. Contact with the seating is maintained chiefly by gravity and these meters must, therefore, be kept upright.

They read correctly at a flow rate of about 20 l/min, under-reading below this and over-reading above it. However, after recent calibration the error should not amount to more than a few per cent. Dry gas meters will respond with reasonable accuracy to unidirectional tidal flow and are commonly incorporated in the expiratory gas circuit. It should be remembered, however, that the pathway of gas through the meter constitutes the whole bulk of the meter (about 20 litres). Therefore, patients must never be connected directly to breathe to and fro through dry gas meters. Furthermore, with certain gas circuits during intermittent positive pressure, several hundred millilitres of gas may be compressed into a dry gas meter during the inspiratory phase. It is therefore essential to arrange the valves of the circuit in such a way that this Boyle's law effect does not give an erroneous measurement of the tidal volume. A non-rebreathing system is usually satisfactory but circle systems may be used with valves between the patient and the meter (Nunn, 1958a).

The Parkinson and Cowan dry gas meter gives accurate readings for volumes which are multiples of 2·5 litres (the volume required for one cycle of the mechanism). Volumes which are not exact multiples of 2·5 litres may be in error by as much as 250 ml and therefore it is advisable to measure minute volumes over two or three minutes if a reasonable level of accuracy is required. Dry gas meters are not satisfactory for the measurement of a single tidal volume. Errors associated with the use of dry gas meters have been discussed by Cooper (1959).

The Wright respirometer (Figure 77)

This device is a miniature air turbine with moving parts of very low inertia (Wright, 1955). The revolutions are recorded by means of a gear train and dial of the type used in wrist watches. The instrument indicates directly the number of litres which have passed between two successive readings. The respirometer responds to gas flow in one direction only and may therefore be used with tidal flow. The internal volume is only 22 ml and the patients may breathe to and fro through the apparatus with negligible increase in resistance and dead space.

In common with all inferential gas meters the response is dependent on the flow rate, since slip occurs to a greater degree as the flow rate is decreased. The·

instruments are adjusted to give correct readings at 20 l/min continuous flow, or 7 l/min reciprocating flow. Above this figure the response increases to become steady at about 10 per cent high for large minute volumes. At lower flow rates the instrument reads low, being about 10 per cent low at a continuous flow of about 10 l/min or a reciprocating flow of about 3 l/min (sinusoidal flow). However, the performance at low minute volumes is markedly improved when the respiratory waveform departs from sinusoidal (as it usually does during anaesthesia) and when nitrous oxide is inhaled. The performance of the

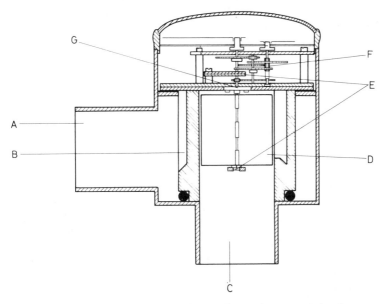

Figure 77. Longitudinal section through the Wright respirometer. (A) Inlet mount. (B) Tangential slots in cylindrical stator ring. (C) Outlet mount. (D) Two-bladed rotor. (E) Jewelled bearings. (F) Gear train. (G) Mercury seal. (Reproduced by permission of British Oxygen Co. Ltd.)

apparatus has been considered in some detail by Nunn and Ezi-Ashi (1962), who reached the conclusion that the accuracy was in excess of clinical requirements. In the event of hypoventilation, the instrument will read low and therefore exaggerate the departure from normality. Its use is thus fundamentally safe. British Oxygen Co. currently supply a version in which the rotation of the vane interrupts a light beam. By means of a photoelectric cell and a counting circuit, the instrument will record tidal volume or minute volume (continuously) on a dial or a digital display. It is also used as the flow transducer in the servo-operated ventilator referred to on page 157.

Miscellaneous dry gas meters

There are on the market a variety of meters (manufactured by Dräger, Monaghan, Bennett, etc.) which are intermediate in size between dry gas meters incorporating bellows and the Wright inferential respirometer. Some of these have been reviewed by Byles (1960).

The integrated pneumotachogram

It has already been pointed out that the integrated pneumotachogram will give an indication of respiratory volume exchange which approaches the accuracy of the spirometer, provided that certain precautions are taken to ensure that calibration is not invalidated by electrical drift or by changes in gas temperature and composition. Once these difficulties have been overcome, the pneumotachograph imposes very little derangement of anaesthetic gas circuits and has even been used successfully in the difficult circumstances of out-patient dental anaesthesia (Smith, 1964b).

Use of rotameters with a Non-rebreathing system

During artificial ventilation certain mechanical ventilators are supplied with a continuous flow of fresh gas which is broken down into tidal volumes, the Manley ventilator being a typical example. Under these circumstances, the patient's minute volume is indicated by the fresh gas flow rate (as shown on the rotameters), provided there are no leaks in the system. This forms a most useful, reliable and reasonably accurate method of determining the minute volume of the patient.

The same principle may be used during spontaneous respiration with a fresh gas reservoir and a valvular non-rebreathing gas circuit, or during artificial ventilation with a device which draws a fixed minute volume from a reservoir. Provided that the reservoir does not become either depleted or overfilled, the flow rate of fresh gas into the reservoir must equal the patient's respiratory minute volume. The particular value of this method of measuring ventilatory exchange is that no additional apparatus is required and, apart from the question of leakage, the accuracy is only limited by that of the rotameters which is normally in excess of the accuracy required for measurement of minute volume for clinical purposes.

Chapter 7 Respiratory Dead Space and Distribution of the Inspired Gas

Anatomical Dead Space
Alveolar Dead Space
Physiological Dead Space
Apparatus Dead Space and Rebreathing
Distribution of the Inspired Gas
Measurement of Dead Space and Distribution of Inspired Gas

The previous chapters have been concerned with the factors which influence the pulmonary ventilation considered as the total quantity of gas which passes into and out of the lungs. So far there has been no detailed consideration of the proportion of the total volume flow which actually takes part in gas exchange.

It was realized in the last century that an appreciable part of each inspiration did not penetrate to those regions of the lungs in which gas exchange occurred and was therefore exhaled unchanged. This fraction of the tidal volume has long been known as the dead space, while the effective part of the minute volume of respiration is known as the alveolar ventilation. The relationship is as follows:

$$\frac{\text{alveolar}}{\text{ventilation}} = \frac{\text{respiratory}}{\text{frequency}} \left(\frac{\text{tidal}}{\text{volume}} - \frac{\text{dead}}{\text{space}} \right)$$

It is often useful to think of two ratios. The first is:

$$\frac{\text{dead space}}{\text{tidal volume}}$$

(often abbreviated to V_D/V_T and expressed as a percentage)

The second useful ratio is:

$$\frac{\text{alveolar ventilation}}{\text{minute volume}}$$

The first fraction is the wasted part of the breath, while the second is the utilized portion of the minute volume. The sum of the two fractions is unity and one may easily be calculated from the other.

Figure 78 shows in diagrammatic form the various components of a single expirate. The first part to be exhaled will be from the *apparatus dead space* if the subject is employing any form of breathing apparatus, as is usually the case during anaesthesia. The next component will be from the *anatomical dead space*, which corresponds to the volume of conducting air passages. Thereafter gas is exhaled from the alveolar level and the diagram shows two representative alveoli.

213

One is perfused and, from this, *'ideal' alveolar gas* is exhaled. The other alveolus is unperfused and so does not permit gas exchange. From this alveolus is exhaled gas approximating in composition to inspired gas. This gas is known as *alveolar dead space gas* and is an important constituent of the expired gas of patients in whom a major part of the lungs are inadequately perfused. This occurs typically after pulmonary embolus but also in patients with emphysema, various forms of heart failure and during anaesthesia. It will be seen in *Figure 78* that the final part of the expirate consists of a mixture of 'ideal' alveolar gas and alveolar dead space gas. A sample of this gas is called an *end-tidal,* or preferably an *end-expiratory* sample. Sometimes, however, it is referred to as a sample of *alveolar gas.* There are thus problems of definition which have not yet been resolved.

Alveolar gas, as defined by Haldane and Priestley (1905) is gas sampled at the end of a forced expiration. Its composition approximates to that of end-expiratory gas since, in a healthy subject, composition changes little between the ends of normal and forced expirations. This interpretation was universal until recently, when it became realized that end-expiratory gas may be actually a mixture of gas from perfused and unperfused alveoli (*Figure 78*). Since only the former takes part in gas exchange, it was felt that it should be distinguished and the term 'ideal' alveolar gas was introduced (Riley et al., 1946). Usage has led to

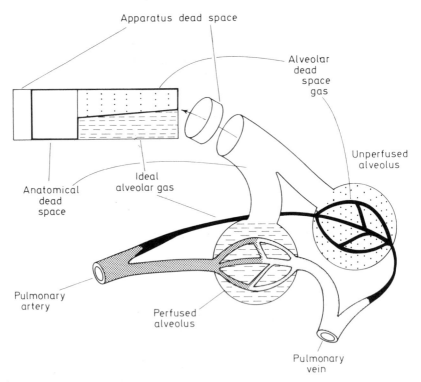

Figure 78. Components of the expired gas of an anaesthetized patient. The rectangle is an idealized representation of a single expirate. The physiological dead space equals the sum of the anatomical and alveolar dead spaces and is outlined in the heavy black line. The alveolar dead space does not equal the volume of the unperfused spaces at alveolar level but only that part of their contents which is exhaled. This varies with the tidal volume

dropping of the qualifying term 'ideal' and nowadays 'alveolar' is usually taken to mean 'ideal alveolar'.

The distinction between 'ideal' alveolar and end-expiratory gas is by no means of theoretical interest alone, but is of considerable importance in patients with a wide range of respiratory disorders and also in the healthy anaesthetized patient. To prevent confusion, when describing gas samples in this book, the unqualified term 'alveolar' is avoided so far as is possible. In the following section, it is used in a simplified statement in which alveolar dead space is ignored and an expirate is considered as consisting simply of (anatomical) dead space gas and alveolar gas. For symbols, the small capital A relates to 'ideal' alveolar gas (e.g. P_{ACO_2} = 'ideal' alveolar P_{CO_2}) while end-expiratory gas is distinguished by a small capital E, suffixed with a prime (e.g. $P_{E'CO_2}$ = end-expiratory P_{CO_2}). The term 'alveolar/arterial P_{O_2} difference' always refers to 'ideal' alveolar gas.

Figure 78 is, of course, purely diagrammatic and it should not be imagined that all alveoli fall into two watertight compartments—perfused and unperfused. There exists an infinite gradation between alveoli with zero blood flow, through those with average blood flow, to those with excessive blood flow. However, it is sometimes helpful from the quantitative standpoint to consider alveoli *as though* they fell into the categories shown in the diagram. This convention is implicit in the definition of the physiological dead space (*see* page 227). Consideration of the full gradation of ventilation/perfusion ratios is postponed to Chapter 9.

ANATOMICAL DEAD SPACE*

The gills of fishes are perfused by a stream of water which enters by the mouth and leaves by the gill slits. All of the water is available for gaseous exchange. Birds and mammals, however, employ tidal ventilation which suffers from the disadvantage that a considerable part of the inspired gas comes to rest in the conducting air passages and is thus not available for gaseous exchange.

This imperfection was understood in the nineteenth century when the volume of the anatomical dead space was calculated from post-mortem casts of the respiratory tract (Zuntz, 1882; Loewy, 1894). The value so obtained was used in the calculation of the composition of the alveolar gas according to the Bohr equation (1891). This was before the concept of alveolar dead space had arisen and at that time alveolar gas simply referred to that part of the expirate which followed the anatomical dead space gas.

The Bohr equation may be simply derived as follows. During expiration all the CO_2 eliminated is contained in the alveolar gas. Therefore:

$$\text{quantity of } CO_2 \text{ eliminated in the alveolar gas} = \text{quantity of } CO_2 \text{ eliminated in the mixed expired gas}$$

that is to say:

$$\text{alveolar } CO_2 \text{ concentration } \textit{multiplied by} \text{ alveolar ventilation} = \text{mixed-expired } CO_2 \text{ concentration } \textit{multiplied by} \text{ minute volume}$$

or, for a single breath:

alv. CO_2 conc. x (tidal volume — dead space)
= mixed-expired CO_2 conc. x tidal volume

---

* Definitions relate to measurement techniques and are postponed to the end of this section (page 220).

Now there is no serious difficulty in measuring the tidal volume and the mixed-expired CO_2 concentration. Therefore the alveolar CO_2 concentration may be derived if the dead space be known or, alternatively, the dead space may be derived if the alveolar CO_2 concentration be known. In the nineteenth century, it was not realized that alveolar gas sampled from normal subjects had a relatively constant composition during the latter part of expiration and could be sampled as end-expiratory gas. Therefore, at that time it was customary to use the Bohr equation for calculation of the alveolar CO_2 concentration, substituting an assumed value for the dead space. After Haldane's historic discovery of the constancy of the alveolar gas (Haldane and Priestley, 1905), the position was reversed and the dead space became the more difficult quantity to measure. Therefore, after 1905, the alveolar CO_2 concentration was measured directly and the Bohr equation used to calculate the dead space.

At this point we must return to the semantic problems surrounding the use of the word alveolar. In the two paragraphs above, the word alveolar refers to that portion of the expirate which follows the anatomical dead space gas, and its composition would be similar to end-expiratory gas. Using the Bohr equation to measure the anatomical dead space, the appropriate value for the 'alveolar CO_2 concentration' is the end-expiratory CO_2 concentration. If the 'ideal' alveolar CO_2 concentration is used, then the value for the dead space yielded by the calculation will be that of the physiological dead space according to the definition in *Figure 78*.

Value for 'alveolar' CO_2 concentration substituted in Bohr equation	Corresponding value obtained for dead space
End-expiratory CO_2 concentration	Anatomical dead space
'Ideal' alveolar CO_2 concentration	Physiological dead space

This distinction between ideal alveolar and end-expiratory gas is fundamental for understanding dead space and is the clue to the controversy which existed for many years between Haldane and Krogh (reviewed by Bannister, Cunningham and Douglas, 1954). In the resting normal conscious healthy subject, the alveolar dead space is very small indeed. Therefore the anatomical and physiological dead spaces are, for practical purposes, identical and there is only a very small difference between the CO_2 concentration of the end-expiratory and the ideal alveolar gas. However, during anaesthesia, in the presence of respiratory disease, after haemorrhage and during exercise the difference becomes appreciable. The clinician, and the anaesthetist in particular are greatly concerned with these states and, therefore, it is appropriate that they should distinguish carefully between the anatomical and physiological dead space, and between the end-expiratory and ideal alveolar gas.

Measurement of the anatomical dead space

The anatomical dead space may be measured in the cadaver by filling the respiratory tract with molten lead, plaster of Paris, wax, Marco resin or simply water. During life, the anatomical dead space is measured as an undergraduate physiological experiment by solution of the Bohr equation using the CO_2

concentration of the end-expiratory gas. The equation given above simplifies into the following familiar form:

$$\frac{\text{anatomical}}{\text{dead space}} = \frac{\text{tidal}}{\text{volume}} \left(\frac{\text{end-expiratory } CO_2 \text{ conc.} - \text{mixed expired } CO_2 \text{ conc.}}{\text{end-expiratory } CO_2 \text{ conc.} - \text{inspired } CO_2 \text{ conc.}} \right)$$

In fact, it is not essential to use CO_2 concentrations and it is perfectly valid to employ oxygen or any tracer gas which may be added for that purpose.

If the CO_2 concentration at the lips is measured continuously with a rapid gas analyser, and then plotted against the volume actually expired, the resulting graph in a normal subject has the form shown in *Figure 79*. The 'alveolar plateau' of CO_2 concentration is not flat but slopes gently. The significance of this is discussed on page 242. It is possible to solve the Bohr equation from values read off the graph but it is simpler to employ the graphical solution

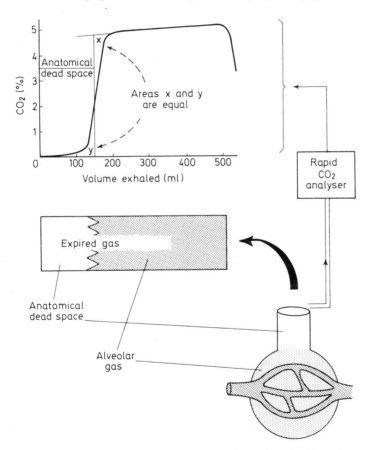

Figure 79. Measurement of the anatomical dead space using carbon dioxide as the tracer gas. If the gas passing the patient's lips is continuously analysed for carbon dioxide concentration, there is a sudden rise to the alveolar plateau level, after the expiration of gas from the anatomical dead space (conducting air passages). If the instantaneous CO_2 concentration is plotted against the volume exhaled (allowing for delay in the CO_2 analyser), a graph similar to that shown above is obtained. A vertical line is constructed so that the two areas x and y are equal. This line will indicate the volume of the anatomical dead space

shown on the diagram. This approach has greatly simplified measurements of anatomical dead space and has now become the standard method. The technique was introduced by Fowler (1948) using a rapid nitrogen analyser to follow a single expiration after the inspiration of 100 per cent oxygen. In his original description of the method Fowler referred to the quantity measured as the physiological dead space, but it is now generally known as anatomical dead space. After 1950, infrared carbon dioxide analysers came into use and DuBois et al. (1952) described the use of a rapid carbon dioxide analyser for measuring the anatomical dead space. It was later shown that identical values for dead space were given by measurement of the expiratory concentration of oxygen, carbon dioxide, nitrogen or helium (Bartels et al., 1954). Choice of the indicator gas now depends largely on the availability of apparatus for measuring the concentration of one of these gases with a sufficiently rapid response (95 per cent response in less than 150 ms). Allowance must, however, be made for the instrumental delay.

Factors influencing the anatomical dead space

The volume of the anatomical dead space is influenced by many factors, some of which are of great importance to the survival of a patient during gross hypoventilation.

Size of the subject must clearly influence the dimensions of the conducting air passages, and Radford (1955) has drawn attention to the fact that the volume of the air passages (in millimetres) approximates to the weight of the subject (in pounds*).

Posture influences many lung volumes, including the anatomical dead space, and Fowler (1950a) quotes the following mean values:

sitting	147 ml
semi-reclining	124 ml
supine	101 ml

Position of the neck and jaw has a pronounced effect on the anatomical dead space, and studies by Nunn, Campbell and Peckett (1959) have indicated the following mean values in three conscious subjects (not intubated):

neck extended, jaw protruded	143 ml
normal position	119 ml
neck flexed, chin depressed	73 ml

It is noteworthy that the first position is that which is sought by anaesthetists to procure the least possible airway resistance. Unfortunately, it also results in the maximum dead space.

Age is usually associated with an increase in anatomical dead space but this may well be associated with an increased incidence of chronic bronchitis which usually results in an enlarged calibre of the major air passages (Fowler, 1950b).

* 1 lb = 0·45 kg.

Lung volume at the end of inspiration affects the anatomical dead space since the volume of the air passages is a function of the lung volume. The effect is not very large, being of the order of 20 ml additional anatomical dead space for each litre increase in lung volume (Shepard et al., 1957).

Tracheal intubation or tracheostomy will bypass the extrathoracic anatomical dead space. This was found to be 72 ml in six cadavers, while the intrathoracic anatomical dead space was found to be 66 ml in three intubated patients (Nunn, Campbell and Peckett, 1959). Intrathoracic anatomical dead space of 12 intubated anaesthetized patients had a mean value of 63 ml (Nunn and Hill, 1960). Between mask-breathing and intubated anaesthetized patients, a difference in total functional dead space of 82 ml has been found by Kain, Panday and Nunn (1969). An undefined part of the difference would have been due to the additional apparatus dead space in the former state. Tracheal intubation or tracheostomy will bypass approximately half of the total anatomical dead space, although this advantage will clearly be lost if a corresponding volume of apparatus dead space is added to the circuit. The improvement conferred by tracheostomy in cases of ventilatory failure is probably due to three factors: (1) reduction in dead space; (2) increased facility for clearing bronchial secretions; and (3) reduction of airway resistance in the pharynx. A fourth advantage accrues from the ease with which intermittent positive pressure ventilation may be instituted when there is a tracheostomy.

Anaesthesia. Loh, Seed and Sykes (1973) reported changes in the anatomical dead space of chloralosed greyhounds; 2 per cent halothane caused a 21 ml increase, 80 per cent nitrous oxide a 17 ml decrease and 1·5 per cent trichloroethylene a 34 ml decrease.

Pneumonectomy will result in a reduction of anatomical dead space if the excised lung was functional (Fowler and Blakemore, 1951).

Hypoventilation results in a marked reduction of the anatomical dead space as measured by Fowler's method. This effect limits the fall of alveolar ventilation resulting from small tidal volumes. It is important in the case of comatose or anaesthetized patients who are left to breathe for themselves when there is either heavy central depression of respiration or partial neuromuscular blockade of the respiratory muscles. Tidal volumes as small as 100 ml are not infrequently recorded and the patients are usually none the worse for this gross physiological trespass.

There are probably two factors which reduce the anatomical dead space during hypoventilation. Firstly, there is a tendency towards streamline or laminar flow of gas through the air passages. Inspired gas advances with a cone front and the tip of the cone penetrates the alveoli before all the gas in the conducting passages has been washed out (*Figure 33*). This, in effect, reduces what we may call the 'functional anatomical dead space' below its value morphologically defined. The reduction of functional anatomical dead space at low tidal volumes was predicted by Rohrer in 1915 and, in the same year, Henderson, Chillingworth and Whitney demonstrated the axial flow of tobacco smoke through glass tubing. The second factor reducing dead space during hypoventilation is the mixing effect of the heart beat which tends to mix all gas lying below the carina. This effect is negligible at normal rates of ventilation, but becomes more marked during hypoventilation and during breath holding. Thus in one hypoventilating patient, Nunn and Hill (1960) found alveolar gas at the carina at the commencement of expiration. A similar effect occurs during breath holding when alveolar gas mixes with dead space gas as far up as the glottis.

In conscious subjects some inspired gas may be detected in the alveoli with tidal volumes as small as 60 ml (Briscoe, Forster and Comroe, 1954). In anaesthetized patients with tidal volumes less than 350 ml, Nunn and Hill (1960) found the 'functional' anatomical dead space to be about one-fifth of the tidal volume, a number of patients having values less than 25 ml at tidal volumes below 250 ml.

Drugs acting on the bronchiolar musculature will affect the anatomical dead space, and an increase has been noted after atropine by Higgins and Means (1915), Severinghaus and Stupfel (1955) and Nunn and Bergman (1964). Nunn and Bergman found a mean increase of 18 ml in six normal subjects, while Severinghaus and Stupfel reported an increase of 45 ml. The latter also reported significant increases with the ganglion-blocking agents hexamethonium and trimetaphan. Histamine caused a small decrease in anatomical dead space.

Hypothermia has been reported to increase the anatomical dead space in dogs (Severinghaus and Stupfel, 1955), but observations by the author (1961a) suggest that there is little significant change in man.

Definition of anatomical dead space

It will now be clear that there are two possible definitions of anatomical dead space.

1. *Morphological definition:* volume of the conducting air passages which are not lined with respiratory epithelium, as measured by casts of the air passages or by geometrical measurements.
2. *Functional definition:* that part of the inspired tidal volume which is expired unchanged at the beginning of expiration, as measured by simultaneous records of expired gas volume and gas composition (synonymous with *series dead space*).

The morphological definition is now seldom used, and the anatomical dead space commonly refers to its functional volume as measured by the method of Fowler (1948).

ALVEOLAR DEAD SPACE

Alveolar dead space may be defined as that part of the inspired gas which passes through the anatomical dead space to mix with gas at the alveolar level, but which does not take part in gas exchange. The cause of the failure of gas exchange is lack of effective perfusion of the spaces to which the gas is distributed at the alveolar level. Parallel dead space (Folkow and Pappenheimer, 1955) is synonymous with alveolar dead space. *Figure 80* shows, in diagrammatic form, some of the possible causes of alveolar dead space. The alveolar dead space is too small to be measured with confidence in healthy supine man but becomes appreciable in many conditions considered below.

Factors influencing alveolar dead space

Hydrostatic failure of alveolar perfusion. The top alveolus in *Figure 80* lies above the level reached by the pressure head of the pulmonary arterial blood. This cause of alveolar non-perfusion probably applies to the supraclavicular parts of the lungs of the normal subject in the upright position. Studies with radioactive gases have clearly shown that the perfusion of the lungs decreases in a linear fashion from the bases to the apices, reaching very low values at the level of the second rib (West, 1962).

Non-perfusion of alveoli will be markedly increased in pulmonary hypotension which occurs in many forms of low-output circulatory failure. The effect is particularly marked in severe haemorrhage which is associated with a great increase in physiological dead space, due to failure of perfusion of a considerable proportion of the ventilated alveoli (Gerst, Rattenborg and Holaday, 1959;

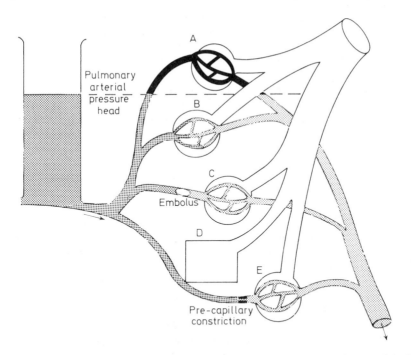

Figure 80. Diagrammatic representation of different forms of alveolar dead space. (A) The uppermost alveolus lies above the pressure head of the pulmonary arterial blood, a normal occurrence in the upright position but more marked in pulmonary hypotension. (B) Normally perfused alveolus. (C) Failure of perfusion due to an embolus lodged in the afferent pulmonary vessel. The embolus may be thrombus, fat, gas or foreign body. (D) An unperfused but communicating air space in parallel with the alveoli. (E) It is not clear to what extent pulmonary vasoconstriction can deprive alveoli of their circulation sufficiently to increase the alveolar dead space

Freeman and Nunn, 1963). It seems likely that similar changes occur after coronary occlusion and perhaps after the administration of atropine, which increases alveolar dead space (Nunn and Bergman, 1964) and is known to reduce the pulmonary arterial pressure (Daly, Ross and Behnke, 1963).

Increases in the alveolar dead space are almost certainly the principal cause of the large increases in physiological dead space reported during anaesthesia with deliberate hypotension (Eckenhoff et al., 1963). The same study found dead space was also influenced by head-up tilt and raised airway pressures, both of which factors would enhance the adverse effects of reduction of cardiac output (and presumably pulmonary arterial pressure) due to the hypotensive agents. These authors reported a number of patients with physiological dead space in excess of 75 per cent of the tidal volume; severe alveolar hypoventilation could easily occur under these circumstances if the anaesthetist was not aware of the effect.

Posture.   In the supine position, the vertical height of the lungs is reduced from about 30 to 20 cm. The gravity-dependent distribution of pulmonary blood flow is still present but in neither position is there direct experimental evidence of a zone which is entirely devoid of perfusion (*see Figure 81*). It would be reasonable to expect that the alveolar dead space is less in the supine than in the upright position. However, it is difficult to demonstrate the alveolar dead space at all in the upright position, and evidence of the effect of change of posture is not available.

In the lateral position it appears that approximately two-thirds of the pulmonary blood flow is distributed to the dependent side. During spontaneous respiration the greater part of the ventilation is also distributed to the lower lung and there is probably little change in alveolar dead space. If, however, the patient is ventilated artificially in the lateral position, ventilation is distributed in favour of the upper lung, particularly in the presence of an open pneumothorax (Nunn, 1961a). Under these conditions, it may be expected that much of the ventilation of the upper lung will constitute alveolar dead space. This interesting problem is discussed in greater detail later in this chapter (page 234).

Pulmonary embolus.   The middle alveolus in *Figure 80* shows obstruction of its afferent vessel due to embolus. Severinghaus and Stupfel (1957) found an increase in alveolar dead space after the intravenous administration of air to dogs. Stein et al. (1961) have obtained clear evidence of an increase in alveolar dead space in dogs after the migration of peripheral thrombi into the pulmonary circulation. Greenbaum et al. (1965) have shown large increases in physiological dead space in two patients with fat emboli from fractured long bones.

Demonstration of an increased physiological dead space would appear to be a valuable clinical test for pulmonary embolus. The method (*see Figure 84*) is suited to the bedside and, in this respect, is clearly far more convenient than either pulmonary angiography or a lung scan. It seems unlikely that the test will yield false negatives and the author has found values for V_D/V_T ratio in excess of 60 per cent in all patients with a known pulmonary embolus. Furthermore, the V_D/V_T has been shown to return to normal values during treatment with heparin or streptokinase. However, the value of the test is marred by a high incidence of false positives. These are patients with various types of circulatory failure who have a high V_D/V_T ratio, presumably as a result of regional pulmonary hypoperfusion due to pulmonary hypotension. Measurements of dead space have thus been disappointing in the differential diagnosis of pulmonary embolus from other conditions with which it may be confused.

Ventilation of non-vascular air space. The next form of alveolar dead space shown in *Figure 80* is the ventilation of an air with no vasculature. This occurs in obstructive lung disease following widespread destruction of alveolar septa and the contained vessels. This is the principal cause of the very marked increase in physiological dead space reported in patients with chronic lung disease (Donald et al., 1952).

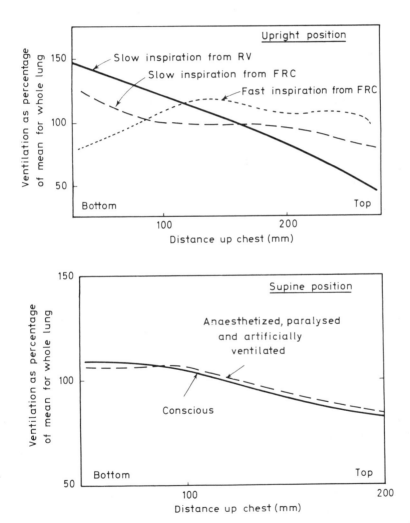

Figure 81. Relative distribution of ventilation in horizontal strata of the lungs. Data for the upright position from West (1962), and Hughes et al. (1972). Data for the supine position from Hulands et al. (1970), comprising inspirations of 1 litre from FRC with normal inspiratory flow rate

Constriction of pre-capillary pulmonary vessels.   The final form of alveolar dead space in *Figure 80* is due to pre-capillary constriction of the pulmonary blood vessels. This cause is rather conjectural. The pulmonary circulation does have some degree of vasomotor control (*see* Chapter 8) but this is far less active than for the systemic circulation.

Obstruction of the pulmonary circulation by external forces.   The anaesthetist is frequently confronted with kinking, clamping or blocking of a pulmonary artery during thoracic surgery. This may be expected to result in an increase in dead space depending on the ventilation of the section of lung supplied by the obstructed vessel.

Anaesthesia.   Although the alveolar dead space is quite small in the normal conscious subject, it seems to be invariably enlarged during general anaesthesia with either spontaneous respiration or artificial ventilation (Nunn and Hill, 1960); similar changes were reported in dogs by Severinghaus and Stupfel in 1957. In anaesthetized man the alveolar dead space averages 70 ml but is markedly influenced by the magnitude of the tidal volume (*Figure 82*).

The cause of the increase in the alveolar dead space during anaesthesia has not so far been satisfactorily explained. One possibility would be a preferential distribution of inspired gas away from the areas perfused by the pulmonary blood flow. Alternatively, there might be a preferential distribution of pulmonary blood flow away from the best ventilated alveoli. Hulands et al. (1970) studied the effect of anaesthesia on the regional distribution of pulmonary perfusion and ventilation using ^{133}xenon as a tracer. This study showed only minor changes following the induction of anaesthesia and paralysis, and did not support the view that the increased alveolar dead space was due to a major diversion of pulmonary blood flow towards the dependent part of the lungs (*see Figure 81*). Their technique, however, only recorded total counts from horizontal strata of the lungs. It is possible that maldistribution occurred within slices of the lungs but this could not be determined by existing techniques.

There are so many factors which influence the size of the alveolar dead space during anaesthesia that very careful experimental design is necessary to determine the effect of any one factor. Usually only the physiological dead space is measured, but it is often possible to be reasonably certain that changes are in the alveolar rather than the anatomical component. For example, it was mentioned in Chapter 5 (page 158) that physiological dead space is greater when the duration of inspiration is reduced. This effect is shown in *Figure 82b*, which also illustrates the further increase when a subatmospheric pressure is used during expiration. It is thought that short inspirations are distributed preferentially to badly perfused alveoli, while a more leisurely rate of inspiration allows time for distribution to better perfused alveoli which, it is postulated, have a longer time constant of inflation.

The effects of duration and depth of anaesthesia may also be considered under the heading of alveolar dead space because any effect is likely to be in the alveolar component. There is no unanimity of opinion on the influence of duration. An early report by Thornton (1960) suggested that there might be a progressive rise of physiological dead space during the course of an anaesthetic, and this was later demonstrated by Askrog et al. (1964). However, this effect was not confirmed by Nunn, Bergman and Coleman (1965), Kain, Panday and

Nunn (1969) or Cooper (personal communication). The reason for the disagreement is not clear but may have been due to progressive changes in some additional factor which was not operative in the studies which found no change. The effect of depth of anaesthesia is not yet established but preliminary observations by Kain, Panday and Nunn (1969) suggested that a relationship might exist, possibly by reduction of pulmonary arterial pressure.

The alveolar component of the physiological dead space will be increased during anaesthesia by any factor which reduces pulmonary flow or pressure. A convincing increase was demonstrated by Eckenhoff et al. (1963) following hypotension induced by ganglion block. It is probably the alveolar component which is principally involved in the positive correlation of physiological dead space with age, which may be observed during anaesthesia (Nunn, Bergman and Coleman, 1965) as in the conscious state (Raine and Bishop, 1963). A review of

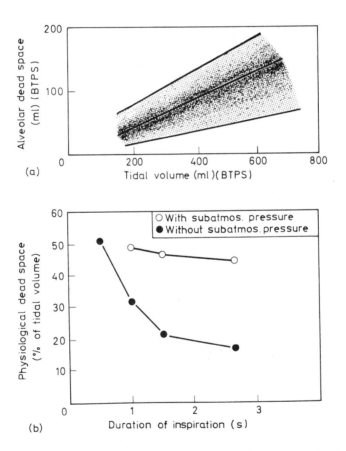

Figure 82. Factors influencing alveolar dead space during anaesthesia. (a) The alveolar dead space as a function of tidal volume in healthy anaesthetized intubated patients. There appears to be no significant difference in this respect between artificial and spontaneous respiration. (b) The effect of the duration of inspiration on the total physiological dead space — the effect being probably on the alveolar component. The use of subatmospheric pressure phase during expiration increases the dead space but variations in the waveform have little effect apart from any influence on duration (after Watson, 1962b)

a number of studies by Cooper (1967) led to the conclusion that, as a rough approximation:

$$\text{VD/VT per cent} = 33 + \frac{\text{age}}{3}$$

(Value of VD was increased artificially by 70 ml to compensate for the volume of the upper respiratory tract bypassed by the endotracheal tube.)

Measurement of the alveolar dead space

The alveolar dead space is measured as the difference between the physiological and anatomical dead spaces determined separately but at the same time. When only the physiological dead space is measured, it is often possible to attribute a large increase in physiological dead space to an increase in the alveolar component, since there are few cicumstances in which the anatomical dead space is greatly enlarged.

The arterial/end-expiratory P_{CO_2} *difference* is a convenient and relatively simple method of assessing the magnitude of the alveolar dead space. In *Figure 78*, expired gas is shown as consisting of four components. The first two, apparatus and anatomical dead spaces, are exhaled in series before the next two which are exhaled in parallel beside one another. Thus the final portion of an expirate consists of a mixture of 'ideal' alveolar gas and alveolar dead space gas. If the patient has an appreciable alveolar dead space, it follows that:

1. it is impossible to sample or analyse 'ideal' alveolar gas;
2. the P_{CO_2} of end-expiratory gas will be less than that of 'ideal' alveolar gas since it is diluted with alveolar dead space gas which is practically free of CO_2.

If, for example, 'ideal' alveolar gas has a P_{CO_2} of 5·3 kPa (40 mm Hg) and the end-expiratory P_{CO_2} is found to be 2·65 kPa (20 mm Hg), it follows that the end-expiratory gas consists of equal parts of 'ideal' alveolar gas and alveolar dead space gas. Thus if the tidal volume is 500 ml and the anatomical dead space 100 ml, the components of the tidal volume would be as follows:

anatomical dead space	100 ml
alveolar dead space	200 ml
'ideal' alveolar gas	200 ml

The physiological dead space would be 100 + 200 = 300 ml and the VD/VT ratio 60 per cent.

In practice, the method has two complications. Firstly, the alveolar dead space gas is not entirely CO_2-free since end-expiratory gas is re-inhaled into the alveolar dead space at the start of inspiration. Secondly, it has been pointed out of that 'ideal' alveolar gas cannot be sampled directly if it is contaminated with alveolar dead space gas. The solution to this difficulty has been to substitute arterial P_{CO_2} for 'ideal' alveolar P_{CO_2}. The rationale of this has been explained in detail by Riley et al. (1946), and is widely accepted. It is based on two premises.

1. There is never a measurable gradient of P_{CO_2} between alveolar gas and blood leaving the pulmonary capillaries.

2. Since the mixed venous/arterial P_{CO_2} difference is small (normally 0·8 kPa or 6 mm Hg), no reasonable degree of venous admixture (shunt) is likely to produce a serious rise in arterial P_{CO_2} above the level in the end-pulmonary capillary blood.

The second premise is only approximately true, since a 33 per cent shunt would raise the arterial P_{CO_2} by about 0·4 kPa (3 mm Hg) if the mixed venous/arterial P_{CO_2} difference were 0·8 kPa (6 mm Hg). Nevertheless, the use of arterial blood for this purpose has proved immensely valuable, and measurement of the arterial/end-expiratory P_{CO_2} difference is probably the most convenient method of estimating the alveolar dead space.

In practice, arterial blood is sampled during the measurement of the end-expiratory P_{CO_2}. The arterial P_{CO_2} is then measured and compared with the end-expiratory value. End-expiratory P_{CO_2} may be measured directly with a rapid analyser sampling from the mouth (infrared or mass spectrometer) or alternatively, end-expiratory gas may be collected for analysis by a variety of techniques (Rahn et al., 1946a; Nunn and Pincock, 1957). A significant positive correlation has been found during anaesthesia between the arterial/end-expiratory P_{CO_2} difference and the alveolar dead space (Nunn and Hill, 1960).

Direct experimentation has confirmed the validity of this approach. Theye and Fowler (1959) and Julian et al. (1960) have performed partial obstruction of the pulmonary arterial bed and shown clearly the resultant increase of arterial/end-expiratory P_{CO_2} difference. However, there is a homeostatic mechanism which deflects ventilation away from unperfused areas of the pulmonary field so that the alveolar dead space resulting from pulmonary arterial obstruction tends to be maximal at first and then decreases (Severinghaus et al., 1961). This change appears to be mediated by an increase in airway resistance of the affected parts, resulting in preferential ventilation of the remaining perfused lung.

The magnitude of the arterial/end-expiratory P_{CO_2} difference is of practical importance if end-expiratory P_{CO_2} is used as an indirect measure of the arterial P_{CO_2}. In the presence of severe respiratory disease with abnormalities of distribution (e.g. emphysema) the difference is so large and variable that measurements of end-expiratory P_{CO_2} are of little value. During anaesthesia the difference appears to be relatively constant in healthy subjects. Ramwell (1958) and Nunn and Hill (1960) were in close agreement on the following points.

1. During anaesthesia, in normal healthy subjects, the arterial/end-expiratory P_{CO_2} difference has a mean value of 0·7 kPa (5 mm Hg) with a range of 0–1·3 kPa (0–10 mm Hg).
2. The magnitude is uninfluenced by the actual level of the P_{CO_2}.
3. The magnitude appears to be similar for spontaneous and artificial ventilation.

Higher levels for arterial/end-expiratory P_{CO_2} difference have been found during thoracic surgery and there was greater variability, values probably being influenced by the degree of expansion of the exposed lung (Nunn, 1961a).

PHYSIOLOGICAL DEAD SPACE

The physiological dead space is defined as that part of the tidal volume which does not participate in gaseous exchange. Nowadays it is universally defined by the Bohr mixing equation with substitution of arterial P_{CO_2} for alveolar P_{CO_2}:

$$\frac{\text{physiological}}{\text{dead space}} = \frac{\text{tidal}}{\text{voulme}} \left(\frac{\text{arterial } P_{CO_2} - \text{mixed-expired } P_{CO_2}}{\text{arterial } P_{CO_2} - \text{inspired } P_{CO_2}} \right)$$

It follows from this equation that the physiological dead space is the functionally ineffective part of the ventilation. Alveolar ventilation is therefore measured as:

$$\frac{\text{respiratory}}{\text{frequency}} \times \left(\frac{\text{tidal}}{\text{volume}} - \frac{\text{physiological}}{\text{dead space}} \right)$$

or alternatively as:

$$\left(1 - \frac{\text{physiological dead space}}{\text{tidal volume}} \right) \times \text{respiratory minute volume}$$

Thus if the physiological dead space is 30 per cent of the tidal volume, (V_D/V_T = 30 per cent), the alveolar ventilation will be 70 per cent of the respiratory minute volume. The use of the V_D/V_T ratio is useful since the ratio tends to remain fairly constant while the actual value for the physiological dead space may vary widely with changing tidal volumes. This approach is radically different from the assumption of a constant 'dead space' which is subtracted from the tidal volume, the difference then being multiplied by the respiratory frequency to indicate the alveolar ventilation.

The proportionality between dead space and tidal volume was first demonstrated by Enghoff in 1931. In a latter publication (1938) he suggested that the dead space be measured by substitution of the arterial P_{CO_2} in Bohr's equation, thus introducing the modern concept of the physiological dead space. He used the term *Volumen inefficax* to stress its functional nature, in contrast to the original term for the dead space—*schädlichen Raum*—which rested on a morphological definition and was akin to the current concept of the anatomical dead space. Enghoff used the term *Inefficax Quotient* to describe V_D/V_T ratio and was able to demonstrate that the ratio remained relatively constant for one individual during hyperventilation and exercise.

In practice, the concept of a relatively constant V_D/V_T ratio simplifies calculations of alveolar ventilation from minute volume, and one easily becomes accustomed to thinking of the alveolar ventilation as a constant fraction of the minute volume.

Factors influencing the physiological dead space

This section summarizes information on the value of the total physiological dead space but reasons for the changes have been considered above in the sections on the anatomical and alveolar dead space.

Age. There is a tendency for V_D and also V_D/V_T ratio to increase with age, with V_D increasing by slightly less than 1 ml per year (Harris et al., 1973). These authors found values for V_D in men of the order of 50 ml greater than in women but the former group had larger tidal volumes and there was a smaller sex difference in the V_D/V_T ratios (33·2–45·1 per cent for men; 29·4–39·4 per cent for women). All subjects were seated. The authors review other studies of normal values for VD/VT ratios which tend to be slightly less than their own values, although there is general agreement that VD/VT increases with age.

Body size. It is evident that VD, in common with other pulmonary volumes, will be larger in larger people. Harris' group recommend correlation with height and report that VD increases by 17 ml for every 10 cm increases in height.

Posture. Craig et al. (1971) showed that VD/VT ratio decreased from a mean value of 34 per cent in the upright position to 30 per cent in the supine position. The study was conducted in a group of 22 subjects, free of cardiovascular disease and aged from 21 to 78 years. The effect of posture was apparent in all subgroups, broken down according to age, smoking habits and closing volume.

Duration of inspiration and breath holding. It is well known that prolongation of inspiration reduces dead space by allowing gas mixing to take place between dead space and alveolar gas. This is shown in *Figure 82.*

Smoking. Craig et al. (1971) showed a highly significant increase in VD/VT ratio of smokers in whom the values were 37 per cent (upright) and 32 per cent (supine), compared with 29 per cent (upright) and 26 per cent (supine) for non-smokers. Smokers were evenly distributed among their age groups.

Pulmonary disease. The previous part of this chapter has considered the enlargement of the alveolar dead space which occurs when parts of the lung are deprived of circulation. Very large increases in VD/VT occur in pulmonary embolus and, to a lesser extent, in pulmonary hypoperfusion and emphysema. Patients with emphysema suffer a further increase in VD/VT ratio following induction of anaesthesia (Pietak et al., 1975).

Anaesthesia. Many studies have now shown that VD/VT ratio of a healthy, anaesthetized intubated patient is of the order of 30–35 per cent whether breathing spontaneously or ventilated artificially. The increase in alveolar dead space is thus approximately offset by the anatomical dead space bypassed by the endotracheal tube. There is always a substantial volume of apparatus dead space in an anaesthetized patient.

Effect of apparatus. Inclusion of normal apparatus dead space raises the total VD/VT ratio to about 46 per cent in intubated patients and about 64 per cent in patients breathing from a mask (Kain, Panday and Nunn, 1969). These values relate to what may be called the total functional dead space which equals the physiological dead space *plus* the apparatus dead space functionally measured. Cooper (1967) added 70 ml of apparatus dead space to his patients as a compensation for the volume of the upper airway bypassed by the endotracheal tube. He obtained a mean value of VD/VT ratio of approximately 50 per cent which is compatible with the measurements quoted above. Thus, when using values of VD/VT ratio from the literature for calculation of the effective part of the tidal volume, it is important to be quite clear whether the author made allowance for apparatus dead space (q.v.). It is no less important in any calculation to take into account the effect of respiratory health, age, haemodynamic state and unusual respiratory frequencies.

Artificial ventilation.   Artificial ventilation itself seems to have little effect upon the VD/VT ratio compared with the value obtained during spontaneous breathing. However, once artificial ventilation is established, VD/VT ratio may be affected by variations in respiratory pressures and phasing (*see Figure 82* and pages 158 et seq.). Suter, Fairley and Isenberg (1975) found that VD/VT was minimized by the optimal value of positive end-expiratory pressure ('best PEEP').

Effects of an increased physiological dead space

Regardless of whether an increase in physiological dead space is due to the anatomical or alveolar components, alveolar ventilation is reduced, unless there is a compensatory increase in minute volume.

Reduction of alveolar ventilation due to an increase in physiological dead space produces changes in the 'ideal' alveolar tensions which are identical to those produced by an equivalent reduction in respiratory minute volume. Alveolar PCO_2 will rise and alveolar PO_2 fall, the two bearing a relationship to one another which is influenced only by the composition of the inspired gas and, to a small extent, the respiratory exchange ratio. The changes may be derived from *Figure 65*, but are shown more clearly on an oxygen–carbon dioxide diagram as in *Figure 83.* Values for the changes in alveolar gas tension may be conveniently determined from the universal alveolar air equation (page 186).

It is almost always possible to counteract the effects of an increase in physiological dead space by a corresponding increase in the respiratory minute volume. If, for example, the minute volume is 10 l/min and the VD/VT ratio 30 per cent, the alveolar ventilation will be 7 l/min. If the patient were then subjected to pulmonary embolism resulting in an increase of the VD/VT ratio to 50 per cent, the minute volume would need to be increased to 14 l/min to

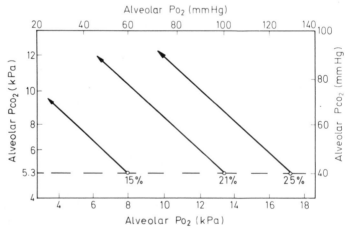

Figure 83. Pathways of changes in alveolar gas tensions during alveolar hypoventilation. The information may be derived from Figure 65. Alveolar hypoventilation may result either from reduction of minute volume or from increase in any component of the dead space. The resultant effect upon both PO_2 and PCO_2 is similar, although the alveolar PO_2 is also influenced directly by the inspired oxygen concentration, which is indicated at the foot of the three lines in the diagram

maintain an alveolar ventilation of 7 l/min. Should the VD/VT increase to 80 per cent, the minute volume would need to be increased to 35 l/min to maintain the alveolar ventilation, and so on. In principle, all that is necessary is to adjust the minute volume until the arterial P_{CO_2} attains the required level. It is, however, impossible to judge what is an adequate ventilation by examination of the expired air if there is a substantial increase in the alveolar dead space.

Measurement of physiological dead space

The measurement of physiological dead space is quite simple and is of considerable value in the management of patients who are ventilated artificially for long periods. Its value lies in the fact that it is the link between respiratory minute volume and alveolar ventilation. It is thus a major factor in defining the total minute volume which is needed to produce a required arterial P_{CO_2} in a particular patient.

Arterial blood and expired air are collected simultaneously over a period of two or three minutes (*Figure 84*). After collection, blood and gas are removed to the laboratory and the P_{CO_2} of each determined. Suitable methods are discussed on page 371.

Provided that the inspired gas is free from carbon dioxide, physiological dead space is indicated by the following form of the Bohr equation:

physiological dead space
$$= \text{tidal volume} \left(\frac{\text{arterial } PCO_2 - \text{mixed-expired gas } PCO_2}{\text{arterial } PCO_2} \right) - \frac{\text{apparatus dead}}{\text{space}}$$

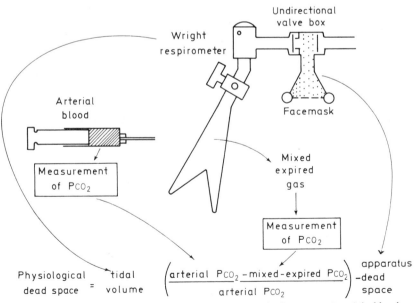

Figure 84. Clinical measurement of physiological dead space. Arterial blood and mixed-expired gas are collected simultaneously over a period of 2–3 minutes. Values for PCO_2 are then substituted in the Bohr equation. Tidal volume is conveniently determined with a Wright respirometer and the apparatus dead space by water displacement

Apparatus dead space includes such items as the facemask and unidirectional valve box. It is usually measured by water displacement and is often found to be surprisingly large. Tidal volume may be determined by a variety of techniques; the Wright respirometer is the most convenient and may easily be incorporated in the gas-collection apparatus (*Figure 84*).

The result is best expressed as the ratio of the physiological dead space to the tidal volume and will be found to be reasonably constant in the same patient under the same circumstances, provided that there is no change in the pulmonary circulation (such as pulmonary embolism). It should, however, be stressed that the physiological dead space is a functional concept defined by its method of measurement. It does not follow that the expired air is actually divided into the watertight compartments shown in *Figure 78*. Scatter of ventilation/perfusion ratios (page 287) undoubtedly contributes to the measured physiological dead space from which it cannot be distinguished by the methods of measurement described in this section.

APPARATUS DEAD SPACE AND REBREATHING

Thus far, we have considered apparatus dead space as though it were always a simple extension of the patient's anatomical dead space and could be treated as such during measurement. This approach is perfectly valid provided that we are only considering endotracheal tubes, mouthpieces and such equipment. A facemask, however, presents a more difficult problem since it is possible that the whole of the gas space under the mask may not be washed out by the tidal volume. Under these conditions we are again confronted by the difference between the morphological and the functional definitions that were noted in relation to anatomical dead space. Usually, only the morphological definition is considered and apparatus dead space is commonly measured by filling with water. Measurement of the functional apparatus dead space may, however, be made by means of a modification of the technique of Fowler (1948) (page 216). In this case, the gas sampling point must lie at the junction between the apparatus dead space and the anatomical dead space; with carbon dioxide being used as the tracer gas, the measurement is made during inspiration. In effect, one measures the volume which must be inhaled through the apparatus dead space before uncontaminated inspired air is reached. Functional apparatus dead space may also be determined by measuring physiological dead space with and without added apparatus dead space and noting the difference.

Concepts of apparatus dead space and rebreathing have been explored in some detail by Nunn and Newman (1964). These authors found the problem far more complicated than might appear at first sight. The principal points which they made are as follows:

1. A variety of gas circuits are in common use by anaesthetists and these circuits impose many different patterns of rebreathing.
2. The gas rebreathed may be end-expiratory gas (as with a simple face-mask), mixed expired gas (as in circuit C described by Mapleson, 1954), or any combination of these gases.
3. Contamination of inspired gas may occur early in inspiration, for example, with the use of simple mouthpieces. However, in other circuits (such as

Ayre's T-piece) contamination may occur late in inspiration. This gas may come to rest in the patient's anatomical dead space and therefore take no part in gas exchange although it has been inhaled into the patient's respiratory tract.

4. If gas exhaled from the patient's anatomical dead space is stored and then re-inhaled (as may occur with the Magill gas circuit), this will not influence gas exchange although, considered in terms of gas volumes, rebreathing has occurred.

5. The effective 'mean inspired gas composition' has two alternative meanings. The first refers to the mean composition of the gas which enters the patient's respiratory tract. The second is restricted to the gas which enters functioning alveoli and so influences gas exchange.

6. 'Mean inspired gas composition' is difficult to measure in the presence of rebreathing. It cannot be derived from a plot of instantaneous gas composition against time, since the required value is the concentration integrated with respect to volume and not to time.

7. An inspiratory gas sampler which will indicate the effective mean inspired gas composition in the presence of changes in inspired gas composition must sample not necessarily at a steady rate, but at a rate which is proportional to the instantaneous inspiratory gas flow rate. Such a device is practicable and has been developed by Bookallil and Smith (1964).

Effects of apparatus dead space

It must be borne in mind that apparatus dead space hampers not only the elimination of carbon dioxide, but also the uptake of oxygen, the uptake of inhalational anaesthetic agents and also their subsequent elimination. Usually these effects are contrary to the patient's interest (unless it is intended to raise the P_{CO_2} to a desirable level by rebreathing).

Generally, the introduction of apparatus dead space or rebreathing affects all these exchanges equally. However, dissociation is possible. A notorious example is the incorrect use of a Waters' canister with the canister connected directly to the endotracheal tube and with fresh gas introduced into the side of the canister distal from the patient, beside the relief valve. Provided the soda-lime is fresh, the apparatus dead space for carbon dioxide consists only of the connections between the patient and the canister. However, for oxygen the apparatus dead space must include in addition the intergranular space of the canister since the patient must breathe through the canister for his expired gas to be recharged with oxygen. The situation is then complex and it is necessary to consider the patient as having two alveolar ventilations: one for carbon dioxide and a second, much smaller one, for oxygen!

Anaesthetists show astonishing ingenuity in 'improving' gas circuits. While these often appear harmless, it sometimes proves that the effects are surprisingly complex and it may become almost impossible to determine the composition of the gas which the patient is inhaling. Control of the gaseous environment is essential for good anaesthesia, and the anaesthetist should know precisely what the patient is breathing at all times. For this reason the author prefers to use gas circuits which avoid rebreathing, appreciating that the control of the gaseous environment is gained at some additional cost in gases and volatile anaesthetic agents. The price appears reasonable (Barton and Nunn, 1975).

DISTRIBUTION OF THE INSPIRED GAS

The distribution of the inspired gas may be considered in a number of contexts. In the first place, it may be considered purely as spatial distribution in relation to anatomical structures. Secondly, it may be considered in relation to the distribution of pulmonary blood, differentiating between the ventilation of unperfused alveoli at one extreme and the failure of ventilation of perfused alveoli at the other extreme. Finally, the distribution of inspired gas may be considered in terms of the rate at which different alveoli fill and empty.

It frequently happens that these distinctions are not clearly made, and confusion may result from a failure to appreciate the precise meaning of the phrase 'distribution of inspired gas' in a particular situation.

Spatial and anatomical distribution of inspired gas

At the time of writing, there is a paucity of information about the spatial distribution of inspired gas and the factors which may influence it. This is largely due to the practical difficulties of measuring the ventilation of different parts of the lungs. The following approaches have been used.

1. Inspection and auscultation of the chest will indicate gross changes in the distribution of the inspired gas such as follow collapse of the greater part of one lung.
2. Chest radiography and screening provide some qualitative information about the relative ventilation of different parts of the lung fields.
3. Bronchospirometry is used to differentiate the ventilation of the two lungs and, to a certain extent, of different lobes.
4. Pneumography provides an indication of the change in circumference of the thorax at different levels. From such measurements it is possible to make some estimate of volume changes.
5. Radioactive tracer gases may be used to study the ventilation of areas of lung over which appropriate counters are placed.
6. Gas expired from different lobes may be sampled at bronchoscopy and analysis will indicate relative ventilation.

Distribution between the two lungs is influenced by posture and by the manner of ventilation. In the normal conscious seated subject, studies with divided airways show that the right lung enjoys a ventilation slightly greater than that of the left side, and this is no doubt associated with the fact that the volume of the right lung is a little greater than that of the left lung (*Table 18*). The supine position is associated with a reduction in the FRC but the relative ventilation of the two lungs is not changed.

In the lateral position the studies of Svanberg (1957) have shown that the lower lung is always better ventilated regardless of the side on which the subject is lying although there remains a tendency towards greater ventilation of the right side (*Table 18*). It appears surprising at first that the lower lung should be better ventilated than the upper since the volume of the lower lung is less, and it is especially liable to collapse (Faulconer, Gaines and Grove, 1946). However, the diminished volume of the dependent lung is associated with the lower diaphragm lying higher in the chest and so being more sharply curved. It will,

Table 18. DISTRIBUTION OF RESTING LUNG VOLUME (FRC) AND VENTILATION BETWEEN THE TWO LUNGS IN MAN

(The first figure is the unilateral FRC (litres) and the second the percentage partition of ventilation)

	Supine		Right lateral (left side up)		Left lateral (right side up)	
	right lung	*left lung*	*right lung*	*left lung*	*right lung*	*left lung*
Conscious man	1·69	1·39	1·68	2·07	2·19	1·38
(Svanberg, 1957)	53%	47%	61%	39%	47%	53%
Anaesthetized man— spontaneous breathing (Rehder and Sessler, 1973)	1·18	0·91	1·03	1·32	1·71	0·79
	52%	48%	45%	55%	56%	44%
Anaesthetized man— artificial ventilation (Rehder et al., 1972)	1·36	1·16	1·33	2·21	2·29	1·12
	52%	48%	44%	56%	60%	40%
Anaesthetized man—thoracotomy (Nunn, 1961a)	—	—	—	—	—	—
	—	—	—	—	83%	17%

Each study refers to separate subjects or patients.

therefore, be able to contract more effectively during inspiration (*Figure 63*). We shall see later that this preferential ventilation of the lower lung accords with increased perfusion of the lower lung so that the ventilation/perfusion ratios of the two lungs are not greatly altered on assuming the lateral position.

Rehder's group from the Mayo Clinic have reported that the preferential ventilation of the lower lung in the lateral position does not occur in the anaesthetized or artificially ventilated human subject (*Table 18*). It is not surprising that this should be the case during artificial ventilation, since the high diaphragm of the lower side no longer confers any advantage in ventilation. In fact, on the contrary, the weight of the mediastinum rests on the lower lung and limits its ability to expand. The studies of Potgieter (1959) showed a considerable reduction in the total compliance of the lower lung-plus-chest wall, when the patient was turned into the lateral nephrectomy position. On the assumption that the ventilation of the two lungs should be in proportion to the static pressure/volume relationships observed by Potgieter, the ventilation of the lower lung would be of the order of 40 per cent of total ventilation which accords reasonably well with the data of Rehder et al. (1972) and also Wulff and Aulin (1972). The preferential ventilation of the upper lung is abolished by the application of PEEP (Rehder, Wenthe and Sessler, 1973).

During anaesthesia with spontaneous breathing, it is by no means obvious why the upper lung should be preferentially ventilated. Rehder and Sessler (1973) ascribed this to the over-all reduction of FRC which follows induction of anaesthesia. This moves each lung down its pressure/volume plot so that the dependent lung moves from a steep part of its curve (with the subject awake) to a flatter part of the curve (after induction of anaesthesia). This is a striking example of anaesthesia producing a relative mismatch of ventilation and perfusion in consequence of mechanical changes, although it must be remembered that the reduction of the FRC following induction of anaesthesia remains unexplained (*see* page 68).

Thoracotomy may result in gross maldistribution of ventilation between the two lungs (*Table 18;* Nunn, 1961a). All depends upon the restraint placed upon the exposed lung. If it is free to expand it will clearly be overventilated as it is not confined by thorax or mediastinum and its total effective compliance is that of the lung itself. If, however, the exposed lung is confined by a retractor, ventilation will be deflected into the dependent and better perfused lung.

Horizontal slices of lung were first studied by West (1962) using a radioactive isotope of oxygen. He found the slices to have different degrees of ventilation with a progressive increase in ventilation (per unit lung volume) the nearer the slices lay to the diaphragm (*see Figure 81*). The original studies were carried out with slow vital capacity inspirations starting from residual volume, but distribution of ventilation must clearly be influenced by a number of additional factors. Firstly, there is the end-expiratory lung volume and the range of lung volume over which the patient breathes. Slow inspirations from FRC to total lung capacity show the same preferential ventilation of the bases but the degree of inequality is reduced and Hughes et al. (1972) report a mean ratio of 1·5 : 1 for basal ventilation compared with apical (*see Figure 81*). The second factor is the rate of inspiration, since regional airway resistance then becomes relatively more important than regional compliance which governs distribution of ventilation during a very slow inspiration. Hughes et al. (1972) showed that fast inspirations from FRC did, in fact, reverse the distribution of ventilation with preferential ventilation of the upper parts of the lungs. Since this is contrary to the distribution of pulmonary blood flow, gas exchange would be impaired and we have already noted that V_D/V_T ratio tends to be increased when the duration of inspiration is short (*see Figure 82*).

Bake et al. (1974) have also studied the effect of inspiratory gas flow rate on distribution of ventilation and found that the preferential ventilation of the dependent parts of the lung was only present at flow rates below 1·5 l/s, starting from FRC. At higher flow rates, distribution was approximately uniform. Normal inspiratory flow rate is substantially less than 1·5 l/s (*see Figure 46*).

Posture affects distribution since *inter alia* the vertical height of the lung is reduced by about 30 per cent in the supine position. The gravitational force generating maldistribution is thus reduced. Hulands et al. (1970) investigated normal tidal breathing in the supine position and found slight preferential ventilation of the posterior slices of the lungs compared with the anterior slices (*see Figure 81*). The inequality was not greatly different from that found by Hughes et al. (1972) in the upright position although the vertical height of the lung was 20 cm compared with 30 cm. Hulands' group also investigated the effect of anaesthesia with paralysis and artificial ventilation but found no significant change in three out of four patients. In the fourth there was a change towards greater uniformity. Brendstrup (1966), in a study of supine subjects, also reported increased uniformity of ventilation between apical and basal zones during anaesthesia with artificial ventilation. These variations are of minor importance in comparison to the gross differences in perfusion which were found and which will be discussed in greater detail in Chapter 9 (page 276).

Changes in the geometrical pattern of expansion of the chest have received little attention until recently. Agostoni (1965) has suggested that tidal volume changes might be related, not only to alterations of the rib cage and abdominal circumferences but also to the ratio of the chest circumference to the dorsoventral diameter. Attention has already been drawn to the gross differences in the volume of the lungs in the lateral position (*see Figure 63*), and the differences in tidal volume referred to above are related to the altered geometry. Emphysematous patients have a rigid chest wall which shows less than the normal change in circumference during breathing. However, limitation of ventilatory capacity and ventilation/perfusion abnormalities are primarily due to pathological changes within the lung parenchyma rather than to the abnormal geometry of chest movement.

Anaesthesia causes profound changes in the geometrical pattern of chest expansion (*see* page 170). The reduction in FRC has been discussed in Chapter 3 (pages 67 eq seq.). Although the diaphragm lies higher in the chest during anaesthesia, Froese and Bryan (1974) showed that, in the anaesthetized supine spontaneously breathing subject, most of the tidal excursion took part in the posterior part of the diaphragm as in the awake supine subject. However, with paralysis and artificial ventilation, tidal excursion of the diaphragm was mainly confined to the anterior part.

Distribution of inspired gas in relation to pulmonary blood flow

We have seen that inspired gas distributed to regions which have no pulmonary capillary blood flow cannot contribute to gaseous exchange and that this fraction of the tidal volume constitutes the alveolar dead space. This was fully appreciated by John Hunter who, in the eighteenth century, wrote:

'In animals where there is no circulation there can be no lungs: for lungs are an apparatus for the air and blood to meet, and can only accord with motion of blood in vessels . . . As the lungs are to expose the blood to the air, they are so constructed as to answer this purpose exactly with the blood brought to them, and so disposed in them as to go hand in hand.'

Measurement of the alveolar dead space as the difference between the physiological and anatomical dead space measures the alveolar dead space *as if* all ventilated alveoli fell into the two categories shown in *Figure 78;* that is to say, normally perfused ('ideal') alveoli and totally unperfused alveoli. In fact, this model does not accord with reality and alveoli exist with a wide spectrum of ventilation/perfusion ratios around the mean value which is normally 0·8 (alveolar ventilation divided by pulmonary blood flow, with both quantities expressed in the same units). Discussion of ventilation/perfusion ratios is postponed until after consideration of the distribution of pulmonary blood flow (Chapter 9) but, at the present time, it should be noted that techniques now exist for the measurement of ventilation at different values of ventilation/perfusion ratio (*see* pages 298 et seq. and *Figure 104*). This permits the distinction between *true* alveolar dead space and the ventilation of *relatively* underperfused alveoli (high ventilation/perfusion ratio) and also indicates the degree of scatter of ventilation/perfusion ratios about the mean value.

Distribution of inspired gas in relation to the rate of alveolar filling

We have already seen in Chapter 5 (page 145) that the rate of inflation of the lung is a function of compliance and airway resistance. The product of the compliance and resistance equals the time constant which is:

1. the time required for inflation to 63 per cent of the final volume attained if inflation is prolonged indefinitely;

OR

2. the time which would be required for inflation of the lungs if the initial gas flow rate were maintained throughout inflation (*see Figure 153*).

These considerations apply equally to small areas of the lungs, and in *Figure 26* were shown fast and slow alveoli, the former with a short time constant and the latter with a long time constant.

We may now consider ventilation of the lungs when different parts have different time constants. The diagrams (*Figure 85*) may look as though we are considering different lungs and the reasoning would certainly apply to cases where the time constants of the lungs were different. We are, however, equally concerned with the general situation in which different *functional units* of lung have different time constants, without specifying the size or the anatomical location of these units.

The considerations are fundamentally similar for spontaneous respiration or for artificial ventilation with a constant or sine-wave flow generator (*Figures 57 and 58*). We shall, however, present the problem by considering the special case of passive inflation of the lungs by development of a constant mouth pressure (*see Figure 54*). This simplifies the presentation, although Otis et al. (1956) have chosen to present the subject as illustrated by ventilation of the lungs in response to development of a sinusoidal mouth pressure. Their presentation may be more lucid to those who are familiar with the theory of alternating current.

Let us consider two functional units of equal compliance and resistance (*Figure 85a*). If the mouth pressure is suddenly increased to a constant level, there will be an increase in volume of each lung unit equal to the mouth pressure multiplied by the compliance of the unit. The time course of inflation will follow the wash-in type of exponential function and the time constant will be equal to the product of compliance and resistance of each unit. The time courses will thus be identical, and if the inspiratory phase is terminated at any instant, the pressure in each will be identical since the alveolar pressures will equal volume change divided by compliance of each unit.

Next let us consider two functional units, one of which has half the compliance but twice the resistance of the other (*Figure 85b*). The time constants of the two will thus be equal. If a constant inflation pressure is maintained, the one with the lower compliance will increase in volume by half the volume change of the other. Nevertheless, the pressure build-up within each unit will be identical. Thus, as in the previous example, the relative distribution of gas between the two functional units will be independent of the rate or duration of inflation. If the inspiratory phase is terminated at any point, the pressure in each unit being identical, no redistribution will occur between the different units.

In the next example (*Figure 85c*), the compliances of the two units are identical but the resistance of one is twice that of the other. Therefore, its time constant is double that of its fellow and it will fill more slowly, although the volume increase in both units will be the same if inflation is prolonged indefinitely. Relative distribution between the units is thus dependent upon the rate and duration of inflation. If inspiration is checked by closure of the upper airway after two seconds (for example), the pressure will be higher in the unit with the lower resistance. Gas will then be redistributed from one unit to the other as shown by the arrow in *Figure 85c*.

Figure85d shows a pair of units with identical resistances but the compliance of one being half that of the other. Its time constant is thus half that of its fellow and it enjoys a more rapid time course of inflation. However, since its compliance is half that of the other, the ultimate volume increase will only be half that of the other unit when the inflation is prolonged indefinitely. It will again be seen that the relative distribution of gas between the two units is not constant throughout inflation, and is therefore dependent upon the rate and

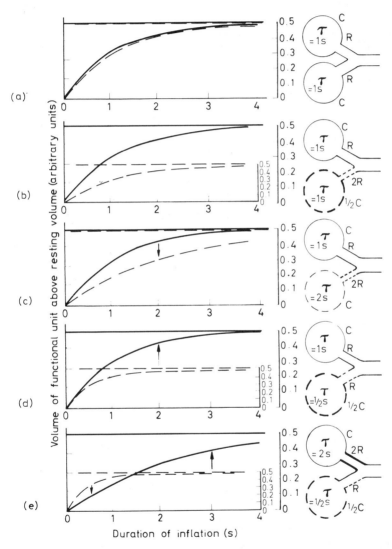

Figure 85. The effect of mechanical characteristics on the time course of inflation of different functional units of the lung when exposed to a sustained constant inflation pressure. The Y co-ordinate is volume change, but a scale showing intra-alveolar pressure is shown on the right. The continuous curve relates to the upper unit and the broken curve to the lower unit, in each case. Separate pressure scales are necessary when the compliances are different. Arrows show the direction of gas redistribution if inflow is checked by closure of the upper airway at the times indicated. See text for explanation of the changes

duration of inflation. Pressure rises more rapidly in the unit with the lower compliance, and if inspiration is checked by closure of the upper airway at 2 seconds (for example) gas will be redistributed from one unit to the other as shown by the arrow in *Figure 85d*.

An interesting and complex situation occurs when one unit has an increased resistance and another a reduced compliance (*Figure 85e*). It will be remembered that this combination was chosen to introduce the concept of fast and slow alveoli in *Figure 26*. In the present example the time constant of one unit is four times that of the other, while the ultimate volume changes are determined by the compliance as in the previous example. When the inflation pressure is sustained, the unit with the lower resistance shows the greater volume change at first, but rapidly approaches its equilibrium volume. Thereafter the other unit undergoes the major volume changes, the inflation of the two units clearly being out of phase with one another. Throughout inspiration, the pressure build-up in the unit with the shorter time constant is always greater and, if inspiration is checked by closure of the upper airway, gas will be redistributed from one unit to the other as shown by the arrows in *Figure 85e*.

If the inflation pressure is sustained indefinitely, the volume change enjoyed by different units of the lungs will depend solely upon their compliance. *If their time constants are equal,* the build-up of pressure in the different units will be identical at all times during inflation and therefore:

1. Distribution of inspired gas will be independent of the rate, duration or frequency of inspiration.
2. Dynamic compliance (so far as it is influenced by considerations discussed in relation to *Figure 26*) will not be affected by changes in frequency.
3. If inspiration is checked by closure of the upper airway, there will be no redistribution of gas within the lungs.

If, however, *the time constants of different units are different,* from whatever cause, it follows that:

1. Distribution of inspired gas will be dependent on the rate, duration and frequency of inspiration.
2. Dynamic compliance will be decreased as respiratory frequency is increased.
3. If inspiration is checked by closure of the upper airway, gas will be redistributed within the lungs.

In the healthy subject, the variations in time constants for different parts of the lung can be demonstrated by the effect on distribution of ventilation of fast and slow inspirations as described above. An increase in scatter of time constants in disease may be shown by an increase in the frequency dependence of compliance (page 76).

Effect of maldistribution of inspired air on gas mixing

This subject is important for two reasons. Firstly, it constitutes the usual method of detecting certain types of maldistribution. Secondly, it has an adverse effect on most forms of inhalation therapy including inhalation anaesthesia.

Various therapeutic manoeuvres require the replacement of the nitrogen in the alveolar gas with a different gas. Examples are the administration of 100 per cent oxygen in severe shunting, the replacement of nitrogen with helium to diminish the resistance to breathing, and finally the replacement of nitrogen with nitrous oxide which is very widely practised in general anaesthesia. In each case the nitrogen is washed out and another gas (oxygen, helium or nitrous oxide) is washed in to replace it. Replacement takes place, not only in the alveolar gas, but in all the tissues of the body and this is relatively more important in the case of the more soluble gases (oxygen being a special case since it is consumed within the body and so can never come into equilibrium between the different tissues). The exchange of gases within the different body compartments is a complex story but we can profitably discuss exchange within the lungs at this stage.

If we ignore, for the time being, the exchange of a gas within the tissue compartments, the wash-in and wash-out of gases in the lungs may be considered as an exponential function (Appendix E). Thus if a patient inhales 100 per cent oxygen, the alveolar nitrogen concentration falls according to a wash-out exponential function (*Figure 152*). If, on the other hand, he inhales a mixture of constant helium concentration, the alveolar helium concentration rises according to a wash-in exponential function (*Figure 153*) towards a plateau concentration equal to that in the inspired gas (the gaseous environment). In each case the time constant* of change of alveolar gas is the same and equals:

$$\frac{\text{functional volume of the lungs}}{\text{alveolar ventilation}}$$

If, for example, the lung volume is 3 litres and the alveolar ventilation is 6 litres/minute, the time constant will be 30 seconds.

This makes an important assumption—that every alveolus is ventilated in proportion to its volume. If this is not the case, we must consider not a single time constant, but a whole family of time constants for different functional units of the lungs. Some will therefore exchange rapidly and some slowly. The over-all picture is that of delayed equilibrium, and after a finite interval (say 7 minutes) it is found that the mixed alveolar gas concentration has not changed as rapidly as would otherwise be expected. It may, furthermore, be shown that the wash-out curve is not that of a simple exponential, but shows two or more components, the areas with short time constants being dominant early and the areas with long time constants being dominant later. Several examples may be cited.

If a patient breathes 100 per cent oxygen, the alveolar nitrogen will normally be reduced to less than 2·5 per cent after 7 minutes. This fall may be delayed by maldistribution. The fall of nitrogen concentration is the basis of the 'nitrogen wash-out test' but the rate of rise of oxygen concentration is often of direct interest to the anaesthetist and others who are concerned with patients with deranged lung function.

We have already considered the helium wash-in method of measurement of functional residual capacity (page 6). Clearly the rate at which equilibrium is attained between spirometer and lungs is also a measure of the equality of distribution. Thus the measurement of functional residual capacity can conveniently be combined with a test of distribution.

---

* This time constant should not be confused with the time constant of lung emptying which equals the product of compliance and resistance.

At a more practical level, all anaesthetists are familiar with the delay in both induction of and recovery from inhalational anaesthesia in patients with advanced lung disease resulting in maldistribution. In cases of emphysema it is as difficult to ensure a rapid induction with inhalational agents as it is to ensure a rapid recovery from inhalational anaesthesia. Eger (1974) has pointed out that ventilation of unperfused alveoli has relatively little effect on the rate of rise of arterial anaesthetic concentrations although pulmonary shunting has an adverse effect, particularly in the case of the less soluble anaesthetics.

Rehder's group at the Mayo Clinic have reported that, during anaesthesia, there is increased uniformity of gas distribution as measured by pulmonary nitrogen clearance (Rehder et al., 1971). The same group also carried out studies with intubation of the main bronchi and showed that uniformity of distribution within each lung was also greater in the anaesthetized subject than in previous studies carried out in conscious subjects. They also showed that anaesthesia resulted in a greater uniformity of nitrogen clearance between dependent and non-dependent lung for patients in the lateral position (Rehder et al., 1972). The same group has recently contributed a most valuable review on the distribution of inspired gas during anaesthesia (Rehder, Sessler and Marsh, 1975).

Effect of maldistribution on the alveolar 'plateau'

If the different functional units of the lung empty synchronously during expiration, the composition of the expired air will be approximately constant after the anatomical dead space gas has been expelled.* This, however, does not occur in maldistribution due to lung disease such as emphysema. In this case, it is usually found that those parts of the lungs which have a defective ventilation for their volume are 'slow', with either high compliance, high resistance or both. Thus they have a prolonged time constant for change of alveolar gas as well as prolonged time constant for emptying and filling. This is hardly surprising since normal respiratory frequencies do not permit uniform distribution in patients with emphysema and, therefore, ventilation is preferentially distributed in favour of the fast alveoli. Since the slow alveoli may well have the larger volume, it will be seen that the two types of maldistribution are linked. Some functional units are slow to fill and empty, and these are hypoventilated for their volume; therefore they are slow to respond to a change in the inspired gas composition. This forms the basis of an important test of maldistribution which, unlike the multi-breath nitrogen wash-out test (described above), will only detect maldistribution if there is sequential emptying of functional units of lung such as we have described above. The test is shown diagrammatically in *Figure 86*. The subject, who has been breathing air, takes a single deep breath of 100 per cent oxygen sufficient to raise the alveolar oxygen concentration to about 50 per cent. The patient then exhales deeply and the nitrogen concentration is measured at the patient's lips. (It would be just as satisfactory to monitor the oxygen concentration, but it happens that it is much easier to measure nitrogen concentrations by an instrument with a sufficiently rapid response.) We may now consider what is found under four different circumstances (*Figure 86a–d*).

---

* During expiration the P_{CO_2} rises slightly while the P_{O_2} falls since the subject is effectively breath holding once expiration commences.

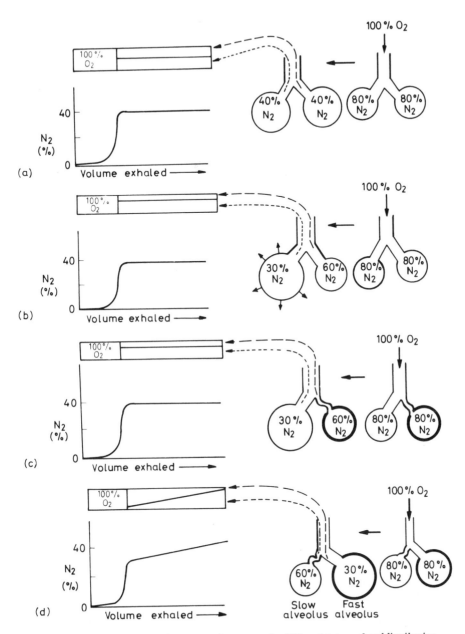

Figure 86. The single-breath nitrogen wash-out test in different types of maldistribution. Reading the diagram from right to left, the subject inhales a deep breath of 100 per cent oxygen and then exhales into a nitrogen meter. (a) Normal subject with uniform distribution. (b) Maldistribution due to non-uniform pull of inspiratory muscles. (c) Maldistribution due to non-uniform mechanical factors in lung units but all having the same time constants. (d) Maldistribution due to non-uniform mechanical factors in lung units resulting in different time constants. Only this type of maldistribution alters the slope of the curve of the expired nitrogen

1. *Figure 86a* shows two identical functional units. Following the inspiration of a single breath of oxygen, the nitrogen concentration in each unit is reduced to the same value and the exhaled nitrogen concentration must therefore remain constant throughout the latter part of expiration.
2. *Figure 86b* shows functional units of identical mechanical properties but which are subjected to unequal forces during inspiration. As a result, the nitrogen concentration is reduced by a greater amount in the better ventilated unit. If expiration is passive, the expirate will consist of the same proportion from each unit throughout expiration. Therefore the exhaled nitrogen concentration will be constant throughout the latter part of expiration, at a value intermediate between that of the two units.
3. *Figure 86c* shows two units of different mechanical properties but which nevertheless have the same time constant. (The unit on the right may be considered as having double the resistance and half the compliance of the unit on the left.) In these circumstances, ventilation will be preferentially distributed to the unit with the higher compliance and lower resistance (*see Figure 85b*). However, if expiration is passive, the expirate will again consist of the same proportion from each unit throughout expiration. Therefore the exhaled nitrogen concentration will remain constant throughout the latter part of expiration as in the previous example.
4. *Figure 86d* has two units with different time constants resulting from different mechanical properties. These are of the type which were used in *Figure 26* to illustrate fast and slow alveoli. During inspiration of finite length, the faster unit will be preferentially ventilated, and its nitrogen concentration will therefore be lower. During expiration, the faster unit empties more rapidly at first while gas from the slower unit forms a proportionately greater part of the end-expiratory gas. Thus the proportion of gas from the two units changes during expiration and the nitrogen concentration rises progressively.

In examples (2) and (3), there is definite maldistribution of inspired gas, but this is not revealed by the single-breath nitrogen test. Only when the time constants of the units differ will the maldistribution be revealed by the test (as in example (4)). This point is frequently glossed over by those who are chiefly concerned with maldistribution caused by lung disease. This is because maldistribution due to the commoner forms of lung disease is usually associated with different time constants and *sequential emptying*. Therefore, under these circumstances the single-breath nitrogen test is a valid method of detection of maldistribution of inspired gas. Anaesthetists, however, may well be confronted with maldistribution which is not associated with changes in time constant, and which could not be demonstrated by the single-breath nitrogen test. Maldistribution of this type might result from the use of the lateral position, intercostal paralysis or from artificial ventilation.

Before leaving the single-breath nitrogen test, two small points may be noted. Firstly, even with perfect distribution the exhaled nitrogen concentration rises slightly during the latter part of the exhalation. This is because oxygen is being consumed in greater volume than carbon dioxide is being produced. Therefore, the alveolar nitrogen concentration always rises slightly as expiration proceeds. (Normal alveolar gas contains 80–81 per cent nitrogen compared with 79 per cent in air.) The upper limit of normal is a rise of 1·5 per cent (more in older subjects) between the exhalation of 750 ml and 1 250 ml after the inhalation of a large breath of oxygen. The second point is that fast alveoli must inhale more than their share of gas lying in the anatomical dead space. Thus the slow alveoli do have a marginal advantage in that their delayed filling results in the uptake of relatively more uncontaminated fresh gas.

MEASUREMENT OF DEAD SPACE AND DISTRIBUTION OF INSPIRED GAS

Most chapters of this book end with a brief account of the principles of the methods of measurement which are relevant to the matters discussed. This chapter has departed from the usual practice since the methods of measurement not only aid the understanding of dead space but actually constitute the definition of certain quantities. It therefore seemed best to mention the methods of measurement as they arose in the text. For convenience, their location is indicated below.

Chapter 8   The Pulmonary Circulation

Pulmonary Blood Volume
Pulmonary Vascular Pressures
Pulmonary Blood Flow
Pulmonary Vascular Resistance
Pulmonary Oedema
Principles of Measurement of the Pulmonary Circulation

The entire blood volume passes through the lungs during each circulation. This is an appropriate arrangement for gas exchange but is no less suitable for the filtering and metabolic functions of the lungs which are considered in Chapter 1.

The flow of blood through the pulmonary circulation is approximately equal to the flow through the whole of the systemic circulation. It therefore varies from about 6 l/min under resting conditions to as much as 25 l/min in severe exercise (Åstrand et al., 1964). Although the flow rates are similar in the two systems, the pressures are greatly different, pulmonary arterial pressures being approximately one-sixth of systemic. The pulmonary vascular resistance is thus much less than that of the systemic circulation and consequently the pulmonary circulation has little ability to vary the distribution of blood flow within the lung fields. This is in marked contrast to the systemic circulation which is able to vary the distribution of blood flow within very wide limits in response to the changing requirements of the individual. We shall see that the pulmonary circulation, lacking the power of selective distribution, is very markedly affected by gravity with a preponderance of circulation in the dependent parts of the lung fields.

The distribution of the pulmonary blood flow has important consequences for gaseous exchange. We have seen in the last chapter that failure of perfusion of parts of the lung prevents exchange occurring with the gas which ventilates those parts, and it is convenient to consider the ventilation of unperfused regions as dead space ventilation. Localized failure of ventilation means that blood perfusing such parts cannot participate in gas exchange and thus constitutes venous admixture similar in effect to a right-to-left shunt. The two abnormalities are fundamentally similar but the resemblance is masked by the fact that blood flow is continuous while gas flow is tidal. It is helpful to represent both flows as continuous and to consider the lungs as a black box* with a gas inflow and outflow and a blood inflow and outflow (*Figure 87*). The object of this black box is to achieve equilibrium of oxygen and carbon dioxide tensions between

* According to current usage, a 'black box' is a process or device, whose internal workings are not understood by the operator, but whose function is important and may be studied in detail without appreciation of the internal mechanism.

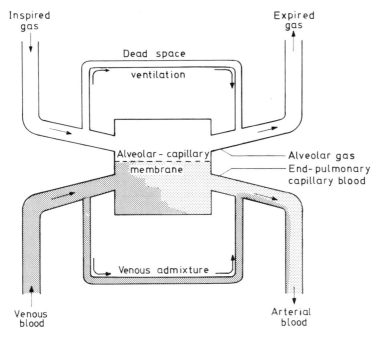

Figure 87. In this functional representation of gas exchange in the lungs, the flow of gas and blood is considered as a continuous process with movement from left to right. Under most circumstances, equilibrium is obtained between alveolar gas and end-pulmonary capillary blood, the gas tensions in the two phases being almost identical. However, alveolar gas is mixed with dead space gas to give expired gas. Meanwhile, end-pulmonary capillary blood is mixed with shunted venous blood to give arterial blood. Thus both expired gas and arterial blood have gas tensions which differ from those in alveolar gas and end-pulmonary capillary blood

the two outflow streams. However, the plumbing of neither side is perfect and in each case the effluent is contaminated with a part of the corresponding inflow. The precise mechanism by which this takes place is often difficult to determine, but it may be possible to obtain valuable guidance on the management of patients by considering the lung as though it functions in the manner shown in *Figure 87.*

PULMONARY BLOOD VOLUME

Haemodynamic considerations

As a first approximation the right heart pumps blood into the pulmonary circulation, while the left heart pumps away the blood which returns from the lungs. Therefore, provided that the output of the two sides is the same, the pulmonary blood volume will remain constant. However, very small differences in the outputs of the two sides will result in large changes in pulmonary blood volume if they are maintained for more than a few beats. Harris and Heath (1962) have pointed out that if the stroke output of the left ventricle were persistently to exceed that of the right ventricle by 0·1 ml, the lungs would become exsanguinated within two hours. The mechanism which prevents this happening is not understood, but Starling's law of the heart is probably concerned.

When we leave our first approximation and attempt to get nearer to the truth, we see that the relationship between the inflow and outflow of the pulmonary circulation is really rather complicated. *Figure 88* is a summary of some of the relevant anatomical features. The lungs receive a significant quantity of blood from the bronchial arteries which usually arise from the arch of the aorta. Blood from the bronchial circulation returns to the heart in two ways. From a plexus around the hilum, blood from the pleurohilar part of the bronchial circulation returns to the systemic veins via the azygos veins, and this fraction may thus be regarded as normal systemic flow neither arising from nor returning to the pulmonary circulation. However, another fraction of the bronchial circulation, distributed more peripherally in the lung, passes through post-capillary anastomoses to join the pulmonary veins, constituting an admixture of venous blood with the arterialized blood from the alveolar capillary networks (Marchand, Gilroy and Wilson, 1950).

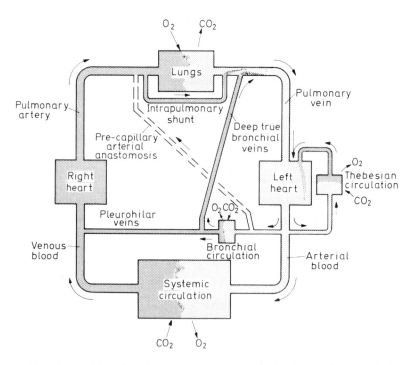

Figure 88. Schema of bronchopulmonary anastomoses and other forms of venous admixture in the normal subject. Part of the bronchial circulation returns venous blood to the systemic venous system (pleurohilar veins) while another part returns venous blood to the pulmonary veins and so constitutes venous admixture. Other forms of venous admixture are the Thebesian circulation of the left heart and flow through atelectatic parts of the lungs. The existence of pre-capillary bronchopulmonary anastomoses in the normal subject is controversial. It will be clear from this diagram why the output of the left heart must be slightly greater than that of the right heart

The paragraph above relates to the normal subject. The situation may be further complicated when blood flows through pre-capillary anastomoses from the bronchial arteries to the pulmonary arteries. The communications have been called 'sperr arteries' meaning muscular vessels which act as sluice gates. These anastomoses are thought to be present in the normal subject (Verloop, 1948; von Hayek, 1960), but they are of definite functional importance in cases of pulmonary oligaemia. This has been demonstrated after experimental ligation of a branch of the pulmonary artery in dogs (Cockett and Vass, 1951), but congenital pulmonary atresia is the most important natural cause of the condition. It should be noted that arterial bronchopulmonary anastomoses achieve the same purpose as a Blalock–Taussig operation.

The catalogue of abnormal communications between the pulmonary and systemic circulations can be continued almost indefinitely, and the reader is referred to the treatise of Aviado (1965). It is not unusual for aberrant pulmonary veins to drain into the right atrium. Furthermore, flow may be reversed through normally occurring channels. Thus, in pulmonary venous hypertension due to mitral stenosis, pulmonary venous blood may traverse the bronchial venous system to gain access to the azygos system.

Factors influencing pulmonary blood volume

The quantity of blood within the pulmonary circulation is 10–20 per cent of total blood volume, between 0·5 and 1·0 litre. The volume fluctuates during the cardiac cycle since inflow exceeds outflow during systole. It is also likely that the cyclical pressure changes caused by respiration will influence pulmonary blood volume which has been found to decrease during a Valsalva manoeuvre, and during positive pressure breathing (Fenn et al., 1947). Conversely, pulmonary blood volume is increased during negative pressure breathing (Slome, 1965).

Posture. A great many authors, cited by Harris and Heath (1962), are agreed that pulmonary blood volume is directly influenced by posture. When a subject changes from the supine to the erect position the pulmonary blood volume falls by 27 per cent, a change which is of the same order as the decrease in cardiac output under the same circumstances. It is thought that both changes are due to pooling of blood in dependent parts of the systemic circulation.

Drugs. Since the systemic circulation has much greater vasomotor activity than the pulmonary circulation, it is to be expected that an over-all increase in the tone of capacity vessels will squeeze blood from the systemic into the pulmonary circulation. This may result from the administration of vaso-constrictor drugs, from release of endogenous catecholamines or by passive compression of the body in a G-suit. Conversely, it seems likely that pulmonary blood volume would be diminished when systemic tone is diminished, as for example by sympathetic ganglion blockade. Large decreases in pulmonary blood volume have been reported during spinal anaesthesia, but increases sometimes occurred when the patient was in the Trendelenburg position (Johnson, 1951). In general it may be said that vasoactive drugs produce a complementary relationship between pulmonary and systemic blood volumes.

Left heart failure.   Pulmonary venous hypertension (due, for example, to mitral stenosis) would be expected to result in an increased pulmonary blood volume. There has, however, been difficulty in the experimental demonstration of any significant change.

Anaesthesia.   There have been few studies of the effect of general anaesthesia on pulmonary blood volume. Johnson (1951) found no significant changes when patients received premedication of morphine and scopolamine. Light ether anaesthesia (stage III, plane 2) was associated with a small increase of pulmonary blood volume (+40 ml) which was not statistically significant. Deep anaesthesia (stage III, plane 3) was associated with a significant fall of pulmonary blood volume (−160 ml). Barbiturate anaesthesia reduced the pulmonary blood volume in all patients by a mean value of 340 ml, but only half this change was found when curare was used in addition to the barbiturate. All measurements were carried out prior to the commencement of surgery when there had been no significant changes in total blood volume.

The extent of the 'pulmonary blood volume'

The measurement of pulmonary blood volume is difficult, and lacks the precision which is obtainable in the measurement of many other circulatory variables.* Harris and Heath (1962) have reviewed the available methods which must lie outside the scope of the present volume. Here it is sufficient to say that they are indirect and most techniques actually measure the 'central blood volume', an indefinite quantity which, apart from the pulmonary vascular system, includes the chambers of the heart and also certain parts of the systemic vascular system depending upon the placement of the catheters used in the measurement technique. Pulmonary capillary volume may be calculated from measurements of diffusing capacity (page 325) and this technique yields values of the order of 80 ml.

In view of the difficulties in measurement, it is perhaps fortunate that pulmonary blood volume is of limited interest from the clinical standpoint, and can often be estimated with sufficient accuracy from the density of the vascular markings seen in a chest radiograph. Considerably greater importance attaches to pulmonary vascular pressures and flow, which are considered in the next two sections of this chapter.

PULMONARY VASCULAR PRESSURES

Pulmonary arterial pressure is only about one-sixth of systemic arterial pressure, although the capillary and venous pressures are not greatly different for the two circulations (*Figure 89*). There is thus only a small pressure drop along the pulmonary arterioles and consequently little possibility for active regulation of the distribution of the pulmonary circulation. There is also little damping of the arterial pressure wave and the pulmonary capillary blood flow is markedly pulsatile.

* Measurement techniques are outlined in the section starting on page 267.

Consideration of pulmonary vascular pressures carries a special difficulty in the selection of the reference pressure. Systemic pressures are customarily measured with reference to ambient atmospheric pressure. Thus a systolic pressure of 16 kPa (120 mm Hg) implies a pressure of 16 kPa above atmospheric (i.e. an absolute pressure of $16 + 101$ kPa or $120 + 760 = 880$ mm Hg). This approach is not always satisfactory when considering the pulmonary circulation because it gives us insufficiently precise information about the important

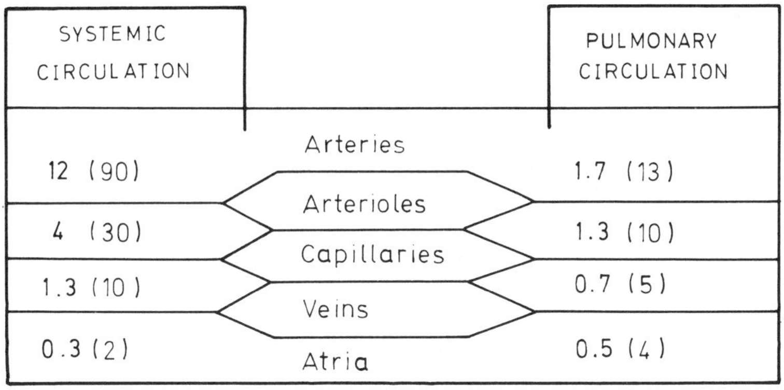

SYSTEMIC CIRCULATION		PULMONARY CIRCULATION
12 (90)	Arteries	1.7 (13)
4 (30)	Arterioles	1.3 (10)
1.3 (10)	Capillaries	0.7 (5)
0.3 (2)	Veins	0.5 (4)
	Atria	

Figure 89. Comparison of pressure gradients along the systemic and pulmonary circulations. (Mean pressures relative to atmosphere kPa with mm Hg in parentheses)

pressure gradient between the inside of pulmonary capillaries and the extravascular space. Neither does it tell us anything about the pressure gradients which cause the blood to flow onwards against the pulmonary vascular resistance into the left atrium. We therefore require to distinguish between pressures within the pulmonary circulation expressed in the three different forms listed below. Measurement techniques may be adapted to indicate these pressures directly (*Figure 90*).

Intravascular pressure is the pressure at any point in the circulation relative to atmosphere. This is the customary way of expressing pressures in the systemic circulation.

Transmural pressure is the difference in pressure between the inside of a vessel and the tissue surrounding the vessel. In the case of the larger pulmonary vessels, the outside pressure is the intrathoracic pressure (commonly measured as the oesophageal pressure as in *Figure 90*). In the case of the capillaries, the outside pressure is closer to alveolar pressure, but its precise value is difficult to determine since the relevant space is the interstitial space between the alveolar membrane and the capillary membrane (*Figures 5 and 6*). The pressure in this space is probably intermediate between alveolar and intrathoracic.

The capillary transmural pressure gradient would drive fluid out of the circulation were it not prevented by the osmotic pressure of the plasma proteins, normally about 3·3 kPa (25 mm Hg). Should this pressure be exceeded by the transmural pressure, pulmonary oedema results and may grossly interfere with gas exchange (*see* page 264).

Driving pressure is the difference in pressure between one point in the circulation and another point downstream. The driving pressure of the pulmonary circulation as a whole is the pressure difference between pulmonary artery and left atrium. This is the pressure which overcomes the flow resistance and should be used for determination of vascular resistance.

These differences are far from being solely academic. The capillary transmural pressure gradients may be markedly influenced by the intra-alveolar pressure which may be raised by positive pressure respiration and reduced by the use of a subatmospheric pressure phase during expiration. The former is thus beneficial and the latter detrimental in threatened pulmonary oedema. However, the intracapillary pressure is directly influenced by changes in alveolar pressure (page 253) and account must therefore be taken of the induced change in intravascular pressure.

The difference between pulmonary arterial intravascular pressure (relative to atmosphere) and the pulmonary driving pressure is of importance in distinguishing between different causes of pulmonary hypertension. If the primary lesion is a raised left atrial pressure, the pulmonary arterial intravascular pressure will be raised but the driving pressure will not be increased unless there is a

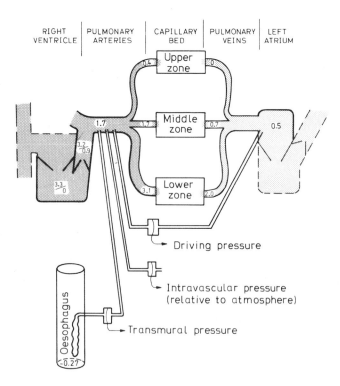

Figure 90. Normal values for pressures in the pulmonary circulation relative to atmosphere (kPa). Systolic and diastolic pressures are shown for the right ventricle and pulmonary trunk. Note the effect of gravity on pressures at different levels in the lung fields. Three differential manometers are shown connected to indicate driving pressure, intravascular pressure and transmural pressure

secondary rise in pulmonary vascular resistance. Left atrial pressure is measured by one of four possible techniques.

1. Wedge pressures are obtained by advancing the cardiac catheter into the pulmonary artery until it impacts. Alternatively, a Swan–Ganz catheter may be used.
2. The left atrium may be punctured by a needle at bronchoscopy.
3. The atrial septum may be pierced from a catheter in the right atrium.
4. A catheter may be passed retrogradely from a peripheral systemic artery.

Typical normal values within the pulmonary circulation are shown in *Figure 90.* The effect of gravity on the pulmonary vascular pressures may be seen, and it will be clear why pulmonary oedema is most likely to occur in the lower zones of the lungs where the intravascular pressures and the transmural pressure gradients are highest.

Factors influencing pulmonary vascular pressures

Posture. It is difficult to study the effect of change of posture on pulmonary blood pressure, since the actual levels of pressure are so low that they are markedly influenced by movement of the reference level. However, it seems likely that the upright position is associated with a lower pulmonary arterial pressure in patients with pulmonary hypertension (Donald et al., 1953). Wedge pressures are also reduced. Intrathoracic pressure is also lower in the upright position, so it is unlikely that capillary transmural pressure is greatly affected.

Exercise results in an increased pulmonary blood flow and, with moderate exercise, the pulmonary arterial pressure is raised in the supine but not the upright position (Dexter et al., 1951). Even in the supine position, the pressure tends to return to the resting level if the exercise is continued (Sancetta and Rakita, 1957).

Intra-alveolar pressure changes up to about 1·1 kPa (8 mm Hg) normally cause an equal change in pulmonary arterial pressure (Lenfant and Howell, 1960). There is a rise in pressure during a Valsalva manoeuvre and cyclical changes occur during spontaneous respiration with pressures higher during expiration and lower during inspiration. Information is required on the magnitude of the effect of lung inflation on pulmonary intracapillary pressure. Since small rises in alveolar pressure cause an equal rise in pulmonary arterial intravascular pressure, there should be no reduction in capillary transmural pressure gradient unless the capillary pressure fails to rise as much as the arterial pressure. With larger changes in alveolar pressure it is known that the rise in pulmonary arterial pressure is less than the rise in alveolar pressure and the disparity may be greater in patients with circulatory disorders. In certain pathological conditions tending towards the production of pulmonary oedema, the intravascular pulmonary capillary pressure will be considerably higher than the alveolar pressure. Elevation of the mean alveolar pressure (by IPP ventilation with or without PEEP) will not necessarily raise the capillary pressure under these conditions, and will therefore reduce the transmural pressure gradient. Favourable results in the treatment of pulmonary oedema by intermittent positive pressure suggest that this is so (Greene, Dameron and Bush, 1952).

Hypoxia.   Breathing of low concentrations of oxygen is associated with a rise in pulmonary arterial pressure which is related to the resultant arterial saturation (Fritts et al., 1960). A fall of saturation to 77 per cent results in a rise of pressure of the order of 0·7 kPa (5 mm Hg). Driving pressure is increased proportionately more than the pulmonary blood flow, and therefore the pulmonary vascular resistance is increased. However, the increased resistance cannot be precisely related to the oxygen saturation of the blood which perfuses the lung. Pulmonary hypertension is one of the principal manifestations of residence at high altitude and it has been suggested that high-altitude pulmonary oedema may be caused by consequent stretching of the arteriolar endothelium with resultant increase in permeability to plasma.

It is thought that the hypoxic stimulus must arise in the alveoli or the pulmonary capillaries, since the response is identical during foward and retrograde perfusion of the lungs (Duke, 1954). Nevertheless, the mechanism of this response remains obscure. Any generalized or humoral mechanism is discounted by the production of a unilateral increase in pulmonary vascular resistance when a gas mixture deficient in oxygen is breathed by one lung only (*see* below). Most workers are agreed that sympathetic denervation or sympathetic blockade by drugs are equally ineffective in preventing the rise of pulmonary arterial pressure due to hypoxia, and West, Dollery and Naimark (1964) obtained a typical response in an isolated dog lung preparation. Whatever the mechanism of this response, it is clear that it has potential teleological significance as a means of diverting the pulmonary blood flow away from regions in which the oxygen tension is low. The subject is discussed at great length by Aviado (1965).

Hyperoxia has little effect upon pulmonary arterial pressure in the normal subject, but many authors have reported a fall in patients with chronic pulmonary disease. This is not always accompanied by a proportionate fall of pulmonary blood flow and, in such cases, oxygen reduces the pulmonary vascular resistance, presumably by withdrawal of the effect of hypoxia.

Drugs.   Acetylcholine has been used extensively in studies of the pulmonary circulation. When introduced into the pulmonary artery, the rate of hydrolysis is so rapid that the drug is destroyed before it can act upon the systemic circulation. Acetylcholine results in a relaxation of vasomotor tone, causing the pulmonary arterial pressure to fall by an amount which depends on the tone present before the administration of the drug. The response to acetylcholine may thus be used as an indicator of the degree of vasomotor tone that exists in the pulmonary circulation. Small falls of pressure occur in the normal subject but much greater falls occur in hypoxic subjects and those with pulmonary hypertension resulting from congenital heart disease, emphysema or mitral stenosis (Harris and Heath, 1962). A number of references cited by these authors concur in the view that atropine does not affect pulmonary arterial pressure and is without vasomotor action of the pulmonary circulation. However, Daly, Ross and Behnke (1963) reported a fall in pressure following 2 mg of atropine (intravenously), and Nunn and Bergman (1964) suggested that this might be a cause of the increase in alveolar dead space which they found to follow the administration of atropine. Sympathomimetic drugs which act primarily upon the α receptors result in an increase in pulmonary arterial pressure, while those drugs which act primarily upon the β receptors cause a fall of pressure, particularly when this is elevated. Ganglion-blocking agents generally cause a fall in pressure and this has also been noted in the case of aminophylline. The effects of drugs have been extensively reviewed by Harris and Heath (1962) and Aviado (1965) to whom reference should be made.

Anaesthesia. During anaesthesia, there may be many factors which alter the pulmonary vascular pressures. These include alteration in blood-gas tensions, changes in mean alveolar pressure, cardiac output and blood volume. However, there is little convincing evidence that anaesthesia *per se* has any major effect on pulmonary vascular pressures. There is certainly no evidence of a reduction in pulmonary arterial pressure which might be invoked to explain the increased alveolar dead space. Studies such as those of Johnson (1951) have tended to report small increases in pulmonary arterial pressure during anaesthesia but these may well be caused by catecholamine release or by other factors mentioned above. During artificial ventilation, especially with PEEP, left atrial pressure is elevated and there is an equivalent increase in pulmonary arterial (intravascular) pressure. Perhaps the most important effect of anaesthesia is upon the vasoconstrictor response to hypoxia, and this is considered below in relation to pulmonary vascular resistance (page 262).

Disease. Many forms of pulmonary and cardiac disease are associated with a rise in pulmonary vascular pressures and these conditions are of considerable practical concern to the anaesthetist. Mitral stenosis and incompetence are the principal conditions leading to an elevation of pressure in the left atrium. It will be clear that the maintenance of the pulmonary driving pressure requires a corresponding increase of the pulmonary arterial pressure, and there must be a rise of pulmonary capillary pressure as well. In many cases of mitral stenosis, there is a secondary increase in pulmonary vascular resistance which results in further elevation of the pulmonary arterial pressure. The cause of this change is unknown. The work of the right ventricle is increased and, in severe cases, increased vascular resistance limits the benefit accruing from mitral valvotomy since the mitral valve is no longer the only site of increased resistance to the circulation. Pulmonary vascular resistance rises in many forms of chronic lung disease (cor pulmonale) and also in cases of pulmonary embolus. In a small number of patients the change appears to be primary and analogous to systemic hypertension.

Pulmonary hypertension may result from an increased pulmonary blood flow. However, following pneumonectomy, the remaining lung, if healthy, appears to be able to take the entire resting pulmonary blood flow without rise in pulmonary arterial pressure. The most important pathological cause of increased flow is left-to-right shunting through a patent ductus arteriosus, atrial or ventricular septal defects. Under these circumstances the pulmonary circulation is greater than the systemic circulation and may be sufficient to result in pulmonary hypertension, even with normal vascular resistance. However, secondary changes commonly result in an increase in vascular resistance, causing a further rise in pulmonary arterial pressure.

Pulmonary hypotension results from pulmonary atresia and, as we have seen, this induces an increased flow through pre-capillary anastomoses from the bronchial circulation, collateral flow sometimes being as great as one litre per minute.

PULMONARY BLOOD FLOW

Total pulmonary blood flow is approximately equal to cardiac output and is a topic which belongs to the field of circulation rather than respiration. We shall not therefore consider pulmonary blood flow in any more detail than is necessary for an understanding of the changes in pulmonary vascular pressure and resistance. Pulmonary gas exchange is, however, greatly influenced by the distribution of pulmonary blood flow, and Chapter 9 will be devoted to this important subject.

Methods for the measurement of pulmonary blood flow are outlined at the end of this chapter, but at this stage it should be pointed out that the older methods of measurement of cardiac output (Fick and dye) measure the pulmonary capillary blood flow, together with the venous admixture (*see Figure 87*). On the other hand, the body plethysmograph measures only the pulmonary blood flow. In this method, the alveoli are filled with nitrous oxide at a concentration of about 15 per cent, and the amount of nitrous oxide taken up by the blood is measured by whole body plethysmography. If the mean alveolar P_{N_2O} and the solubility of nitrous oxide in blood are known, it is possible to calculate the pulmonary blood flow on the assumption that the alveolar P_{N_2O} equals the arterial P_{N_2O} and the mixed venous P_{N_2O} is zero. The method may be used to measure the instantaneous capillary blood flow, which is found to be pulsatile.

PULMONARY VASCULAR RESISTANCE

Vascular resistance is an expression of the relationship between driving pressure and flow, as in the case of resistance to gas flow (*see Figure 32*). There are, however, important differences. It will be remembered that when gases flow through rigid tubes the flow is laminar, or turbulent, or a mixture of the two. In the first case pressure increases in direct proportion to flow rate and the resistance remains constant (Poiseuille's law). In the second case pressure increases according to the square of the flow rate, and the resistance increases with flow. When the type of flow is mixed, the pressure rises in proportion to the flow rate raised to a power between one and two, typical examples being shown in *Figure 38*.

The circumstances differ in the case of blood since the tubes through which the blood flows are not rigid, but tend to expand as flow is increased, particularly in the pulmonary circulation. Consequently the resistance tends to fall as flow increases and the plot of pressure against flow rate may be neither linear nor curved-with-the-concavity-upwards, but curved-with-the-concavity-downwards. As an added complication, blood is a non-Newtonian fluid (due to the presence of the corpuscles) and its viscosity varies with the shear rate and therefore its linear velocity through tubes. The situation is thus two degrees more complicated than in the case of gas flow, although the practical importance of these points should not be exaggerated. In fact, regardless of these considerations, there is a widespread convention that vascular resistance should be expressed as though the vessels were rigid and Poiseuille's law was obeyed.

Resistance is usually expressed in the form directly analogous to electrical resistance which is used for laminar gas flow (*see Figure 32*):

$$resistance = \frac{driving\ pressure}{flow\ rate}$$

In the case of the pulmonary circulation, the driving pressure is the difference in mean pressures between pulmonary artery and left atrium. Sometimes the pressure in the left atrium is measured directly, but more often the 'wedge pressure' taken at cardiac catheterization is considered to be representative of pulmonary venous pressure. Flow rate is usually taken as cardiac output.

Vascular resistance is expressed in units derived from those which are used for expression of pressure and flow rate. The appropriate SI units will probably be kilopascal litre^{-1} minute (kPa l^{-1}min). Using conventional units, vascular resistance may be expressed in units of mm Hg litre^{-1} minute (mm Hg l^{-1}min). In absolute CGS units, vascular resistance is usually expressed in units of dynes/square centimetre per cubic centimetre/second (dyn sec cm^{-5}). Normal values for the pulmonary circulation in the various units are as follows:

	Driving pressure	*Pulmonary blood flow*	*Pulmonary vascular resistance*
SI units	1·2 kPa	5 l/min	0·24 kPa l^{-1} min
Conventional units	9 mm Hg	5 l/min	1·8 mm Hg l^{-1} min
Absolute CGS units	12 000 dyn/sq. cm	83 cu. cm/sec	144 dyn sec cm^{-5}

The measurement of pulmonary vascular resistance is important not only in the diagnosis of the primary cause of pulmonary hypertension, but also for the detection of increased pulmonary vascular resistance which often develops in patients in whom the primary cause of pulmonary hypertension is raised left atrial pressure.

Localization of the pulmonary vascular resistance

It will be recalled that by far the greatest part of the systemic resistance is within the arterioles, along which the pressure falls from a mean value of about 12 kPa (90 mm Hg) down to about 4 kPa (30 mm Hg) (*Figure 89*). This pressure drop largely obliterates the pulse pressure wave, and the capillary flow is not pulsatile to any great extent. In the pulmonary circulation, the pressure drop along the arterioles is very much smaller than in the systemic circulation, being probably only of the order of 0·4 kPa (3 mm Hg). A further pressure drop of about 0·7 kPa (5 mm Hg) occurs along the length of the pulmonary capillaries (*Figure 89*). Thus the pulmonary capillary bed constitutes about 60 per cent of the total vascular resistance of the pulmonary circulation, in contrast to the systemic capillary bed which constitutes only 25 per cent of the total vascular resistance of the systemic circulation. Thus in the pulmonary circulation, the capillaries play the major role in governing vascular resistance and the distribution of the pulmonary blood flow.

Recruitment and distension in the pulmonary capillary bed

As the pulmonary blood flow increases from the resting level of about 5 l/min to exercise levels of the order of 20 l/min, there is proportionately a much smaller rise in pulmonary arterial pressure. Therefore, the vascular resistance is substantially reduced at the higher flow rate, implying an increase in the total cross-sectional area of the pulmonary capillary bed which is the major source of vascular resistance. This is achieved mainly by recruitment of new capillaries with opening of new passages in the network lying in the alveolar septa (*see Plate 5*). Sections cut in lungs rapidly frozen while perfused with blood have shown that the number of open capillaries increases with rising pulmonary arterial pressure, particularly in the mid-zone of the lung (Glazier et al., 1969; Warrell et al., 1972). It seems likely that individual pulmonary capillaries show a spread of opening pressures and the sequence of recruitment in the face of increasing pressure may be a purely physical phenomenon (West, 1974).

In addition to recruitment, it would be surprising if there were not an element of distension in the capillaries in response to increased transmural pressure gradient, since these vessels appear devoid of any vasomotor control. Sobin et al. (1972) have determined the distensibility of the capillary vessels and reported the diameter increasing from 5 to 10 μm as the transmural pressure increased from 0·5 to 2·5 kPa (5 to 25 cm H_2O). Distension plays the major role in zone 3 where most of the capillaries are already open (Glazier et al., 1969).

Effect of inflation of the lung

The mechanism of the effect of inflation of the lung on the pulmonary vessels is extremely complex, but the quantitative effect on pulmonary vascular resistance has recently been clarified. Much confusion and dispute has arisen in the past and it appears that this has, to a large extent, been due to failure to appreciate that pulmonary vascular resistance must be derived from driving pressure and not from pulmonary arterial or transmural pressure. This is very important since inflation of the lungs normally influences the pressure in the oesophagus, pulmonary artery and left atrium.

When pulmonary vascular resistance is correctly calculated from the driving pressure, there is reasonable agreement that, in the open-chested or isolated preparation, the pulmonary vascular resistance is minimal at an inflation pressure of the order of 0·5–1 kPa (5–10 cm H_2O)* (*Figure 91*). Change in inflation pressure may have very little effect upon resistance but the usual response is for the resistance to increase markedly with a rise of pressure and, to a lesser extent, with a fall of pressure. The response to complete collapse (zero inflation pressure) is variable, the mean change being of the order of a 50 per cent increase, probably due to kinking of larger blood vessels. There is certainly no massive increase in resistance as a result of acute collapse, and there are therefore no grounds to support the comforting myth that circulation immediately ceases through an *acutely* collapsed lung or section of a lung. Indeed, this fallacy has been directly exploded by Björk (1953) and by Aviado (1960). In *long-standing* collapse, the circulation is reduced but this is due to structural changes in the vessels.

* 1 kilopascal (1 kPa) is approximately equal to 10 centimetres of water (10 cm H_2O).

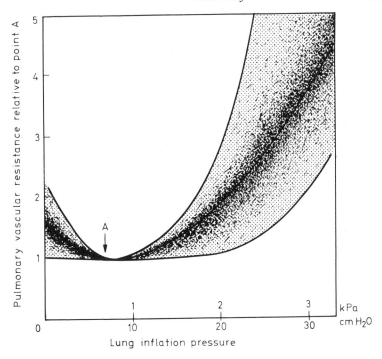

Figure 91. The mean and range of the response of pulmonary vascular resistance to changes in lung inflation pressure, relative to the resistance at the point A corresponding to the FRC. The diagram is composite and incorporates results reported by Burton and Patel (1958) for open-chested rabbits, Banister and Torrance (1960) for isolated cats' lungs, and Whittenberger et al. (1960) for open-chested dogs

Although it is possible to determine the gross effect of inflation of the lungs upon pulmonary vascular resistance, it is less easy to discover the mechanism of this effect. It seems likely that inflation of the lungs increases the calibre and the volume of the larger blood vessels. This is achieved by the tethering effect of surrounding lung tissue which is sufficient to develop substantial subatmospheric pressures in the large vessels during expansion of the isolated non-perfused lung (Howell et al., 1961). However, opposite changes occur in the smaller vessels which are collapsed as the lung is expanded by inflation.

The vascular weir

The interplay of alveolar pressure, flow rate and vascular resistance is best considered by dividing the lung field into three zones (West, Dollery and Naimark, 1964; West and Dollery, 1965). In the upper zone (zone 1 of *Figure 92*), the pressure within the arterial end of the collapsible vessels is less than the alveolar pressure, and therefore insufficient to open the vessels which remain collapsed. The behaviour of these vessels is similar to that of a Starling resistor (*see Figure 36*). Provided the pressure outside the tube exceeds the pressure inside, there can be no flow regardless of the venous pressure, which is thus irrelevant: this is the condition in the uppermost parts of the lungs of the human subject in the upright position. The situation is analogous to a weir in which the upstream water level is below the top of the weir.

In the mid-zone (zone 2 of *Figure 92*), the pressure at the arterial end of the collapsible vessels exceeds the alveolar pressure and, under these conditions, a collapsible vessel, behaving like a Starling resistor, permits flow in such a way that the flow rate depends upon the arterial/alveolar pressure difference. (Resistance in the Starling resistor is concentrated at the point marked with the arrow in *Figure 92*.) The larger the difference, the more widely the collapsible vessels will open and the lower will be the vascular resistance. Note that the venous pressure is still not a factor which affects flow or vascular resistance. This condition is still analogous to a weir with the upstream depth (head of pressure) corresponding to the arterial pressure, and the height of the weir corresponding to alveolar pressure. Clearly the flow of water over the weir depends solely on the difference in height between the top of the weir and the upstream water level. The depth of water below the weir (analogous to venous pressure) cannot influence the flow of water over the weir unless it rises above the height of the weir.

In the lower zone (zone 3 of *Figure 92*) of the lungs the pressure in the venous end of the capillaries is above the alveolar pressure, and under these conditions a collapsible vessel behaving like a Starling resistor will be held wide open and the flow rate will, as a first approximation, be governed by the arterial/venous pressure difference (the driving pressure) in the normal manner for the systemic circulation. However, as the intravascular pressure increases in

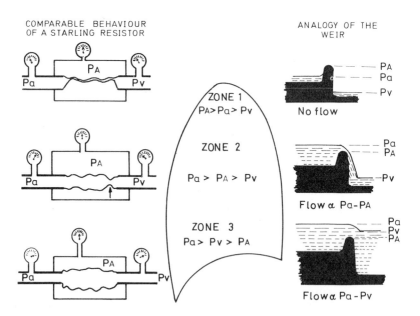

Figure 92. The effect of gravity upon pulmonary vascular resistance is shown by comparison with a Starling resistor (left) and with a weir (right). Pa, pressure in pulmonary artery; PA pressure in alveoli; Pv, Pressure in pulmonary vein (all pressures relative to atmosphere). This analogy does not illustrate zone 4 in which perfusion is reduced, apparently due to interstitial pressure acting on the larger vessels (Hughes et al., 1968). See text for full discussion

relation to the alveolar pressure, the collapsible vessels will be further distended and their resistance will be correspondingly reduced. Returning to the analogy of the weir, the situation is now one in which the downstream water level has risen until the weir is completely submerged and offers little resistance to the flow of water, which is largely governed by the difference in the water level above and below the weir. However, as the levels rise further, the weir is progressively more and more submerged and what little resistance it offers to water flow is still further diminished. The concept of the weir is particularly helpful and was introduced by Permutt and Riley (1963) as the 'vascular waterfall'. Portrayal of a weir instead of a waterfall permits representation of zone 3 conditions.

To the three-zone model shown in *Figure 92*, Hughes et al. (1968) have added a fourth zone of reduced blood flow in the most dependent parts of the lung. This reduction in blood flow appears to be due to compression of the larger blood vessels by increased interstitial pressure. This effect is more pronounced at reduced lung volumes. It is not shown in the weir analogy.

So far we have not mentioned the critical closing pressure of the pulmonary vessels (Burton, 1951). Current views suggest that the vessels of the lungs collapse at a pressure which is very close indeed to the alveolar pressure; that is to say that their critical closing pressure is extremely low (West and Dollery, 1965). The observations of these authors (and those reported by West, Dollery and Naimark in 1964) suggest that pulmonary blood flow ceases in any region where the alveolar pressure is in excess of the pressure at the arterial end of the collapsible vessels but that it recommences as soon as the vascular pressure exceeds the alveolar pressure. Simple hydrostatic considerations thus seem to define the amount of lung which is not perfused.

If the lungs are passively inflated by positive pressure, the pulmonary capillaries would clearly collapse if the pulmonary vascular pressures were to remain unchanged. In fact, the pulmonary vascular pressures normally rise by an amount almost exactly equal to the change in alveolar pressure up to inflation pressures of about $1 \cdot 1$ kPa (8 mm Hg) (Lenfant and Howell, 1960). Beyond this the rise in intravascular pressure is less than the rise in alveolar pressure and the cut-off by the mechanism of the Starling resistor operates over a larger area of the lung field. This has been demonstrated as an increase in physiological dead space during positive pressure breathing (Bitter and Rahn, 1956; Folkow and Pappenheimer, 1955). One might therefore expect that the physiological dead space for anaesthetized patients would be greater during artificial ventilation than during spontaneous respiration; the author, however, has been unable to demonstrate this (Nunn and Hill, 1960).

Chemical factors

Reference has been made above (page 254) to the effect of various chemical factors on pulmonary arterial pressure. This effect is principally mediated through changes in pulmonary vascular resistance and we may here note that pulmonary vascular resistance is increased by hypoxia (Fritts et al., 1960), acidaemia (Thilenius and Derenzo, 1972), histamine and 5-hydroxytryptamine. Acetylcholine causes a reduction in pulmonary vascular resistance.

Anaesthesia

There is as yet no convincing evidence that anaesthesia *per se* has any direct effect on pulmonary vascular resistance, but the circumstances of anaesthesia may be associated with changes in P_{CO_2}, pH and alveolar pressure, all of which are known to influence pulmonary vascular resistance. There is, however, interesting new evidence that anaesthetic concentrations of halothane, diethyl ether and trichloroethylene diminish the hypoxic-vasoconstrictor response in isolated, perfused cat lungs (Sykes et al., 1973). Trichloroethylene has also been shown to have this effect in the intact dog but at the rather high inspired concentration of 1 per cent (Sykes et al., 1975). This work raises the possibility that anaesthesia, by suppression of the reflex, prevents the tendency towards redistribution of pulmonary blood flow to better ventilated areas, and that this contributes to the observed increase in alveolar/arterial P_{O_2} difference which follows the induction of anaesthesia.

Structural factors which influence pulmonary vascular resistance

Organic obstruction of pulmonary blood vessels is important in a wide variety of conditions. Obstruction from within the lumen may be caused by emboli (thrombus, fat or gas) or by thrombosis (e.g. the chicken fat thrombus formed when death is imminent). Obstruction arising within the vessel wall is probably the cause of eventual reduction of flow through collapsed areas, and medial hypertrophy causes an increase in vascular resistance in certain cases of pulmonary hypertension due to obstruction of the outflow tract (e.g. mitral stenosis). Kinking of vessels may cause partial obstruction during extreme reduction of lung volume (*Figure 91*). Obstruction arising from outside the vessel wall may be due to a variety of pathological conditions (tumour, abscess, etc.) or to surgical manipulations during thoracotomy. Finally, vessels may be destroyed in emphysema and certain inflammatory conditions, causing a reduction in the total pulmonary vascular bed and an increase in vascular resistance.

PULMONARY OEDEMA

(see reviews by Fishman, 1972 and Staub, 1974)

Pulmonary oedema is defined as an increase in pulmonary extravascular water, which occurs when transudation (or exudation) exceeds the capacity of lymphatic drainage. In severe manifestations, it interferes with pulmonary gas exchange and constitutes a grave threat to life. It is all too common in the intensive therapy situation.

Sequence of development

Whatever the aetiology of pulmonary oedema, the sequence of fluid accumulation seems to be the same. Four stages may be described (*Figure 93*).

1. *Interstitial pulmonary oedema.* The earliest stage consists of an increase in interstitial fluid without alveolar flooding. At least with the light microscope, this is first detected as a 'cuffing' by distended lymphatics around the branches of the bronchi and pulmonary arteries (*see Plate 2* of Staub, Nagano and Pearce, 1967). Fluid also accumulates in the interstitial space of the alveolar septa, but this can only be demonstrated by electron microscopy in the early stages (Fishman, 1972; Szidon, Pietra and Fishman, 1972).

In a later stage of interstitial pulmonary oedema, the peribronchial and perivascular cuffing becomes more marked and is probably responsible for the characteristic butterfly pattern visible on chest radiography. Thickened alveolar septa become visible on light microscopy but the details can only be seen by electron microscopy. Cottrell et al. (1967) reported that, in haemodynamic pulmonary oedema (caused by an excessive transudation pressure gradient), the expansion of the interstitial space is not symmetrical on the two sides of the pulmonary capillary but is concentrated on the 'service' side which contains the collagen fibrils (*see Figure* 7). On the opposite ('active') side of the capillary, the capillary endothelium tends to remain in apposition with the alveolar epi-

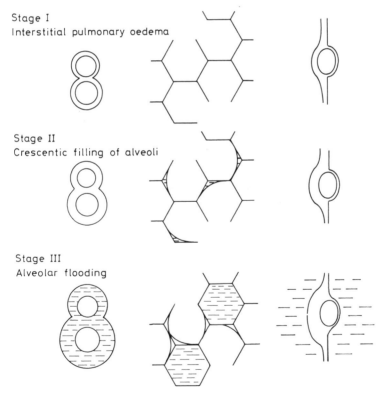

Stage I
Interstitial pulmonary oedema

Stage II
Crescentic filling of alveoli

Stage III
Alveolar flooding

Figure 93. Stages in the development of pulmonary oedema. On the left is shown the development of the cuff of distended lymphatics around the branches of the bronchi and pulmonary arteries. In the middle is the appearance of the alveoli by light microscopy (fixed in inflation). On the right is the appearance of the pulmonary capillaries by electron microscopy. The active side of the capillary is to the right. For an explanation of the stages, see text

thelium, with no great increase in the total thickness of the alveolar-capillary membrane. It would thus seem that gas exchange should continue normally at this stage, which is fortunate for the patient. Physical signs are generally absent in purely interstitial pulmonary oedema.

2. *Crescentic filling of alveoli.*   In the next stage of pulmonary oedema, interstitial oedema of the alveolar septa is increased and fluid begins to pass into the alveolar lumen where it first appears as crescents in the angles between adjacent septa. There is still no flooding and interference with gas exchange should not be gross.

3. *Alveolar flooding.*   In the third stage, there is alveolar flooding which is quantal. Some alveoli are totally flooded while others, frequently adjacent, have only the crescents described above or else no fluid at all in the lumen. It seems likely that fluid accumulates up to a point at which there is a critical radius of curvature when surface tension effects sharply increase the transudation pressure gradient. This would produce flooding on an all-or-none basis for each individual alveolus.

Clearly, there can be no effective gas exchange in a flooded alveolus and the over-all defect of gas exchange presents as a venous admixture with a slight increase in physiological dead space. Râles can be heard on auscultation and the lung fields show over-all opacity in the chest radiograph. The condition can often be distinguished from other forms of pathological venous admixture by the rapidity of development and response to treatment.

4. *Froth in the air passages.*   The fourth and final stage of pulmonary oedema consists of alveolar flooding that is so extensive that fluid spills into the air passages which become filled with froth. Characteristically, the froth is pink-stained from erythrocytes which pass into the alveolar lumen. Under these conditions, there is gross interference with gas exchange and there is imminent danger of death.

Aetiology of pulmonary oedema

Intravascular pulmonary capillary pressure is normally about 1 kPa (7·5 mm Hg) above alveolar pressure. Staub (1974) reviewed the evidence for his belief that the interstitial space around the capillaries has a pressure which cycles positive and negative with breathing but, on average, equals the alveolar pressure. However, Meyer, Meyer and Guyton (1968) carried out direct measurements of interstitial pressure with implanted capsules and reached the conclusion that the pressure was 1·3 kPa (10 mm Hg) below atmospheric. This would mean enhanced transudation from the capillaries to the interstitial space but not onwards into the alveolar lumen.

The hydrostatic transmural pressure difference tending to produce transudation is offset by the osmotic pressure of the plasma proteins (3·3 kPa or 25 mm Hg) which tends to retain fluid in the intravascular compartment. There is a considerable measure of agreement that pulmonary oedema develops in dogs when the left atrial pressure exceeds about 3 kPa (22·5 mm Hg).

The balance between hydrostatic pressure gradient and protein concentration gradient can be disturbed under a variety of circumstances and these form the basis for the classification of the aetiology of pulmonary oedema.

Increased pulmonary capillary transmural pressure gradient (haemodynamic pulmonary oedema).   This is the most important group of causes of pulmonary oedema. Absolute hypervolaemia may arise from overtransfusion, excessive and rapid administration of other blood volume expanders or from accidental access of irrigation fluids through open venous channels in hollow organs, as for example during prostatectomy. Relative redistribution of the blood volume to the lungs may occur from use of the Trendelenburg position or occlusive limb torniquets. Vasopressor mechanisms and drugs act on the systemic circulation to a greater extent than on the pulmonary circulation and this has resulted in pulmonary oedema.

A rise in pulmonary venous pressure leading to an increased pulmonary capillary pressure may occur in any form of left heart failure, including left ventricular failure, arrhythmias, mitral valve lesions and rare conditions such as atrial myxoma. Excessively high pulmonary blood flow may cause a critical rise in pulmonary capillary pressure and this may result from left-to-right cardiac shunts, anaemia or, rarely, as a result of exercise. Finally, the transmural pressure gradient may be increased by the use of subatmospheric airway pressure when using a 'negative phase' during IPP ventilation (page 159) or by incorrect clearance of secretions by intratracheal suction. At all times, intravascular pressures are higher in the dependent parts of the lung, and pulmonary oedema usually appears first in these areas.

Decreased plasma protein osmotic pressure.   This is seldom the primary cause of pulmonary oedema. However, a reduced level of plasma proteins decreases the critical level of the capillary transmural pressure gradient at which transudation occurs (Guyton and Lindsey, 1959). Low plasma albumin levels are not uncommon in gravely ill patients and are frequently seen in patients undergoing intensive therapy. In such patients, left atrial pressures should always be considered in relation to the plasma albumin levels.

Increased pulmonary capillary permeability.   Fulminating pulmonary oedema may very quickly follow damage to the capillary endothelium caused by a wide variety of agents. These include the response to acids, particularly inhaled gastric contents resulting in Mendelson's syndrome (1946). A very similar condition follows the inhalation of nitrogen dioxide (Greenbaum et al., 1967a) and a variety of war gases, including chlorine and phosgene. Experimentally the condition may be produced in animals by the intravenous injection of oleic acid or alloxan. A very similar condition occurs in oxygen toxicity (page 426) and in 'shock lung' (page 296).

The special feature of increased permeability is loss of protein into the interstitial space and the lumen of the alveoli. This clearly impedes resorption of the fluid and may also leave behind a shell of protein lining the alveoli, with a histological appearance similar to the hyaline membrane of the infant respiratory distress syndrome. It is characterized by extreme reduction in compliance and gross interference with gas exchange.

Lymphatic obstruction.   This is a theoretical cause of pulmonary oedema but one which seems to be of little importance in practice.

Miscellaneous causes. 'Neurogenic' pulmonary oedema may follow head injuries or other cerebral lesions. It has been demonstrated that it may be prevented in the experimental animal by pulmonary vagal block (as in an autotransplanted lung) but the mechanism remains a mystery.

Acute exposure to altitude may cause pulmonary oedema. It is now known that there may be substantial pulmonary arterial hypertension although the wedge pressure may remain normal (Hultgren and Grover, 1968). It is possible that this form of pulmonary oedema may be due to mechanical stretching of the vascular endothelium, resulting in increased permeability to plasma proteins (Szidon, Pietra and Fishman, 1972). This may also provide the explanation of pulmonary oedema occurring in Gram-negative septicaemia which appears to cause pulmonary venous constriction in the dog (Kuida et al., 1958).

Diamorphine overdosage occasionally causes pulmonary oedema and it has been suggested that this may be secondary to pulmonary hypertension caused by hypoxaemia.

Diagnosis of pulmonary oedema

It has been explained above that the interstitial phase of pulmonary oedema usually produces no clinical signs and diagnosis from the chest radiograph is often difficult. It is only when alveolar flooding commences that physical signs are present and, at this stage, the alveolar/arterial Po_2 gradient is usually increased. What is required is an *in vivo* method of measurement of lung water. In the past the most hopeful approach has been the double indicator method yielding a pair of dye curves (page 271). One indicator is chosen to remain within the circulation while the other diffuses into the interstitial fluid. Staub (1974) discusses the limitation of these methods and there is widespread agreement that they are technically very difficult and that a high level of accuracy is required to demonstrate small changes in lung water. Measurement of thoracic electrical impedance is an alternative approach but one which is also beset with difficulties. Only rarely will control measurements before the onset of oedema be available.

There are a variety of methods of determining lung water in post-mortem specimens. Simple lung weight is useful. In the author's hospital, it is the practice to fix the lungs in inflation with formalin vapour at $37^\circ C$ (Wright et al., 1974). The lung may then be examined radiographically and sections prepared for microscopy. Oedema fluid is clearly visible in stained sections.

Pathophysiology of pulmonary oedema

Reference has been made above to the physiological dysfunctions arising from various degrees and types of pulmonary oedema. In summary, it may be said that interstitial oedema does not generally interfere with gas exchange although it may be possible to demonstrate a reduction in pulmonary compliance. Even when crescents of fluid are present in the corners of the alveoli, gas exchange is likely to remain normal. Quantal flooding, however, presents as a pulmonary shunt with the magnitude of the shunt reflecting the extent of the flooding. Pulmonary compliance is markedly reduced. When frothing commences, there is interference with ventilation of alveoli which have not been flooded and there is a massive increase in shunt characterized by gross arterial hypoxaemia. The hypoxic drive to respiration and perhaps stimulation of the J receptors (page 55) produces hyperventilation which prevents or minimizes the development of hypercapnia. Eventually, however, the interference with alveolar ventilation is sufficient to cause the P_{CO_2} to rise, particularly if the administration of oxygen has given some protection from hypoxaemia.

Physiological principles of treatment of pulmonary oedema

The highest priority is to restore the arterial P_{O_2} and oxygen enrichment of the inspired gas takes first place. In severe cases, 100 per cent oxygen is required. In the presence of frothing, artificial ventilation will be required to raise the alveolar P_{O_2}, but suction should first be employed to remove as much froth as possible. The second line of treatment is to drive the oedema fluid back into the circulation; IPP ventilation, preferably with PEEP, may achieve spectacular results within a few minutes, particularly when the cause is raised pulmonary capillary pressure. It seems that this improvement is mainly due to elevation of the mean alveolar pressure with reduction of the transmural pressure gradient. However, reduction of cardiac output may also be helpful. Redistribution of blood volume to the periphery may be accomplished by application of venous occlusive cuffs to the limbs and placing the patient in the head-up position. Morphine may exert its beneficial effect by inducing peripheral vasodilatation. The third line of treatment is directed towards aetiological factors, such as hypervolaemia, left ventricular failure, hypoproteinaemia, etc.

The exudative type of pulmonary oedema is much more difficult to treat. The measures outlined above afford symptomatic relief but increased permeability of capillary endothelium may be intractable. Furthermore, protein may remain in the alveoli and form a 'hyaline' membrane.

PRINCIPLES OF MEASUREMENT OF THE PULMONARY CIRCULATION

Detailed consideration of haemodynamic measurement techniques must lie outside the scope of this book. The following section presents only the broad principles of measurement such as may be required for an understanding of respiratory physiology.

Pulmonary blood volume

Reference has already been made to the review of Harris and Heath (1962) for methods of measurement of pulmonary blood volume. Available methods are based on the technique used for measurement of cardiac output by dye dilution (*see* page 270). In essence, the dye is injected into a central vein and its concentration is recorded in samples aspirated from some point in the systemic arterial tree. Cardiac output is determined by the method described below, and then the interval is measured between the time of the injection of the dye and the mean arrival time of the dye at the sampling point. Cardiac output is multiplied by this time interval to indicate the amount of blood lying between injection and sampling sites. Assumed values for the extrapulmonary blood are then subtracted to indicate the intrapulmonary blood volume.

It is not at all easy to obtain satisfactory results with this method. The 'mean arrival time of the dye' is difficult to determine and the correction for the extrapulmonary blood volume can be little more than an inspired guess but may be improved by injection into the pulmonary artery with sampling from the left ventricle. It may be better to omit the correction and use the term 'central blood volume' which implies an appropriate lack of definition.

Pulmonary capillary blood volume may be measured as a byproduct of the measurement of pulmonary diffusing capacity, and the method is discussed in Chapter 10.

Pulmonary vascular pressures

Pressure measurements within the pulmonary circulation are almost always made with electronic differential pressure transducers. These invariably have a diaphragm which is deformed by a pressure difference across it. The movement of the diaphragm may be transduced to an electrical signal in a variety of ways. Its movement may influence special resistors of which the resistance is a function of their length (strain gauge). The diaphragm may form one plate of a capacitor of which the other plate is fixed. As the diaphragm is moved the distance between the plates changes and this alters the capacitance of the device (capacitance manometer). Finally, the diaphragm may be linked to the core of a coil whose inductance is thus altered by movements of the diaphragm (inductance manometer). It is relatively simple for changes in resistance, capacitance or inductance to be detected, amplified and displayed as indicative of the pressures across the diaphragm of the transducer.

The space on the reference side of the diaphragm is in communication with atmosphere, oesophageal balloon or left atrial blood, as the case may be (*Figure 90*). The other side of the diaphragm is filled with a liquid (usually heparanized saline) which is in direct communication with the blood of which the pressure is being measured.

If the system is to have the ability to respond to rapid changes of pressure, damping must be reduced to a minimum. This requires the total exclusion of bubbles of air from the manometer and connecting tubing, and the intravascular cannula must be unobstructed. Damping does not influence the measurement of mean pressure but reduces the apparent systolic pressure and increases the apparent diastolic pressure. The basic principles of pressure transducers have been reviewed by Leraand (1962) and sources of error in their use have been described by Crul (1962) and Kelman (1971).

These methods do not measure absolute pressure and can only be used for comparison with a primary standard (such as a column of mercury of known height). Electrical signals are often used as secondary standards, but must be checked at intervals against primary standards.

Electrical manometry yields a plot of instantaneous pressure against time (*Figure 94a*). From this it is often necessary to calculate the mean pressure. This is *not* simply:

$$\frac{\text{systolic pressure} + \text{diastolic pressure}}{2}$$

since the duration of diastole is greater than that of systole and therefore the effective or integrated mean must be weighted in favour of the diastolic pressure. Mean pressure is often taken to be one-third of the way from diastolic to systolic pressure (i.e. diastolic plus one-third of pulse pressure), but it is more correctly derived from assessing the area under the instantaneous pressure curve. A rectangle is then constructed with length equal to the duration of one cardiac cycle and area equal to the area under the pressure curve over the same time interval. The height of the rectangle indicates the mean pressure.

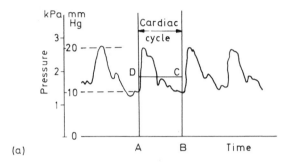

(a)

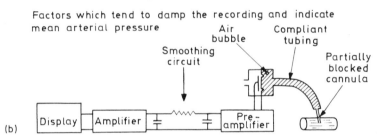

(b)

Figure 94. Determination of mean pulmonary arterial pressure. (a) An actual trace of instantaneous intravascular pulmonary arterial pressure during four cardiac cycles. For the second cycle, a rectangle has been constructed (ABCD) which has an area equal to that under the curve over the same time interval. The height of the rectangle (AD) indicates the effective integrated mean pressure. It will be seen to be approximately equal to diastolic pressure plus one-third of pulse pressure. (b) Factors which tend to damp the recording of instantaneous pressure (i.e. lower the indicated systolic pressure and raise the indicated diastolic pressure) tending towards an indication of the integrated mean pressure. Some of these factors are accidental (e.g. air bubble or blocked cannula) but others (e.g. smoothing circuit) may be employed deliberately to avoid the tedious method of calculation of mean pressure shown in (a)

More simply, the mean pressure may be determined by damping the measurement (or display) of the instantaneous pressure. This may be done on the actual measurement system (e.g. by allowing the intravascular cannula to become partly occluded) or by electrical means. These methods are illustrated in *Figure 94b*. It should be noted that it is generally easier to measure mean pressure than instantaneous pressure. Exactly similar considerations apply to the determination of mean intrathoracic pressure (page 124). In the case of the intrathoracic pressure, the relevant cycle is, of course, that of respiration and not the heart beat.

Pulmonary blood flow

The total flow of blood through the pulmonary circulation may be measured by four groups of methods, each of which contains many variants (Kelman, 1971).

The Fick principle states that the amount of oxygen picked up from the respired gases equals the amount added to the blood which flows through the lungs. Alternatively, the amount of carbon dioxide exhaled equals the amount lost by the blood which flows through the lungs. In the case of oxygen it is evident that the oxygen uptake of the subject must equal the product of pulmonary blood flow and arteriovenous oxygen content difference. This is conveniently expressed in Pappenheimer symbols (*see* Appendix C):

$$\dot{V}_{O_2} = \dot{Q} \, (Ca_{O_2} - C\bar{v}_{O_2})$$

therefore

$$\dot{Q} = \frac{\dot{V}_{O_2}}{Ca_{O_2} - C\bar{v}_{O_2}}$$

All the quantities on the right-hand side can be measured, although determination of the oxygen content of the mixed venous blood requires catheterization of the right ventricle or preferably the pulmonary artery.

Interpretation of the result is less easy. The calculated value includes the intrapulmonary arteriovenous shunt, but the situation is complicated beyond the possibility of easy solution if there is appreciable extrapulmonary admixture of venous blood (*see Figure 88*).

Indirect methods avoid right heart catheterization by calculating the composition of mixed venous blood by measurement of changes in composition of rebreathed gas. This is only practicable in the case of carbon dioxide, and determination of mixed venous Pco_2 is described in Chapter 11. Unfortunately, the derivation of mixed venous CO_2 content is not sufficiently accurate for the method to be a satisfactory alternative to the direct Fick method.

One important source of error is of particular concern to the anaesthetist. Between the pulmonary capillaries and the apparatus for measurement of oxygen consumption is a large volume of gas, comprising the subject's lungs, air passages, mouthpiece, valve box, etc. The method requires that the amount of oxygen in this volume remain constant throughout the period of measurement (1–5 minutes). Clearly both the volume of the space and the composition of its content must not be allowed to vary, and this can usually be achieved when the subject is breathing air. If the concentration of oxygen is allowed to alter during the period of measurement, a considerable error may be introduced. Thus if a patient breathing nitrous oxide and oxygen is connected to a closed-circuit spirometer containing oxygen for the measurement of oxygen uptake, nitrous oxide will pass from the patient to the spirometer and change both the total gas volume and its composition. This difficulty may be overcome, but only by quite elaborate methodology (Nunn and Pouliot, 1962). Measurement of oxygen consumption is discussed at the end of Chapter 12.

Dye dilution. Currently the most popular technique for measurement of cardiac output is by dye dilution. Measurement can be repeated up to at least 20 times at three-minute intervals with dye and indefinitely with a thermal indicator.

An indicator substance is suddenly introduced into a large vein and its concentration is measured continuously at a sampling site in the systemic arterial tree. *Figure 95a* shows the method as it is applied to continuous non-circulating flow as, for example, of fluids through a pipeline. In the top right-hand corner is shown the sudden injection of the bolus of dye. It is carried downstream past a sampling point where some of the fluid in the pipe is drawn through a device which performs a continuous analysis of the concentration of the dye in the

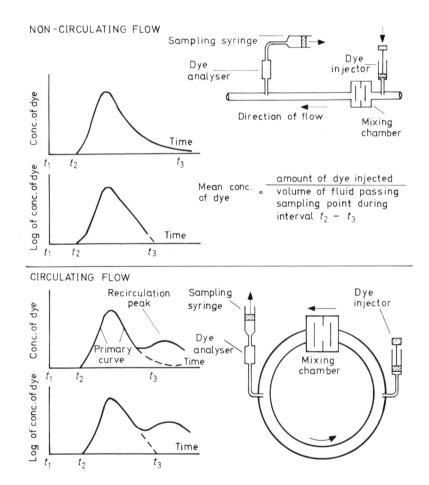

$$\text{Mean conc. of dye} = \frac{\text{amount of dye injected}}{\text{volume of fluid passing sampling point during interval } t_2 - t_3}$$

Figure 95. Measurement of flow by dye dilution. (a) shows the measurement of continuous non-circulating flow rate of fluid in a pipeline. The bolus of dye is injected upstream and its concentration is continuously monitored downstream. The relationship of the relevant quantities is shown in the equation. Mean concentration of dye is determined from the area under the curve as shown in Figure 94. (b) indicates the more complicated situation when recirculation occurs and the front of the circulating dye laps its own tail, giving a recirculation peak. Reconstruction of the primary curve is based on extrapolation of the primary curve before recirculation occurs. This is facilitated by the fact that the down curve is exponential and therefore a straight line on a logarithmic plot

fluid. The concentration is displayed on the Y axis of the graph against time on the X axis. The dye is injected at time t_1 and is first detected at the sampling point at time t_2. The uppermost curve shows the form of a typical curve. There is a rapid rise to maximum concentration followed by a decay which is exponential wash-out in form (see Appendix E), reaching insignificant levels at time t_3. The second graph shows the concentration (Y axis) on logarithmic co-ordinates. Under these circumstances the exponential part of the decay curve becomes a straight line (*see Figure 152*). If we consider only the part of the graph between times t_2 and t_3, it is evident that:

mean concentration of dye

$$= \frac{\text{amount of dye injected}}{\text{volume of fluid flowing past sampling point during the interval } t_2 - t_3}$$

$$= \frac{\text{amount of dye injected}}{\text{flow rate of fluid} \times \text{time interval } t_2 - t_3}$$

This equation may now be rearranged to show the flow rate of the fluid:

$$\text{flow rate of fluid} = \frac{\text{amount of dye injected}}{\text{mean concentration of dye} \times \text{time interval } t_2 - t_3}$$

Now the denominator of the right-hand side will be indicated by the area under the curve, and the flow rate may thus be readily calculated provided that the calibration of the dye analyser has been established.

Figure 95b shows the more complicated situation when fluid is flowing round a circuit. Under these conditions, the front of the dye-laden fluid may lap its own tail so that a recirculation peak appears on the graph before the primary peak has decayed to insignificant levels. This commonly occurs when cardiac output is determined in man, and steps must be taken to reconstruct the tail of the primary curve as it would have been had recirculation not taken place. To do this we make use of the fact that the exponential wash-out phase has usually been entered before the recirculation peak appears. This is clearly shown in the lowermost of the four graphs. On the logarithmic plot, it is possible to detect the point at which the recirculation peak appears and the initial part of the down curve may be extrapolated in a straight line. This is replotted on a linear scale (graph three) and the area of the reconstructed primary curve determined. For technical details of the method, reference should be made to Kinsman, Moore and Hamilton (1929), Zierler (1962) and Kelman (1966c).

Many different indicators have been used for the dye dilution technique, but currently the most satisfactory appears to be 'coolth'. A bolus of cold saline is injected and the dip in temperature is recorded downstream with the temperature record corresponding to the dye curve. No blood sampling is required and temperature is measured directly with a thermometer mounted on the catheter. The 'coolth' is dispersed in the systemic circulation and therefore there is no recirculation peak to complicate the calculation. The thermal method is particularly suitable for repeated measurements.

Direct measurements of intravascular flow rate.   The instantaneous flow through a blood vessel may be measured with an electromagnetic flowmeter probe in the form of a cuff attached directly to the blood vessel. The method is clearly of limited application to man but this has had important application in animal studies. They may be used, for example, for comparisons of left and right pulmonary artery blood flows, which would be very difficult to make by any other means. The *velocity* of blood flow in a vessel may be measured by the Doppler shift using ultrasound. This can only be translated into *flow rate* if the diameter of the vessel is known. Practical difficulties arise in being sure that the signal arises solely from the vessel under consideration.

Methods based on uptake of inert tracer gases. A modified Fick method of measurement of cardiac output may be employed with fairly soluble inert gases such as acetylene (Grollman, 1929). With this technique, a single breath of a dilute acetylene mixture is taken and held. It is then exhaled and the alveolar (or more correctly end-expiratory) concentration of acetylene determined. Analysis of volume and composition of expired gas permits measurement of acetylene uptake. Since the duration of the procedure does not permit recirculation, it may be assumed that the mixed venous concentration of acetylene is zero. The Fick equation then simplifies to the following:

acetylene uptake = cardiac output x arterial acetylene concentration

The arterial acetylene concentration is derived from the assumption that the arterial acetylene tension equals the alveolar acetylene tension which is directly measured on the expired gas. Content is derived from tension using an assumed value for the solubility coefficient of acetylene in blood. This method entirely avoids sampling of blood and does not therefore require cannulation of vessels, a feature which appeals to the subjects.

The technique outlined above had fallen into disuse for a variety of reasons principally concerned with technical difficulties in making the various measurements. The idea behind the method has come back into prominence following the introduction of the body plethysmograph which has already been mentioned on page 134, in connection with the measurement of airway resistance. Its use in the determination of cardiac output is for the measurement of the uptake of the tracer gas (usually nitrous oxide at the present time). The subject inhales a mixture of about 15 per cent nitrous oxide, and holds his breath with his mouth open. Nitrous oxide uptake is measured directly from the fall of the pressure within the box, and the arterial nitrous oxide content is derived from the alveolar nitrous oxide tension and the solubility coefficient in blood in exactly the manner described above for acetylene (Lee and DuBois, 1955).

The methods of the fourth group outlined above have the following characteristics in common.

1. They measure pulmonary capillary blood flow, excluding any flow through shunts. This is in contrast to the Fick and dye methods.
2. The assumption that the tension of the tracer gas is the same in end-expiratory gas and arterial blood is invalid in the presence of disorders of blood and gas distribution within the lungs.
3. Some of the tracer gas dissolves in the tissues lining the respiratory tract and is carried away by blood perfusing these tissues. The indicated blood flow is therefore higher than the actual pulmonary capillary blood flow.

When the body plethysmograph is used to measure the tracer gas uptake, it is possible to detect pulsatile uptake synchronous with systole. This is taken as evidence that pulmonary capillary blood flow is pulsatile.

Chapter 9   Distribution of the Pulmonary Blood Flow

Anatomical Maldistribution of Pulmonary Blood Flow
The Concept of Venous Admixture
Forms of Venous Admixture
Increased Scatter of V/Q Ratios
Anaesthesia
Principles of Assessment of Distribution of Pulmonary Blood Flow

Maldistribution of pulmonary blood flow is the commonest cause of impaired oxygenation of the arterial blood. The pulmonary blood flow is probably never distributed evenly to all parts of the lung field and the degree of non-uniformity is usually much greater than is the case for inspired gas. Uneven distribution may be present between the two lungs and between different lobes but always between successive horizontal slices of the lungs. These differences can be measured and are discussed in this chapter under the heading of 'Anatomical maldistribution' since the relevant zones of lung can be defined anatomically.

Maldistribution may also occur diffusely between tiny zones of lung which cannot be defined anatomically. The chief manifestation of this type of maldistribution is impairment of oxygenation of arterial blood, and the effect can be quantified in physiological terms although the disorder can seldom be explained in morphological terms.

Maldistribution of pulmonary perfusion is only relevant to the oxygenation of blood in so far as it is related to the distribution of ventilation. If, for example, all perfusion and all ventilation were confined to one lung, gas exchange could be normal. If, however, perfusion were confined to one lung and ventilation to the other, the results would be disastrous. It is useful, therefore, to consider ventilation/perfusion ratios—in this example zero for the first lung and infinity for the second. In general, the smaller the scatter of regional ventilation/perfusion ratios, the better is the gas exchange. Wide scatter about the mean and particularly areas with ratios of infinity or zero, cause less efficient gas exchange.

It is often convenient to consider abnormalities of ventilation/perfusion relationships as if the resultant defects were entirely due to increased alveolar dead space and/or increased venous admixture or pulmonary shunting. The concept of alveolar dead space has been considered in Chapter 7; the concept of venous admixture is considered below.

ANATOMICAL MALDISTRIBUTION OF PULMONARY
BLOOD FLOW

Distribution between the two lungs

Use of a divided airway (such as a Carlen's tube) has permitted accurate estimation of the partition of the tidal volume between the two lungs. Unfortunately, no method of comparable simplicity exists to study the partition of the pulmonary blood flow in man. It might at first sight appear that a Carlen's tube would permit solution of the Fick equation for the two lungs separately. This, however, would require sampling of the blood leaving the two lungs separately, and this could probably be contrived if it were not for the fact that each lung drains through two pulmonary veins. Representative sampling therefore requires blood to be sampled from each vein in proportion to its flow rate and this is not feasible. It is, however, possible to make a rough and ready estimate of the pulmonary venous oxygen content and this enables an approximate idea of unilateral flow to be obtained from the unilateral oxygen consumption, which is easily derived by using a Carlen's tube and a pair of bronchospirometers.

An alternative approach is to label the pulmonary circulation (with radioactive macroaggregates or [133]xenon dissolved in saline) and then to observe the activity in the two lung fields, either with suitably collimated counters or with a gamma camera. In animals, it is possible to implant electromagnetic flow probes around left and right branches of the pulmonary artery and so to obtain a continuous record of left and right lung blood flow.

Defares et al. (1960) have studied supine subjects using an indirect method based on the Fick principle using CO_2 and obtained values for unilateral flow which agree closely with the distribution of ventilation observed by Svanberg (1957) in the supine position (*see Table 18*).

In the lateral position there is an increased perfusion of the dependent lung, as would be expected from considerations of the effect of gravity on the pulmonary circulation (page 276). In the dog, with its narrow chest, the effect is not large, and Rehder, Theye and Fowler (1961) reported only small increases in perfusion of the dependent lung when dogs were turned from the supine to the lateral position. Surprisingly, the effect was reversed when the thorax was opened.

In man the thorax is of the order of 30 cm in lateral diameter and so, in the lateral position, the column of blood in the pulmonary circulation exerts a hydrostatic pressure which is high in relation to the mean pulmonary arterial pressure. A fairly gross maldistribution is therefore to be expected with much of the upper lung comprising zone 2 and much of the lower lung comprising zone 3 (*see Figure 92*). Using the [133]xenon technique, Kaneko et al. (1966) showed uniform high perfusion of the dependent lung (apparently in zone 3) but with reduced perfusion of the upper lung which appeared to be mainly in zone 2. There was no evidence of the existence of a zone 1 (absent perfusion).

The increased perfusion of the lower lung is advantageous during thoracic surgery in the lateral position. Surgical intervention frequently limits or prevents ventilation of the exposed (upper) lung. Ventilation is thus deflected to the lower lung which presumably receives most of the pulmonary circulation. Gas exchange is undoubtedly impaired (page 436) but the effects are mitigated by the gravitationally imposed distribution of the pulmonary circulation. Nevertheless, the high perfusion of the dependent lung, combined with its low relative lung volume (*see Figure 63*), cause the dependent lung to be at increased risk of absorption collapse (Potgieter, 1959).

Distribution in horizontal slices of the lung

In the previous chapter, it was shown how the pulmonary vascular resistance is mainly in the capillary bed and is governed by the relationship between alveolar, pulmonary arterial and pulmonary venous pressures. *Figure 92* presented the concept of the vascular weir with pulmonary vascular resistance decreasing and pulmonary blood flow increasing with distance down the lung, until zone 4 is entered where there is increased alveolar vascular resistance in larger vessels apparently due to increased interstitial pressure. This results in reduced perfusion of the most dependent part of the lung.

The first studies with radioactive gases took place at total lung capacity and showed flow increasing progressively down the lung in the upright position (West, 1963). However, it was later found that there was a significant reduction of flow in the most dependent parts of the lung (zone 4) which became progressively more important as lung volume was reduced from total lung capacity towards the residual volume (Hughes et al., 1968). *Figure 96* is redrawn from the work of Hughes' group and shows that pulmonary perfusion (per alveolus) is, in fact, reasonably uniform in the normal tidal range. However, the dependent parts of the lung contain more but smaller alveoli than the apices at FRC and the perfusion *per unit lung volume* is still increased at the bases.

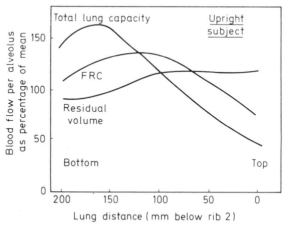

Figure 96. Pulmonary perfusion per alveolus as a percentage of that expected if all alveoli were equally perfused. At total lung capacity, perfusion increases down to 150 mm, below which perfusion is slightly decreased (zone 4). At FRC, zone 4 conditions apply below 100 mm, and at residual volume the perfusion gradient is actually reversed. It should be noted that perfusion has been calculated per alveolus. *If shown as perfusion* per unit lung volume, *the non-uniformity at total lung capacity would be the same because alveoli are all the same size at total lung capacity. At FRC there are more but smaller alveoli at the bases and the non-uniformity would be greater. (Data are redrawn from Hughes et al. (1968))*

In the *supine* position the differences in blood flow between apices and bases are replaced by differences between anterior and posterior aspects. Over the 200 mm (20 cm) height of the lung field in the average supine adult, the perfusion *per unit lung volume* increases progressively, with the most dependent parts receiving approximately double the perfusion of the uppermost parts at FRC (Kaneko et al., 1966; Hulands et al., 1970). However, as in the upright position, the dependent parts of the lungs contain more but smaller alveoli, and perfusion *per alveolus* is almost uniform down the lung (Kaneko et al., 1966). Zones 1 and 4 conditions were not observed in these studies.

The effect of *anaesthesia, paralysis* and *artificial ventilation* on distribution of perfusion was studied by Hulands et al. (1970). They found no major change in the distribution of perfusion in four subjects studied before and after induction of anaesthesia. There was no evidence of failure of perfusion (zone 1) in the upper parts of the lung, which might have provided a plausible explanation of the increased alveolar dead space observed during anaesthesia. Nothing was found which would explain the increased alveolar/arterial Po_2 difference observed during anaesthesia.

THE CONCEPT OF VENOUS ADMIXTURE

Nomenclature of venous admixture

Venous admixture refers to the degree of admixture of mixed venous blood with pulmonary end-capillary blood which would be required to produce the observed difference between the arterial and pulmonary end-capillary Po_2. (Pulmonary end-capillary Po_2 is usually taken as equal to ideal alveolar Po_2 — *see* Chapter 10.) The calculation is shown in *Figure 97*. Note that the venous admixture is not the *actual* amount of venous blood which mingles with the arterial blood but the *calculated* amount which would be required to produce the arterial blood-gas picture. The difference is due to the contribution to the arterial blood of blood from alveoli having a V/Q ratio of more than zero but less than the normal value. The strict quantitative basis of the calculation is also destroyed by the admixture of bronchial and Thebesian venous blood of unknown oxygen content. *Venous admixture* is thus a convenient index but does not define the anatomical pathway of shunt.

Anatomical shunt, frank shunt or shunt (unqualified).   These terms refer to the amount of venous blood which mingles with the pulmonary end-capillary blood on the arterial side of the circulation. The terms embrace bronchial and Thebesian venous blood flow and also admixture of mixed venous blood caused by atelectasis, bronchial obstruction, congenital heart disease with right-to-left shunting, etc. This excludes blood draining any alveoli with V/Q ratio of more than zero.

Pathological shunt is sometimes used to describe the forms of anatomical shunt which do not occur in the normal subjct.

Physiological shunt is, unfortunately, used in two senses. In the first sense it is used to describe the degree of venous admixture which occurs in a normal

healthy subject. Differences between the actual measured venous admixture and
the 'physiological shunt' thus indicate the amount of venous admixture which
results from the disease process. In its alternative sense, physiological shunt is
synonymous with venous admixture and is derived from the mixing equation
(*Figure 97*) in a manner exactly analogous to the derivation of the physiological
dead space from Bohr's equation. It is then possible to subtract the anatomical
shunt from the physiological shunt and so derive some idea of the malfunction
due to abnormal ventilation/perfusion ratios. This is comparable to the
derivation of alveolar dead space.

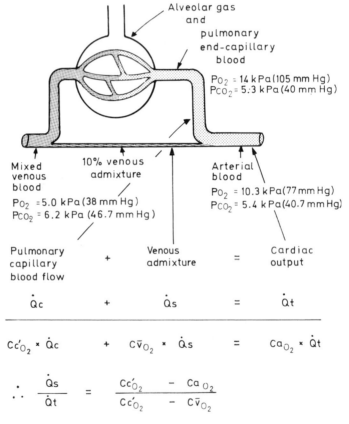

*Figure 97. A schematic representation of venous admixture. It makes the simplifying
assumption that all the arterial blood has come either from alveoli with normal V/Q ratio or
from a shunt. This is never true but it forms a convenient method of quantifying venous
admixture and can be used as a basis for oxygen therapy. The shunt equation is similar to
the Bohr equation and is based on the axiomatic relationship that the total amount of
oxygen in one minute's flow of arterial blood equals the sum of the amount of oxygen in
one minute's flow through the pulmonary capillaries and the amount of oxygen in one
minute's flow through the shunt. Amount of oxygen in one minute's flow of blood equals
the product of the blood flow rate and the concentration of oxygen in the blood. $\dot{Q}t$, total
cardiac output; $\dot{Q}c$, pulmonary capillary blood flow; $\dot{Q}s$, flow of blood through shunt; Ca_{O_2},
concentration of oxygen in arterial blood; Cc'_{O_2}, concentration of oxygen in pulmonary
end-capillary blood; $C\bar{v}_{O_2}$, concentration of oxygen in mixed venous blood*

Physiological dead space	Physiological shunt (calculated venous admixture)
=	=
anatomical dead space	anatomical shunt
+	+
alveolar dead space ('dead-space-like effect' due to areas of increased ventilation/perfusion ratio).	'shunt-like effect' due to areas of decreased ventilation/perfusion ratio.

The author tends to retreat in the face of alternative definitions of important terms. In this case, there is no hardship in avoiding the term 'physiological shunt'. In its first sense 'normal degree of venous admixture' seems unequivocal, while in its second sense it can easily be replaced by 'calculated venous admixture', both terms being self-explanatory.

Effects of venous admixture

Qualitatively, it will be clear that venous admixture reduces the over-all efficiency of gas exchange and results in arterial blood-gas tensions which are closer to those of mixed venous blood than would otherwise be the case. Quantitatively, the effect is simple provided that we consider the *contents* of gases in blood. Considering a simple anatomical shunt such as that shown in *Figure 97* we may take as an example:

pulmonary end-capillary oxygen content	20 vols %
mixed venous blood oxygen content	10 vols %

It will be clear that a 50 per cent venous admixture will result in an arterial oxygen content of 15 vols per cent, a 25 per cent venous admixture will result in an arterial oxygen content of 17·5 vols per cent, and so on. The calculation is based on the conservation of mass:

the amount of oxygen flowing in the arterial system in each minute	=	the amount of oxygen leaving the pulmonary capillaries in each minute	+	the amount of oxygen flowing through the venous admixture in each minute

For each term in this equation the amount of blood flowing per minute may be expressed as the product of the blood flow rate and the oxygen content of the blood flowing in the vessel. In the case of the pulmonary capillary blood flow, this equals $\dot{Q}c$ *times* Cc'_{O_2} and so on (the symbols are explained in *Figure 97* and Appendix C). *Figure 97* shows how the equation may be cleared and solved for the ratio of the venous admixture to the cardiac output. The final equation has a form similar to that of the Bohr equation for the physiological dead space (page 228).

To calculate the venous admixture, it is first necessary to determine the gas contents of the arterial, pulmonary end-capillary and mixed venous blood. In practice these are usually measured or calculated as oxygen tensions, and content is then derived from the oxygen dissociation curve and the oxygen capacity of the blood, allowance being made for dissolved oxygen. Conversely, if we know the degree of venous admixture, the effect on arterial blood-gas *contents* may be easily calculated. If, hower, we require to know the effect on arterial blood Po_2, we must undertake the tiresome calculation of tension from content using the oxygen dissociation curve and the oxygen capacity of the blood.*

The shape of the oxygen dissociation curve looms very large in any consideration of venous admixture. If a normal subject has a pulmonary end-capillary Po_2 of 14 kPa (105 mm Hg) (the normal value) and a venous admixture of 5 per cent of his cardiac output, the consequent reduction of his arterial oxygen content or saturation is too small to be measured easily (*Table 19*). However, due to the flatness of the oxygen dissociation curve in this range, there is a considerable fall in arterial Po_2 which may be detected without difficulty.

Table 19. EFFECT OF 5 PER CENT VENOUS ADMIXTURE
ON THE DIFFERENCE BETWEEN ARTERIAL AND
PULMONARY END-CAPILLARY BLOOD LEVELS OF
CARBON DIOXIDE AND OXYGEN

	Pulmonary end-capillary blood	*Arterial blood*
CO_2 content (vols %)	49·7	50·0
Pco_2 (kPa)	5·29	5·33
Pco_2 (mm Hg)	39·7	40·0
O_2 content (vols %)	19·9	19·6
O_2 saturation (%)	97·8	96·8
Po_2 (kPa)	14·0	12·0
Po_2 (mm Hg)	105	90

It has been assumed that the arterial/venous oxygen content difference is 4·5 vols per cent and that the haemoglobin concentration is 14·9 g per cent. Typical changes in Po_2 and Pco_2 have been shown for a 10 per cent venous admixture in *Figure 97*.

The effect of this degree of venous admixture on arterial CO_2 content is similar in magnitude to that of oxygen content. However, due to the relative steepness of the CO_2 dissociation curve in this range the effect on arterial Pco_2 is also very small and is far less than the change in arterial Po_2 (*Table 19*). Two conclusions may be drawn.

1. Arterial Po_2 is the most useful blood-gas measurement for the detection of venous admixture.
2. Venous admixture reduces the arterial Po_2 markedly, but has relatively little effect on arterial Pco_2 or the content of either CO_2 or O_2, unless the venous admixture is large.

Quite large degrees of venous admixture are needed to produce clinically recognizable reduction of arterial oxygen content, and elevations of Pco_2 are seldom seen. It is, in fact, more usual for venous admixture to *lower* the Pco_2 indirectly since the resultant lowering of the Po_2 commonly causes hyper-

* These calculations may be expedited by the use of the computer-written tables produced by Kelman and Nunn (1968) although they are based on an oxygen capacity of 1·39 ml/g of haemoglobin, a value which now appears to be too high (*see* page 401).

ventilation, which more than compensates for the slight elevation of P_{CO_2} which would otherwise result from the venous admixture (*see Figure 66*).

Since the effect of venous admixture on arterial P_{O_2} is so markedly influenced by the slope of the dissociation curve, it will clearly depend upon the section of the dissociation curve which is concerned in a particular situation. Thus if the pulmonary end-capillary P_{O_2} is high (above 40 kPa (300 mm Hg) where the curve is flat), venous admixture causes a very marked fall in arterial P_{O_2} (approximately 2·3 kPa (17 mm Hg) for 1 per cent venous admixture). If, however, the pulmonary end-capillary P_{O_2} is low (below 9·3 kPa (70 mm Hg) where the curve is steep), venous admixture has relatively little effect on arterial P_{O_2} (*see Figure 131* in Chapter 12). It would probably be wrong to consider this from the teleological standpoint, but it is nevertheless convenient to remember that a given degree of venous admixture causes a greater fall of P_{O_2} in the better oxygenated patients and a smaller fall in the less well oxygenated patients.

Effects of scatter of V/Q ratio

The healthy lung receives each minute an alveolar ventilation of about 5 litres and a pulmonary blood flow of about 6 litres. This gives an over-all ventilation/perfusion (V/Q) ratio of 5 : 6 or about 0·85, a figure which is close to, but not directly related to, the respiratory exchange ratio. Not all alveoli have the same V/Q ratio as the mean value for the lungs as a whole.

West's monograph (1965) depicts a spread of V/Q ratios in horizontal slices of the lungs ranging from 3·3 at the top of the lung to 0·63 at the bottom for healthy upright subjects. The variation in regional perfusion was substantially greater than the variation in ventilation. The spread of V/Q ratios is influenced by many factors which alter the distribution of either ventilation or perfusion or both. These have been considered above and in Chapter 7, but include posture, lung volume, inspiratory gas flow rate and age.

It is important to remember that West's original data relate to a slow vital capacity inspiration and not to normal tidal breathing. Hulands et al. (1970) studied supine subjects, breathing at a normal inspiratory flow rate from FRC and found, when they were conscious, a spread of V/Q ratios from 1·0 at the top of the lung down to 0·5 at the bottom. The spread was slightly increased during anaesthesia, paralysis and artificial ventilation to 1·3 at the top and 0·5 at the bottom of the lung.

The study of horizontal strata of the lung does not give the full picture of the spread of ventilation/perfusion ratios, but only the part of maldistribution which is gravity-dependent. It tells us nothing about inhomogeneity within slices of the lung and nothing about areas of alveolar dead space and intrapulmonary shunts which are spread diffusely through the lung fields. It thus seems likely that in the normal subject the true spread of ventilation/perfusion ratios is greater than is indicated by study of horizontal strata, and this is certainly true in diseases such as emphysema.

Scatter of V/Q ratios or, more precisely, areas of very low V/Q ratio are often considered as though they constitute a shunt. This is partly because the arterial blood gases present a common picture which cannot easily be distinguished, and partly because it is a convenient approach in the clinical situation. Quantification of the effect of an increased scatter of V/Q ratios is tedious but an example should help to clarify the general principles. *Figure 98* represents an imaginary patient in whom we may consider the functioning alveoli as falling into three groups (which might perhaps correspond to three horizontal strata), each group having its own V/Q. The figure also shows the percentage contribution that each group makes to the mixed alveolar gas and the pulmonary end-capillary blood. The Po_2 of the alveolar gas in each group has been calculated from the V/Q ratio* and it is assumed that the pulmonary end-capillary Po_2 equals the alveolar Po_2 in each group. The pulmonary end-capillary oxygen saturation of

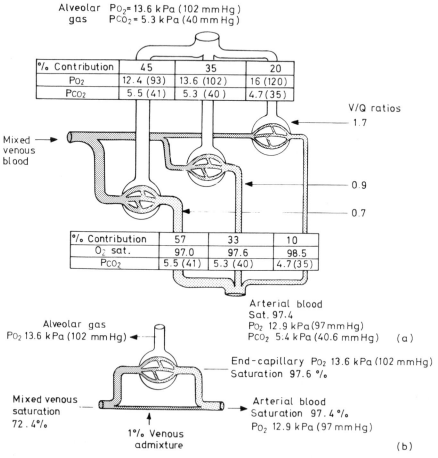

Figure 98. Alveolar/arterial PO_2 difference caused by scatter of V/Q ratios and its representation by an equivalent degree of venous admixture. (a) shows scatter of V/Q ratios corresponding roughly to the three zones of the lung in the normal upright subject. Mixed alveolar gas PO_2 is calculated with allowance for the volume contribution of gas from the three zones. Arterial saturation is similarly determined and the PO_2 derived. There is an alveolar/arterial PO_2 difference of 0·7 kPa (5 mm Hg). (b) shows an entirely imaginary situation which would account for the difference. This is a useful method of quantifying the functional effect of scatter of V/Q ratios but should be carefully distinguished from the actual situation

* The imaginary patient is breathing air and the mixed venous blood has the normal gas contents.

each group has then been determined from the oxygen dissociation curve. Saturation can easily be converted into content, and the saturation of the mixed arterial blood has been determined making allowance for the different volume contributions of blood from the three zones. Arterial Po_2 was derived from the arterial saturation, using the dissociation curve. Mixed alveolar Po_2 was determined by a similar procedure but without the necessity of using the dissociation curve (since Po_2 of a gas is directly proportional to the oxygen content provided that the barometric pressure remains constant).

It will be seen that the saturation of the mixed arterial blood (97·4 per cent) is less than the arithmetic mean of the saturations from the three groups (97·7 per cent). This is partly due to the curvature of the oxygen dissociation curve (*see* below) but also because the group of alveoli with the lowest saturation makes the largest contribution to the arterial blood. As a result of these two effects the arterial Po_2 is always less than the alveolar Po_2, and in this example there is an alveolar/arterial Po_2 difference of 0·7 kPa (5 mm Hg). In contrast, the scatter of Pco_2 between the three groups of alveoli is small and alveolar/arterial Pco_2 difference is only 0·1 kPa (0·6 mm Hg). This is mainly because the mixed venous/arterial Pco_2 difference is small.

It is only possible to measure the V/Q ratios of different parts of the lung by the use of sophisticated techniques. Most investigators in this field can only make a simplified assessment based on measurement of the following oxygen levels: (1) alveolar Po_2; (2) arterial Po_2 and saturation; (3) mixed venous Po_2 and saturation; (4) oxygen capacity of the patient's blood.

These measurements are not by themselves sufficient to calculate the spatial scatter of V/Q ratios as shown in *Figure 98a.* Therefore, there has arisen a useful convention according to which the investigator *pretends* that all functioning alveoli have the same V/Q ratio but that there is a shunt (zero V/Q ratio). This *entirely imaginary* situation is shown in *Figure 98b.* In this example a calculated venous admixture of 1 per cent has been shown, which would produce the same alveolar/arterial Po_2 difference that results from the scatter of V/Q ratios shown in the real situation in *Figure 98a.* This is a useful method of quantifying the functional effect of scatter of V/Q ratios but should be carefully distinguished from the true situation. The calculation of the 1 per cent venous admixture in *Figure 98b* is not a measurement of true shunt in the patient, but is a calculation of *the amount of venous admixture which would be required to produce the observed alveolar/arterial Po_2 difference*, which is actually caused by the scatter of V/Q ratios shown in *Figure 98a* and which, in most laboratories, cannot be measured directly.

Effect of mean alveolar Po_2. Overventilated alveoli fail to compensate for underventilated alveoli in the maintenance of the arterial oxygen level. There are two reasons for this. The first is shown in *Figure 98* and arises from the fact that the relatively underventilated alveoli usually contribute more blood than the relatively overventilated alveoli to the mixed arterial blood. The second reason is that, due to the shape of the oxygen dissociation curve, the overventilated alveoli cannot return blood with a saturation of much more than 98·5 per cent saturation, and so cannot offset the contribution of desaturated blood from the underventilated alveoli. Asmussen and Nielsen (1960) have pointed out that this effect will be more pronounced if the mean alveolar Po_2 is depressed to the tension corresponding to the bend of the dissociation curve. This is a Po_2 of about 6·7 kPa (50 mm Hg), which is encountered only in fairly severe underventilation or during the inhalation of oxygen mixtures of less than 20 per cent. This effect is illustrated in *Figure 99* where the mean alveolar Po₂ is reduced to 10·7 kPa (80 mm Hg).

It follows from the latter consideration that the degree of calculated venous admixture which is equivalent in effect to a fixed degree of scatter of V/Q ratio will depend upon the actual level of the alveolar Po₂. At high levels of alveolar Po₂ the effect of V/Q scatter will be small since blood from all alveoli will be close to 100 per cent saturation, even if the V/Q ratios vary widely and the alveolar/arterial Po₂ difference due to V/Q scatter is therefore sharply reduced.

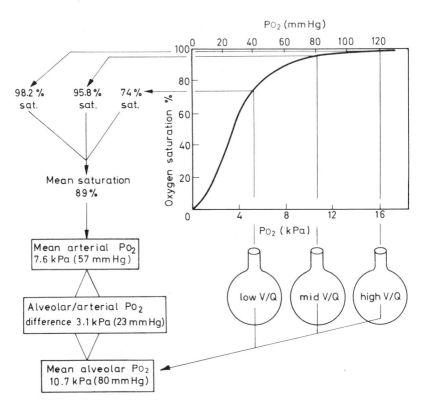

Figure 99. Alveolar/arterial Po₂ *difference caused by scatter of V/Q ratios resulting in oxygen tensions around the bend of the oxygen dissociation curve. The diagram shows the effect of three groups of alveoli with* Po₂ *values of 5·3, 10·7 and 16·0 kPa (40, 80 and 120 mm Hg). Ignoring the effect of the different volumes of gas and blood contributed by the three groups, the mean alveolar* Po₂ *is 10·7 kPa. However, due to the bend of the dissociation curve, the saturations of the blood leaving the three groups are not proportional to their* Po₂. *The mean arterial saturation is, in fact, 89 per cent and the* Po₂ *therefore is 7·6 kPa. The alveolar/arterial* Po₂ *difference is thus 3·1 kPa. The actual difference would be somewhat greater since gas with a high* Po₂ *would make a relatively greater contribution to the alveolar gas, and blood with a low* Po₂ *would make a relatively greater contribution to the arterial blood. In this example a calculated venous admixture of 27 per cent would be required to account for the scatter of V/Q ratios in terms of the measured alveolar/arterial* Po₂ *difference, at an alveolar* Po₂ *of 10·7 kPa*

At normal levels of alveolar P_{O_2} the situation is as shown in *Figure 98*. When the alveolar P_{O_2} is less than normal, scatter of V/Q ratios appears as an even larger venous admixture as the alveolar P_{O_2} falls towards 6·7 kPa (50 mm Hg). In the example in *Figure 99* (alveolar P_{O_2} 10·7 kPa or 80 mm Hg), the scatter of V/Q ratios produces an effect equivalent to a venous admixture of 27 per cent.

Combined effects of alveolar dead space, scatter of V/Q ratios and shunt

Figure 100 portrays an imaginary patient with disordered pulmonary function breathing gas containing 21 per cent oxygen. Ten per cent of the alveolar ventilation is distributed to unperfused alveoli where the V/Q ratio is infinity. This alveolar dead space gas mingles with gas from perfused alveoli during expiration. The mixed alveolar gas from the three perfused alveoli has a composition whose derivation has been shown in *Figure 98*. The end-expiratory gas consists of mixed gas from perfused alveoli diluted with air from the alveolar dead space during expiration. *Figure 98* also showed the derivation of the gas tensions of the mixed pulmonary end-capillary blood and the values are the same as those in *Figure 100*.

The alveolar/arterial gas tension gradients have been considered in *Figure 98*. Further gas tension gradients exist between mixed pulmonary end-capillary blood and arterial blood; these gradients are due to the shunt which has the value of 10 per cent of pulmonary blood flow in this example; the influence of the shunt of P_{CO_2} and P_{O_2} has been explained in *Figure 97*.

The whole series of gradients of P_{CO_2} and P_{O_2} between air and arterial blood have been tabulated below *Figure 100*. The following general conclusions may be drawn.

1. *Ambient gas/end-expiratory* P_{O_2} and P_{CO_2} gradients are of comparable magnitude and are influenced primarily by ventilation, being low at high minute volume.
2. *End-expiratory/mixed alveolar* P_{O_2} and P_{CO_2} gradients are of comparable magnitude and are influenced mainly by alveolar dead space ventilation.
3. *Mixed alveolar/mixed end-capillary* P_{CO_2} gradient is usually negligible. The P_{O_2} gradient is appreciable and a function of scatter of V/Q ratios (*Figures 98 and 99*).
4. *Mixed end-capillary/arterial* P_{CO_2} gradient is usually negligible unless the shunt is very large. The P_{O_2} gradient is appreciable and a function of the magnitude of the shunt* (*Figure 97*).

It is impossible to sample the mixed alveolar gas from the perfused alveoli (uncontaminated with gas from the alveolar dead space), and similarly mixed pulmonary end-capillary blood can only be sampled after admixture with shunted blood to form arterial blood. Therefore, direct measurement of P_{CO_2} and P_{O_2} of mixed alveolar gas and mixed end-capillary blood is not possible.

---

* The end-capillary/arterial P_{O_2} gradient is also increased when the mixed venous/arterial P_{O_2} gradient is increased and this is a function of low cardiac output in relation to O_2 consumption.

This is shown in *Figure 100* as a black box from within which samples cannot ordinarily be collected. The internal workings of the black box must be deduced from samples taken from outside it, that is to say, mixed venous and arterial blood, inspired, expired and end-expiratory gas.

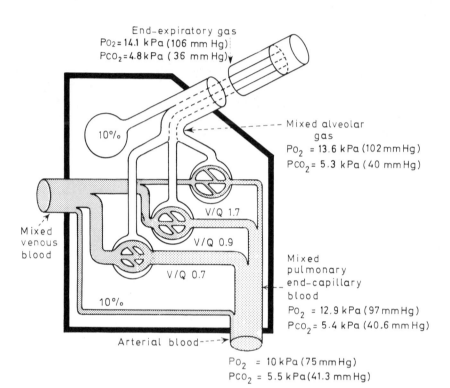

End-expiratory gas
$PO_2 = 14.1$ kPa (106 mm Hg)
$PCO_2 = 4.8$ kPa (36 mm Hg)

10%

Mixed alveolar
gas
$PO_2 = 13.6$ kPa (102 mm Hg)
$PCO_2 = 5.3$ kPa (40 mm Hg)

V/Q 1.7

V/Q 0.9

Mixed
venous
blood

V/Q 0.7

Mixed
pulmonary
end-capillary
blood
$PO_2 = 12.9$ kPa (97 mm Hg)
$PCO_2 = 5.4$ kPa (40.6 mm Hg)

10%

Arterial blood

$PO_2 = 10$ kPa (75 mm Hg)
$PCO_2 = 5.5$ kPa (41.3 mm Hg)

Figure 100. Schematic representation of an imaginary but typical anaesthetized patient breathing air, to show combined functional effects of alveolar dead space, scatter of V/Q ratios and shunt. Ten per cent of the alveolar ventilation is distributed to unperfused alveoli (V/Q infinity); 10 per cent of the mixed venous blood passes through unventilated spaces (V/Q zero). Ventilated and perfused alveoli are considered as falling into three groups whose ventilation/perfusion ratios vary as in the normal upright subject. Gas tensions show a continuous gradient from air to arterial blood, but the effects of the different abnormalities on PCO_2 and PO_2 show striking quantitative differences

	PO_2		PCO_2	
	kPa	*(mm Hg)*	*kPa*	*(mm Hg)*
Air	20	(150)	0	(0)
End-expiratory gas	14·1	(106)	4·8	(36·0)
Mixed alveolar gas (not contaminated with alveolar dead space gas)	13·6	(102)	5·3	(40·0)
Mixed pulmonary end-capillary blood (not contaminated with shunted blood)	12·9	(97)	5·4	(40·6)
Arterial blood	10·0	(75)	5·5	(41·3)

The 'Riley' method of analysis of distribution abnormalities

Without sampling from within the black box, it might appear an impossible task to quantify the errors of distribution shown in *Figure 100*. However, Riley and his co-workers, in a brilliant series of papers, have suggested an approach which is of great practical value although it does not pretend to offer a precise definition of the nature of malfunction (Riley et al., 1946; Riley and Cournand, 1949; Riley and Cournand, 1951; Riley, Cournand and Donald, 1951).

The 'Riley' approach ignores the scatter of V/Q ratios and considers the lung as a three-compartment model—ventilated but unperfused alveoli (alveolar dead space), perfused and ventilated alveoli ('ideal' alveoli), and perfused but unventilated alveoli (venous admixture or shunt) (*Figure 101*). The small gradient in Pco_2 caused by scatter of V/Q ratio and shunt is ignored and it is assumed that the 'ideal' alveolar Pco_2 equals the arterial Pco_2. The 'ideal' alveolar Po_2 may then be calculated on the assumption that the respiratory exchange ratios of 'ideal' alveolar and expired gas are the same (the latter may

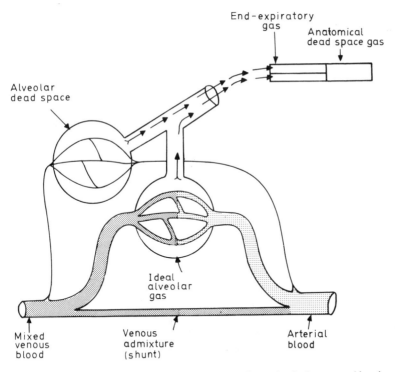

Figure 101. The assessment of the efficiency of gas exchange in the lungs considered as a black box. The lung is imagined to consist of three functional units: (1) alveolar dead space, (2) 'ideal' alveoli, and (3) venous admixture or shunt. Gas exchange occurs only in the 'ideal' alveoli. The measured alveolar dead space consists of true alveolar dead space together with a component caused by V/Q scatter. The measured venous admixture consists of true venous admixture (shunt) together with a component caused by V/Q scatter. Note that 'ideal' alveolar gas is exhaled contaminated with alveolar dead space gas (if present). Under such circumstances it is not possible to sample 'ideal' alveolar gas, the Po_2 of which is therefore derived indirectly

easily be measured). This calculation is performed with any of a number of forms of the alveolar air equation (*see* pages 307 et seq.).*

If we embark on a 'Riley' analysis of the imaginary patient in *Figure 100*, we start by assuming that the 'ideal' alveolar P_{CO_2} is 5.5 kPa (41.3 mm Hg). This is, in fact, too high but by an insignificant amount. We next calculate the 'ideal' alveolar P_{O_2}, to be 13.5 kPa (101 mm Hg), a value which is very close to the mixed alveolar P_{O_2}. Using these values in conjunction with the measured end-expiratory gas tension, we would calculate the alveolar dead space ventilation to be 13 per cent of the alveolar ventilation. Similarly, by comparing our calculated 'ideal' alveolar P_{O_2} with the measured arterial P_{O_2} we would derive a calculated venous admixture of 11 per cent of pulmonary blood flow. Each of these estimates is higher than the corresponding malfunctions built into the model. However, the 'Riley' analysis makes no estimate of the scatter of V/Q ratios, and the enhanced values of calculated alveolar dead space and shunt include the equivalent effect of the scatter of V/Q ratios which is not measured. *Table 20* shows how very accurately this is done.

Table 20. DETECTION OF PULMONARY MALDISTRIBUTION BY THE 'RILEY' METHOD OF ANALYSIS

	Malfunction built into the model patient shown in Figure 100	*Malfunction which would be indicated by 'Riley' method of analysis*
Alveolar dead space ventilation	10%	13%
Scatter of V/Q ratios	Approx. equal to that found in normal upright subjects	Not estimated
Shunt	10%	11%

The scatter of V/Q ratios which is not estimated by the 'Riley' method of analysis, appears as enhanced values for dead-space-like effect and shunt effect.

Although the 'Riley' analysis does not give a precise estimate of what is going on inside the black box of the lungs, it gives a most valuable quantification of the degree of abnormality as though it were all due to alveolar dead space or shunt. It is then reasonable to go ahead and treat the patient on this basis. Thus the minute volume may be increased to allow for ventilation which is wasted in the alveolar dead space, and the inspired oxygen concentration may be increased to restore the arterial P_{O_2} when this has been decreased by 'shunt effect'. This is done by raising the oxygen content of the pulmonary end-capillary blood until there is sufficient surplus oxygen to saturate the shunted blood. Full restoration of arterial P_{O_2} by this means is not possible if the shunt is large (*Figure 102*). A simplified practical approach has been described by Benatar, Hewlett and Nunn (1973).

Distinction between shunt and scatter of V/Q ratios

The 'Riley' analysis described in the section above makes no distinction between shunt and scatter of V/Q ratios. The great majority of publications on venous admixture in clinical practice similarly draw no distinction and authors

* This paragraph constitutes the definition of the 'ideal' alveolar gas.

may attribute their findings to either shunt or scatter of V/Q ratios, often with little evidence to support their preference. In fact, the distinction is far from simple and has been attempted by very few workers.

The most satisfactory approach would be to measure the shunt and scatter of V/Q ratios directly by the techniques outlined at the end of this chapter. However, the methods are elaborate and few workers possess the facilities for their use. Instead it is commoner to measure the calculated venous admixture at different levels of alveolar P_{O_2} and, from these results, to attempt a deduction of the relative contribution of shunt and scatter of V/Q ratios to the total calculated venous admixture measured at the different values of alveolar P_{O_2}.

The distinction is made possible by the difference in slope of the oxygen dissociation curve at different values of P_{O_2}. This is the reason why a given degree of scatter of V/Q ratios appears as though it were a venous admixture of different magnitude at different levels for alveolar P_{O_2}. As an example, let us consider a patient with particularly gross scatter of V/Q ratios in whom, while breathing air, 65 per cent of the arterial blood is derived from alveoli with P_{O_2} 9·3 kPa (70 mm Hg), and 10 per cent from alveoli with P_{O_2} 18·7 kPa (140 mm Hg). This gross degree of scatter of V/Q ratios would produce an alveolar/arterial P_{O_2} gradient of about 3·6 kPa (27 mm Hg). If this gradient were due to a shunt, it would correspond to a shunt of about 10 per cent. Now if the patient were to breathe an oxygen concentration of 60 per cent or more, blood leaving even the worst ventilated alveoli would still be almost fully saturated and the functional defect would then correspond to a shunt of only 1 per cent. If, however, the patient were to breathe about 16 per cent oxygen, the alveolar/arterial P_{O_2} gradient would then correspond to a shunt of about 50 per cent. Thus if measurements of the calculated venous admixture were found to be 50 per cent while breathing 16 per cent oxygen, 10 per cent while breathing air and 1 per cent while breathing 100 per cent oxygen, we might reasonably infer the patient had hardly any true shunt but a serious degree of scatter of V/Q ratio. If, alternatively, the calculated venous admixture were found to be 10 per cent regardless of the concentration of oxygen inspired, we could infer that this was a true shunt and there was no appreciable scatter of V/Q ratios. It is more likely that we should find a calculated venous admixture of (say) 60 per cent during the inhalation of 16 per cent oxygen, 20 per cent while breathing air and 11 per cent while inhaling 100 per cent oxygen. We could then infer that there was a true shunt of about 10 per cent together with a serious degree of scatter of V/Q ratio.

This approach rests upon an assumption of doubtful validity, that the true shunt is uninfluenced by the concentration of oxygen which the patient is breathing. Clearly, the P_{O_2} may influence the pulmonary vasculature and also the presence of 100 per cent oxygen may result in absorption atelectasis. Furthermore, from the practical point of view the procedure is laborious and few estimates of this nature have been performed. Cole and Bishop (1963) and Nunn and Bergman (1964) showed, in conscious subjects, a significant increase in calculated venous admixture at lower values of alveolar P_{O_2} and their results accord roughly with the degree of scatter of V/Q ratios which is believed to occur in man. In anaesthetized man breathing spontaneously, Nunn (1964) showed raised values for calculated venous admixture with low values for alveolar P_{O_2}, and this suggests the presence of a significant degree of scatter of V/Q ratios under these conditions.

The iso-shunt diagram

If we consider arterial P_{CO_2}, haemoglobin and arterial/mixed venous oxygen content difference to be constant, the arterial P_{O_2} is determined mainly by the inspired oxygen concentration and venous admixture considered in the context of the Riley analysis (*Figure 101*). The relationship between inspired oxygen concentration and arterial P_{O_2} is a matter for constant attention in such situations as intensive therapy, and it has been found a matter of practical convenience to prepare a graph of the relationship at different levels of venous admixture (Benatar, Hewlett and Nunn, 1973). The arterial/mixed venous oxygen content difference is often unknown in the clinical situation and therefore the diagram has been prepared for an assumed content difference of 5 ml oxygen/100 ml of blood. Iso-shunt bands have then been drawn on a plot of arterial P_{O_2} against inspired oxygen concentration (*Figure 102*). The bands are sufficiently wide to encompass all values of P_{CO_2} between 3·3 and 5·3 kPa (25–40 mm Hg) and haemoglobin levels between 10 and 14 g/100 ml. Normal barometric pressure is assumed. Since calculation of the venous admixture requires knowledge of the actual arterial/mixed venous oxygen content difference, the iso-shunt lines in *Figure 102* refer to the 'virtual shunt' which is defined as the calculated shunt on the basis of an assumed value of the arterial/mixed venous oxygen content difference of 5 ml/100 ml.

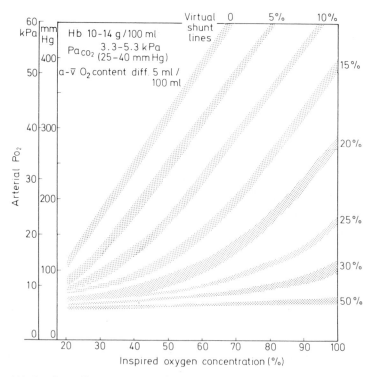

Figure 102. Iso-shunt diagram. On co-ordinates of inspired oxygen concentration (abscissa) and arterial P_{O_2} (ordinate), iso-shunt bands have been drawn to include all values of Hb, $P_{a_{CO_2}}$ and a-v̄ oxygen content difference shown above. (Redrawn from Benatar, Hewlett and Nunn (1973) by courtesy of the Editor of British Journal of Anaesthesia)

In practice, the iso-shunt diagram is useful for adjusting the inspired oxygen concentration to obtain a required level of arterial P_{O_2}. For example, if a patient is found to have an arterial P_{O_2} of 30 kPa (225 mm Hg) while breathing 90 per cent oxygen, he has a virtual shunt of 20 per cent and, if it is required to attain an arterial P_{O_2} of 10 kPa (75 mm Hg), this should be achieved by reducing the inspired oxygen concentration to 45 per cent. Ideally, the new value for arterial P_{O_2} should be checked by direct measurement but, in practice, use of the iso-shunt chart simplifies the process of attaining a satisfactory level of arterial P_{O_2} and reduces the number of measurements which will be required. Resolution of conditions such as a pulmonary oedema, infection or collapse is shown by a reduction of the virtual shunt which may therefore be used as an indication of progress.

If the defective oxygenation of the arterial blood is due primarily to scatter of V/Q ratios, rather than a shunt, then the plot of the patient's arterial P_{O_2} against inspired oxygen concentration will cross the iso-shunt lines rising towards the right of the graph (King et al., 1974). This may be observed and the appropriate conclusions drawn. The iso-shunt chart is, in fact, useful for demonstrating that the changes of arterial P_{O_2} in a particular patient cannot be explained simply in terms of shunt. In practice, however, the plot of most patients accords fairly well with the iso-shunt lines. Harris et al. (1974) found the virtual shunt of normal subjects to be almost constant with inspired oxygen concentration in the range 21–100 per cent, although it was reduced by *deep breaths* of 100 per cent oxygen. Virtual shunt was increased as expected during the inhalation of 14 per cent oxygen. In contrast, Cole and Bishop (1967) found a fall in alveolar/arterial P_{O_2} difference (and therefore virtual shunt) when inspired oxygen concentration was increased from 82·5 to 99·5 per cent.

FORMS OF VENOUS ADMIXTURE

Venae cordis minimae (Thebesian veins)

Some small veins of the left heart drain directly into the chambers of the left heart and so mingle with the arterial blood. The oxygen content of this blood is probably very low, and, therefore, the flow (believed to be about 0·3 per cent of cardiac output; Ravin, Epstein and Malm, 1965) causes an appreciable fall in the mixed arterial oxygen tension. It was thought by Cole and Bishop (1963) that the venae cordis minimae constitute the major part of the venous admixture in healthy man.

Bronchial veins

Figure 88 shows that a part of the venous drainage of the bronchial circulation passes by way of the deep true bronchial veins to reach the pulmonary veins. It is uncertain how large this component is in the healthy subject but is probably less than 1 per cent of cardiac output. In bronchial disease and coarctation of the aorta, the flow through this channel may be greatly increased, and in bronchiectasis and emphysema may be as large as 10 per cent of cardiac output. Under these circumstances it becomes a major cause of arterial desaturation.

Congenital heart disease

Right-to-left shunting in congenital heart disease is the cause of the worst examples of venous admixture. In patients with pulmonary atresia, right-to-left shunting is often present at all times. When there are abnormal communications· between right and left hearts without pulmonary atresia, shunting will normally be from left to right unless the pulmonary arterial pressure is raised above that of the systemic circulation. In that event the shunt is reversed and venous admixture occurs. Although there is usually a progressive tendency to reversal as a result of hypertrophic changes in the pulmonary arterioles, sudden reversal may occur as a result of increases in alveolar pressure. This may occur during anaesthesia, and in the author's experience has followed artificial ventilation, and straining during induction of anaesthesia with irritant inhalational agents.

Atelectasis and pulmonary collapse*

It is uncertain whether there is some slight degree of atelectasis in the normal subject. Measured by modern analytical methods, the alveolar/arterial Po_2 difference can to a large extent be accounted for by the venous drainage from the Thebesian and bronchial circulation. Therefore the normal flow through atelectatic lung is likely to be very small if present at all. However, under pathological circumstances, venous admixture through collapsed areas of lung may be a large fraction of the total pulmonary blood flow and a most important cause of hypoxaemia.

Causes of collapse.   Fundamentally there are two causes of collapse. The first is loss of the pressure gradient across the wall of the alveolus, with consequent collapse of the alveolus due to its own elasticity. This is seen at thoracotomy when the intrathoracic pressure rises to atmospheric: unless the alveolar pressure is maintained above atmospheric (e.g. by artificial ventilation) the lung will quickly collapse. Less complete collapse is caused by pneumothorax or by loss of integrity of the chest wall, such as may result from thoracoplasty or crushed chest injuries.

The second cause of collapse is obstruction of the air passages with absorption of the sequestered gases. The obstruction may be due to any cause (pages 111 et seq.) such as retained secretions and the use of bronchial blockers. No less important is the obstruction of the smaller air passages which occurs when expiration is carried to the residual volume (*Figure 23* and page 70). Reduction of lung volume below the functional residual capacity normally occurs during anaesthesia, but the lung volume may be further reduced as a result of expiratory muscle activity (e.g. coughing) or the use of subatmospheric airway pressures (e.g. 'negative phase' used during artificial ventilation). Velasquez and Farhi (1964) have demonstrated increased venous admixture in dogs ventilated artificially with a subatmospheric expiratory pressure, while Nunn et al. (1965b) produced severe degrees of collapse in healthy conscious subjects merely by forced expiration while breathing 100 per cent oxygen.

---

* The term 'atelectasis' refers to lung tissue which has never become aerated. Acquired de-aeration is therefore more correctly termed 'collapse'.

When gases are sequestered by airway obstruction, they exchange with the gases carried in the mixed venous blood, the rate and direction of change being governed by the difference in tensions between the trapped alveolar gas and the mixed venous blood. Alveolar Pco_2 is normally only about 0·8 kPa (6 mm Hg) below the level in the mixed venous blood. Therefore rather small quantities of carbon dioxide will pass from mixed venous blood into sequestered alveolar gas until its Pco_2 equals that of the mixed venous blood. The Po_2 of alveolar gas, on the other hand, will usually be much higher than that of mixed venous blood (*see Table 34*) and therefore oxygen is rapidly absorbed from sequestered alveoli until the Po_2 equals that of mixed venous blood.

If the patient has been breathing 100 per cent oxygen prior to obstruction, the alveoli will contain only oxygen, carbon dioxide and water vapour. Since the last two together normally amount to less than 13·3 kPa (100 mm Hg), the alveolar Po_2 will usually be greater than 88 kPa (660 mm Hg) so long as the alveoli contain any gas at all. Now, the oxygen saturation of the mixed venous blood can seldom rise above 90 per cent and its Po_2 is usually less than 8 kPa (60 mm Hg). In consequence, there will be an alveolar/mixed venous Po_2 gradient which is almost certainly over 80 kPa (600 mm Hg). Absorption of oxygen will thus be rapid and collapse will quickly occur (*Figure 103*).

The situation is much more favourable if the patient is breathing air since most of the alveolar gas is then nitrogen which is at a tension only about 0·5 kPa

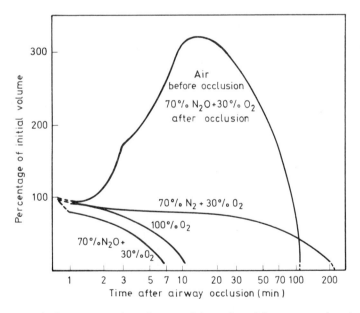

Figure 103. The lower curves show the rate of absorption of the contents of sections of the lung whose air passages are obstructed, resulting in sequestration of the contents. The upper curve shows the expansion of the sequestered gas when nitrous oxide is breathed by a patient who has recently suffered regional airway obstruction while breathing air. In all other cases, it is assumed that the inspired gas is not changed after obstruction has occurred. Similar considerations apply to gas sequestered in other parts of the body, and the data apply to pneumothorax, gas emboli and air introduced during pneumoencephalography. (Reproduced from Webb and Nunn (1967) by courtesy of the authors and the Editor of Anaesthesia)

below that of mixed venous blood (Klocke and Rahn, 1961). Alveolar P_{N_2} rises above that of the mixed venous blood as oxygen is absorbed from the alveoli. Absorption is thus slow and collapse occurs more slowly. The relationship between inspired oxygen concentration, V/Q ratio and alveolar instability is considered below (*Figure 105*).

If nitrous oxide is present in the sequestered alveoli, absorption will usually be more rapid than would be the case with the same concentration of nitrogen (*Figure 103*). There are two reasons for this. Firstly, nitrous oxide is much more soluble in blood than nitrogen, and secondly, the mixed venous tension of nitrous oxide is usually much less than the alveolar tension, except after a long period of inhalation.

When the inspired gas composition is changed *after* obstruction occurs, the pattern of absorption is altered. Consider, for example, a patient who has been breathing a nitrous oxide/oxygen mixture and who, immediately after sequestration, returns to breathing air. There will then be a gradient of tension for nitrous oxide from alveolus to blood and for nitrogen from blood to gas. Therefore, nitrous oxide will pass out of the alveolus and nitrogen will pass into it. Since, however, nitrous oxide is so much more soluble than nitrogen, the rate at which it leaves the alveolus will exceed the rate at which nitrogen passes in and collapse will rapidly supervene. The converse is more complex. If the patient has been breathing air at the time of obstruction and the inspired gas is then changed to a nitrous oxide/oxygen mixture, the tension gradients will be the opposite of those in the preceding example. Therefore, nitrous oxide will pass into the alveolus faster than the nitrogen is absorbed. Consequently, the volume of the gas trapped in the alveolus will increase and, provided that this does not release the obstruction, the alveolus will ultimately increase to about three times the initial volume. Later on, as more nitrogen is absorbed, the nitrous oxide tension in the sequestered gases rises above its tension in the mixed venous blood and absorption takes place, slowly at first and then more quickly until total atelectasis results. The sequence of events is shown in *Figure 103* for which the data have been prepared by forward integration (Webb and Nunn, 1967).

These changes are important to the anaesthetist. Exactly similar considerations apply to gas trapped in any part of the body including pneumothorax, air introduced in the course of pneumoencephalography and gas emboli. Changes in the volume of any of these may be of critical importance to a patient. Special attention should be paid to the possibility of loculi of air increasing in volume when a patient inhales nitrous oxide. A recent air encephalogram is an absolute contraindication to the use of nitrous oxide, and its use in a patient with a pneumothorax may result in a tension pneumothorax if thoracic pressures are not carefully monitored. Air emboli will increase in size and are more dangerous during the inhalation of nitrous oxide (Munson and Merrick, 1967).

The diagnosis of collapse may be made on physical signs but reliance is usually placed on chest radiography. When collapse occurs in the upright position, it is usually most marked in the basal segments where it may be detected without difficulty. However, in the supine position, collapse is more likely to occur in the dorsal parts of the lungs where the blood flow is likely to be relatively greater. Areas of collapse will thus be spread out in a plane parallel to the radiograph, and consequently difficult to recognize (Prys-Roberts et al., 1967b). Furthermore, it must be remembered that the collapse is of tissue with a very low density. Therefore a large area of lung will produce only a small area of shadow. Nor is this the whole story. Diagnosis of collapse in the unconscious patient is often made with portable x-ray apparatus, and the quality of the picture is further impaired by the inability of the patient to take a deep inspiration. These factors combine to make it extraordinarily difficult to detect collapse by radiography in an anaesthetized patient (Bendixen, Hedley-Whyte and Laver, 1963; Nunn, 1964; Hamilton et al., 1964).

Collapse diminishes the functional volume of the lung and so will reduce the compliance (page 80). A reduction in compliance has therefore been used by many groups of workers to indicate the development of collapse (Butler and Smith, 1957; Bendixen, Hedley-Whyte and Laver, 1963; Velasquez and Farhi, 1964). The practical value of compliance as an indication of collapse is limited by the wide scatter of the normal values of compliance in the anaesthetized patient. However, it is probably valid to interpret an acute fall in pulmonary compliance as an increase in the degree of collapse. Unfortunately, this requires control measurements made on the patient prior to collapse and these will seldom be available.

If we assume that pulmonary collapse is the most likely cause of a very large venous admixture found during anaesthesia, then the demonstration of venous admixture is probably the simplest and most satisfactory method of diagnosing collapse under these conditions. Venous admixture is assessed by measurement of the alveolar/arterial Po_2 difference, but it must be stressed that this quantity is also influenced by the level of mixed venous oxygen content (page 392). The diagnosis of collapse is fairly certain if the alveolar/arterial Po_2 difference is diminished by hyperinflation of the lung.

The author and his colleagues (unpublished) compared changes in chest x-ray, FRC and arterial Po_2 in a series of healthy subjects who acquired absorption collapse by breathing oxygen at residual volume in the sitting position. There was little to choose between the three methods in their ability to detect minimal collapse which, when present at all, was detected by all three methods. Chest radiography suffers the disadvantage that it is far less satisfactory when collapse has occurred in the supine position, while the other two methods are only useful if control observations are available before collapse has occurred.

Pulmonary infection

In the days when lobar pneumonia was common, it was a familiar sight to see a patient hyperventilating but deeply cyanosed. The hypoxaemia was due to a large shunt through the lobe which was affected by the pneumonic process. It seems likely that the infection increased the blood flow through the affected lobe above its normal value.

Although lobar pneumonia is now rare, bronchopneumonia is still relatively common, particularly in the elderly, and also, on occasion, after operation and in patients undergoing prolonged artificial ventilation. Under these conditions, pulmonary infection is a common cause of venous admixture and the alveolar/arterial Po_2 difference is a useful aid to diagnosis and assessment of progress.

Pulmonary oedema

Pulmonary oedema has been considered in detail in the previous chapter (pages 262 et seq.). Once alveolar flooding has occurred, perfusion through the affected alveoli constitutes venous admixture and the alveolar/arterial P_{O_2} difference increases. When froth enters the bronchial tree there is failure of ventilation of whole regions of the lungs and venous admixture reaches high levels, resulting in gross hypoxaemia.

Post-traumatic respiratory insufficiency ('shock lung', traumatic wet lung, congestive atelectasis, etc.)

It has been known since World War II that pulmonary function may be impaired by trauma which does not appear to involve the lung directly, and in cases without fat embolism. The earliest signs are hyperventilation with reduction of P_{CO_2} and marked reduction of P_{O_2}. At first there may be no characteristic physical signs or chest radiographic appearance but, in due course, evidence of pulmonary oedema may develop. The blood-gas findings suggest an increased V_D/V_T ratio and shunt. Dyspnoea ensues and high concentrations of oxygen are required to maintain a satisfactory arterial P_{O_2}. Pulmonary compliance is reduced, and airway resistance increased. Artificial ventilation may be required together with inspired oxygen concentrations which are high enough to carry the additional hazard of pulmonary oxygen toxicity.

It is probable that this syndrome is multifactorial. There may be unnoticed direct trauma to the lungs from blast or direct force applied to the thorax which may leave no obvious signs. There may be pulmonary capillary damage with extravasation of blood or plasma into the alveoli and loss of surfactant due to injury, dysfunction or destruction of type II alveolar cells (Henry et al., 1967). Both these factors may decrease the pulmonary compliance. Wardle (1974) has reviewed the evidence for microembolization of the lung by platelet aggregates as one aspect of disseminated intravascular coagulation with the lung acting as the filter of the circulation (page 21). Apart from the direct effect of the embolization (which would explain the increased V_D/V_T), the platelet aggregates release bronchoconstrictors including histamine, bradykinin, serotonin (5-HT) and catecholamines. This can result in areas of hypoventilation and collapse (explaining the shunt and arterial hypoxaemia). As the condition develops, infection may become an important factor with focal bronchopneumonia or even septicaemia.

To these natural developments of trauma we must add a range of possible iatrogenic complications. Overhydration or overtransfusion may increase lung water and further difficulties may arise from interference with coagulation resulting from massive transfusions. Old stored blood also results in microembolization of the lungs. The administration of inspired oxygen concentrations in excess of 60 per cent may cause pulmonary oxygen toxicity. This difficult subject is discussed in Chapter 12 but it may be mentioned here that very high concentrations of oxygen are only required, and should only be given, when there is gross failure of oxygenation in the lung. In most patients, there is then such complicated pulmonary pathology that it is virtually impossible to define that part of the final pathological picture which may be ascribed to pulmonary oxygen toxicity.

Finally, we should note those injuries which have a specific effect upon pulmonary function. Apart from such obvious conditions as open pneumothorax and flail chest, it is important to be aware of the possibility of fat embolism in any patient with a skeletal injury and even in some patients who have only soft tissue injury. Pulmonary oedema is well known as a complication of head injury (page 266).

Respiratory distress syndrome (hyaline membrane)

Apart from neonatal respiratory distress syndrome (page 75), there are a variety of severe pulmonary disorders, including trauma, oedema, and infection, often requiring prolonged artificial ventilation, which may lead to the deposition of a fibrinous sheath lining the alveoli. The condition is plain to see in sections obtained at autopsy and could presumably be detected by lung biopsy. However, in adults during life, the diagnosis may be difficult. There is no specific appearance in the chest radiograph and the blood-gas picture does not distinguish the condition from bronchopneumonia, pulmonary oedema or collapse. Increased stiffness of the lungs may be noticed in a patient on artificial ventilation and thereafter diagnosis rests chiefly on exclusion of other possible explanations of the blood-gas changes which may be severe and life-threatening.

Pulmonary embolus

The primary effect of pulmonary embolus is to produce a large alveolar dead space. However, this is usually accompanied by demonstrable venous admixture which is probably due to spasm of air passages (*see* above) and often to superadded infection. These changes are particularly marked with fat embolism (Prys-Roberts et al., 1970).

Pulmonary neoplasm

Any pulmonary neoplasm is likely to cause a shunt as its venous drainage mingles with the pulmonary venous blood. With bronchial or secondary carcinoma, the flow through the neoplasm may be high, resulting in appreciable arterial hypoxaemia. Pulmonary haemangioma is rare but may first present as an unexplained venous admixture.

Pulmonary arteriovenous shunts

The existence of potential channels has been demonstrated by von Hayek (1960). The channels are 'sperr' arteries, structurally similar to those linking the pulmonary and bronchial arteries (page 249), and forming a T-network allowing blood to flow from bronchial artery to pulmonary artery, or from pulmonary artery to bronchial veins (and thence to pulmonary veins) according to the relaxation of these muscular vessels. There is also the possibility of direct shunting through the giant capillaries below the pleura. Although these possibilities exist, very little is known of the role of these vessels in the regulation of the pulmonary circulation (Krahl, 1964). It is, however, not without interest that von Hayek suggested that, when open, these communications might take as much as 20 per cent of the total pulmonary blood flow. Nevertheless, the functional significance of these potential shunts remains in doubt, but it is certain that flow through them must be negligible in the healthy conscious subject.

Evidence of passage of blood through pulmonary arteriovenous anastomoses has largely been obtained from injection of tracer substances into the pulmonary artery, clearly of limited application in anaesthetized patients. Tobin and Zariquiey (1950) have demonstrated the passage through perfused animal lungs of glass beads up to 0·5 mm in diameter. More convincing have been *in vivo* cinefluorography studies of Thorotrast injected into the pulmonary artery of dogs (Rahn, Stroud and Meier, 1952; Rahn, Stroud and Tobin, 1952). Injected material reached the pulmonary veins so rapidly that it could not all have passed through the pulmonary capillaries. However, the significance of pulmonary arteriovenous shunts, or even their existence, has not been universally accepted and there have been a number of studies which have failed to demonstrate the passage of glass beads larger than 0·05 mm diameter. For a review of this difficult subject the reader is referred to the monograph of Aviado (1965, page 943).

Niden and Aviado (1956) have themselves obtained evidence which strongly supports the existence of arteriovenous communications in the anaesthetized dog after embolization with glass beads. Injection into the pulmonary artery of 8 g of glass beads (0·125 mm diam.) resulted in a sharp rise of pulmonary arterial pressure which was due primarily to an increase in pulmonary vascular resistance, caused both by obstruction of the vascular bed and also by reflex pulmonary vasoconstriction. (Crossed circulation experiments showed an increase in pulmonary vascular resistance in a lung which was perfused from another dog and so spared the embolization which affected the lung in the donor dog.) After embolization, beads of diameter 0·42 mm passed through the lungs, and the ease with which they passed was directly related to the pulmonary arterial pressure. Hypoxia increased the passage of beads, presumably due to the rise in pulmonary arterial pressure which it caused. This would accord with the gross degree of shunting found by Cater et al. (1963) during the ventilation of dogs with 100 per cent nitrogen. Of the greatest interest was the pulmonary venous oxygen saturation in Aviado's study. As successive injections of beads raised the pulmonary arterial pressure, there was an immediate and progressive lowering of the pulmonary venous oxygen saturation. This change could only be due to shunting and, in combination with the evidence of the passage of the glass beads, is strongly suggestive of the opening of arteriovenous shunts.

INCREASED SCATTER OF V/Q RATIOS

We have above (page 281) considered how increased scatter of V/Q ratios may interfere with arterial oxygenation and may, in fact, be considered as if it were venous admixture (Riley analysis). This is particularly true of areas of low V/Q ratio which may arise in a variety of conditions. The new technique developed by West's group (page 306) permits measurement of the distribution of ventilation and perfusion to lung units of different V/Q ratios and indicates in the normal young subject a logarithmic Gaussian distribution of ventilation and perfusion with 95 per cent limits at V/Q ratios of about 0·3 and 3·0 (Wagner et al., 1974). Areas of zero and infinite V/Q ratios are not discernible but the method does not measure the extrapulmonary venous admixture which must be present. The spread of V/Q ratios increases with advancing ages and, in particular, there appears a 'shelf' of perfusion distributed over the range of V/Q ratios 0·01–0·1 (*Figure 104*). This probably represents gross underventilation of dependent areas of the lungs due to airway closure. It will be recalled (page 70) that closing capacity increases with age and, in due course, encroaches on the tidal range. Conditions which reduce the FRC would also produce areas of hypoventilation.

The spread of V/Q ratios is also increased in a number of pathological conditions, including pulmonary oedema and pulmonary embolus (Wagner et al., 1975). In chronic bronchitis and emphysema, Briscoe and Cournand (1962) have postulated a bimodal distribution into fast alveoli with a high V/Q ratio and slow alveoli with a low V/Q ratio (*see Figure 26*).

West's group has shown that, in older subjects and in those with patho-logically increased scatter of V/Q ratios, there may be substantial blood flow to areas of lung with V/Q ratios in the range 0·01–0·1 (West, 1975). These grossly hypoventilated areas are liable to collapse if the patient breathes a high concentration of oxygen. If the V/Q ratio is 0·05 or less, it follows that ventilation cannot supply the oxygen which is removed by the perfusing venous

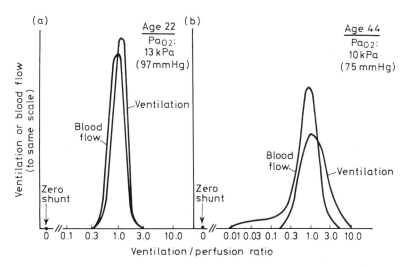

Figure 104. The distribution of ventilation and blood flow in relation to ventilation/ perfusion ratios in two normal subjects. (a) shows a male aged 22 years with typical narrow spread and no measurable intrapulmonary shunt or alveolar dead space. This accords with the high arterial PO₂ while breathing air. (b) shows the wider spread in a male aged 44 years. Note in particular the 'shelf' of blood flow distributed to alveoli with V/Q ratios in the range 0·01–0·1. There is still no measurable intrapulmonary shunt or alveolar dead space. However, the appreciable distribution of blood flow to underperfused alveoli is sufficient to reduce the arterial PO₂ to 10 kPa (75 mm Hg) while breathing air. (Redrawn from Wagner et al. (1974) by courtesy of the authors and the Editor of the Journal of Clinical Investigation)

blood, assuming an arterial/mixed venous oxygen content difference of 5 ml/100 ml (i.e. 0·05 ml/ml). Absorption collapse would then be inevitable. Wagner et al. (1974) have actually demonstrated the conversion of a 'shelf' of low V/Q ratios to a true shunt when awake subjects breathe 100 per cent oxygen (*Figure 105*), and Dantzker, Wagner and West (1975) have discussed the theoretical basis of the interplay between V/Q ratios and inspired oxygen concentration in the production of absorption collapse. The critical V/Q ratio for production of absorption collapse increases from 0·001 to 0·05 as the inspired gas is changed from air to 100 per cent oxygen (*Figure 105*). Areas of very low V/Q ratio develop if the lung volume is reduced to residual volume, and absorption collapse may easily be produced under these circumstances by breathing 100 per cent oxygen (Nunn et al., 1965b). Apart from considerations of pulmonary oxygen toxicity, the danger of absorption collapse is a cogent

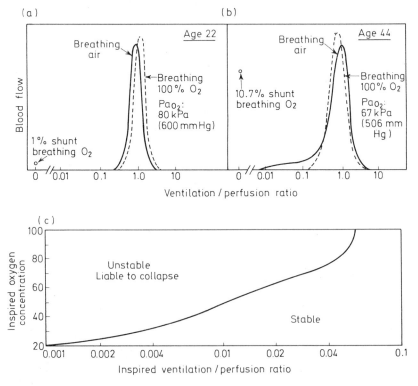

Figure 105. Inspiration of 100 per cent oxygen causes collapse of alveoli with very low ventilation/perfusion ratios. (a) shows the minor change in the distribution of blood flow (in relation to V/Q ratio) when a young subject breathes oxygen. Collapse is minimal and a shunt of 1 per cent develops. (b) shows the changes in an older subject with a 'shelf' of blood flow distributed to alveoli with very low V/Q ratios. Breathing oxygen causes collapse of these alveoli and this is manifested by disappearance of the shelf and appearance of an intrapulmonary shunt of 10·7 per cent. (c) relates the inspired oxygen concentration to the inspired V/Q ratio which is critical for absorption collapse. (Redrawn from Wagner et al. (1974) by courtesy of the authors and the Editor of the Journal of Clinical Investigation, *and from Dantzker, Wagner and West (1975) by courtesy of the authors and the Editor of the* Journal of Applied Physiology)

reason for avoiding excessively high oxygen concentrations in any patient believed to have areas of very low V/Q ratio.

ANAESTHESIA

The alveolar/arterial Po_2 difference is increased during routine uncomplicated anaesthesia in all except young adults and children. The changes in Po_2 are discussed in Chapter 12 (pages 434 et seq.) but it is appropriate at this point to consider how far the changes are due to venous admixture or to increased scatter of V/Q ratios. It seems unlikely that the primary dysfunction is a reduction of diffusing capacity (Chapter 10) but a reduction of cardiac output will magnify the fall of arterial Po_2 with either venous admixture or areas of very low V/Q ratio. This is because a reduction of cardiac output will, other things being equal, lower the mixed venous saturation and so enhance reduction of the arterial Po_2 due to venous admixture (Kelman et al., 1967).

A great many studies have demonstrated that the arterial Po_2 during anaesthesia is less than would be expected for the inspired oxygen concentration. Mean results from eight studies have been plotted on the iso-shunt diagram which was presented in *Figure 102*. The results (in *Figure 106*) show a remarkable consistency and, whether respiration was spontaneous or artificial, the mean values are closely grouped along the 10 per cent shunt line throughout the range of inspired oxygen. The iso-shunt diagram assumes an arterial/mixed venous oxygen content difference of 5 ml/100 ml which clearly may not be the case for many individual patients represented in *Figure 106*. Special attention should therefore be paid to those few studies in which the percentage venous admixture was directly determined from a knowledge of the mixed venous oxygen saturation. Such studies present a considerable ethical and technical challenge meriting discussion in some detail.

Marshall et al. (1969) studied ten patients before and during anaesthesia with spontaneous respiration of halothane vaporized in oxygen. Arterial and mixed venous blood gases, cardiac output and respiratory minute volumes were directly measured before, during and after anaesthesia. There was a reduction in cardiac output during anaesthesia but this was insufficient to explain the whole of the fall in arterial Po_2. The venous admixture increased threefold during anaesthesia but had almost returned to control values three hours after anaesthesia. Michenfelder, Fowler and Theye (1966) avoided pulmonary artery catheterization by back-calculating the mixed venous oxygen content from the cardiac output, arterial oxygen content and oxygen consumption using the Fick equation (page 270). Pre-anaesthetic measurements were not made but, during inhalational anaesthesia with artificial ventilation, abnormally high values for venous admixture were observed, according well with those of Marshall. A third study by Price et al. (1969) reported observations before and during anaesthesia with halothane or cyclopropane, spontaneous and artificial ventilation and at two levels of inspired oxygen concentration. This study, too, reported substantial increases in venous admixture with all types of anaesthesia compared with control observations in conscious subjects. Values for venous admixture from these three studies are summarized in *Table 21*, and values for arterial Po_2 are plotted along with other less detailed studies in *Figure 106*. Their values for arterial Po_2 accord very well with the other studies and this provides strong inferential evidence that an increased venous admixture is a usual feature of routine anaesthesia.

Hulands et al. (1970) studied the effect of anaesthesia, paralysis and artificial ventilation on the distribution of ventilation/perfusion ratios in horizontal strata of the lungs. This was in the course of the study of distribution of perfusion in horizontal strata to which reference has been made above (page 277). They found only minor increases in the spread of V/Q ratios and nothing to explain the increased alveolar/arterial Po_2 difference associated with routine anaesthesia. This study did not investigate spread of V/Q ratios *within* horizontal strata and, at the time of writing, it is not known whether there are any changes in distribution of V/Q ratios as would be shown by the method of West as displayed in *Figure 104*. For the present, we can only say that the measured

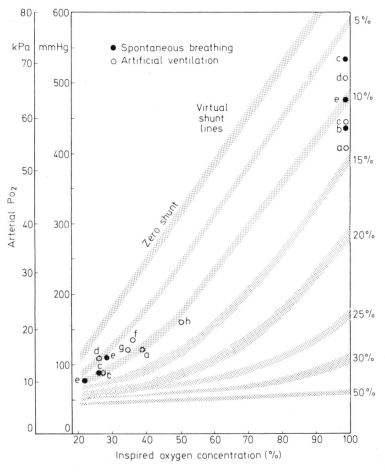

Figure 106. Mean values for arterial Po_2 are plotted against inspired oxygen concentrations for 15 published studies of anaesthetized patients, using the same co-ordinates as in Figure 102. (a) Michenfelder, Fowler and Theye, 1966; (b) Marshall et al., 1969; (c) Price et al., 1969; (d) Nunn, Bergman and Coleman, 1965; (e) Nunn, 1964; (f) Hewlett et al., 1974c; (g) Theye and Tuohy, 1964a; (h) Gold and Helrich, 1967

venous admixture is usually increased to about 10 per cent anaesthesia and that this is presumably due to development of a shunt or to areas of very low V/Q ratio or to a mixture of the two.

It might be expected that the distinction between shunt and areas of low (but not zero) V/Q ratio might be made by inspection of *Figure 106*. If the primary dysfunction was a shunt then values would be expected to fall along a shunt line. In fact, they do follow the 10 per cent shunt line very closely, and these observations accord fully with the hypothesis that anaesthesia results in the appearance of a shunt of about 10 per cent of the pulmonary blood flow. If the primary dysfunction of anaesthesia were the development of areas of low V/Q ratio, then values for arterial P_{O_2} at different values of inspired oxygen concentration should indicate a high 'shunt' at low inspired oxygen concentration and a lower 'shunt' at high inspired oxygen concentrations for the reasons given above (page 283). In fact, this is clearly not the case, suggesting at first sight that the dysfunction is a true shunt rather than an increased scatter of V/Q ratios. However, there is the further possibility of a dual type of dysfunction with increased spread of V/Q ratios as the primary defect but with areas of low V/Q converted to true shunts by absorption collapse when the patients breathe high concentrations of oxygen. The mechanism of this has been discussed above (page 291). The data shown in *Figure 106* could then be interpreted as follows. Up to an inspired oxygen of 50 per cent, values for arterial P_{O_2} are compatible with areas of low (but not zero) V/Q ratio. At high inspired oxygen concentrations, values for arterial P_{O_2} indicate true shunt caused by collapse of

Table 21. VALUES FOR PULMONARY VENOUS ADMIXTURE MEASURED DURING ANAESTHESIA IN MAN

Reference	*Circumstances*	F_{IO_2} (%)	$\dot{Q}s/\dot{Q}t$ (%)
Michenfelder, Fowler and	Artificial ventilation	40*	10·2
Theye (1966)	Inhalational anaesthesia	100*	13·7
Price et al. (1969)	Conscious controls	25	5·9
	before anaesthesia	100	3·1
	Halothane anaesthesia	25	18·9
	spontaneous respiration	98·5	6·1
	Halothane anaesthesia	25	15·1
	artificial ventilation	98·5	11·1
	Conscious controls	25	2·5
	before anaesthesia	80	2·0
	Cyclopropane anaesthesia	25	11·3
	(spont. and artif. vent.)	80	7·9
	Halothane + N₂O anaesth.	28	10·0
	(spont. and artif. vent.)		
Marshall et al. (1969)	Conscious controls	100	4·4
	before anaesthesia		
	Halothane anaesthesia	100*	12·1
	30 minutes after induction		
	3½ hours after induction	100*	14·8
	30 minutes after anaesthesia	100	6·5
	3 hours after anaesthesia	100	5·2

* These values were slightly reduced by the addition of unspecified concentrations of halothane or other inhalational anaesthetics.

those areas. This has been demonstrated for older, unanaesthetized subjects with airway closure, in whom the 'shelf' of low V/Q ratios converts to a true shunt when they breathe 100 per cent oxygen (*see Figure 105*).

It has proved difficult to determine the fundamental respiratory dysfunction which occurs so consistently during anaesthesia. We may, however, be reasonably certain that there is a reduction in lung volume below the FRC (page 67) and, in all except young patients, this will reduce the tidal range below the closing capacity. This will produce either airway closure and therefore a shunt, or at least areas of relative underventilation (low V/Q ratio) which may be converted to collapse by the breathing of 100 per cent oxygen. Collapse as the fundamental dysfunction was advanced by Bendixen, Hedley-Whyte and Laver (1963) but more recent studies have been unable to demonstrate a reduction of the alveolar/arterial Po_2 gradient by hyperventilation (Panday and Nunn, 1968).

Finally, there remains the possibility that anaesthesia results in the opening of arteriovenous anastomoses in the lungs (pages 20 and 297). This has been neither demonstrated nor disproved.

PRINCIPLES OF ASSESSMENT OF DISTRIBUTION OF PULMONARY BLOOD FLOW

Measurement of unilateral pulmonary blood flow

Reference has been made to the considerable difficulty of measuring unilateral blood flow in the intact subject. Direct measuring devices may be attached to, or inserted into, the left and right pulmonary arteries, but clearly such methods are of limited application to the human subject. Most attempts to measure unilateral pulmonary blood flow in the human subject are based on an endeavour to apply the Fick principle using oxygen as the indicator gas. Divided airway techniques such as the Carlen's catheter enable the investigator to measure unilateral oxygen uptake and unilateral ventilation. The pulmonary arterial blood is common to both lungs and the only remaining problem is the measurement of the oxygen content of the blood draining each lung separately. This cannot be determined directly. Even if it were feasible to cannulate pulmonary veins, it would not be possible to sample proportionately from the two pulmonary veins which drain each lung. Their flow rate and oxygen content are both likely to be different, at least in the upright position. The usual approach is to measure the end-expiratory Po_2 and assume that the pulmonary venous Po_2 is less than this by a certain amount. Alternatively, the 'ideal' alveolar Po_2 may be calculated for each lung indirectly from its end-expiratory Pco_2. Clearly these approaches are very indirect, although it is feasible to calculate the likely error of the technique. The error is less than might be imagined since the shape of the oxygen dissociation curve limits the likely range of pulmonary venous oxygen content (in contrast to tension). Elaborate attempts have been made to assess the validity of observations which have been made (Defares et al., 1960).

On a simpler plane, some estimate of blood flow may be obtained from measurements of unilateral ventilation and oxygen uptake. Clearly, if the ventilation of the two lungs is similar and the oxygen uptake differs, it may be assumed that the blood flow rates differ by approximately the same extent.

However, because ventilation and blood flow alter the pulmonary venous oxygen content, it is impossible to make a precise assessment of blood flow from the simple measurements made with the bronchospirometer.

A semi-quantitative estimate of the distribution of pulmonary blood flow between the two lungs may be made by injection of a suitable radioactive tracer into a vein and subsequently counting over the lung fields. A γ radiation emitter is required and two different methods may be employed. Firstly, a relatively insoluble gas such as [133]xenon may be dissolved in saline and injected into a systemic vein. The xenon is evolved in the lungs and may be counted in the alveolar gas. It is rapidly cleared by pulmonary ventilation and the method is therefore only suitable if counting can be completed during a breath hold. The second method is to inject labelled particles which have a diameter greater than about $50\,\mu$m and so lodge in the pulmonary circulation. They can then be counted at leisure without the limitation of breath-holding time. Different isotopes with different energy levels of radiation can be used at different times to study changes in the pulmonary circulation and the lung fields are then counted for different energy levels. Counts may be obtained by stationary or moving scintillation counters and graphical representation of the circulation may be presented as a lung scan or by means of a gamma camera.

It is possible to deflect the pulmonary blood flow away from one lung, and so to study the ability of the other lung to take the whole of the pulmonary circulation. This may be achieved by inflation of a balloon on the end of a cardiac catheter within one branch of the pulmonary artery (Carlens, Hanson and Nordenström, 1951). It is also possible to combine this procedure with bronchial occlusion and so to reproduce the cardiorespiratory effects of pneumonectomy (Nemir et al., 1953).

Measurement of pulmonary lobar blood flow

By intubation, the right upper lobe bronchus may be isolated in man (Mattson and Carlens, 1955), and the oxygen consumption of this lobe may therefore be estimated. It is found to be considerably less than proportionate to its ventilation and this indicates a low rate of perfusion.

End-expiratory gases sampled from different lobes at bronchoscopy will give some qualitative indication of blood flow, although precise calculation of flow is not possible. A simple estimate of ventilation/perfusion ratio may be obtained from the respiratory exchange ratio (Armitage and Taylor, 1956). A more complete assessment has been made by the simultaneous analysis of a number of gases exhaled from various bronchi, using a mass spectrometer at bronchoscopy (Hugh-Jones and West, 1960).

Measurement of perfusion in horizontal slices of the lung

Reference has been made above to techniques for estimating unilateral pulmonary blood flow, using radioactive tracers. These techniques were, in fact, first employed for studying the blood flow to horizontal slices of the lung and were introduced for this purpose by West (1962).

Measurement of the scatter of ventilation/perfusion ratios

For many years, the degree of scatter of ventilation/perfusion ratios about the mean was a matter for speculation. The Riley three-compartment analysis (*Figure 101*) is still widely used as a substitute for direct measurement. West's introduction of a method of measurement of ventilation and perfusion in horizontal slices of the lung made it possible to quantify the scatter of V/Q ratios in these slices although it was realized that further inequalities would probably exist within the slices themselves. Nevertheless, his method of analysis was a milestone in pulmonary physiology. A new technique, more recently developed by West's group, now permits the display of a continuous distribution of both ventilation and perfusion in terms of functional units covering the full spectrum of V/Q ratios from zero to infinity. Examples have been shown in *Figures 104 and 105.*

The technique has been described by Wagner, Saltzman and West (1974). It employs a range of tracer gases ranging from very soluble (e.g. acetone) to very insoluble (e.g. sulphur hexafluoride). Saline is equilibrated with these gases and infused intravenously at constant rate. After about 20 minutes a steady state is achieved and samples of arterial blood and mixed expired gas are collected. Levels of the tracer gases in the arterial blood are then measured by gas chromatography (Wagner, Naumann and Laravuso, 1974) and levels in the mixed venous blood are derived by use of the Fick principle. It is then possible to calculate the retention of each tracer in the blood passing through the lung and the elimination of each in the expired gas. Retention and elimination are related to the solubility coefficient of each tracer in blood and then, by numerical analysis, it is possible to compute a distribution curve for pulmonary blood flow and alveolar ventilation respectively in relation to the spectrum of V/Q ratios. In practice, a number of finite values of V/Q are employed. The range of V/Q ratios between 0·005 and 100 is divided equally on a logarithmic scale into 48 compartments which, together with zero (shunt) and infinity (alveolar dead space) make 50 in all.

The technique is sophisticated and laborious. It is hardly likely to become widely employed in the foreseeable future. However, the results shown in *Figures 104 and 105* indicate the enormous potential of the method. It is expected that it will indicate the precise nature of the disturbances of gas exchange in a wide range of diseases and special conditions, including anaesthesia.

Measurement of venous admixture

The usual method of calculation of venous admixture is by solution of the equation shown in *Figure 97.* It has been explained above that when the alveolar P_{O_2} is less than about 27 kPa (200 mm Hg), scatter of V/Q ratios contributes appreciably to the total calculated venous admixture. This effect is maximal when the alveolar P_{O_2} is within the range 6·7–10·7 kPa (50–80 mm Hg). When the subject breathes a high oxygen concentration, the calculated venous admixture contains only a small component due to scatter of V/Q ratios. Nevertheless, the calculated quantity still does not indicate the precise value of shunted blood since some of the shunt consists of blood of which the oxygen content is unknown (e.g. from bronchial veins and venae cordis minimae). The calculated venous admixture is thus at best an index rather than a precise measurement of contamination of arterial blood with venous blood.

In the equation shown in *Figure 97*, some of the quantities on the right-hand side are amenable to direct measurement. The arterial and mixed venous oxygen contents may be derived by sampling and analysis. Arterial blood may be drawn from any convenient systemic artery, but the mixed venous blood must be withdrawn from the right ventricle or pulmonary artery. A Swan–Ganz catheter is suitable for this purpose. Blood in the right atrium is not perfectly mixed, and blood from inferior and superior venae cavae and coronary sinus forms separate streams. The major problem is, however, measurement of alveolar P_{O_2}. If *Figure 101* is studied in conjunction with *Figure 97*, it will be seen that the 'alveolar' P_{O_2} required for measurement of venous admixture is the 'ideal' aveolar P_{O_2} and not the end-expiratory P_{O_2} since the end-expiratory gas is contaminated with alveolar dead space gas if this is present.

The alveolar air equation. 'Ideal' alveolar gas cannot be sampled and its P_{O_2} must be derived by indirect means (page 287). Derivation of the 'ideal' alveolar P_{O_2} was first suggested by Benzinger (1937) and later by Rossier and Méan (1943). It was finally formulated with greater precision by Riley et al. (1946).

Derivation of the 'ideal' alveolar P_{O_2} is based on the following considerations.

1. Quite large degrees of venous admixture or V/Q scatter cause relatively little difference between P_{CO_2} of 'ideal' alveolar gas (or pulmonary end-capillary blood) and arterial blood (*Table 19*). Therefore 'ideal' alveolar P_{CO_2} is approximately equal to arterial P_{CO_2}.
2. The respiratory exchange ratio of ideal alveolar gas (in relation to inspired gas) equals the respiratory exchange ratio of mixed expired gas (again in relation to inspired gas).

From these considerations it is possible to derive an equation which indicates the 'ideal' alveolar P_{O_2} in terms of arterial P_{CO_2}, inspired gas P_{O_2}, respiratory exchange ratio or related quantities. As a very rough approximation, the oxygen and carbon dioxide in the alveolar gas replace the oxygen in the inspired gas. Therefore, very approximately:

$$\text{alveolar } P_{O_2} \doteqdot \text{inspired } P_{O_2} - \text{arterial } P_{CO_2}$$

This is not sufficiently accurate for use except in the special case considered below. In practice three corrections are required to overcome errors due to the following factors: (*a*) usually, less CO_2 is produced than oxygen is consumed (respiratory exchange ratio); (*b*) the respiratory exchange ratio produces a secondary effect due to the fact that the expired volume does not equal the inspired volume; (*c*) the inspired and expired gas volumes may also differ because of inert gas exchange.

We may now see how corrections are applied to produce successive improvements in the accuracy of the equation.

1. The simplest practicable form of the equation is that suggested by Benzinger (1937) and Rossier and Méan (1943). It makes correction for

the principal effect of the respiratory exchange ratio (*a*), but not the small supplementary error due to the difference between the inspired and expired gas volumes which results from the respiratory exchange ratio (*b*):

$$\text{alveolar } P_{O_2} = \text{inspired } P_{O_2} - \frac{\text{arterial } P_{CO_2}}{\text{respiratory exchange ratio}}$$

This form is suitable for rapid bedside calculations of alveolar P_{O_2}, when great accuracy is not required.

2. One stage more complicated is an equation which allows for differences in the volume of inspired and expired gas due to the respiratory exchange ratio, but still does not allow for differences due to the exchange of inert gases. This equation exists in various forms, all algebraically identical:

$$\text{alveolar } P_{O_2} = P_{IO_2} - \frac{P_{aCO_2}}{R}(1 - F_{IO_2}(1 - R))*$$

(derived from Riley et al., 1946)

This equation is suitable for use whenever the subject has been breathing the inspired gas mixture long enough for the inert gas to be in equilibrium. It is unsuitable for use when the inspired oxygen concentration has recently been changed, when the ambient pressure has recently been changed (e.g. during hyperbaric oxygen therapy), or when the inert gas concentration has recently been changed (e.g. soon after the start or finish of a period of inhaling nitrous oxide. It will thus be clear that this form of the alveolar air equation has only limited application to those patients with whom an anaesthetist is likely to be concerned. These considerations have been discussed in detail by Nunn (1963).

3. Perhaps the most satisfactory form of the alveolar air equation is that which was advanced by Filley, MacIntosh and Wright (1954). This equation makes no assumption that inert gases are in equilibrium and allows for the difference between inspired and expired gas from whatever cause. It also proves to be very simple in use and does not require the calculation of the respiratory exchange ratio:

$$\text{alveolar } P_{O_2} = P_{IO_2} - P_{aCO_2}\left(\frac{P_{IO_2} - P_{\bar{E}O_2}}{P_{\bar{E}CO_2}}\right)$$

If the alveolar P_{O_2} is calculated separately according to the last two equations, the difference (if any) will be that due to inert gas exchange. This affords a method of study of such phenomena as so-called diffusion anoxia (Fink, Carpenter and Holaday, 1954).

Calculation of alveolar P_{O_2} of a patient breathing 100 per cent oxygen.   When the inspired oxygen concentration approximates to 100 per cent the 'ideal' alveolar gas contains only oxygen and carbon dioxide. Under these special circumstances a very simplified form of the alveolar air equation is applicable:

$$\text{alveolar } P_{O_2} = \text{inspired } P_{O_2} - \text{arterial } P_{CO_2}$$

* Symbols are listed in Appendix C.

In general this form should only be used when the inspired oxygen concentration exceeds 90 per cent. It is also applicable to patients breathing air who have a respiratory exchange ratio of exactly 1·0.

The critical reader will have seen that the measurement of venous admixture is a very artificial affair, based on a number of simplifications and assumptions which are only partly true. Before dismissing the whole subject in scorn, it should be realized that this approach, imperfect though it may be, has opened an extremely difficult field to quantification. It will be seen in Chapter 12 that, even if we do not know precisely what we are measuring, the measurement of venous admixture is of very considerable practical value in prognosis and therapy.

Distinction between shunt and the effect of V/Q scatter

Shunt and scatter of V/Q ratios will each produce an alveolar/arterial Po_2 difference from which a value for venous admixture may be calculated. It is, however, often impossible to say from the measurements whether the disorder is a true shunt or else an excessive scatter of V/Q ratios. Three methods are available for distinction between the two conditions.

If the inspired oxygen concentration is altered, the effect on the arterial Po_2 will depend upon the nature of the disorder. If oxygenation is impaired by a large shunt, the arterial Po_2 will always rise by less than the inspired Po_2. If, however, the disorder is due to scatter of V/Q ratios, the arterial Po_2 will rise by more than or approximately the same amount as the inspired Po_2. This subject is discussed on page 291.

Measurement of the alveolar/arterial P_{N_2} difference is a specific method for quantification of V/Q scatter, since the P_{N_2} difference is entirely uninfluenced by a true shunt. The method has not come into general use, particularly with patients who are not in a state of complete nitrogen equilibrium which is a prerequisite of the method. Furthermore, the method is technically difficult, requiring the measurement of P_{N_2} to an accuracy which is not easily obtainable. The method is lucidly presented by Rahn and Farhi (1964).

West's analysis of distribution of blood flow in relation to V/Q ratio is the best method of distinction between shunt and areas of low V/Q ratio (*see* above).

Inserted at reprinting of this edition

Effect of anaesthesia on continuous distribution of ventilation/perfusion ratios

Dueck, Rathbun, Clausen and Wagner ((1977) Abstracts of Scientific Papers, Annual Meeting of the American Society of Anesthesiologists, 223) used a modification of the technique of Wagner, Saltzman and West (1974) to investigate the effect of anaesthesia on the continuous distribution of ventilation/perfusion ratios in man (*see* pages 298–301 and 306). Patients were studied awake and then following the induction of anaesthesia with paralysis and tracheal intubation. Following induction of anaesthesia there were large increases in both intrapulmonary shunt and also perfusion of regions with very low $\dot{V}a/\dot{Q}$. These results would be compatible with a reduction in lung volume.

Chapter 10   Diffusion

FUNDAMENTALS OF THE DIFFUSION PROCESS

Diffusion of a gas is a process by which a net transfer of molecules takes place from a zone in which the gas exerts a high partial pressure to a zone in which it exerts a lower partial pressure. The mechanism of transfer is the random movement of molecules and the term excludes transfer by mass movement of gas in response to a total pressure difference (as occurs during expiration). The partial pressure (or tension) of a gas in a gas mixture is the pressure which it would exert if it occupied the space alone (equal to total pressure multiplied by fractional concentration). The tension of a gas in solution in a liquid is defined as being equal to the tension of the same gas in a gas mixture which is in equilibrium with the liquid.

Typical examples of diffusion are shown in *Figure 107*. In each case there is a net transfer of oxygen from one zone to another in response to a tension gradient. We may note certain points which are common to all three examples.

1. Total pressure differences play no significant part in gas transfer.
2. Gas transfer results from the random movement of the molecules and is therefore dependent on temperature.
3. Gas molecules pass in each direction but at a rate proportional to the tension of the gas in the zone which they are leaving. The *net* transfer of the gas is the difference in the number of molecules passing in each direction, and is thus proportional to the difference in tension between the two zones.
4. In a static situation, such as the example in *Figure 107a*, the process of diffusion proceeds to equilibrium, when there will be no difference between the tension of the gas in the two zones. There will then be no *net* transfer of the gas, although molecules will continue to pass in both directions but at the same rate.

Conditions are not static for oxygen and carbon dioxide in the living body since oxygen is constantly being consumed while carbon dioxide is being produced. Therefore, static equilibrium cannot be attained as in the case of the open bottle of oxygen in *Figure 107a*. Instead, a dynamic equilibrium is attained with a cascade of oxygen tensions from 21 kPa (160 mm Hg) in dry air, down to

1–3 kPa at the site of consumption in the mitochondria (*see* Chapter 12). The maintenance of these tension gradients is, in fact, a characteristic of life.

These considerations do not apply to gases and vapours which are not metabolized, such as nitrogen, nitrous oxide and volatile anaesthetic agents. In these cases, there is always a tendency towards a static equilibrium at which all

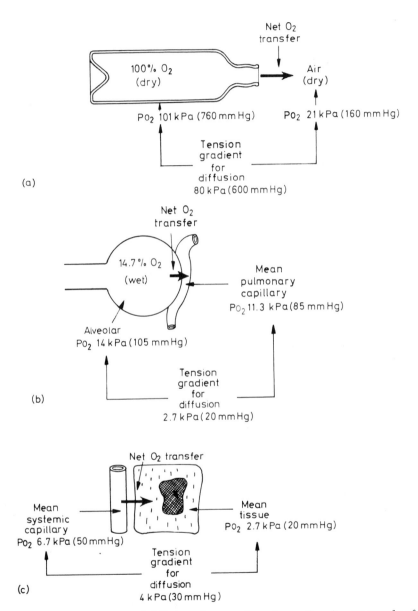

Figure 107. Three examples of diffusion of oxygen. In each case there is a net transfer of oxygen from left to right in accord with the tension gradient. (a) Oxygen passes from one gaseous phase to another. (b) Oxygen passes from a gaseous phase to a liquid phase. (c) Oxygen passes from one liquid phase to another

tissue tensions become equal to the tension of the particular gas in the inspired air. This is attained in the case of nitrogen and would also be attained with an inhalational agent if it were administered for a very long time.

Resistance to diffusion

In each of the examples shown in *Figure 107*, there is a finite resistance to the transfer of the gas molecules. In *Figure 107a*, the resistance is concentrated at the restriction in the neck of the bottle. Clearly, the narrower the neck, the slower will be the process of equilibration with the outside air. In *Figure 107b*, the site of the resistance to diffusion is less circumscribed but includes the alveolar-capillary membrane, the diffusion path through the plasma, and the delay in combination of oxygen with the reduced haemoglobin in the erythrocyte. In *Figure 107c*, the resistance commences with the delay in the release of oxygen by haemoglobin, and includes all the interfaces between the erythrocyte cell membrane and the site of oxygen consumption in the cell (the mitochondria). There may then be an additional component in the rate at which oxygen enters into chemical combination.

There is a clear analogy between the diffusion of gases in response to a partial pressure gradient and the passage of an electrical current in response to a potential difference in an electrical circuit. Diffusing capacity is analogous to conductance (inverse of resistance):

$$\text{diffusing capacity} = \frac{\text{net rate of gas transfer (ml/min)}}{\text{partial pressure gradient (kPa or mm Hg)}}$$

$$\text{conductance} = \frac{\text{current flow (amps)}}{\text{potential difference (volts)}}$$

It will be recalled that the unit of electrical conductance is the *mho*. The usual biological unit of diffusing capacity has been ml/min/mm Hg, but in SI units will probably be ml min^{-1}kPa^{-1}. Alternatively, the quantity of oxygen may be expressed in millimoles and the second may replace the minute.

The size of gas molecules limits their ability to diffuse, and small molecules diffuse more easily than large molecules. Graham's law states that the rate of diffusion of a gas is inversely proportional to the square root of its density. This means that only large differences in density have any marked effect on the rate of diffusion within a gas phase. Thus, nitrous oxide has a density of 1·4 times that of oxygen, but the rate of gaseous diffusion of oxygen is only 1·2 times that of nitrous oxide.

When a gas is diffusing into or through an aqueous phase, the solubility of the gas in water becomes an important factor and the diffusing capacity under these circumstances is considered to be directly proportional to the solubility. Nitrous oxide would thus be expected to have about 20 times the diffusing capacity of oxygen in crossing a gas/water interface. High solubility does not confer an increased 'agility' of the gas in its negotiation of an aqueous barrier, but simply means that, for a given tension, more molecules of the gas are present in the liquid.

Apart from these factors, inherent in the gas, the resistance to diffusion is related directly to the length of the diffusion path and inversely to the area of interface which is available for diffusion. In the case of the lungs, for example, the diffusion path extends from the gas side of the alveolar membrane to some unspecified reference point within the erythrocyte. The area of interface probably corresponds to the total area of pulmonary capillary endothelium in contact with alveolar lining membrane. It is important to remember that the pulmonary diffusing capacity is as much a measure of the area of the interface as it is of the thickness of the tissues which comprise the diffusion path.

The diffusing capacity of oxygen in the lung is markedly influenced by the rate of combination of oxygen with reduced haemoglobin. Clearly, if this is slow, it will retard the whole process of oxygen transfer and similar considerations apply to release of carbon dioxide from chemical combination.

Tension and concentration gradients

In gas mixtures at the same total pressure, the tension of any component gas is directly proportional to its concentration. Therefore, when we consider a gas diffusing from one gas mixture to another, the tension gradient of the gas between the two mixtures will be directly proportional to the concentration gradient. This is not the case when a gas in solution in a liquid diffuses into a different liquid. When gases are in solution, the tension they exert is directly proportional to their concentration in the solvent but inversely to the solubility of the gas in the solvent. Thus, if water and oil have the same concentration of nitrous oxide dissolved in each, the tension of nitrous oxide in the oil will be only one-third of the tension in the water since the oil/water solubility ratio is about 3 : 1. If the two liquids are shaken up together, there will be a net transfer of nitrous oxide from the water to the oil until the tension in each phase is the same. At that time the concentration of nitrous oxide in the oil will be about three times the level in the water. Under all circumstances, the direction and rate of diffusion are governed by tension gradients and it is therefore more useful to consider *tensions* rather than *concentrations* in relation to movement of gases and vapours from one compartment of the body to another. The same units of pressure may be used in gas, liquid and lipoid phases.

DIFFUSION OF OXYGEN WITHIN THE LUNGS

It is now widely accepted that oxygen passes from the alveoli into the pulmonary capillary blood by a passive process of diffusion according to physical laws. For a long time this view was contested by a school of thought which believed that oxygen was actively secreted into the blood. A similar process was known to occur in the swim-bladders of certain fish, so the postulated mechanism was certainly feasible, but proof of secretion depended on the demonstration of an arterial Po_2 which was higher than the alveolar Po_2. In the earlier years of this century a great controversy raged, with active secretion being upheld by Bohr and Haldane while the Kroghs and Barcroft took the opposite view. Much of the difficulty hinged on the analytical problems and on the sampling of representative alveolar gas, particularly under the conditions of exercise. Finally the day was won by the diffusion school although it was for some time contended that secretion might play a part in adaptation to altitude. The idea of active transport of oxygen has recently been revived in relation to cytochrome P-450 (page 381).

There is now strong evidence for believing that diffusion equilibrium is very nearly achieved for oxygen during the normal pulmonary capillary transit time in the resting subject.* Therefore, under these circumstances, the uptake of oxygen is limited by pulmonary blood flow and not by diffusing capacity. However, under conditions of exercise while breathing gas mixtures deficient in oxygen, the diffusing capacity becomes important and may actually limit the oxygen uptake.

The diffusion path

The gas space within the alveolus

In the past there has been some doubt as to the degree of gas mixing which occurs within the alveolus. Some believed that gaseous diffusion would not be sufficiently rapid to maintain equality of gas composition between the core (freshly charged with inspired gas) and the periphery of the alveolus (where the oxygen concentration would be lowest, due to uptake by the pulmonary capillaries). 'Layering' of gas would clearly be a factor limiting the uptake of oxygen, and would impose a tension gradient between the centre of the alveolus and the alveolar-capillary membrane.

Georg et al. (1965) have demonstrated unequal mixing of helium and the heavy gas, sulphur hexafluoride, within the alveolus. However, it seems unlikely that non-uniformity within a single alveolus is an important factor under normal conditions. At functional residual capacity, the diameter of the average human alveolus is of the order of 200 μm (Wiebel and Gomez, 1962), and it is likely that mixing is almost instantaneous over the very small distance from the centre to the periphery. Precise calculations are impossible on account of the complex geometry of the alveolus, but the over-all efficiency of gas exchange within the lungs suggests that mixing must be complete within less than 10 ms (Forster, 1964b). Therefore, in practice it is usual to consider alveolar gas as uniformly mixed within a single alveolus.

The alveolar-capillary membrane

Electron microscopy has revealed details of the actual path between alveolar gas and pulmonary capillary blood, shown in *Figures 4–6*. Each alveolus is completely lined with epithelium which, with its basement membrane, is about 0·2 μm thick, except where its nuclei bulge into the alveolar lumen. Beyond the basement membrane is a tissue space which is very thin where it overlies the capillaries, particularly on the active side: elsewhere it is thicker and contains collagenous and elastic fibres and lymphatics. The pulmonary capillaries are lined with endothelium, also with its own basement membrane, which is approximately the same thickness as the alveolar epithelium, except where it is expanded to enclose the endothelial nuclei. The total thickness of the active part of the alveolar-capillary membrane is thus about 0·5 μm. This arrangement is shown in *Figure 6*.

* In the resting subject, blood passes through the pulmonary capillaries in about 0·75 second. Transit time decreases as the cardiac output rises (*Table 22*).

Pulmonary capillaries

Weibel (1962) has suggested a mean diameter of 7 μm for the human pulmonary capillary. This is similar to the diameter of the erythrocyte which is therefore forced into close proximity with the alveolar-capillary membrane. The pulmonary capillary network is seen by studying thick sections, which will occasionally reveal a face view of an alveolar septum. The space between the capillaries is normally less than the diameter of the capillaries themselves (*Figure 4*).

Diffusion within the blood

Since the diameter of the erythrocytes is so close to that of the capillaries, the diffusion path through plasma may be very short indeed. Furthermore, since the diameter of the erythrocyte is about 14 times the thickness of the alveolar-capillary membranes, it is clear that the diffusion path within the erythrocyte is likely to be much longer than the path through the alveolar-capillary membrane, although the shape of the erythrocyte does tend to concentrate the cell mass at the periphery. Even so, the rim has a thickness of about 2·5 μm, and the diffusion path within it is still large compared with the alveolar-capillary membrane. Once within the cell, diffusion of oxygen is aided by mass movement of the haemoglobin molecules caused by the deformation of the erythrocyte as it passes through the capillary bed. Other factors may be involved since oxygen diffuses through a layer of haemoglobin solution more rapidly than through a layer of water which might be expected to offer less resistance (Hemmingsen and Scholander, 1960).

Uptake of oxygen by haemoglobin

The greater part of the oxygen which is taken up in the lungs enters into chemical combination with haemoglobin. This chemical reaction takes a finite time and forms an appreciable part of the total resistance to the transfer of oxygen. Indeed, it now appears that the reaction of oxygen with haemoglobin is sufficiently slow to be the limiting factor in the rate of transfer of oxygen from the alveolar gas into chemical combination within the erythrocyte. This important discovery by Staub, Bishop and Forster in 1961 resulted in an extensive reappraisal of the whole concept of diffusing capacity, since it followed that measurements of 'diffusing capacity' did not necessarily give an indication of the degree of permeability of the alveolar-capillary membrane. It will be seen below that methods exist for analysing the diffusing capacity of carbon monoxide into two components, one through the alveolar-capillary membrane and the other within the pulmonary blood. The latter component is determined by the pulmonary capillary volume and the rate of chemical combination of carbon monoxide with haemoglobin.

Quantification of the diffusing capacity for oxygen

Diffusing capacity of a gas is defined as the rate of its transfer, divided by the tension gradient across the interface. The rate of transfer of oxygen is simply the

ARP—11*

oxygen uptake, which may be easily measured. The tension gradient is from alveolar gas to pulmonary blood where the relevant tension is the mean pulmonary capillary P_{O_2}.

$$\frac{\text{Oxygen diffusing}}{\text{capacity}} = \frac{\text{oxygen uptake}}{\text{alveolar } P_{O_2} - \text{mean pulmonary capillary } P_{O_2}}$$

The alveolar P_{O_2} can be derived with some degree of accuracy (page 307) but there are serious problems in estimating the mean capillary P_{O_2}.

Changes of P_{O_2} in the pulmonary capillary

It is clearly impossible to make a direct measurement of the mean P_{O_2} of the pulmonary capillary blood, and therefore attempts have been made to derive this quantity indirectly from the presumed changes of P_{O_2} which occur as blood passes through the pulmonary capillaries.

The earliest analysis of the problem was made by Bohr (1909). He made the assumption that, at any point along the pulmonary capillary, the rate of diffusion of oxygen was proportional to the P_{O_2} difference between the alveolar gas and the pulmonary capillary blood at that point. If, for example, the alveolar P_{O_2} is 13·3 kPa (100 mm Hg) and blood enters the pulmonary capillaries at P_{O_2} of 5·3 kPa (40 mm Hg), the rate of transfer of oxygen at the arterial end of the capillary will be 60 times as great as it will be at that point in the capillary where the P_{O_2} has reached 13·2 kPa (99 mm Hg). Using this approach it is possible to construct a graph of capillary P_{O_2}, plotted against the time the blood has been in the pulmonary capillary, provided that the following quantities are known: (1) alveolar P_{O_2}; (2) pulmonary arterial P_{O_2} (= mixed venous P_{O_2}); (3) pulmonary end-capillary P_{O_2}; (4) haemoglobin dissociation curve.

Once the curve has been drawn (*Figure 108*), it is relatively easy to derive the effective or integrated mean pulmonary capillary P_{O_2}. This is similar to the technique for the determination of the effective mean intrathoracic or arterial blood pressure, and the graphical method of determination has already been shown in *Figure 47*. The mean pulmonary capillary P_{O_2} is the height of a rectangle whose area is equal to that under the curve and whose length corresponds to the total pulmonary capillary transit time. The actual procedure for deriving the curve is known as the Bohr integration procedure and, for reasons given below, is now largely of historical interest. Those who are interested in the actual mechanics of the operation will find it expounded by Comroe et al. (1962, page 353). Alternatively, graphs have been prepared to do the arithmetic. These graphs are not published but are referred to by Riley, Cournand and Donald (1951).

The Bohr integration procedure was shown to be invalid when it was found that the fundamental assumption was untrue. The rate of transfer of oxygen is *not* proportional to the alveolar/capillary P_{O_2} gradient at any point along the capillary. It would no doubt be true if the transfer of oxygen were a purely physical process (as in the case of nitrous oxide, for example) but the transfer is actually limited by the chemical combination of oxygen with haemoglobin, which is sufficiently slow to comprise the greater part of the total resistance to transfer of oxygen.

In vitro studies of the rate of combination of oxygen with haemoglobin have shown that this is not directly proportional to the P_{O_2} gradient for two distinct reasons.

1. The combination of the fourth molecule of oxygen with the haemoglobin molecule ($Hb_4(O_2)_3 + O_2 \rightleftharpoons Hb_4(O_2)_4$) has a much higher velocity constant than that of the combination of the other three molecules (Staub, Bishop and Forster, 1961). This is discussed further on page 404.

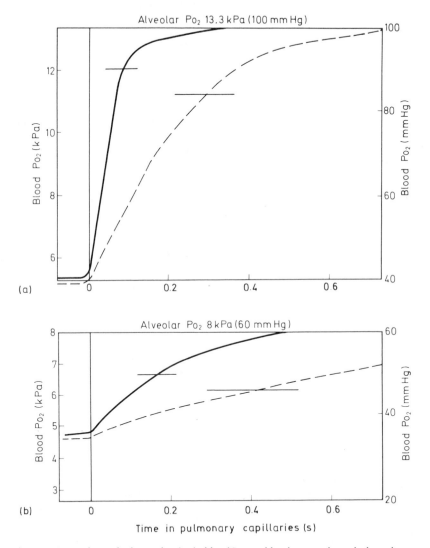

Figure 108. Each graph shows the rise in blood P_{O_2} as blood passes through the pulmonary capillaries. The horizontal line at the top of the graph indicates the alveolar P_{O_2} which the blood P_{O_2} is approaching. In (a) the patient is breathing air, while in (b) the patient is breathing about 14 per cent oxygen. The broken curve shows the rise in P_{O_2} calculated according to the Bohr procedure on an assumed value for the alveolar/end-capillary P_{O_2} gradient. The continuous curve shows the values obtained by forward integration (Staub, 1963a). Horizontal bars indicate mean pulmonary capillary P_{O_2} calculated from each curve

2. As the capillary oxygen saturation rises, the number of molecules of reduced haemoglobin diminishes and the velocity of the forward reaction must therefore diminish by the law of mass action. This depends upon the haemoglobin dissociation curve and is therefore not a simple exponential function of the actual P_{O_2} of the blood.

When these two factors are combined it is found that the resistance to 'diffusion' due to chemical combination of oxygen within the erythrocyte is fairly constant up to a saturation of about 80 per cent (P_{O_2} 6 kPa = 45 mm Hg). Thereafter, it falls very rapidly to become zero at full saturation (Staub, Bishop and Forster, 1962). These authors proceeded to elaborate the Bohr integration procedure to allow for changes in the rate of combinations of haemoglobin with oxygen. Assuming traditional values for the alveolar/end-capillary P_{O_2} difference, they obtained a curve lying to the left of the original Bohr curve shown in *Figure 108*. This indicated a mean pulmonary capillary P_{O_2} higher than had previously been believed, and therefore an oxygen diffusing capacity which was substantially higher than the accepted value. The situation is actually one degree more complicated still, since quick-frozen sections prepared by Staub have shown that the colour of haemoglobin is beginning to alter to the red colour of oxyhaemoglobin within the pulmonary arterioles before the blood has entered the pulmonary capillaries.

Uncertainties about the pulmonary end-capillary P_{O_2}

Both the classical and the modified Bohr integration procedures for calculation of mean capillary P_{O_2} depend critically on the precise value of the pulmonary end-capillary P_{O_2}, and the constructed curve is considerably influenced by very small variations in the value which is assumed. It is therefore appropriate to consider how this value is derived, because it can never be measured directly. Some readers may be content with the simple statement that it is now realized that the pulmonary end-capillary P_{O_2} *cannot* be satisfactorily derived from the arterial P_{O_2}. Others may be interested to read the following paragraphs which explain how it was once thought that it could be done.

The previous chapter has explained how a shunt causes a difference between the P_{O_2} of pulmonary end-capillary and arterial blood. This difference falls to very small values when the alveolar P_{O_2} is reduced to less than about 9·3 kPa (70 mm Hg). Now it happens that the alveolar/end-capillary P_{O_2} difference caused by resistance to diffusion behaves in exactly the opposite way. When the alveolar P_{O_2} is low, the mixed venous P_{O_2} is not reduced by an equal amount because it falls along the steep part of the dissociation curve. Therefore the alveolar/mixed venous P_{O_2} difference is much less than it is when the patient has a normal alveolar P_{O_2}. Consequently, the transfer of oxygen is slower and the alveolar/end-capillary P_{O_2} difference is greater when the alveolar P_{O_2} is low. Riley et. (1946) therefore suggested that alveolar and arterial P_{O_2} should be compared when the subject was breathing first air and then 11 per cent oxygen. At the alveolar P_{O_2} of the first pair of observations, the component of the alveolar/arterial P_{O_2} difference due to resistance to diffusion would be small and the total difference would thus be largely due to venous admixture: under the conditions of the second pair of observations, the component of the difference due to venous admixture would become small while the difference due to resistance to diffusion would be appreciable. It was assumed that both the diffusing capacity and the venous admixture would remain the same while breathing air and 11 per cent oxygen. Typical normal values obtained by this approach were as follows.

	breathing air	*breathing 11% oxygen*
Venous admixture component	1·2 kPa (9 mm Hg)	0·1 kPa (1 mm Hg)
'Diffusion' component	0·1 kPa (1 mm Hg)	1·2 kPa (9 mm Hg)
Total alveolar/arterial PO_2 difference	1·3 kPa (10 mm Hg)	1·3 kPa (10 mm Hg)

Unfortunately, the two-level oxygen study made two assumptions which are now known to be incorrect. Firstly, the component of the alveolar/arterial PO_2 difference due to venous admixture does not fall to small values when the alveolar PO_2 is reduced, because a considerable part of it is now known to be due to regional scatter of ventilation/perfusion ratios (*Figure 98*), and this component actually increases as the alveolar PO_2 falls (*Figure 99*).

The second fallacy is that the resistance to diffusion should be uninfluenced by the actual level of arterial PO_2. It has been explained above that the major part of the resistance to 'diffusion' is due to the rate of chemical combination of oxygen with haemoglobin and we have seen the rate of combination is very markedly influenced by the actual level of PO_2.

The present position of the two-level oxygen method may be summarized as follows.

1. It is not possible to derive the alveolar/end-capillary PO_2 gradient by the two-level method or, indeed by any other known method.
2. Were it possible to derive the alveolar/end-capillary PO_2 gradient, it would still be very difficult to derive the mean pulmonary capillary PO_2 because of the important and variable influence of the rate of combination of oxygen with haemoglobin.

We are thus at least two stages away from the possibility of measuring the mean pulmonary capillary PO_2 and therefore cannot, in the present state of knowledge, measure the diffusing capacity of oxygen. Measurements reported in the earlier literature were based on false assumptions and cannot therefore be regarded as valid.

'Forward integration and let the chips fall where they may' (Staub, personal communication)

The preceding paragraphs have brought us to the position where we can appreciate that it might be possible to derive the mean pulmonary capillary PO_2 if we knew the end-capillary PO_2. However, we cannot derive the end-capillary PO_2 and seem unlikely to be able to do so in the foreseeable future. A new and entirely opposite approach was made by Staub in a most important paper in 1963 (a). Staub started from what was known about the behaviour of oxygen in the pulmonary capillary and, beginning at the pulmonary arterial end, calculated the PO_2 of the capillary blood progressively along the capillary until he was able to give an estimate of the remaining alveolar/capillary PO_2 gradient at the end of the capillary. This procedure of forward integration was thus the reverse of the classical approach which, starting from the alveolar/end-capillary PO_2 gradient, worked backwards to see what was happening along the capillary.

It is useful to list Staub's assumptions.

1. The ability of oxygen to penetrate the alveolar-capillary membrane was taken to be 1·23 times that of carbon monoxide, which is measured more readily (*see* page 332). The ratio of 1·23 expresses the difference in density and water solubility of the two gases.
2. The volume of blood in the pulmonary capillaries was taken to be 86 ml in

resting subjects, the value being derived from studies with carbon monoxide (*see* below).

3. Staub used his own previously published data on the rate of uptake of oxygen by blood (Staub, Bishop and Forster, 1961, 1962).

4. It was assumed that distribution of ventilation and perfusion was ideal.

Staub's forward integrations gave startling results. They suggested that alveolar/end-capillary Po_2 gradients were very much smaller than had previously been thought. Papers by Asmussen and Nielsen (1960) and Thews (1961) had presaged much of Staub's conclusion and, at the time of writing, there is no strong dissent from his view which is a radical departure from what was believed prior to 1963. The results of Staub's calculations are summarized in *Table 22*.

Table 22. VALUES FOR THE ALVEOLAR/END-CAPILLARY PO_2 GRADIENT SUGGESTED BY THE FORWARD INTEGRATION PROCEDURE OF STAUB (1963a)

Conditions	Capillary transit time (s)	Alveolar/end-capillary PO_2 gradient	
		kPa	mm Hg
Resting subject ($\dot{V}O_2$ = 270 ml/min)			
Breathing air (PA_{O_2} = 13·3 kPa = 100 mm Hg)	0·760	0·000 000 001	0·000 000 01
Breathing low oxygen (PA_{O_2} = 6·3 kPa = 47 mm Hg)	0·636	0·03	0·2
Moderate exercise ($\dot{V}O_2$ = 1 500 ml/min)			
Breathing low oxygen (PA_{O_2} = 7·3 kPa = 55 mm Hg)	0·476	0·5	4·0
Heavy exercise ($\dot{V}O_2$ = 3 000 ml/min)			
Breathing air (PA_{O_2} = 16 kPa = 120 mm Hg)	0·496	<0·000 1	<0·001
Breathing low oxygen (PA_{O_2} = 7·9 kPa = 59 mm Hg)	0·304	2·1	16·0

Abbreviations: $\dot{V}O_2$ oxygen consumption; PA_{O_2}, alveolar PO_2.

Importance of the capillary transit time. It is convenient at this point to stress the importance of the capillary transit time as a factor determining both the pulmonary end-capillary Po_2 and also the diffusing capacity. It will be seen from *Figure 108a* that, if the capillary transit time is reduced below 0·2 second, there will be an appreciable gradient between the alveolar and end-capillary Po_2. Other things being equal, this will result in hypoxaemia. Since the diffusion gradient from alveolar gas to mean pulmonary capillary blood will be increased (and perhaps the oxygen consumption reduced), the oxygen diffusing capacity must be less than it would be with a normal capillary transit time.

The *mean* pulmonary capillary transit time equals the pulmonary capillary blood volume divided by the pulmonary blood flow (approximately equal to cardiac output). This gives a normal time of the order of 0·8 second with a subject at rest. However, there appears to be a wide range of values on either side of the mean, and times as short as 0·1 second have been suggested (McHardy,

1972). Blood from capillaries with the shortest time will yield desaturated blood and this will not be compensated by blood from capillaries with longer than average transit times, since capillary P_{O_2} probably reaches its maximum in about 0·2 second. Therefore a wide spread of transit times will increase the alveolar/arterial P_{O_2} gradient. This effect is rather similar to that of the spread of V/Q ratios shown in *Figure 99* and it may be described as due to a spread of D/Q ratios. The concept of spread of D/Q ratios as a potential cause of hypoxaemia was proposed in two important papers by Piiper, Haab and Rahn (1961) and Piiper (1961). It also applies, of course, to reduced diffusing capacity due to causes other than diminished capillary transit time.

Possible causes of a reduction in oxygen 'diffusing capacity'

At this stage, it is helpful to consider the possible causes of a reduction in the value of the oxygen diffusing capacity as defined by the equation on page 316.

1. In the section above, it has been explained how a reduction in capillary transit time may reduce the diffusing capacity. The mean transit time is reduced when the cardiac output is raised (as in anaemia or exercise) and the scatter of transit times may be increased in a number of diseases of the lungs.
2. The total area of the alveolar-capillary membrane may be reduced by any disease process or surgery which removes a substantial number of alveoli. In fact, occlusion of blood flow through one lung has little effect on the alveolar/arterial P_{O_2} difference in patients, even with pulmonary fibrosis (Stanek et al., 1967), but emphysema is thought to reduce the diffusing capacity mainly by destruction of alveolar septa.
3. A reduction in pulmonary capillary blood volume, sufficient to leave a substantial part of the lung unperfused, must reduce the diffusing capacity since the functioning interface is reduced in area.
4. Pulmonary congestion may reduce diffusing capacity by increasing the length of the diffusion pathway for oxygen within the pulmonary capillaries.
5. Severe maldistribution of ventilation relative to perfusion results in a physiological dysfunction which presents many of the features of a reduction in diffusing capacity. If, for example, most of the ventilation is distributed to the left lung and most of the pulmonary blood flow to the right lung, then the effective interface must be reduced. Minor degrees of maldistribution greatly complicate the interpretation of a reduced diffusing capacity and a distinction between maldistribution and a true reduction of diffusing capacity cannot be made by simple means.
6. At first sight, the most obvious cause of reduced diffusing capacity would seem to be an impediment at the alveolar-capillary membrane itself, which might either be thickened or else have its permeability to gas transfer reduced by some chemical abnormality. The term 'alveolar/capillary block' was introduced by Austrian et al. (1951) to describe a syndrome characterized by reduced lung volume, reasonably normal ventilatory capacity, hyperventilation and normal arterial P_{O_2} at rest, but with desaturation on exercise. A reduced diffusing capacity suggested an

impermeability of the alveolar-capillary membrane, which was supported by the light microscopy appearance in such conditions as scleroderma, sarcoidosis, asbestosis, pulmonary fibrosis and pulmonary oedema. Evidence for such a condition at the magnification offered by electron microscopy has proved elusive. We have described elsewhere how interstitial pulmonary oedema tends to accumulate on the inactive side of the pulmonary capillary, leaving the active side relatively normal in appearance and thickness (page 263). This suggests that diffusion across the membrane should remain normal in spite of the presence of considerable pulmonary oedema. Something rather similar has been described for idiopathic interstitial pulmonary fibrosis (Hamman-Rich syndrome or fibrosing alveolitis). Electron microscopy showed that collagen was deposited on one side of the capillaries. Where capillaries were in contact with the alveolar membrane on the other (active) side of the capillary, the alveolar-capillary membrane was normal in appearance and thickness (Gracey, Divertie and Brown, 1968).

It will be seen that the measured oxygen-diffusing capacity may be influenced by many factors which are really nothing to do with diffusion *per se*. In fact, there is considerable doubt whether a true defect of diffusion (e.g. by a thickened alveolar-capillary membrane) is ever the limiting factor in transfer of oxygen from the inspired gas to the arterial blood. In view of these considerations, Cotes (1975) has suggested that the term 'diffusing capacity' be abandoned and replaced by the term 'transfer factor' which implies that factors other than just diffusion may be involved. The symbol T may be used instead of D but the definition and methods of measurement remain the same. It is unfortunate that the term transfer factor has an entirely different meaning in immunology.

The cause of hypoxaemia, previously thought to be due to alveolar/capillary block

The previous section suggests that a true impairment of diffusion is either never or seldom the limiting factor in the transfer of oxygen to the arterial blood. This must be reconciled with the fact that alveolar/capillary block is a well recognized clinical entity, characterized by dyspnoea, hyperventilation (usually with reduced Po_2), cyanosis on exercise (if not at rest) and with radiological evidence of widespread involvement of the lungs by any of a wide variety of pathological processes. The syndrome is clearly distinguished from obstructive airway disease and the FEV/VC ratio is normal or only slightly reduced although the vital capacity itself may be substantially reduced. The syndrome of alveolar/capillary block may be due to a wide variety of diseases, including asbestosis, fibrosing alveolitis and alveolar cell carcinoma. Pulmonary fibrosis may have a known aetiology but otherwise is described as idiopathic interstitial fibrosis (fibrosing alveolitis or Hamman–Rich syndrome). Finally, interstitial pulmonary oedema presents a rather similar picture.

When doubts were cast on the validity of the classical concept of impaired diffusing capacity, Finley, Swenson and Comroe (1962) studied a group of patients previously diagnosed as having alveolar/capillary block and found that, in each case, the arterial hypoxaemia could be explained by disturbances of distribution without the need to invoke an alveolar/end-capillary P_{O_2} gradient.

A similar but more sophisticated study has been carried out by Arndt, King and Briscoe (1970). They investigated 10 patients with the clinical syndrome of alveolar/capillary block. Arterial oxygenation was studied at different inspired oxygen concentrations and the results analysed in terms of a two-compartment lung model (*see Figure 26*). In 2 patients (alveolar cell carcinoma and idiopathic interstitial pulmonary fibrosis), hypoxaemia was present at rest while breathing air and could be explained by the existence of large shunts. In the next 4 patients (sarcoidosis, sarcoidosis with pulmonary fibrosis, desquamative interstitial pneumonia, and eosinophilic granuloma), hypoxaemia could be explained in terms of the 'slow compartment' having a low V/Q ratio (mean value 0·39) and yet sufficient perfusion (mean value 27 per cent of total pulmonary perfusion) to explain the hypoxaemia. This would correspond to a well marked 'shelf' of the type shown for blood flow in *Figure 104a*. Arndt and his co-workers were then left with 4 patients (interstitial pulmonary oedema, sarcoidosis with pulmonary fibrosis and systemic sclerosis with pulmonary fibrosis) in whom there was no appreciable shunt and with identical V/Q ratios in fast and slow alveolar compartments. Therefore, within the limits of their method of analysis, there were no demonstrable grounds for believing that maldistribution interfered with oxygenation of the arterial blood. In fact, this group had a mean arterial oxygen saturation of 96 per cent when breathing air at rest, although this presumably fell on exercise. All 10 patients had severe reductions in their diffusing capacity (measured for carbon monoxide, *see* below), with gross reduction for the slow compartment. It would appear that this was the only remaining cause of desaturation on exercise in the last group of 4 patients.

DIFFUSION OF CARBON MONOXIDE WITHIN THE LUNGS

The diffusion of carbon monoxide has been studied in detail because it is one of the few gases for which measurement of the diffusing capacity is feasible. Measurement of the carbon monoxide diffusing capacity is a routine pulmonary function test which is sensitive to a range of conditions in which other tests yield normal values. It does in fact provide an index which shows that something is wrong and changes in the index provide a useful indication of progress of the disease. However, it is much more difficult to explain a reduced diffusing capacity in terms of the underlying physiology (*see* below).

The outstanding difficulty in the measurement of the oxygen diffusing capacity is derivation of the mean pulmonary capillary P_{O_2}. Turning away from this intractable problem, it was reasonable to consider measuring the diffusing capacity of carbon monoxide as a substitute for oxygen, since the affinity of carbon monoxide for haemoglobin is so high that, for all practical purposes, the tension of the gas in the pulmonary capillary blood remains at zero throughout the usual procedures for measurement of the carbon monoxide diffusing capacity. The formula for calculation of this quantity then simplifies to the following:

$$\text{diffusing capacity for carbon monoxide} = \frac{\text{carbon monoxide uptake}}{\text{alveolar } P_{CO}}$$

(Compare with equation for oxygen, page 316.) The mean pulmonary capillary P_{CO_2} is deleted from the equation because it is equal to zero. There are no insuperable difficulties in the measurement of either of the quantities on the right-hand side of the equation, and the methods are outlined at the end of the chapter.

The diffusion path for carbon monoxide

Diffusion of carbon monoxide within the alveolus, through the alveolar-capillary membrane and through the plasma is governed by the same factors which apply to oxygen and have been outlined above. The quantitative difference is due to the different vapour density and water solubility of the two gases. These factors indicate that the rate of diffusion of oxygen up to the point of entry into the erythrocyte is 1·23 times the corresponding rate for carbon monoxide. It will be remembered that the rate of diffusion is directly proportional to water solubility of the gas and inversely to the square root of the vapour density (Graham's law).

Uptake of carbon monoxide by haemoglobin

At equilibrium the *affinity* of haemoglobin for carbon monoxide is about 250 times as great as for oxygen. Nevertheless, it does not follow that the *rate* of combination of carbon monoxide with haemoglobin is faster than the rate of combination of oxygen with haemoglobin and it is, in fact, rather slower (Forster, 1964a). The reaction is slower still when oxygen is displaced from oxyhaemoglobin according to the equation:

$$CO + HbO_2 \rightarrow O_2 + HbCO$$

Thus the reaction rate of carbon monoxide with haemoglobin is reduced when the oxygen saturation of the haemoglobin is high. The inhalation of different concentrations of oxygen thus causes changes in the reaction rate of carbon monoxide with the haemoglobin of a patient. Use has been made of this fact to study different components of the resistance to diffusion of carbon monoxide in man.

Quantification of the components of the resistance to diffusion of carbon monoxide

When two resistances are arranged in series, the total resistance of the pairs is equal to the sum of the two individual resistances. Diffusing capacity is analogous to conductance, which is the reciprocal of resistance. Therefore when considering the diffusing capacity of a pair of structures in series, both of which offer resistance to diffusion, the reciprocal of the diffusing capacity of the total system equals the sum of the reciprocals of the diffusing capacities of the two components:*

* Adding of reciprocals has already been encountered in the summation of compliances (page 87).

$$\frac{1}{\substack{\text{total diffusing capacity}\\\text{for CO}}} = \frac{1}{\substack{\text{diffusing capacity of CO}\\\text{through the alveolar-}\\\text{capillary membrane}}} + \frac{1}{\substack{\text{'diffusing capacity' of CO}\\\text{within the erythrocyte}}}$$

The second component on the right-hand side is not really a matter of diffusion, since the limiting factor to the passage of carbon monoxide within the erythrocyte is the rate of chemical combination with haemoglobin (exactly as in the case of oxygen). This 'diffusing capacity' within the erythrocyte is equal to the product of the pulmonary capillary blood volume and the rate of reaction of carbon monoxide with haemoglobin (θco), a parameter which varies with the oxygen saturation of the haemoglobin. The equation may now be rewritten:

$$\frac{1}{\substack{\text{total}\\\text{diffusing}\\\text{capacity}\\\text{of CO}}} = \frac{1}{\substack{\text{diffusing capacity}\\\text{of CO through the}\\\text{alveolar-capillary}\\\text{membrane}}} + \frac{1}{\left(\substack{\text{pulmonary}\\\text{capillary}\\\text{blood}\\\text{volume}}\right) \times \left(\substack{\text{reaction rate}\\\text{of CO with}\\\text{haemoglobin}\\(\theta\text{co})}\right)}$$

The usual symbols for representation of this equation are as follows:

$$\frac{1}{\text{DL}_{CO}} = \frac{1}{\text{DM}_{CO}} + \frac{1}{\text{Vc} \times \theta_{CO}}$$

The term DM_{CO} equals $0\cdot80 \, \text{DM}_{O_2}$ under similar conditions (*see Table 24*).

Table 23. VALUES OBTAINED BY VARIOUS METHODS OF MEASUREMENT OF DIFFUSING CAPACITY (TRANSFER FACTOR) OF CARBON MONOXIDE (DATA FROM FORSTER, 1964b)

Technique of measurement	*Total diffusing capacity for CO*		*Membrane component of diffusing capacity*		*Pulmonary capillary blood volume*
	$ml \, min^{-1} \, kPa^{-1}$	$ml/min/mm \, Hg$	$ml \, min^{-1} \, kPa^{-1}$	$ml/min/mm \, Hg$	(ml)
Steady state	113	15	195	26	73
Single breath	225	30	428	57	79
Rebreathing	203	27	300	40	110

The total diffusing capacity for carbon monoxide may be readily measured by the techniques outlined at the end of this chapter; θco may be determined, at different values of oxygen saturation, by *in vitro* studies. This leaves two unknowns—the diffusing capacity through the alveolar-capillary membrane and the pulmonary capillary blood volume. By repeating the measurement of total diffusing capacity at different values of θco (obtained by inhaling different concentrations of oxygen and so varying the oxygen saturation of the haemoglobin), it is possible to obtain two simultaneous equations with two unknowns. It is then possible to solve and derive values for the following.

1. Total diffusing capacity of carbon monoxide at different levels of oxygenation of the blood.

2. Diffusing capacity of the alveolar-capillary membrane (presumably independent of oxygenation).
3. Pulmonary capillary blood volume.
4. The 'diffusing capacity' of carbon monoxide within the erythrocyte at different values of oxygen saturation.

This elegant approach was introduced by Roughton and Forster (1957). Although the original data appeared to undergo an unreasonable amount of manipulation, confidence in the whole operation is engendered by the observed fact that the total diffusing capacity of carbon monoxide is undoubtedly reduced by the inhalation of high concentrations of oxygen. Furthermore, the change occurs very quickly and it would be unreasonable to expect that it was due to changes in the alveolar-capillary membrane. The technique yields normal values for pulmonary capillary blood volume within the range 60–110 ml. These appear astonishingly small, but morphometric studies by Weibel (1962) have indicated a value of about 100 ml at a lung volume of 2·5 litres. This approximates to the functional residual capacity of the human lung in the supine position.

Normal values obtained by various methods of measurement of the carbon monoxide diffusing capacity have been collected by Forster (1964b) as shown in *Table 23.*

Interpretation of the carbon monoxide diffusing capacity

Factors which may affect the oxygen diffusing capacity have been described above. Similar considerations apply to the carbon monoxide diffusing capacity and it will be clear that a low value does not necessarily imply a thickened impermeable alveolar-capillary membrane. It does, in fact, indicate that there is an impediment to oxygen transfer from inspired gas to arterial blood other than hypoventilation. In some cases, it will be clear that the reduced 'diffusing capacity' (or 'transfer factor') is due to a shunt or to well perfused areas of low V/Q ratio (*see* above). However, the present consensus of opinion is that there remain some patients in whom the main defect of oxygen transfer cannot be explained by maldistribution and in whom it is probably reasonable to believe that it is due to a diffusion defect or perhaps to an abnormally wide scatter of diffusion/perfusion ratios. Even this does not mean that the patient has a thickened impermeable membrane. For reasons given above, the defect may be due to short capillary transit time or to excessive destruction of the alveolar-capillary membrane. The effective area of the membrane may also be reduced by pulmonary hypoperfusion.

Having said all this, the carbon monoxide diffusing capacity remains an extremely valuable diagnostic aid. It has the advantage of being sensitive. It shows changes long before these are reflected in altered blood-gas values or other simple tests of pulmonary function. It is, in fact, the most sensitive test of function which is generally available. The test also provides a most useful *numerical index* which may be observed during the course of a disease as a guide to deterioration or response to treatment, even if the physiological basis of the index is not precisely known. It is most useful in patients with the alveolar/capillary block syndrome (*see* above).

Certain non-pathological factors influence diffusing capacity:

Body size influences diffusing capacity directly. This is inevitable since alveolar/capillary gas tension gradients are not greatly different in different species or in different-sized individuals while, of course, gas exchange volumes vary directly with size.

Lung volume. Diffusing capacity is markedly increased when the lung volume is increased (Gurtner and Fowler, 1971).

Exercise results in an increase in diffusing capacity and some workers believe that the increase proceeds to a plateau value which is known as the maximal diffusing capacity (Riley et al., 1954).

Age results in a diminution of both the diffusing capacity and the maximal diffusing capacity.

Posture. Diffusing capacity is substantially increased when the subject is supine rather than standing or sitting (Ogilvie et al., 1957). This change is explained in part by the increase in pulmonary blood volume, and the improvement in the uniformity of distribution of perfusion of the lungs.

Anaesthesia. Bergman (1970) reported no significant change in the carbon monoxide diffusing capacity (steady state method) following the induction of anaesthesia and paralysis (*d*-tubocurarine).

Cytochrome P-450. There is some evidence that the transfer of carbon monoxide (and perhaps oxygen) across the placenta and the alveolar-capillary membrane is partially facilitated by binding to cytochrome P-450 (page 380). Both gases are known to bind to cytochrome P-450. It has been shown that the carbon monoxide diffusing capacity (steady state method) is reduced in man by administration of the antihistamine diphenhydramine which, it has been suggested, may interfere with carrier transfer of gases by cytochrome P-450 (Sumner and Gurtner, 1973). Evidence for cytochrome P-450 acting as a carrier in the placenta is considered on page 38).

DIFFUSION OF CARBON DIOXIDE WITHIN THE LUNGS

Carbon dioxide has a much higher water solubility than oxygen and, although its vapour density is greater, it may be calculated to penetrate an aqueous membrane about 20 times as rapidly as oxygen. Therefore it was formerly believed that diffusion problems could not exist for carbon dioxide because the patient would have succumbed from hypoxia before hypercapnia could attain measurable proportions. All of this ignored the fact that chemical reactions of the respiratory gases were sufficiently slow to limit the rate of diffusion. Attention was therefore turned to the rate of release of carbon dioxide from its chemical combination in the pulmonary arterial blood.

The carriage of carbon dioxide in the blood is discussed in Chapter 11, but for the moment it is sufficient to say that the essential reactions in the release of carbon dioxide in the pulmonary capillaries are as follows.

1. Release of some carbon dioxide from carbamino carriage.
2. Conversion of bicarbonate ions to carbonic acid followed by dehydration to release molecular carbon dioxide.

It will be remembered that the latter reaction involves the movement of bicarbonate ions across the erythrocyte membrane (Hamburger effect) but its rate is probably limited by the dehydration of carbonic acid. This reaction would be very slow indeed if it were not catalysed by carbonic anhydrase which is present in abundance in the erythrocyte. The important limiting role of the rate of this reaction was elegantly shown in a study by Cain and Otis (1961) of the effect on carbon dioxide transport of inhibition of carbonic anhydrase. This resulted in a large increase in the arterial/alveolar P_{CO_2} gradient corresponding to a gross decrease in the apparent 'diffusing capacity' of carbon dioxide.

Although the rate of release of carbon dioxide from whole blood is not precisely known, it is likely to be of the same order as for oxygen (Forster, 1964b).

Equilibrium is probably very nearly complete within the normal pulmonary capillary transit time. However, even if it were not so, it would be of little significance since the mixed venous/alveolar P_{CO_2} difference is itself quite small (about 0·8 kPa or 6 mm Hg). Therefore an end gradient as large as 20 per cent of the initial difference would still be too small to be of any importance and, indeed, could hardly be measured by modern analytical methods.

Hypercapnia is, in fact, never caused by decreased 'diffusing capacity' except when carbonic anhydrase is inhibited by drugs. Under pathological conditions, hypercapnia may always be explained by other causes, usually an inadequate alveolar ventilation for the metabolic rate of the patient.

The assumption that there is no measurable difference between the P_{CO_2} of the alveolar gas and the pulmonary end-capillary blood is used when the alveolar P_{CO_2} is assumed equal to the arterial P_{CO_2}. The assumption is also made that there is no measurable difference between end-capillary and arterial P_{CO_2}. We have seen in the last chapter (page 278) that this is only partly true and a large shunt will cause an arterial/end-capillary P_{CO_2} gradient of up to 1 kPa.

DIFFUSION OF 'INERT' GASES WITHIN THE LUNGS

In the biological sense, inert gases are those which do not undergo chemical changes within the body. This definition includes nitrogen, helium and most of the anaesthetic gases and vapours. Diffusion of these gases is as important to the diver as it is to the anaesthetist, and is an essential consideration in the pharmacokinetics of the inhalational anaesthetic agents.

Since the substances are carried in the blood by purely physical means, their diffusing capacity consists only of the membrane component and there is no limitation due to chemical reaction as in the case of oxygen, carbon monoxide and carbon dioxide. Their diffusing capacities are therefore governed primarily by their water solubilities, and the diffusing capacities of the anaesthetic agents are all very much higher than for oxygen. Heavy molecules such as chloroform, halothane and methoxyflurane result in a high vapour density, but the effect of this is more than offset by their water solubility which is also very high and influences the diffusing capacity in direct proportion. It will be remembered that vapour density only affects diffusing capacity inversely according to its square root, so that its influence is relatively unimportant. Physical properties influencing diffusing capacity are set out in *Table 24*.

Table 24. THE INFLUENCE OF PHYSICAL PROPERTIES ON THE DIFFUSION OF GASES THROUGH A GAS/LIQUID INTERFACE

Gas	Density relative to oxygen	Water solubility relative to oxygen	Diffusing capacity relative to oxygen
Oxygen	1·00	1·00	1·00
Carbon monoxide	0·88	0·75	0·80
Nitrogen	0·88	0·515	0·55
Carbon dioxide	1·37	24·0	20·5
Nitrous oxide	1·37	16·3	14·0
Helium	0·125	0·37	1·05
Ether	2·30	580	380
Halothane	5·07	27·3	12·1

Whatever the small differences between the diffusing capacity of different anaesthetic agents, the important point is that they are all high enough for there to be virtually complete equilibrium between alveolar and end-capillary anaesthetic gas tensions at all times during induction of anaesthesia and recovery. Only very small gradients of partial pressure have been found between end-expired gas and arterial blood (Eger and Bahlman, 1971). The actual value of the pulmonary diffusing capacity is thus irrelevant to the pharmacokinetics of the agent. Uptake from the lungs is *blood-flow limited* rather than *diffusion limited*. In this way they differ from carbon monoxide and resemble oxygen and carbon dioxide.

Since the diffusing capacity of anaesthetic agents is irrelevant to their rate of uptake, it follows that relative insolubility in no way slows down the rate of onset of anaesthesia. In fact, on the contrary, the more soluble the agent, the greater the quantity which must be transferred to the arterial blood to build up the required tension for narcosis. Therefore, contrary to what might be expected from considerations of diffusing capacity, the more soluble an anaesthetic agent the slower will be the induction of anaesthesia and recovery.

DIFFUSION OF GASES IN THE TISSUES

In the case of oxygen there is a series of tension gradients from ambient air to the mitochondria of the cells, the site of oxygen consumption and the point at which the P_{O_2} is lowest (page 383). The series of tension gradients for carbon dioxide is in the reverse direction with the highest values in the mitochondria and the lowest in ambient air.

During induction, anaesthetic gases and vapours diffuse outwards from the capillaries until the tissues reach tension-equilibrium with the incoming blood. During recovery, gases and vapours leave the tissues until zero tension is attained.

Oxygen

Oxygen leaves the systemic capillaries by the reverse of the process by which it entered the pulmonary capillaries. After leaving the tissue capillaries, oxygen passes to its site of utilization in the mitochondria by diffusion, although possibly aided by protoplasmic streaming.

Diffusion paths are much longer in tissues than in the parenchyma of the lung. In well vascularized tissue, such as brain, each capillary serves a zone of radius about 20 μm, but the corresponding distance is about 200 μm in skeletal muscle and greater still in fat and cartilage.

It is impracticable to talk about mean tissue Po_2 since this varies from one organ to another and must also depend on perfusion in relation to metabolic activity. Furthermore, within an organ there must be some cells occupying favourable sites towards the arterial ends of capillaries, while others must be content with accepting oxygen from the venous ends of the capillaries where the Po_2 is lower. This is well demonstrated in the liver where the centrilobular cells must exist at a lower Po_2 than their fellows at the periphery of the lobule. Even within a single cell, there is no uniformity of Po_2. Not only are there 'low spots' around the mitochondria, but those mitochondria nearest to the capillaries presumably enjoy a higher Po_2 than those lying further away.

Figure 109 shows a model in which an area of tissue is perfused by three parallel capillaries. Vertical height indicates Po_2 which falls exponentially along the line of the capillaries, with troughs lying in between the capillaries. Five 'low

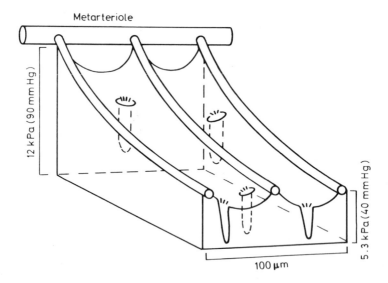

Figure 109. Diagrammatic representation of PO_2 within the tissues. The vertical axis represents the actual PO_2; in the horizontal plane is represented the course of three parallel capillaries from the metarteriole to the point of entry into the venule (not shown). The PO_2 falls exponentially along the course of each capillary with a trough of PO_2 between the capillaries. The pits represent the low spots of PO_2 from about 12 kPa (90 mm Hg) in the tissue close to the arterial end of the capillaries down to less than 1 kilopascal at the mitochondria near the venous end of the capillaries. This is the simplest of many possible models of tissue perfusion

spots' corresponding to mitochondria are shown. This diagram makes no pretence to histological accuracy but merely illustrates the difficulty of talking about the 'mean tissue Po_2' which is not an entity like the arterial or mixed venous Po_2.

There is uncertainty about the actual Po_2 within a mitochondrion. It is known that oxidative phosphorylation will continue down to a Po_2 of about 0.1 kPa (1 mm Hg) (page 380) and some mitochondria may habitually operate at this level. Others, particularly those close to the arterial end of the capillaries, may have a much higher Po_2. Capillary/tissue Po_2 gradients probably range from about 3–5 kPa (22–38 mm Hg).

Since the oxygen consumption of a mitochondrion is probably fairly constant and the geometric layout of its diffusion path for oxygen is also relatively static, it follows that the Po_2 gradient from capillary to a particular mitochondrion must also remain fairly constant. This follows from the general equation for diffusing capacity. Nevertheless, there must be a broad spectrum of different Po_2 gradients for the many mitochondria of a cell.

Carbon dioxide

Little is known about the magnitude of carbon dioxide gradients between the mitochondria and the tissue capillaries. It is, however, thought that the tissue/venous Pco_2 gradient can be increased by two methods. The first is by inhibition of carbonic anhydrase which blocks the uptake of carbon dioxide by the blood. The second is by hyperoxygenation of the arterial blood caused by breathing 100 per cent oxygen at high pressures. If the Po_2 of the arterial blood exceeds about 300 kPa (2250 mm Hg), the dissolved oxygen will be sufficient for the usual tissue requirements. Therefore no significant amount of oxyhaemoglobin will be dissociated and reduced haemoglobin is not available for the carbamino carriage of carbon dioxide, for which it is more efficient than oxyhaemoglobin. This results in partial blocking of the uptake of carbon dioxide by the blood. This theory was advanced by Gessell (1923) as an explanation of the cause of oxygen convulsions. However, it seems likely that the alternative method of carbon dioxide carriage as bicarbonate would be able to function quite adequately in the absence of the facilitated carbamino carriage.

Inert gases and anaesthetic agents

Inert gases will ultimately attain equilibrium in the tissues because, unlike oxygen, they are not constantly being consumed which must result in permanent tension gradients.* The rate of attaining equilibrium with inert gases depends upon the perfusion of the tissue relative to its bulk and the solubility of the agent in the tissue. There is an important distinction between well perfused and poorly perfused tissues. The former are those tissues in which all parts of the cells come into rapid equilibrium with the inert gas carried in the arterial blood, so that the tension of the gas in blood leaving the tissue may be considered equal

---

* Certain anaesthetic agents, including halothane, diethyl ether and methoxyflurane, undergo biotransformation and therefore would never come into true equilibrium.

to the mean tension of the gas in the tissue. Well perfused tissues include brain, heart and liver. Poorly perfused tissues are those in which inert gases tend to diffuse slowly, forming tension gradients in the form of the cylinders and cones which were considered in the case of oxygen, above. Less well perfused tissues include fat, cartilage and, to a certain extent, resting muscle. The practical importance is that the tension of the gas in the venous blood draining the tissue does not give a representative value for the mean tissue tension, being higher during loading and lower during unloading of the agent. This greatly complicates measurement of exchange and also theoretical consideration of long-term changes in tissue levels. Appreciation of this problem has been of the greatest importance in establishing techniques for avoidance of bends after prolonged dives.

There is now evidence that anaesthetics diffuse across tissue boundaries in accord with partial pressure gradients. The quantitative significance of this is not known (Eger, 1974).

PRINCIPLES OF METHODS OF MEASUREMENT OF CARBON MONOXIDE DIFFUSING CAPACITY

All the methods are based on the general equation:

$$\text{Dco} = \frac{\dot{V}\text{co}}{\text{PAco} - \text{P}\bar{\text{c}}\text{co}}$$

In each case it is usual to assume that the mean tension of carbon monoxide in the pulmonary capillary blood (P$\bar{\text{c}}$co) is effectively zero. It is, therefore, only necessary to measure the carbon monoxide uptake ($\dot{V}$co), and the alveolar carbon monoxide tension (PAco). The diffusing capacity indicated (Dco) is the total diffusing capacity including that of the alveolar capillary membrane and the component due to the reaction of carbon monoxide with haemoglobin.

The steady state method

The subject breathes a gas mixture containing about 0·3 per cent carbon monoxide for about a minute. After this time, expired gas is collected when the alveolar Pco_2 is steady by the mixed venous Pco_2 has not yet reached a level high enough to require consideration in the calculation.

The carbon monoxide uptake ($\dot{V}$co) is measured in exactly the same way as oxygen consumption by the open method (page 444): the amount of carbon monoxide expired ($\dot{V}$E x F$\bar{\text{e}}$co) is subtracted from the amount of carbon monoxide inspired ($\dot{V}$I x Fico). The alveolar Pco is calculated from the form of the alveolar air equation derived by Filley, MacIntosh and Wright (1954):

$$\text{PAco} = \text{Pico} - \text{PAco}_2 \frac{\text{Fico} - \text{F}\bar{\text{e}}\text{co}}{\text{F}\bar{\text{e}}\text{co}_2}$$

Rewritten for oxygen, this equation has proved of great value for the calculation of the alveolar Po_2 under the circumstances of general anaesthesia, and is discussed in Chapter 9 (page 308). Measurement of inspiratory and expiratory carbon monoxide and expiratory carbon dioxide concentrations presents no serious difficulty, and infrared analysis has proved satisfactory. Measurement of alveolar P_{CO_2} is more difficult and is discussed in Chapter 11.

For present purposes, it is sufficient to say that the usual method is to sample arterial blood and assume that the alveolar P_{CO_2} is equal to the arterial P_{CO_2}. This is not strictly true in the presence of maldistribution. As an alternative, some workers measure the end-expiratory P_{CO_2} although this, too, does not equal the arterial P_{CO_2} in the presence of maldistribution (page 286). Finally, it is possible to derive the alveolar P_{CO_2} from the mixed venous P_{CO_2} by the rebreathing technique, assuming a reasonable value for the mixed venous/alveolar P_{CO_2} difference (page 373).

The single-breath method

This method has a long history of progressive refinement. The patient is first required to exhale maximally. He then draws in a vital-capacity breath of a gas mixture containing about 0·3 per cent carbon monoxide and about 10 per cent helium. The breath is held for 10 seconds and a gas sample is then taken after the exhalation of the first 0·75 l, which is sufficient to wash out the patient's dead space. The breath-holding time is sufficient to overcome maldistribution of the inspired gas.

It is assumed that no significant amount of helium has passed into the blood and, therefore, the ratio of the concentration of helium in the inspired gas to the concentration in the end-expiratory gas, multiplied by the volume of gas drawn into the alveoli during the maximal inspiration, will indicate the total alveolar volume during the period of breath holding. The alveolar P_{CO} at the commencement of breath holding is equal to the same ratio multiplied by the P_{CO} of the inspired gas mixture. The end-expiratory P_{CO} is measured directly.

From these data, together with the time of breath holding, it is possible to calculate the carbon monoxide uptake and the mean alveolar P_{CO}. A neat mathematical solution is available, and the interested reader is referred to Cotes (1975). Methodology has been discussed in detail by Bates, Macklem and Christie (1971).

The rebreathing method

Somewhat similar to the single-breath method is the rebreathing method by which a gas mixture containing about 0·3 per cent carbon monoxide and 10 per cent helium is rebreathed rapidly from a rubber bag. The bag and the patient's lungs are considered as a single system, with gas exchange occurring in very much the same way as during breath holding. The calculation proceeds in a similar way to that for the single-breath method.

Measurement of oxygen diffusing capacity

For reasons which were developed in this chapter, it now appears that the measurement of oxygen diffusing capacity is based on assumptions which can no longer be considered valid. Therefore, the method is not described here but reference may be made to Comroe et al. (1962).

Chapter 11   Carbon Dioxide

Carbon dioxide is the end product of aerobic metabolism. It is produced in the cells and almost entirely in the mitochondria where the P_{CO_2} is highest. From its point of origin there are a series of tension gradients as carbon dioxide passes through the cytoplasm, and the extracellular fluid into the blood. In the lungs the P_{CO_2} of the blood entering the pulmonary capillaries is higher than the alveolar P_{CO_2}, and therefore carbon dioxide diffuses from the blood into the alveolar gas. Carbon dioxide finally passes into the expired air where it mixes with the ambient air.

Abnormal levels of carbon dioxide have important physiological effects throughout the body. There are many clinical situations in which the P_{CO_2} must be maintained at the optimal level.

CARRIAGE OF CARBON DIOXIDE IN BLOOD

In physical solution

Carbon dioxide belongs to the group of gases with moderate solubility in water. This group includes many of the anaesthetic gases, and the solubility of carbon dioxide is rather greater than that of nitrous oxide. According to Henry's law of solubility:

$$P_{CO_2} \times \text{solubility coefficient} = CO_2 \text{ concentration in solution} \quad \ldots (1)$$

The solubility coefficient of carbon dioxide (α) is expressed in units of $\text{mmol } l^{-1} \text{ kPa}^{-1}$ (or mmol/l/mm Hg). The value depends on temperature, and values are listed in *Table 25*. The contribution of dissolved carbon dioxide to the total carriage of the gas in blood is shown in *Table 26*.

As carbonic acid

In solution carbon dioxide hydrates to form carbonic acid:

$$CO_2 + H_2O \rightleftharpoons H_2CO_3 \qquad \ldots (2)$$

Table 25 VALUES FOR SOLUBILITY OF CARBON DIOXIDE IN PLASMA AND FOR
pK' AT DIFFERENT TEMPERATURES (VALUES FROM SEVERINGHAUS,
STUPFEL AND BRADLEY, 1956a, b)

Temperature ($°C$)	Solubility of CO_2 in plasma		pK'		
	$mmol\ l^{-1}\ kPa^{-1}$	$mmol/l/mm\ Hg$	at pH 7·6	at pH 7·4	at pH 7·2
40	0·216	0·0288	6·07	6·08	6·09
39	0·221	0·0294	6·07	6·08	6·09
38	0·226	0·0301	6·08	6·09	6·10
37	0·231	0·0308	6·08	6·09	6·10
36	0·236	0·0315	6·09	6·10	6·11
35	0·242	0·0322	6·10	6·11	6·12
33	0·253	0·0337	6·10	6·11	6·12
30	0·272	0·0362	6·12	6·13	6·14
25	0·310	0·0413	6·15	6·16	6·17
20	0·359	0·0478	6·17	6·19	6·20
15	0·416	0·0554	6·20	6·21	6·23

The equilibrium of this reaction is far to the left under physiological conditions. Published work shows some disagreement on the value of the equilibrium constant, but it seems likely that less than 1 per cent of the molecules of carbon dioxide are in the hydrated form. It should be mentioned that there is a rather misleading medical convention by which both forms of carbon dioxide in equation (2) are sometimes shown as carbonic acid. Thus the term H_2CO_3 may, in some situations, mean the total concentrations of dissolved CO_2 and H_2CO_3 and, to avoid confusion, it is preferable to use $αPco_2$ as in equation (7) below. This does not apply to equations (4) and (5) below, where H_2CO_3 has its correct meaning.

It would be theoretically more correct to indicate the thermodynamic activities rather than concentrations, the two quantities being related as follows:

$$\frac{activity}{concentration} = activity\ coefficient$$

At infinite dilution the activity coefficient is unity but, in physiological concentrations, it is significantly less than unity. In practice it is usual to work in concentrations,* and values for the various equilibrium constants are adjusted accordingly, as indicated by a prime after the symbol thus—K'. This is one of the reasons why these 'constants' are not in fact constant but should be considered as parameters which vary slightly under physiological conditions.

The reaction of carbon dioxide with water (equation 2) is non-ionic and slow, requiring a period of minutes for equilibrium to be attained. This would be far too long for the time available for gas exchange in pulmonary and systemic capillaries were the reaction not speeded up enormously in both directions by the enzyme carbonic anhydrase which is present in erythrocytes but not in plasma. In addition to its role in the respiratory transport of carbon dioxide, this enzyme is concerned with the transfer and accumulation of hydrogen and bicarbonate ions in secretory organs including the kidney.

Carbonic anhydrase is a zinc-containing enzyme of low molecular weight,

* The glass electrode responds to hydrogen ion activity and not concentration.

discovered by Meldrum and Roughton (1933). It is inhibited by a large number of unsubstituted sulphonamides (general formula $R-SO_2NH_2$). Sulphonilamide is an active inhibitor but the later antibacterial sulphonamides are substituted ($R-SO_2NHR'$), and therefore inactive. Other active sulphonamides include the thiazide diuretics and various heterocyclic sulphonamides, of which acetazolamide is the most important. This drug produces complete inhibition at 5–20 mg/kg in all organs and has no other pharmacological effects of importance. Acetazolamide has been much used in the study of carbonic anhydrase and has revealed the surprising fact that it is not essential to life. With total inhibition, Pco_2 gradients between tissues and alveolar gas are increased. Pulmonary ventilation is increased and alveolar Pco_2 is decreased. The serious student is referred to the important review of carbonic anhydrase by Maren (1967).

As bicarbonate ion

The largest fraction of carbon dioxide in the blood is in the form of bicarbonate ion which is formed by ionization of carbonic acid:

$$H_2CO_3 \rightleftharpoons H^+ + HCO_3^- \rightleftharpoons 2\,H^+ + CO_3^{\,-} \qquad \ldots(3)$$

$$\underset{\substack{\text{first} \\ \text{dissociation}}}{} \quad \underset{\substack{\text{second} \\ \text{dissociation}}}{}$$

The second dissociation occurs only at high pH (above 9) and is not a factor in the carriage of carbon dioxide by the blood. The first dissociation is, however, of the greatest importance within the physiological range. The pK_1' is about 6·1 and carbonic acid is about 96 per cent dissociated under physiological conditions (Morris, 1968).

According to the law of mass action:

$$\frac{[H^+] \times [HCO_3^-]}{[H_2CO_3]} = K_1' \qquad \ldots(4)$$

where K_1' is the equilibrium constant of the first dissociation. The subscript 1 indicates that it is the first dissociation, and the prime indicates that we are dealing with concentrations rather than the more correct activities.

Rearrangement of equation (4) gives the following:

$$[H^+] = K_1' \frac{[H_2CO_3]}{[HCO_3^-]} \qquad \ldots(5)$$

The left-hand side is the hydrogen ion concentration, and this equation is the non-logarithmic form of the Henderson–Hasselbalch equation (Henderson, 1909). The concentration of carbonic acid cannot be measured and the equation may be modified by replacing this term with the total concentration of dissolved CO_2 and H_2CO_3, most conveniently quantified as αPco_2 as described above. The equation now takes the form:

$$[H^+] = K' \frac{\alpha Pco_2}{[HCO_3^-]} \qquad \ldots(6)$$

The new constant K' is the *apparent* first dissociation constant of carbonic acid and includes a factor which allows for the substitution of total dissolved carbon dioxide concentration for carbonic acid.

The equation is now in a useful form and permits the direct relation of plasma hydrogen ion concentration, Pco_2 and bicarbonate concentration, all quantities which can be measured. The value of K' cannot be derived theoretically and is determined experimentally by simultaneous measurements of the three variables. Under normal physiological conditions, if $[H^+]$ is in nmol/l, Pco_2 in kPa, and HCO_3 in mmol/l, the value of the combined parameter $(\alpha K')$ is about 180. If Pco_2 is in mm Hg, the value of the parameter is 24. This equation is very simple to use and has been strongly recommended by Campbell (1962).

Those who prefer to use the pH scale may follow the approach of Hasselbalch (1916) and take logarithms of the reciprocal of each term in equation (6) with the following familiar result:

$$pH = pK' + \log \frac{[HCO_3^-]}{\alpha Pco_2} = pK' + \log \frac{[CO_2] - \alpha Pco_2}{\alpha Pco_2} \qquad \ldots (7)$$

where pK' has an experimentally derived value of the order of 6·1 but variable with temperature and pH (*Table 25*). $[CO_2]$ refers to the total concentration of carbon dioxide in all forms (dissolved CO_2, H_2CO_3 and bicarbonate) as indicated by Van Slyke analysis.

It is sometimes useful to clear equation (7) for Pco_2:

$$Pco_2 = \frac{[CO_2]}{\alpha\{antilog\,(pH - pK') + 1\}} \qquad \ldots (8)$$

It is important to remember that $[CO_2]$ refers to the carbon dioxide concentration in plasma and not whole blood.

Carbamino carriage

Amino groups have the ability to combine directly with carbon dioxide thus:

$$\begin{array}{ccccc} H & & H & & H \\ | & & | & & | \\ R-N-H + CO_2 & \rightleftharpoons & R-N-C-OH & \rightleftharpoons & R-N-C-O^- + H^+ \\ & & \| & & \| \\ & & O & & O \end{array}$$

In a protein, the amino groups involved in the peptide linkages between amino-acid residues cannot combine with carbon dioxide. Carbamino carriage is therefore restricted to the one terminal amino group in each protein and to the side chain amino groups in lysine and arginine. The terminal amino groups are the most effective at physiological pH, and one binding site per protein monomer is more than sufficient to account for the quantity of carbon dioxide carried as a carbamino compound.

Only very small quantities of carbon dioxide are carried in carbamino compounds with plasma protein. Almost all is carried by haemoglobin, and reduced haemoglobin is about 3·5 times as effective as oxyhaemoglobin (*Figure 110*). The actual Pco_2 has very little effect upon the quantity of carbon dioxide carried in this manner, throughout the physiological range of Pco_2 (Ferguson, 1936).

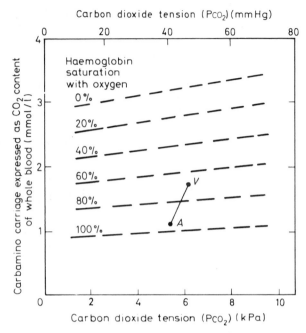

Figure 110. The broken lines on the graph indicate the carbamino carriage of carbon dioxide at different levels of saturation of haemoglobin with oxygen (15 g Hb/100 ml blood). It will be seen that this has a far greater influence on carbamino carriage than the actual PCO_2 *(abscissa). A represents arterial blood (95 per cent saturation and* PCO_2 *5·3 kPa or 40 mm Hg); V represents mixed venous blood (70 per cent saturation and* PCO_2 *6·1 kPa or 46 mm Hg). Note that the arterial/venous difference in carbamino carriage is large in relation to the actual level of carbamino carriage, and accounts for about a third of the total arterial/venous blood* CO_2 *content difference (see Table 26). (These values have not been drawn from a single publication but present the mean of values reported from a number of studies)*

The Haldane effect.   Although the amount of carbon dioxide carried in the blood in carbamino carriage is small (*Table 26*), the *difference* between the amount carried in venous and arterial blood is about a third of the total arterial/venous difference. This accounts for the major part of the Haldane effect which is the difference in the quantity of carbon dioxide carried, at constant PCO_2, in oxygenated and reduced blood (*Figure 111*). The remainder of the effect is due to the increased buffering capacity of reduced haemoglobin which is discussed below. It is interesting to recall that when the Haldane effect was described by Christiansen, Douglas and Haldane (1914) they believed that the whole effect was due to altered buffering capacity: carbamino carriage was not proved until much later (Ferguson and Roughton, 1934).

Formation of carbamino compounds does not require the dissolved carbon dioxide to be hydrated and so is independent of carbonic anhydrase. The reaction is very rapid and would be of particular importance in a patient who had received a carbonic anhydrase inhibitor. The arterial/venous difference in carbamino carriage is lost in certain regions of the body when a patient inhales 100 per cent oxygen at a pressure of about 3 atmospheres absolute, since the oxygen dissolved in the arterial blood is then sufficient for metabolic requirements and very little reduced haemoglobin appears in the venous blood.

Table 26 NORMAL VALUES FOR CARBON DIOXIDE CARRIAGE IN BLOOD

	Arterial blood (Hb 95% sat.)	Mixed venous blood (Hb 70% sat.)	Arterial/venous difference
Whole blood			
pH	7·40	7·367	−0·033
P_{CO_2} (kPa)	5·3	6·1	+0·8
(mm Hg)	40·0	46·0	+6·0
Total CO_2 (mmol/l)	21·5	23·3	+1·8
(vols %)	48·0	52·0	+4·0
Plasma (mmol/l)			
Dissolved CO_2	1·2	1·4	+0·2
Carbonic acid	0·0017	0·0020	+0·0003
Bicarbonate ion	24·4	26·2	+1·8
Carbamino CO_2	Negligible	Negligible	Negligible
Total	25·6	27·6	+2·0
Erythrocyte fraction of 1 litre of blood			
Dissolved CO_2	0·44	0·51	+0·07
Bicarbonate ion	5·88	5·92	+0·04
Carbamino CO_2	1·10	1·70	+0·60
Plasma fraction of 1 litre of blood			
Dissolved CO_2	0·66	0·76	+0·10
Bicarbonate ion	13·42	14·41	+0·99
Total in 1 litre of blood (mmol/l)	21·50	23·30	+1·80

These values have not been drawn from a single publication but represent the mean of values reported in a large number of studies.

Gessell (1923) suggested that the loss of the arterial/venous difference in carbamino carriage of carbon dioxide under these conditions resulted in tissue retention of carbon dioxide, and was a major factor in the cerebral toxic effects produced by high tensions of oxygen. It is, however, unlikely that this would cause a rise of tissue P_{CO_2} greater than 1 kilopascal (7·5 mm Hg), and it is known that such a rise can be tolerated without any of the symptoms characteristic of oxygen toxicity. Furthermore, administration of carbonic anhydrase inhibitors does not produce a condition resembling oxygen toxicity.

The reader who is interested in advances in carbamino carriage is referred to reviews by Roughton (1964) and Kilmartin and Rossi-Bernardi (1973).

Effect of buffering power of proteins on carbon dioxide carriage

Amino and carboxyl groups concerned in peptide linkages have no buffering power. Neither have most side chain groups (e.g. in lysine and glutamic acid) since their pK values are far removed from the physiological range of pH. In contrast is the imidazole group of the amino acid histidine which is almost the only effective buffer in the normal range of pH. Imidazole groups constitute the major part of the considerable buffering power of haemoglobin, each molecule of which contains 38 histidine residues. The buffering power of plasma proteins is less and is proportional to their histidine content.

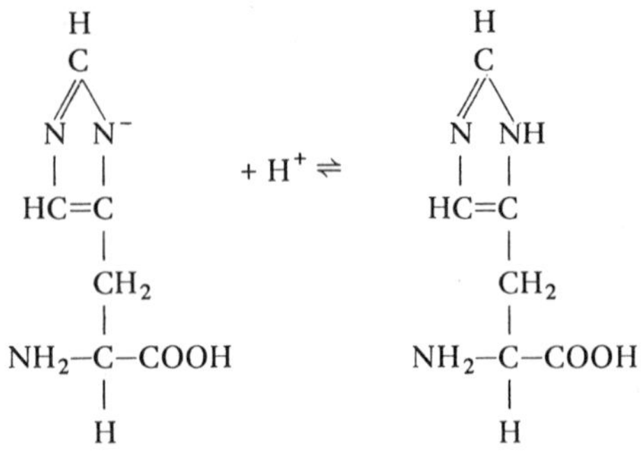

$$
\begin{array}{ccc}
\text{Basic form} & +\,H^+ \rightleftharpoons & \text{Acidic form}
\end{array}
$$

Basic form of histidine   Acidic form of histidine

The four haem groups of a molecule of haemoglobin are attached to the corresponding four amino-acid chains by means of one of the histidine residues on each chain (page 401). The following is a section of a β chain of human haemoglobin:

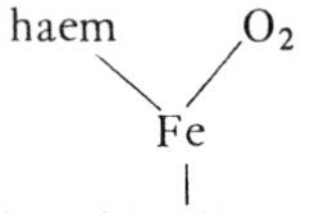

haem O_2

Fe

—leucine—histidine—cysteine—aspartic acid—lysine—leucine—histidine—valine—
  91   92   93   94   95   96   97   98

The figures indicate the position of the amino-acid residue in the chain. The histidine in position 92 is one to which a haem group is attached. The histidine in position 97 is not. Both have buffering properties but the dissociation constant of the imidazole groups of the four histidine residues to which the haem groups are attached is strongly influenced by the state of oxygenation of the haem. Reduction causes the corresponding imidazole group to become more basic. The converse is also true: in the acidic form of the imidazole group of the histidine, the strength of the oxygen bond is weakened. Each reaction is of great physiological interest and both effects were noticed many decades before their mechanisms were elucidated.

1. *The reduction of haemoglobin causes it to become more basic.* This results in increased carriage of carbon dioxide as bicarbonate, since hydrogen ions are removed permitting increased dissociation of carbonic acid (first dissociation of equation 3). This accounts for a part of the Haldane effect, the other and greater part being due to increased carbamino carriage (*see above*).

2. *Conversion to the basic form of histidine causes increased affinity of the corresponding haem group for oxygen.* This is, in part, the cause of the Bohr effect (page 400).

Total reduction of the haemoglobin in blood would raise the pH by about 0·03 pH units if the P_{CO_2} were held constant at 5·3 kPa (40 mm Hg), and this would correspond roughly to the addition of 3 mmol of base to 1 litre of blood. The normal degree of desaturation in the course of the change from arterial to mixed venous blood is about 25 per cent, corresponding to a pH rise of about 0·007 if P_{CO_2} remains constant. In fact P_{CO_2} rises by about 0·8 kPa (6 mm Hg), which would cause a fall of pH of 0·040 units if the oxygen saturation were to

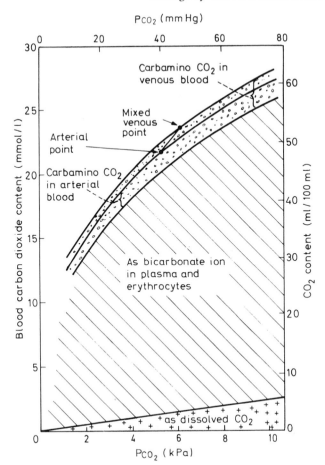

Figure 111. Components of the carbon dioxide dissociation curve for whole blood. Dissolved CO_2 and bicarbonate ion vary with P_{CO_2} but are little affected by the state of oxygenation of the haemoglobin. (Increased basic properties of reduced haemoglobin causes slight increase in formation of bicarbonate ion.) Carbamino carriage of CO_2 is strongly influenced by the state of oxygenation of haemoglobin but hardly at all by P_{CO_2}. (These values have not been drawn from a single publication but represent the mean of values reported in a large number of studies)

remain the same. The combination of a rise of P_{CO_2} of 0·8 kPa and a fall of saturation of 25 per cent thus results in a fall of pH of 0·033 units (*Table 26*).

Transfer of carbon dioxide across cell membranes

It may readily be demonstrated in the laboratory that membranes made of most plastic materials e.g. polytetrafluorethylene or Teflon) permit the free diffusion of carbon dioxide, but will not permit the passage of hydrogen ions. This is, in fact, the principle of the CO_2-sensitive electrode (page 373).

Selectivity of a somewhat similar type exists across cell membranes in the living body. These membranes are relatively impervious to hydrogen ions, but permit the rapid diffusion of carbon dioxide. Therefore, the intracellular hydrogen ion concentration is relatively uninfluenced by changes in extracellular pH, but can be altered by perfusion with a solution containing dissolved carbon dioxide. The carbon dioxide passes through the membrane and inside the cell is able to hydrate and ionize, thus producing hydrogen ions. This property is unique to carbon dioxide which is the only substance, normally present in the blood, able to alter the intracellular pH in this manner.

The passage of carbon dioxide through the cell membrane to release hydrogen ions within the cell is reminiscent of the seige of Troy (Virgil, 19 B.C.). The city of Troy is analogous to the cell and its walls were impervious to Greek soldiers (hydrogen ions). However, the wooden horse (carbon dioxide) passed through the walls without difficulty and once within the city (cell) was able to release the Greek soldiers (hydrogen ions).

This effect of carbon dioxide is of immense physiological importance, and probably accounts for many of the effects of carbon dioxide which are thought to be specific, in contrast to its effect of reducing the blood pH. Chapter 2 describes how this mechanism is thought to underlie the effect of carbon dioxide on the respiratory centre.

Distribution of carbon dioxide within the blood

Table 26 shows the form in which carbon dioxide is carried in normal arterial and mixed venous blood. Although the amount carried in solution is small, most of the carbon dioxide enters and leaves the blood as CO_2 itself (*Figure 112*). Within the plasma there is little combination of carbon dioxide for three reasons. Firstly, there is no carbonic anhydrase in plasma and therefore carbonic acid is only formed very slowly. Secondly, there is little buffering power in plasma to promote the dissociation of carbonic acid. Thirdly, it is thought that the formation of carbamino compounds by plasma proteins is not great, and is presumably almost identical for arterial and venous blood.

Carbon dioxide can, however, diffuse freely into the erythrocyte where two courses are open. Firstly, carbamino compounds may be formed with haemo-globin, not so much because the Pco_2 is raised, but rather because the oxygen saturation is likely to be reduced at the same time as the Pco_2 is rising (*see* above). The second course is hydration and dissociation. Hydration is greatly facilitated by the presence of carbonic anhydrase in the erythrocyte, and dissociation is facilitated by the presence of the imidazole groups on the histidine residues of the haemoglobin, particularly reduced haemoglobin. In this way considerable quantities of bicarbonate ion are formed and these are able to diffuse into the plasma in exchange for chloride ions which diffuse in the opposite direction (Hamburger, 1918).

Dissociation curves of carbon dioxide

Figure 111 shows the classical form of the dissociation curve of carbon dioxide relating blood content to tension. Recently, there has been much greater interest in curves which relate any pair of the following: (1) plasma bicarbonate concentration; (2) Pco_2; (3) pH. These three quantities are related by the

Henderson–Hasselbalch equation and therefore the third variable can always be derived from the other two. For this reason the three possible plots may be used interchangeably and selection is largely a matter of custom or convenience. There is some doubt about the nomenclature of the plots. A plot of plasma $[CO_2]$ against P_{CO_2} is not really a dissociation curve, and a plot of plasma $[HCO_3^-]$ against pH (*Figure 113*) is not really a titration curve since in each case the relevant concentration is in plasma and not blood. The difference however, is not very great, and the general shape of the curve is much the same as when the ordinate is expressed as concentration in blood. With current analytical techniques a plot of P_{CO_2} (logarithmic) against pH has special attractions (*Figure 114*), and is best described as a CO_2 equilibration curve (Siggaard-Andersen, 1964).

It is important to appreciate that, if the P_{CO_2} of an entire patient is altered and the pH changes are not the same as those of a blood sample whose P_{CO_2} is

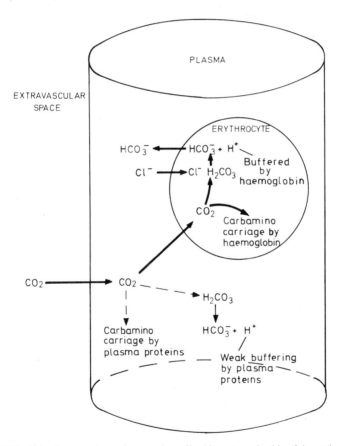

Figure 112. This diagram shows how carbon dioxide enters the blood in molecular form. Within the plasma, there is only negligible carbamino carriage due to the structure of the plasma proteins and a slow rate of hydration to carbonic acid due to the absence of carbonic anhydrase. The greater part of the carbon dioxide diffuses into the erythrocytes where conditions for carbamino carriage are much more favourable. In addition, hydration to carbonic acid occurs rapidly in the presence of carbonic anhydrase and subsequent ionization is promoted by the buffering capacity of haemoglobin for the hydrogen ions

altered *in vitro*. This is because the blood of a patient is in continuity with the extracellular fluid (of very low buffering capacity) and also with intracellular fluid (of high buffering capacity). Bicarbonate ions pass rapidly and freely across the various interfaces, and experimental studies have shown the following changes to occur in the arterial blood of an intact subject when the P_{CO_2} is acutely changed.

1. The arterial pH reaches a steady state within minutes of establishment of the new level of P_{CO_2}.
2. The change in arterial pH is intermediate between the pH changes obtained *in vitro* with plasma and whole blood after the same change in P_{CO_2}. That is to say the *in vivo* change in pH is greater than the *in vitro* change in the patient's blood when subjected to the same change in P_{CO_2}.

Numerous studies have been carried out in animals, and there is indication of some species differences (Shaw and Messer, 1932). Studies in conscious man

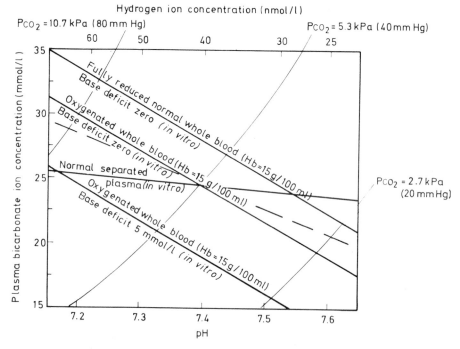

Figure 113. This graph shows a number of CO_2 equilibration curves plotted on the co-ordinates pH/[HCO_3^-]. (Isobars are shown for P_{CO_2} 10·7, 5·3, 2·7 kPa = 80, 40 and 20 mm Hg.) For most biological fluids, the plot is linear over the physiological range. pH = 7·40, P_{CO_2} = 5·3 kPa (40 mm Hg) and HCO_3^- = 24·4 mmol/l is the accepted normal point through which all curves for normal oxygenated blood or plasma pass. The steepest curve passing through that point is the curve of normal oxygenated whole blood; the flattest is that of plasma, both curves being obtained in vitro. The broken curve describes blood of haemoglobin 10 g per cent equilibrated in vitro, or alternatively the arterial blood (Hb = 15 g per cent) equilibrated in vivo of a normal anaesthetized patient whose P_{CO_2} is acutely changed (Prys-Roberts, Kelman and Nunn, 1966). The uppermost curve is that of reduced but otherwise normal blood equilibrated in vitro. The lowermost curve is that of oxygenated blood with a metabolic acidosis (base deficit) of 5 mmol/l equilibrated in vitro

show *in vivo* changes close to the *in vitro* changes obtained in plasma (Cohen Brackett and Schwartz, 1964). Prys-Roberts, Kelman and Nunn (1966) studied step changes of PCO_2 in anaesthetized patients and obtained *in vivo* dissociation curves of similar slope of those which would be obtained with the patient's blood *in vitro* if the haemoglobin concentration were reduced by a third (*Figures 113 and 114*). These curves permit calculation of the very small error in

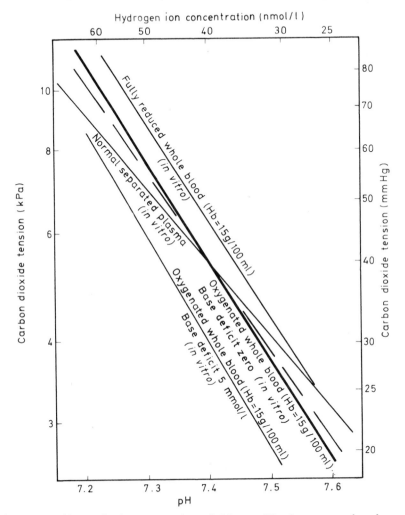

Figure 114. This graph shows a number of CO_2 equilibration curves plotted on the co-ordinates pH/log PCO_2. For most biological fluids the plot is linear over the physiological range. pH = 7·40 and PCO_2 = 5·3 kPa (40 mm Hg) is the accepted normal value through which all curves for normal oxygenated blood or plasma pass. The steepest curve passing through this point is that of normal oxygenated blood; the flattest is that of plasma, both curves being obtained in vitro. *The broken curve describes blood of haemoglobin 10 g per cent, equilibrated* in vitro, *or alternatively the arterial blood, equilibrated* in vivo *(Hb = 15 g per cent), of a normal anaesthetized patient whose PCO_2 is acutely changed (Prys-Roberts, Kelman and Nunn, 1966). The uppermost curve is that of reduced but otherwise normal blood equilibrated* in vitro. *The lowermost curve is that of oxygenated blood with a metabolic acidosis (base deficit) of 5 mmol/l, equilibrated* in vitro

estimation of base excess in patients whose PCO_2 is far outside the normal range. The measured base excess will be about 2 mmol/l low (apparent metabolic acidosis) if blood is sampled when the PCO_2 is 10·7 kPa (80 mm Hg), and the measured base excess will be about 2 mmol/l high (apparent metabolic alkalosis) if blood is sampled when the PCO_2 is 2·7 kPa (20 mm Hg). Values of PCO_2 outside these limits are comparatively rare and a correction factor can easily be applied if necessary.

For further details of acid–base balance, the reader is referred to the monographs of Davenport (1958) and Siggaard-Andersen (1964). An excellent chapter has been contributed by Woodbury (1965), and Nunn (1962c) has reviewed the methods of presentation of acid–base data. Reference should also be made to Campbell (1962), Campbell and Dickinson (1960) and Huckabee (1961).

FACTORS INFLUENCING THE CARBON DIOXIDE TENSION IN THE STEADY STATE

In common with other catabolites, the level of carbon dioxide in the body fluids depends upon the balance between production and elimination. There is a

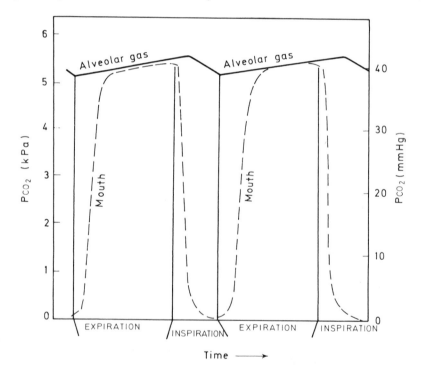

Figure 115. Changes in alveolar and mouth PCO_2 during the respiratory cycle. The alveolar PCO_2 is shown by a continuous curve, and the mouth PCO_2 (as determined by a rapid analyser) by the broken curve. The mouth PCO_2 falls at the commencement of inspiration but does not rise during expiration until the anatomical dead space gas is washed out. The alveolar PCO_2 rises during expiration and also during the early part of inspiration until fresh gas penetrates the alveoli after the anatomical dead space is washed out. The alveolar PCO_2 then falls until expiration commences. This imparts a saw-tooth curve to the alveolar PO_2.

continuous gradient of P_{CO_2} from the mitochondria (the site of production of carbon dioxide) through the cytoplasm, the venous blood, the alveolar gas and thence by way of expired air to dispersal in the ambient air. The P_{CO_2} in all cells is not identical, but is lowest in tissues with the lowest metabolic activity and the highest perfusion (e.g. skin) and highest in tissues with the highest metabolic activity for their perfusion (e.g. the myocardium). Therefore the P_{CO_2} of venous blood differs from one tissue to another, and the mixed venous P_{CO_2} is the integrated mean for the body as a whole.

In the pulmonary capillaries, carbon dioxide passes into the alveolar gas and this causes the alveolar P_{CO_2} to rise steadily during expiration. During inspiration, the inspired gas dilutes the alveolar gas and the P_{CO_2} falls by about 0·4 kPa. This imparts a saw-tooth curve to the alveolar P_{CO_2} when it is plotted against time. One section of this curve may be determined from the carbon dioxide concentration determined at the mouth with a rapid analyser (*Figure 115*). The amplitude of the oscillations of aveolar P_{CO_2} is increased during exercise and this has implications in the control of breathing (page 37).

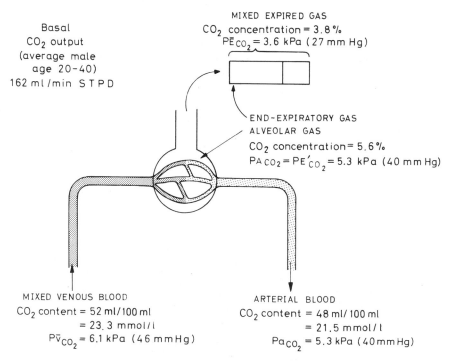

Figure 116. Normal values of CO_2 levels in the healthy unanaesthetized subject. These normal values are rounded off and ignore the small difference in P_{CO_2} between end-expiratory gas, alveolar gas and arterial blood. Actual values of P_{CO_2} depend mainly on alveolar ventilation but the differences depend upon maldistribution; the alveolar/end-expiratory P_{CO_2} difference depends on alveolar dead space and the very small arterial/alveolar P_{CO_2} difference on shunts. Scatter of V/Q ratios makes a small contribution to both alveolar/end-expiratory and arterial/alveolar P_{CO_2} gradients. The arterial/mixed venous CO_2 content difference is directly proportional to CO_2 output and inversely proportional to cardiac output. Secondary symbols: E, mixed expired; E', end-expiratory; A, alveolar; a, arterial; v̄, mixed venous

On the arterial side, the blood leaving the pulmonary capillary has a Pco_2 which is very close to that of the alveolar gas and, therefore, varies with *time* in the same manner as the alveolar Pco_2. There is also a *regional* variation depending upon the ventilation/perfusion ratio of different parts of the lung. This exerts a marked effect upon regional Pco_2, which is inversely related to the ventilation/perfusion ratio (*see Figure 98*). The mixed arterial Pco_2 is the integrated mean of blood from different parts of the lung, and a sample drawn over several seconds will average out the cyclical variations resulting from respiration.

When discussing factors influencing the level of carbon dioxide, it is more convenient to consider tension than content. This is because carbon dioxide always moves in accord with tension gradients even if they are in the opposite direction to concentration gradients. Also, the concept of tension may be applied with equal significance to gas and liquid phases: content has a rather different connotation in the two phases. Furthermore, it seems likely that the effects of carbon dioxide (e.g. upon respiration) are a function of tension rather than content. Normal values for tension and content are shown in *Figure 116*.

Each factor which influences the Pco_2 has already been mentioned in this book and it only remains in this chapter to draw them together, illustrating their relationship to one another. The following section may, therefore, be used either as an introduction to the subject or as a summary.

It is convenient first to summarize the factors influencing the alveolar Pco_2 and then to consider the factors which influence the relationship between the alveolar and the arterial Pco_2.

The alveolar Pco_2 ($PAco_2$) (Figure 117)

Carbon dioxide is constantly being added to the alveolar gas from the pulmonary blood and removed from it by the alveolar ventilation. The concentration of carbon dioxide is simply equal to the ratio of the two, provided carbon dioxide is not inhaled.

$$\text{alveolar } CO_2 \text{ concentration} = \frac{\text{carbon dioxide output}}{\text{alveolar ventilation}}$$

This axiomatic relationship is the basis of all the methods of predicting the Pco_2 and is, in fact, a form of the Bohr equation. Derivations from this equation have been presented in Chapter 6 and we may note the following equation which describes the principal factors influencing the alveolar Pco_2:

$$\begin{array}{c}\text{alveolar} \\ Pco_2\end{array} = \begin{array}{c}\text{dry} \\ \text{barometric} \\ \text{pressure}\end{array} \left(\begin{array}{c}\text{mean} \\ \text{inspired } CO_2 \\ \text{concentration}\end{array} + \frac{CO_2 \text{ output}}{\text{alveolar ventilation}} \right)$$

The equation is shown in graph form in *Figure 118*. Prediction of Pco_2 from ventilation has been discussed on page 186.

The dry barometric pressure is not a factor of much importance in the determination of alveolar Pco_2, and normal variations of barometric pressure at sea level are unlikely to influence the Pco_2 by more than 0.3 kPa (2 mm Hg). At high altitude, the hypoxic drive to ventilation lowers the Pco_2.

The mean inspired CO_2 concentration is a more difficult concept than it appears at first sight, and has been considered in relation to apparatus dead space on page 232. For the present we may note that the effect of inspired carbon dioxide on the alveolar P_{CO_2} is additive. If, for example, a patient breathes gas with P_{CO_2} 4·0 kPa (30 mm Hg or 4·2 per cent of an atmosphere), the alveolar P_{CO_2} will be raised 4·0 kPa above the level it would be if there were no carbon dioxide in the inspired gas, other factors remaining the same. The barometric pressure is the only limit to the elevation of P_{CO_2} which may be obtained by the inhalation of carbon dioxide mixtures. Arterial tensions of over 27 kPa (200 mm Hg) may be produced by a few breaths of 30 per cent carbon dioxide.

Carbon dioxide output is equal to carbon dioxide production in a steady state. However, during unsteady states, output may be quite different from production (Nunn and Matthews, 1959). For example, during acute hypoventilation, the output may temporarily fall to very low figures until the alveolar carbon dioxide concentration has risen. Conversely, acute hyperventilation results in a transient increase in carbon dioxide output. A sudden fall in cardiac output decreases the carbon dioxide output until the carbon dioxide concentration in the mixed venous blood rises. The unsteady state is considered in more detail later.

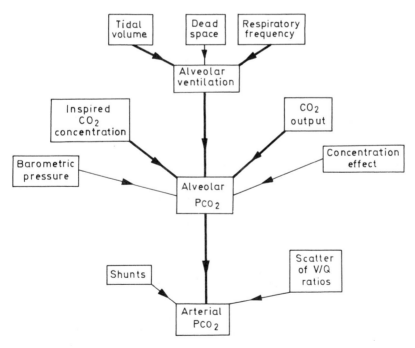

Figure 117. Summary of factors which influence P_{CO_2}; the more important ones are indicated with the thicker arrows. In the steady state, the carbon dioxide output of an anaesthetized patient usually lies within the range 100–200 ml/min and the alveolar P_{CO_2} is largely governed by the alveolar ventilation, provided that the inspired carbon dioxide concentration is zero. The barometric pressure is the only limit to the elevation of P_{CO_2} which may be brought about by the inhalation of gas mixtures containing CO_2. See text for explanation of the concentration effect

Alveolar ventilation, for the present purposes, means the product of the respiratory frequency and the difference between the tidal volume and the physiological dead space (page 228). It is subject to gross departures from normal in certain disease states. These changes are considered elsewhere (page 190).

With gas circuits which result in rebreathing, it is possible for the fresh gas inflow rate to replace the alveolar ventilation in the relationship defined in the equation above. With the alveolar ventilation considerably in excess of the fresh gas inflow rate, the latter may then be used to control the level of the P_{CO_2} (Scholfield and Williams, 1974).

The concentration effect.   Apart from the factors shown in the equation above and in *Figure 118,* the alveolar P_{CO_2} is influenced by what is, for want of a better name, known as the concentration effect. This is caused by a sudden

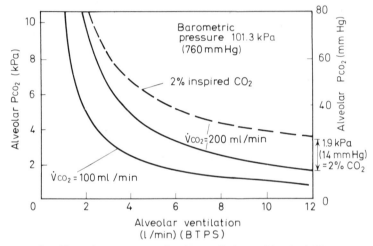

Figure 118. The effect of CO_2 output, alveolar ventilation and inspired CO_2 concentration on alveolar P_{CO_2}. The lower continuous curve shows the relationship between ventilation and alveolar P_{CO_2} for a carbon dioxide output of 100 ml/min (STPD). The upper continuous curve shows the relationship when the carbon dioxide output is 200 ml/min (STPD). The broken curve represents the relationship when the carbon dioxide output is 200 ml/min and there is an inspired CO_2 concentration of 2 per cent. Two per cent CO_2 is equivalent to about 1·9 kPa (14 mm Hg) and each point on the broken curve is 1·9 kPa above the upper of the two continuous curves. The continuous curves are rectangular hyperbolas with identical asymptotes (zero alveolar P_{CO_2} and zero alveolar ventilation). The broken curve is also a rectangular hyperbola but the horizontal asymptote is P_{CO_2} 1·9 kPa (14 mm Hg) which is the tension in the inspired gas

change in the net transfer of inert gases across the alveolar-capillary membrane. This is only likely to have an important effect on carbon dioxide at the end of an anaesthetic when large quantities of nitrous oxide are passing from the body stores into the alveolar gas, and a much smaller quantity of nitrogen is returning to its accustomed place in the body. This leads to a dilution of the alveolar carbon dioxide. The fall in P_{CO_2} is probably small but may be sufficient to cause a transient reduction in ventilation when nitrous oxide is withdrawn at the end of an operation.(*See also* page 388.) The reverse effect occurs at the start of nitrous oxide inhalation.

The end-expiratory P_{CO_2}

In the normal, healthy, conscious subject, the end-expiratory gas consists almost entirely of alveolar gas. If, however, appreciable numbers of alveoli are ventilated but not perfused, they will contribute a significant quantity of CO_2-free gas from the alveolar dead space to the end-expiratory gas (*see Figure 78*). As a result the end-expiratory P_{CO_2} (end-tidal or Haldane–Priestley sample) will have a lower P_{CO_2} than that of the alveoli which are perfused. Gas cannot be sampled selectively from the perfused alveoli, but Chapter 9 explains how the arterial P_{CO_2} usually approximates closely to the mean value of the perfused alveoli in spite of scatter of ventilation/perfusion ratios (*see Figure 100*). It is, therefore, possible to compare the arterial P_{CO_2} with the end-expiratory P_{CO_2} to demonstrate the existence of an appreciable proportion of unperfused alveoli. Studies during anaesthesia have, for example, shown an arterial/end-tidal P_{CO_2} gradient of about 0·7 kPa (5 mm Hg) in patients without lung disease (Ramwell 1958; Nunn and Hill, 1960).

The alveolar/arterial P_{CO_2} *Gradient*

For reasons which have been discussed in Chapter 10, we may discount the possibility of any significant gradient between the P_{CO_2} of alveolar gas and pulmonary end-capillary blood. Arterial P_{CO_2} may, however, differ slightly from the mean alveolar P_{CO_2} as a result of shunting or scatter of ventilation/perfusion ratios. The magnitude of the gradient has been considered in Chapter 9 where it was shown that a shunt of 10 per cent will only cause an alveolar/arterial P_{CO_2} gradient of about 0·08 kPa (0·6 mm Hg). Since the normal degree of ventilation/perfusion ratio scatter causes a gradient of the same order, neither can be considered to cause a significant gradient and, for practical purposes, there is an established convention by which the arterial and alveolar P_{CO_2} values are taken to be identical. It is only in exceptional patients that the gradient is likely to exceed 0·3 kPa (2 mm Hg).

The table accompanying *Figure 100* shows the gradients in P_{CO_2} between air and arterial blood in imaginary but typical anaesthetized patients with 10 per cent alveolar dead space effect, 10 per cent shunt and the normal degree of scatter of ventilation/perfusion ratios. Much the largest part of the arterial/end-expiratory P_{CO_2} gradient is due to the component between the true mean alveolar gas and the end-expiratory gas caused by alveolar dead space, or a dead-space effect produced by areas of very high V/Q ratio.

The arterial P_{CO_2}

The normal range

There are 7 studies of healthy subjects with in-dwelling arterial cannulas reported by various authors from 5 countries. Pooled results show a mean of 5·1 kPa (38·1 mm Hg) with 95 per cent limits (2 s.d.) of ± 1·0 kPa (7·6 mm Hg). Five per cent of normal patients will lie outside these limits and it is therefore preferable to refer to this as the reference range rather than the normal range. There is no evidence that P_{CO_2} is influenced by age unless the patient goes into respiratory failure.

Hypocapnia (respiratory alkalosis)

Low values of Pco_2 are very commonly found. This may be due to voluntary hyperventilation resulting from arterial puncture and it is sometimes better to insert a cannula, returning for the sample when the patient has settled. Persistently low values may now be due to an excessive respiratory drive resulting from one of the following causes.

Hypoxaemia is a common cause of hypocapnia, occurring in congenital heart disease with right-to-left shunting, residence at high altitude, pulmonary collapse or consolidation and any other condition which reduces the arterial Po_2 below about 8 kPa (60 mm Hg). The pathway of Pco_2/Po_2 changes in shunting is shown in *Figure 66*.

Metabolic acidosis produces a compensatory hyperventilation (air hunger) which minimizes the fall in pH which would otherwise occur. This is a pronounced feature of diabetic ketosis and severe haemorrhagic shock. Arterial Pco_2 values below 3 kPa (22·5 mm Hg) are not uncommon.

Mechanical abnormalities of the lung may drive respiration through the vagus, resulting in moderate reduction of the Pco_2. Thus conditions such as pulmonary fibrosis and asthma are usually associated with a low to normal Pco_2 until the patient passes into respiratory failure.

Hypotension may drive respiration directly but, in cases of haemorrhage, metabolic acidosis is usually a more important factor.

Hysteria, head injuries and various neurological disorders may result in hyperventilation.

This list is not exhaustive but serves to show the wide range of conditions which may result in hyperventilation. More than one factor may operate at the same time. Reference may be made to Chapter 2, in which control of breathing is considered.

Hypercapnia (respiratory acidosis)

It is uncommon to encounter an arterial Pco_2 above the normal range in a healthy subject. Any value of more than 6 kPa (45 mm Hg) should be considered abnormal. Values up to 6·7 kPa (50 mm Hg) may be attained by breath holding but, by breathing mixtures of carbon dioxide in oxygen, the normal subject may attain a Pco_2 of 10 kPa (75 mm Hg) without ill effect. Higher values, whether due to inhalation of carbon dioxide or to hypoventilation, result in confusion and loss of consciousness. While breathing air, it is not possible for a hypoventilating patient to have a Pco_2 in excess of about 13 kPa (100 mm Hg) because, at that level of ventilation, the accompanying hypoxaemia will become critical (*see Figure 66*). Pco_2 values in excess of 13 kPa can only occur in patients breathing oxygen-enriched gas mixtures and the condition can therefore be regarded as iatrogenic.

Pathological causes of hypoventilation leading to hypercapnia have been considered in Chapter 6 (pages 190 et seq). In respiratory medicine, the commonest cause of hypercapnia is chronic bronchitis. The type of patient known as the blue bloater has reduced ventilatory capacity combined with reduced ventilatory response to carbon dioxide. It is an intractable, progressive condition which renders the patient a poor risk for anaesthesia and surgery (Milledge and Nunn, 1975). Fortunately, it is becoming far less common in Great Britain. In other chest diseases, including asthma and emphysema (pink puffers) the rise in P_{CO_2} is generally late and may be terminal.

In patients with chronic bronchitis, respiratory failure is accompanied by dyspnoea, and hypercapnia may frequently be diagnosed on clinical grounds. The skin is usually flushed and the pulse is full and bounding with occasional extrasystoles. The blood pressure is often raised but this is not always the case. Muscle twitchings and a characteristic flap of the hands are seen as the P_{CO_2} approaches the level at which coma occurs. Convulsions may occur. It would, however, be quite wrong to believe that hypercapnia can always be diagnosed on clinical examination. It may be quite impossible to detect at the bedside, particularly when it is due to a neurological failure of ventilation such as depression of the 'respiratory centre', poliomyelitis or polyneuritis. It is also impossible to be certain of the P_{CO_2} in cases of crushed chest. If there is the least doubt, it is essential to measure the P_{CO_2}, preferably by arterial puncture and one of the methods of analysis outlined at the end of this chapter.

Exogenous hypercapnia results from inhalation of carbon dioxide from a source outside the patient. As a rough approximation, the arterial P_{CO_2} is raised by an amount equal to the P_{CO_2} of the inspired gas mixture. Thus the use of 5 per cent carbon dioxide in the inspired gas raises the P_{CO_2} by approximately 4·8 kPa (36 mm Hg) at sea level while the inhalation of 30 per cent carbon dioxide will raise the arterial P_{CO_2} above 28·5 kPa (214 mm Hg). An account of the use of this gas mixture in psychiatry has been given by Meduna (1958). The new elevated level of P_{CO_2} is attained within one or two minutes.

The rate of change of P_{CO_2} under various circumstances is considered below (page 354).

Carbon dioxide levels during anaesthesia

From the above discussion of factors which influence carbon dioxide levels it will be clear that, during anaesthesia, the principal factors must be the inspired carbon dioxide concentration, the carbon dioxide output and the alveolar ventilation, the last being a function of the total ventilation and the physiological dead space.

The concentration of carbon dioxide in the inspired gas is normally zero but may be raised accidentally or intentionally to any concentration. Accidental administration of about 30 per cent carbon dioxide has been described for endogenous carbon dioxide by Schultz et al. (1960), and for exogenous carbon dioxide by Prys-Roberts, Smith and Nunn (1967). The only difference between the two conditions is that the increase of P_{CO_2} due to exogenous carbon dioxide may be very much more rapid than when the patient's own carbon dioxide is allowed to accumulate.

Carbon dioxide output in the anaesthetized patient is reasonably constant *during the steady state* and is likely to be within 50 ml/min of the values shown in *Table 15*. Unsteady states are considered in the next section. They may cause wide temporary disparities between the carbon dioxide output and the carbon dioxide production which probably remains fairly constant.

The minute volume may vary widely during anaesthesia. The lower limits are reached during spontaneous respiration with either deep anaesthesia or partial neuromuscular blockade, when minute volumes as low as 1·95 l/min have been recorded (Nunn, 1958a). On the other hand, during artificial ventilation, very high minute volumes may be attained and values in excess of 20 l/min are common. Nunn (1958a) has demonstrated the effect of changes in ventilation on the P_{CO_2} of patients under routine anaesthesia and Figure 5 in that article may be compared with *Figure 118*.

The effects of anaesthesia upon the various subdivisions of the dead space have been discussed in Chapter 7. It is a reasonable working rule that the alveolar ventilation of a healthy, intubated anaesthetized patient is two-thirds of the total minute volume (excluding ventilation of the apparatus dead space; Nunn and Hill, 1960). *Including* apparatus dead space, aveolar ventilation approximates half the minute volume of intubated patients but only one-third of the minute volume of patients breathing from a mask (Kain, Panday and Nunn, 1969).

It will be apparent from the paragraphs above that, during anaesthesia, the arterial P_{CO_2} may lie anywhere between 2 and, say, 30 kPa (15–255 mm Hg), largely according to the whim of the anaesthetist. In fact, it generally lies between 2·7 and 4·7 kPa (20–35 mm Hg) during anaesthesia with artificial ventilation, and between 5·3 and 8·7 kPa (40–65 mm Hg) during anaesthesia with spontaneous respiration. However, levels as high as 21·3 kPa (160 mm Hg) are apparently accepted by some anaesthetists in the course of routine anaesthesia (Birt and Cole, 1965).

During thoracotomy, values as high as 31·5 kPa (236 mm Hg) were recorded by some anaesthetists in the days before general appreciation of the value of artificial ventilation in patients with an open thorax (Ellison, Ellison and Hamilton, 1955). With artificial ventilation, normal or subnormal values for arterial P_{CO_2} may be attained during thoracic surgery without excessively large minute volumes, 7 l/min being sufficient in most cases (Nunn, 1961a).

CARBON DIOXIDE STORES AND THE UNSTEADY STATE

The quantity of carbon dioxide in the body is very large (about 120 litres), much of it being in the form of carbonates in bone or dissolved in lipids. Even the aqueous body fluids contain about 500 ml of carbon dioxide per litre. In contrast, all body fluids (except blood) contain considerably less oxygen than 2 ml/l, and even arterial blood contains only about 200 ml of oxygen per litre.

Because of the vast amount of carbon dioxide in the body, the total quantity can only be changed very slowly when ventilation is altered out of accord with metabolic requirements. However, the body is not a single compartment but consists of an infinite number of compartments, each of which has its own time course of change of P_{CO_2} in response to a change in ventilation. As a simplification, it is reasonably satisfactory to represent the body as though it consisted of three compartments. *Figure 119* shows a hydrostatic analogy in which the depth of water represents PCO_2, and the volume of water corresponds to volume of carbon dioxide. The production of CO_2 in the tissues is represented by the variable flow of water from the supply tank into three lower tanks which represent the body compartments.

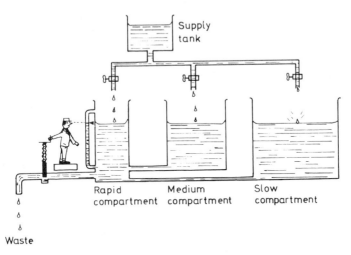

Figure 119. A hydrostatic analogy of the elimination of carbon dioxide. See text for full discussion

The rapid compartment represents circulating blood, brain, kidneys and other well perfused tissues which are at a PCO_2 slightly higher than that of alveolar gas and tend to follow a similar time course during changes of PCO_2. The medium compartment represents skeletal muscle (in the resting state) and other parts of the body with a moderate blood flow. This tank is quite large and is connected to the rapid compartment by a relatively narrow pipe; therefore, sudden changes in the level of water in the rapid tank will produce only gradual changes in the water level in the medium tank. (For example, during acute hyperventilation, the muscle PCO_2 falls more slowly than that of alveolar gas.) The slow compartment represents fat and bone and other tissues with a very large capacity for carbon dioxide, but which are only able to change their carbon dioxide level slowly. In the case of fat, this is because of poor blood supply while, in the case of bone, it is because of the slow process by which carbon dioxide is released from carbonates. It will be clear from the diagram that the level of water can change only very slowly in the slow compartment.

The elimination of carbon dioxide by alveolar ventilation is represented by the outflow pipe which is controlled by a tap operated by a man observing the level in the rapid compartment. He represents the 'respiratory centre', which controls alveolar ventilation in accord with the PCO_2 of the arterial blood (*inter alia*). If the outlet valve is suddenly opened widely (hyperventilation) while the inflow is unchanged, the levels will all fall to a new equilibrium level. That in the rapid compartment will start to fall rapidly as soon as the valve is opened, with those in the other tanks lagging behind. As the level in the 'fast' tank falls, the outflow rate slackens and the transfer of water from the medium and slow compartments to the rapid compartment then becomes appreciable in relation to the outflow. The final approach to the equilibrium level in the rapid compartment is then very slow.

If we plot the level of water in the rapid tank against time, during a sudden opening of the outlet valve, the graph will be analogous to the change in arterial Pco_2 produced by a sudden increase in ventilation (not associated with an increase in metabolism). The wash-out curve in each case is rather complex, being a compound of a number of exponential functions each with its own time constant (Appendix E). In fact, the changes can usually be adequately expressed as though there were only two compartments and two exponentials. As a further simplification we may sometimes consider the situation as though it were a single-compartment system represented by a single exponential. In fact such a simplified plot would not be so very different from the more accurate three-compartment model, and a practised eye and very careful measurements are needed to demonstrate the wash-out of multi-compartment systems.

If we may be permitted to talk of the human body as though it were a single-compartment system, we might go so far as to talk about the half-time of the system, which is the time required for the Pco_2 to fall half-way to its final value after a step increase in ventilation (*Figur 152*). This has been studied by Fahri and Rahn (1955a), and Nunn and Matthews (1959), and is of the order of 3–4 minutes in man. *Figure 120* (solid circles) shows a typical example of the time course of the fall of Pco_2, in this case following a step increase of ventilation from 3·3 to 14 l/min in an anaesthetized paralysed patient. The slow component of change cannot be detected against the background scatter of the experimental observations after 20 minutes.

It has been realized only comparatively recently that the time course of the increase of Pco_2 following step decrease of ventilation does not necessarily follow the mirror image of the time course of decrease of Pco_2 when ventilation is increased. In fact, the rate of rise is much slower than the rate of fall, which is fortunate for patients in asphyxial situations. In the event of total respiratory arrest, the rate of rise of arterial Pco_2 is of the order of 0·4–0·8 kPa/min (3–6 mm Hg/min), which is the resultant of the rate of production of carbon dioxide and the capacity of the body stores to accommodate the carbon dioxide which is produced. Returning to the hydrostatic analogy in *Figure 119*, it will be clear that, if the outflow pipe is totally obstructed, the rate of rise of water will be the resultant of the inflow from the supply tank and the capacity of the tanks. The most important of these is the capacity of the rapid compartment because the changes in the other tanks are too slow to influence matters in an acute asphyxial situation. It happens that the maximal rate of rise is much slower than the rate of fall which can occur when the outflow valve is opened widely.

During acute hypoventilation in an anaesthetized patient, the rate of rise of arterial Pco_2 will always be less than the maximal rate in apnoea, and the study of Nunn (1964) suggested that the measurable rate of rise of Pco_2 during hypoventilation was unlikely to be complete in an hour. Sullivan, Patterson and Papper (1966) showed that the time course of rise was indeed very much slower than the known rate of fall of Pco_2 when ventilation was increased, and half-changes required about 15–20 minutes (open circles in *Figures 120*). The time course of rise of Pco_2 after step reduction of ventilation is faster when the previous level of ventilation has been of short duration (Ivanov and Nunn, 1968).

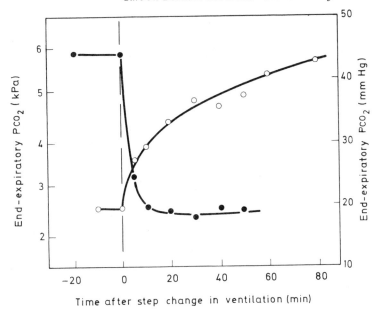

Figure 120. Time course of changes in end-expiratory PCO_2 *following step changes in ventilation. The solid circles indicate the changes in end-expiratory* PCO_2 *which followed a step change in ventilation from 3·3 to 14 l/min. The open circles show the change following a step change in ventilation from 14 to 3·3 l/min in the same patient. During the fall of* PCO_2, *half the total change is completed in about 3 minutes. During the rise of* PCO_2, *half-change takes approximately 16 minutes*

The practical significance of the difference in time courses shown in *Figure 120* is that hyperventilation of an anaesthetized patient causes a rapid fall in PCO_2, with the new low level attained, for all practical purposes, within about 10 minutes. On the other hand, if a patient is permitted to hypoventilate, the PCO_2 will rise to a new high level but the change will not be precipitate. For example, if a patient hypoventilates at 3 litres per minute during an operation lasting one hour, we may expect the PCO_2 to rise towards a level of about 9·3 kPa (70 mm Hg), which is the predicted steady-state level of PCO_2, appropriate allowance being made for apparatus dead space. However, the PCO_2 will only have risen from 5·3 to about 7·3 kPa (40 to about 55 mm Hg) by the end of the first 15 minutes, and is probably only about 8·3 kPa (63 mm Hg) at the end of the operation. Clearly, prediction of PCO_2 will be of very limited value after acute reductions in ventilation, and it must be remembered that prediction does not claim to indicate the actual PCO_2, but the PCO_2 which will be attained if the level of ventilation is maintained (Nunn, 1960a).

Ivanov and Nunn (1969) compared the rapidity with which PCO_2 could be elevated in a hyperventilated patient. As described above, reduction of minute volume was too slow a method to be used in an acute situation. Hypoventilation with a low fresh gas inflow into a circle system without soda-lime was the fastest practicable method without using exogenous carbon dioxide. This technique was more effective than simple hypoventilation and achieved a mean rate of rise of PCO_2 of about 0·4 kPa/min (3 mm Hg/min). However, even this did not compare with the rate of rise of P_{CO_2} attainable by the use of exogenous carbon dioxide. The use of an inspired gas mixture containing 5 per cent carbon dioxide elevated the P_{CO_2} by 2·3 kPa (17·3 mm Hg) in 2 minutes, most of the change occurring in the first minute.

Laparoscopy with carbon dioxide as the inflating gas seems at first sight to carry a hazard of exogenous carbon dioxide intoxication. However, a number of studies have now shown that the elevation of P_{CO_2} is minimal provided that pulmonary ventilation is properly maintained (Kelman et al., 1972). Surprisingly, the elevation of P_{CO_2} appears to be greater if nitrous oxide is used as the inflating gas.

It will be seen in Chapter 12 that, unlike the P_{CO_2}, the P_{O_2} changes very quickly after changes in ventilation. Consequently, changes in ventilation are followed by temporary changes in the respiratory exchange ratio although, if the ventilation is held constant, the respiratory exchange ratio must eventually return to the level determined by the metabolic process of the body. Carbon dioxide stores have been reviewed by Farhi (1964).

APNOEIC MASS-MOVEMENT OXYGENATION
(formerly known as DIFFUSION RESPIRATION)

When a patient becomes apnoeic, the alveolar gas tends to come into equilibrium with the mixed venous blood which continues to perfuse the lungs. Assuming normal initial values for the composition of the alveolar gas and mixed venous gas tensions, this would entail a rise of P_{CO_2} from 5·3 to 6·1 kPa (40 to 46 mm Hg) and a fall of P_{O_2} from 14 to 5·3 kPa (105 to 40 mm Hg). The *volume* of gas which would require to cross the alveolar-capillary membrane is directly proportional to the gas tension change. Ignoring changes in the composition of the mixed venous blood and assuming an average FRC, equilibration of alveolar gas with mixed venous blood would require the output of 21 ml of carbon dioxide and the uptake of 230 ml of oxygen at normal lung volume. The small quantity of carbon dioxide could be transferred in a few seconds, but 230 ml of oxygen would require more than a minute under basal conditions. Therefore, carbon dioxide would come into equilibrium within one circulation time while oxygen would take much longer. Thus for practical purposes, carbon dioxide does reach equilibrium while oxygen is always *tending towards* equilibrium but never reaching it, since the mixed venous P_{O_2} is always lower than the arterial P_{O_2} after the blood has passed through the systemic circulation. There are no appreciable body stores of oxygen, and therefore the arterial/mixed venous oxygen content difference must remain fairly constant.

What actually happens in apnoea depends upon the patency of the airway and the composition of the ambient gas if the airway is patent.

With airway occlusion the pattern of change is close to that described above. There is a rapid attainment of equilibrium between alveolar and mixed venous P_{CO_2}. The arterial, alveolar and mixed venous P_{CO_2} values remain close together and rise gradually at the rate of about 0·4–0·8 kPa/min (3–6 mm Hg/min), with more than 90 per cent of the metabolically produced carbon dioxide passing into the body stores. Alveolar P_{O_2} falls rapidly towards the mixed venous P_{O_2} which itself falls continuously as the arterial P_{O_2} decreases. The lung volume falls by the difference between the oxygen uptake and the carbon dioxide output.

Initially the rate would be 230 − 21 = 209 ml/min. The change in alveolar Po_2 may be calculated, and gross hypoxia supervenes after about 90 seconds if the experiment follows air breathing and starts at the functional residual capacity.

With patent airway and air as ambient gas the oxygen is initially taken up and the carbon dioxide rises as described above. However, instead of the lung volume falling by the net gas exchange rate (initially 209 ml/min), this amount of ambient gas is drawn in by mass movement down the trachea. If the ambient gas is air, the oxygen in it will be removed but the nitrogen will accumulate and rise above its normal concentration until gross hypoxia supervenes after about 2 minutes. This is likely to occur when the accumulated nitrogen has reached 90 per cent since the alveolar carbon dioxide concentration will then have reached about 8 per cent. Carbon dioxide elimination cannot occur as the mass-movement of gas is down the trachea and this prevents the loss of carbon dioxide by diffusion. Measured at the mouth there is oxygen uptake but no carbon dioxide output; the respiratory exchange ratio is thus zero.

With patent airway and oxygen as the ambient gas the situation is quite different. Oxygen is drawn in by mass-movement and replaces the oxygen which crosses the alveolar-capillary membrane. No nitrogen is added to the alveolar gas, and the alveolar Po_2 only falls as fast as the Pco_2 rises (about 0·4–0·8 kPa/min or 3–6 mm Hg/min). Therefore the patient will not become seriously hypoxic for several minutes. If the patient has been breathing oxygen prior to the respiratory arrest, the starting alveolar Po_2 will be of the order of 88 kPa (660 mm Hg) and therefore the patient can theoretically survive about 100 minutes of apnoea provided he is connected to a supply of 100 per cent oxygen. This, in fact, is true and has been demonstrated in both animals and man (Draper and Whitehead, 1944; Enghoff, Holmdahl and Risholm, 1951; Holmdahl, 1956; Frumin, Epstein and Cohen, 1959). The phenomenon has moved out of the laboratory into clinical anaesthesia (Holmdahl, 1953) and has been used as a practical anaesthetic technique, particularly for bronchoscopy without artificial ventilation (Barth, 1954; Payne, 1962).

With preliminary inhalation of oxygen and an unobstructed supply of oxygen, there is no difficulty in maintaining an adequate arterial Po_2 during at least 20 minutes of apnoeic mass-movement oxygenation. However, the technique causes total retention of carbon dioxide and the arterial Pco_2 rises within the ranges 0·4–0·8 kPa/min (3–6 mm Hg/min). Hypercapnia is thus an inevitable feature of the technique. Arterial Pco_2 as high as 18·7 kPa (140 mm Hg) has been reported by Payne (1962) after 11 minutes (with an initial Pco_2 of 11·1 kPa or 83 mm Hg).

The technique has been modified by numerous workers in an attempt to prevent the rise of Pco_2. However, the problem of anaesthesia for bronchoscopy appears to have been solved by the technique of intermittent inflation with a venturi (page 155).

THE EFFECTS OF CHANGES IN THE CARBON DIOXIDE TENSION

Few subjects in the field of physiology are as complicated as the effects of changes in the carbon dioxide tension. A whole book would be required to do justice to this topic alone, and therefore only a brief outline will be presented at this time. Previous reviews include Brown (1953), the special issue of *Anaesthesiology* of December 1960, Nunn (1962d), Robinson (1962), Tenney and Lamb (1965), and Prys-Roberts (1971).

A number of special difficulties encompass an understanding of the effects of changes in P_{CO_2}. Firstly, there is the problem of species difference, which is a formidable obstacle to the interpretation of animal studies. The second difficulty arises from the fact that carbon dioxide can exert its effect in a number of ways. For example, the so-called 'inert gas' narcotic effect would presumably be produced by carbon dioxide in accord with its physical properties, although it is more likely to exert its effects upon the central nervous system by means of its unique ability to alter the intracellular pH (*see* above). This is quite apart from the fact that a change in P_{CO_2} usually alters the pH of the circulating blood. In addition, it remains possible that carbon dioxide can exert specific effects unrelated to the mechanisms listed above, although this would be difficult to prove. The third difficulty in the understanding of the effects of carbon dioxide arises from the fact that the gas seems to act at many different sites. Sometimes the action of carbon dioxide at different sites produces opposite effects upon a

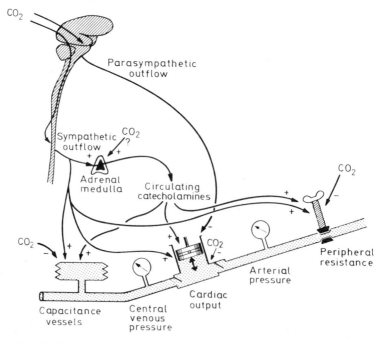

Figure 121. This diagram shows the complexity of the mechanisms by which carbon dioxide may influence the circulatory system. The over-all effect in the anaesthetized patient is an increase in cardiac output which is roughly proportional to the arterial P_{CO_2}. The rise in cardiac output exceeds the rise in blood pressure and this may be described as a fall in peripheral resistance (total). In spite of the rise of cardiac output, there is an increase in central venous pressure. This implies that capacitance vessels are contracted to cause a rise in filling pressure with which the increased cardiac output does not keep pace. In the absence of sympathetic nervous system activity, the direct effect of carbon dioxide upon the myocardium causes a fall of cardiac output and a profound fall in preipheral resistance is also seen. A fall in arterial blood bressure is then inevitable

particular function, and the action of carbon dioxide upon blood pressure (*Figure 121*) is an example of the complexity of the manner in which its effects may be produced.

Effects upon the nervous system

Carbon dioxide has at least five major effects upon the brain.

1. It is the major factor governing the cerebral blood flow.
2. It may be presumed to exert the inert gas narcotic effect in accord with its physical properties which are similar to those of nitrous oxide.
3. It influences the excitability of the neurones, particularly relevant in the case of the reticulo-activating system.
4. It is the main factor influencing the intracellular pH, which is known to have important effects upon the metabolism of the cell.
5. It influences the CSF pressure through changes in cerebral blood flow.

The interplay of these effects is difficult to understand, although the gross changes produced are well established.

Effects on consciousness. Carbon dioxide was used as an anaesthetic by Henry Hill Hickman in 1824, later by Ozanam (1862), and finally by Leake and Waters (1928). Thirty per cent carbon dioxide is sufficient for the production of anaesthesia, and this concentration causes total but reversible flattening of the electroencephalogram (Clowes, Hopkins and Simeone, 1955). Unfortunately, the use of carbon dioxide as an anaesthetic is impaired by the frequent production of convulsions at about the concentration required for anaesthesia (Leake and Waters, 1928). Higher concentrations have been shown to be tolerated in dogs, in whom the tendency to convulsions disappears when the P_{CO_2} rises above about 33·3 kPa (250 mm Hg). Carbon dioxide is at the present time widely used as a routine anaesthetic agent for small laboratory animals.

The effect of varying levels of P_{CO_2} on the susceptibility of a patient to anaesthesia has been widely debated. It has been claimed that hyperventilation and hypocapnia enhance the actions of agents used to produce general anaesthesia (Gray and Rees, 1952) and this is supported by the demonstration of a reduced threshold to the pain of tibial pressure (Clutton-Brock, 1957). These effects have been variously attributed to decreased excitation of the reticulo-activating system or to cerebral hypoxia resulting from the combined effects of cerebral vasconstriction and shift of the oxyhaemoglobin dissociation curve. The reinforcement of anaesthesia by hypocapnia has been challenged by Eisele, Eger and Muallem (1967), who found that, in dogs, the minimal alveolar concentration (MAC) of halothane required for anaesthesia was unaltered by changes of P_{CO_2} within the range 2–12·7 kPa (15–95 mm Hg). Above 12·7 kPa the narcotic effect of carbon dioxide was apparent and the halothane requirement was progressively reduced until, at P_{CO_2} 32·7 kPa (245 mm Hg), anaesthesia was achieved with carbon dioxide alone. These results accord well with observations of patients in ventilatory failure. In these patients carbon dioxide narcosis occurs when the P_{CO_2} rises above 12–16 kPa (90–120 mm Hg) (Westlake, Simpson and Kaye, 1955; Refsum, 1963).

The cause of narcosis by carbon dioxide is not due primarily to its inert gas narcotic effects, because its oil solubility indicates a very much weaker narcotic than it appears to be. It seems likely that the major effect on the central nervous system is by alteration of the intracellular pH with consequent derangements of metabolic processes (Woodbury and Karler, 1960). Eisele's results (Eisele, Eger and Muallem, 1967) showed that the narcotic effect correlated better with cerebrospinal fluid pH than with arterial P_{CO_2}.

Cerebral blood flow rises with P_{CO_2} within the range 3–13 kPa (approximately 20–100 mm Hg). The effect is exerted on the cerebral vascular resistance by means of changes in the extracellular pH in the region of the arterioles. The full response curve is S-shaped (*Figure 122*). The response at very low P_{CO_2} is probably limited by the vasodilator effect of tissue hypoxia, and the response above 16 kPa (120 mm Hg) seems to represent maximal vasodilation since there is little further increase in cerebral blood flow when the P_{CO_2} is raised as high as 59 kPa (440 mm Hg) (Reivich, 1964). The changes shown in *Figure 122* represent the brain as a whole and it is not possible to generalize about regional changes. It should also be remembered that sensitivity to carbon dioxide may be lost in the region of tumours, infarctions or trauma. There is commonly a fixed vasodilatation in these areas giving rise to so-called luxury perfusions (Lassen, 1966). Far from being luxurious, this may give rise to dangerous increases in intracranial pressure. Conversely, some areas of the brain may develop focal ischaemia without the ability to respond to increased P_{CO_2}.

Areas with either luxury perfusion or focal ischaemia may respond to altered P_{CO_2} in the opposite direction to the normal as it is shown in *Figure 122*. Thus a

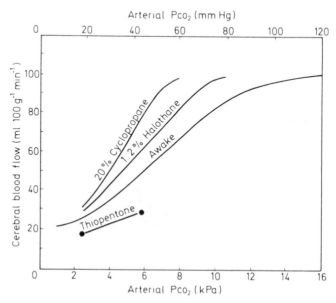

Figure 122. Relationship of cerebral blood flow to arterial P_{CO_2} in awake and anaesthetized patients. Lower concentrations of cyclopropane (5 and 13 per cent) appear to reduce cerebral blood flow (Alexander et al., 1962). Data are drawn from various sources, including Reivich (1964), Lassen (1959), Pierce et al. (1962), Smith and Wollman (1972) and Alexander et al. (1968)

high P_{CO_2} may increase blood flow through normal brain tissue and actually decrease perfusion through ischaemic areas which have lost their response to carbon dioxide. This has been termed the intracerebral steal (Hoedt-Rasmussen et al., 1967). The reverse phenomenon may occur when P_{CO_2} is lowered in patients with an area of luxury perfusion. Vasoconstriction in the surrounding normal tissue may divert blood flow towards the abnormal area of luxury perfusion which has no ability to respond to lowered P_{CO_2}. This has been termed the inverse steal or Robin Hood syndrome (Lassen and Palvalgyi, 1968).

Since hyperventilation is commonly practised during anaesthesia (Gray and Rees, 1952), while other patients are allowed to become severely hypercapnic (Birt and Cole, 1965), it is important to know the extent to which anaesthesia may modify the effect of P_{CO_2} on the cerebral blood flow. Pierce et al. (1962) studied the effect of hyperventilation on human volunteers anaesthetized with thiopentone. At normal levels of P_{CO_2}, cerebral blood blow was reduced in accord with the reduced cerebral oxygen consumption (*Table 27*), but further vasoconstriction occurred with hyperventilation (*Figure 122*), resulting in a substantial fall in jugular venous P_{O_2}. Brain tissue P_{O_2} would undoubtedly have been reduced but there is no convincing biochemical or psychometric evidence that the practice of hyperventilation during anaesthesia results in any significant level of cerebral damage. Inhalation anaesthetics have a direct cerebral vasodilator effect and accentuate the response to P_{CO_2} (*Figure 122*). Valuable reviews have been writted by Lassen (1959) and Smith and Wollman (1972).

Table 27 EFFECTS OF HYPERVENTILATION AND ANAESTHESIA ON CEREBRAL BLOOD FLOW AND OXYGENATION IN MAN

State of patient or subject	Cerebral oxygen consumption (ml 100 g^{-1} min^{-1})	Cerebral blood flow (ml 100 g^{-1} min^{-1})	Internal jugular venous P_{O_2} kPa	mm Hg
Conscious				
Arterial P_{CO_2} 5·3 kPa (40 mm Hg)	3·0	44·0	4·7–5·3	35–40
Arterial P_{CO_2} 2·7 kPa (20 mm Hg)	3·0	22·0	—	—
Anaesthetized:				
thiopentone				
Arterial P_{CO_2} 5·9 kPa (44 mm Hg)	1·5	27·6	4·7	35
Arterial P_{CO_2} 2·4 kPa (18 mm Hg)	1·7	16·4	2·4	18
halothane 1·0%				
Arterial P_{CO_2} 5·5 kPa (41 mm Hg)	2·2*	54·4*	5·3†	40†

Data on the conscious subject from Smith and Wollman (1972).
Data on patients anaesthetized with thiopentone from Pierce et al. (1962).
 * Data on patients anaesthetized with halothane from Christensen, Hoedt-Rasmussen and Lassen (1967).
 † Data on blood from superior sagittal sinus of dogs breathing 2% halothane (derived from oxygen saturation) (McDowall, 1967).

Intracranial pressure tends to rise with increasing P_{CO_2}, probably as a result of cerebral vasodilatation. This has important implications in the management of patients with head injuries and in those undergoing neurosurgery. Hyperventilation has now become one of the standard methods of reducing intracranial pressure after head injury (Shenkin and Bouzarth, 1970) but some patients react in the opposite direction. The author has found it useful to monitor intracranial pressure and ascertain the optimal P_{CO_2} for individual patients with head injuries. Hyperventilation has long been a standard method for controlling brain tension during neurosurgical operations (Marrubini, Rossanda and Tretola, 1964). Halothane and other inhalational anaesthetics may cause a dangerous rise in intracranial pressure in patients with intracranial tumours (Jennett, McDowall and Barker, 1967) but this effect may be partly mitigated by prior induction of hypocapnia, as suggested by Jennett and his co-workers and later confirmed by Adams et al. (1972).

Effects upon the autonomic and endocrine systems

Survival in severe hypercapnia is, to a large extent, dependent on the autonomic response which is therefore one of the most important effects of carbon dioxide. A great many of the effects of carbon dioxide on other systems are, in fact, either due to or influenced by the autonomic response to carbon dioxide. Examples of this multiplicity of mechanism of action are shown in *Figure 121.*

Nahas, Ligou and Mehlman (1960) and Millar (1960) have clearly shown the increase in plasma levels of both adrenaline and noradrenaline caused by an elevation of P_{CO_2} during apnoeic mass-movement oxygenation (*Figure 123*). In moderate hypercapnia, there is a proportionate rise of adrenaline and noradrenaline, but, in gross hypercapnia (P_{CO_2} more than 27 kPa or 200 mm Hg), there is an abrupt rise of adrenaline. Similar, though very variable, changes have been obtained over a lower range of P_{CO_2} in human volunteers inhaling carbon dioxide mixtures (Sechzer et al., 1960).

The relationship between P_{CO_2} and plasma catecholamine levels is considerably influenced by the administration of inhalational anaesthetic agents. Higher levels of adrenaline and noradrenaline are obtained during cyclopropane anaesthesia than in the unanaesthetized subject. Price et al. (1960) reported levels of 10 μg/l with a P_{CO_2} increase to only 10·7 kPa (80 mm Hg) during cyclopropane administration. However, the same group found that plasma catecholamine levels of patients under halothane anaesthesia rose in much the same way as in conscious subjects.

The effect of an increased level of circulating catecholamines is, to a certain extent, offset by a decreased sensitivity of target organs when the pH is reduced (Tenney, 1956). This is additional to the general depressant direct effect of carbon dioxide on target organs. There is also evidence that the anterior pituiary gland is stimulated by carbon dioxide, resulting in increased secretion of ACTH (Tenney, 1960). Acetylcholine hydrolysis is reduced at low pH and therefore certain parasympathetic effects may be enhanced during hypercapnia.

It is generally believed that reduction of P_{CO_2} after a period of hypercapnia results in a further elevation of the plasma catecholamine level (see review by Tenney and Lamb, 1965). However, it is difficult to find experimental evidence for this statement and there is, in fact quite a lot of evidence to suggest the contrary. Millar (1960) showed a rapid fall of both adrenaline and noradrenaline within minutes of reduction of a gross elevation of P_{CO_2} (*Figure 123*). The principal evidence for post-hypercapnic elevation of catecholamine levels seems to be the study of Tenney (1956), in which an auto-bioassay was carried out using the denervated nictitating membrane of cats which were subjected to change of P_{CO_2}. The plasma level of catecholamine was derived from the degree of contraction of the membrane with reference to a single calibrating injection of a known amount of adrenaline: the accuracy of the procedure could thus be influenced by change in the sensitivity of the nictitating membrane which is known to be reduced by the direct action of carbon dioxide, as demonstrated in the same publication. It is therefore possible that the further contraction of the nictitating membrane during fall of P_{CO_2} was due, not to a further increase in catecholamine level, but to the fall of P_{CO_2} raising the sensitivity to the circulating catecholamines, which fell more slowly than the P_{CO_2}.

Some support of the theory of post-hypercapnic elevation of plasma catecholamine levels has been derived from the cardiovascular response to reduction of an elevated P_{CO_2}. This is considered below.

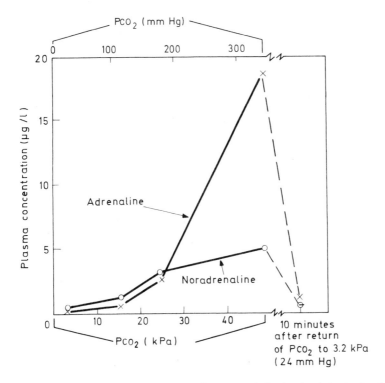

Figure 123. This graph shows the changes in plasma catecholamine levels in the dog during the rise of P_{CO_2} from 2·9 to 45 kPa (22 to 338 mm Hg) in the course of one hour of apnoeic oxygenation. After 10 minutes of ventilation with oxygen, P_{CO_2} returned to 32 kPa (24 mm Hg). Catecholamines were almost back to control values but the adrenaline remained higher than the noradrenaline. (Prepared from Table 4 of Millar, 1960)

Effects upon the respiratory system

Chapter 2 discusses in some detail the role of carbon dioxide in the control of ventilation. In general the maximal stimulant effect is attained within the P_{CO_2} range 13·3–20 kPa (100–150 mm Hg) (Graham, Hill and Nunn, 1960). At higher levels of P_{CO_2} the stimulation is reduced, while at very high levels respiration is depressed and later ceases altogether. Graham, Hill and Nunn (1960) made the curious observation that dogs maintained at a very high tension of carbon dioxide (above 46·7 kPa or 350 mm Hg) eventually started breathing again. The breathing was of a gasping character but was sufficient to maintain life for at least an hour without any artificial assistance to ventilation. The breathing in this state (termed 'supercarbia') is uninfluenced by changes in P_{CO_2} or by vagal section. The P_{CO_2}/ventilation response curve is generally displaced to the right and its slope reduced by the action of anaesthetic agents and other depressant drugs (Severinghaus and Larson, 1965). In profound anaesthesia the response curve may be flat, or even sloping downwards, and carbon dioxide then acts as a respiratory depressant.

Reduction of P_{CO_2} does not always lead to apnoea in the naïve subject, who is unaware of the classical work. However, during anaesthesia, reduction of P_{CO_2} below the threshold value usually does result in apnoea (Fink, 1961). Therefore, to restore spontaneous respiration at the end of an operation in which artificial hyperventilation has been employed, it is necessary either to raise the P_{CO_2} above the apnoeic threshold value or to awaken the patient (Ivanov and Nunn, 1969). References to the respiratory effects of carbon dioxide are given in Chapter 2.

Effects upon oxygenation of the blood

Quite apart from the effect of carbon dioxide upon ventilation, it exerts two other important effects which influence the oxygenation of the blood. Firstly, if the concentration of nitrogen (or other 'inert' gas) remains constant, the concentration of carbon dioxide in the alveolar gas can only increase at the expense of oxygen which must be displaced. Secondly, an increase in P_{CO_2} caused a displacement of the oxygen dissociation curve to the right (page 404); in a patient with gross hypercapnia, Prys-Roberts, Smith and Nunn (1967) reported visibly desaturated arterial blood although the P_{O_2} was 14 kPa (104 mm Hg). Unfortunately, the saturation was not measured but subsequent studies suggested that a value of the order of 90 per cent would be expected.

Effects upon the circulatory system

The effects of carbon dioxide upon the circulation are extraordinarily complicated due to the alternative modes of action upon the different components of the system (*Figure 121*). Many actions are in opposition to each other and, under different circumstances, the over-all effect of carbon dioxide upon certain circulatory functions can be entirely reversed. Special reference should be made to the review by Price (1960).

Myocardial contracility and heart rate are diminished by elevated P_{CO_2} in the isolated preparation (Jerusalem and Starling, 1910). However, in the intact subject the depressant direct action of carbon dioxide is overshadowed by the stimulant effect mediated through the sympathetic system. Blackburn et al. (1972) have clearly shown a positive inotropic effect with increasing P_{CO_2} in the dog and demonstrated that this is prevented by β-adrenergic blockade. Prys-Roberts et al. (1967a) are in agreement with Cullen and Eger (1974) that, in artificially ventilated man, increased P_{CO_2} raises cardiac output and slightly reduces total peripheral resistance so that blood pressure tends to be increased. Cullen and Eger obtained similar results during spontaneous breathing.

At very high levels of P_{CO_2} it is likely that cardiac output falls. Study of a single dog by Severinghaus, Mitchell and Nunn (unpublished) showed a progressive decline of cardiac output with increasing P_{CO_2} in supercarbia (*Table 28*). The response of cardiac output to increased P_{CO_2} is diminished by most anaesthetics and by spinal analgesia (Gregory et al., 1974; and a survey of other studies by Cullen and Eger, 1974).

Table 28 CIRCULATORY CHANGES AT VERY HIGH P_{CO_2} OBSERVED IN A SINGLE DOG BY SEVERINGHAUS, MITCHELL AND NUNN, UNPUBLISHED)

| Time | Arterial blood | | | | | Cardiac output (l/min) | Blood pressure syst/diast | |
| | Pa_{CO_2} | | pH | PO_2 | | | | |
	kPa	mm Hg		kPa	mm Hg		kPa	mm Hg
11.51	6·8	51	7·32	39·2	294	3·14	22·0/15·3	165/115
12.35	52·4	393	6·50	27·2	204	2·34	22·0/14·7	165/110
13.00	62·4	468	6·42	20·3	152	0·98	12·0/ 8·0	90/60
13.15	72·0	540	6·41	16·0	120	0·64	11·3/ 6·0	85/45
14.33	6·4	48	7·28	39·1	293	1·29	15·3/12·7	115/95

The dog breathed spontaneously in the state of 'supercarbia' above a P_{CO_2} of 44·9 kPa (337 mm Hg) which was attained at 12.25.

P_{CO_2} was gradually reduced from 13.16 until 14.33.

Cyclopropane anaesthesia was used when the P_{CO_2} was low.

Anaesthesia was terminated at 14.40 and the dog regained consciousness at 14.55. Recovery was uneventful.

Arrhythmias have been reported in unanaesthetized man during acute hypercapnia but have seldom been of serious import (cases reviewed by Nunn, 1962d, table I). The position is, however, more dangerous under anaesthesia with cyclopropane (Lurie et al., 1958), halothane (Black et al., 1959), and possibly with other agents which have not yet been adequately studied in man. With these anaesthetic agents it appears that arrythmias will always occur above a 'P_{CO_2} arrhythmic threshold' which is reported to be surprisingly constant for a particular patient under particular conditions. The mean value is 9·9 kPa (74 mm Hg) for cyclopropane and 12·3 kPa (92 mm Hg) for halothane. Multifocal ventricular extrasystoles have been reported and the danger of ventricular fibrillation cannot be discounted. This has not deterred the anaesthetists studied by Birt and Cole (1965). In their series, values for arterial P_{CO_2} rose as high as 21·3 kPa (160 mm Hg), and 17 of the 22 patients developed arrythmias, 4 showing multifocal ventricular extrasystoles. Nevertheless, no one seems to have condemned the technique which is apparently widely used. However, there remains the possibility that cases of ventricular fibrillation have occurred but not been reported. Most investigators have found that arrhythmias (short of ventricular fibrillation) have little effect upon the blood pressure and appear to do the patient no obvious harm.

It should be noted that Graham, Hill and Nunn (1960) raised the P_{CO_2} of a series of dogs to 73·3 kPa (550 mm Hg) and found no arrhythmias regardless of whether the dogs were receiving cyclopropane or halothane. This is a good example of the importance of species difference and shows the error which may arise from extrapolation of evidence from animal experiments to man.

Arrhythmias caused by elevated P_{CO_2} in anaesthetized patients occur at catecholamine levels which are above normal, but which are not *per se* high enough to cause arrhythmias. It therefore seems that arrhythmias are caused by the increased sensitivity of the heart to carbon dioxide in addition to or instead of elevation of plasma catecholamine levels (Price et al., 1958).

There is widespread acceptance of the work of Brown and Miller (1952) that ventricular fibrillation may follow the sudden reduction of a high P_{CO_2} in dogs. Graham, Hill and Nunn (1960) and Millar (1960) were quite unable to confirm these observations after precipitous falls of P_{CO_2} caused by ventilation with oxygen. They suggest that in the study of Brown and Miller, the dogs may have suffered hypoxia caused by ventilation with air in the presence of a high P_{CO_2}. Enquiries by the author over a period of 17 years have only revealed one case of ventricular fibrillation which occurred in an anaesthetized patient during rapid reduction of an elevated P_{CO_2}. The subject has been reviewed by Prys-Roberts, Smith and Nunn (1967). It is difficult, if not impossible to disprove a dangerous causal relationship of this type and the reader must draw his own conclusions.

Blood pressure is generally raised as P_{CO_2} increases in both conscious and anaesthetized patients (*see* above). However, the response is variable and centainly cannot be relied upon as an infallible diagnostic sign of hypercapnia. At very high levels of P_{CO_2} the blood pressure declines (*Table 28*) and appears to be the cause of death if the condition of supercarbia persists for much more than an hour (Graham, Hill and Nunn, 1960). Hypotension accompanies an elevation of P_{CO_2} if there is blockade of the sympathetic system by ganglioplegic drugs or spinal blockade (Payne, 1958b).

There is general agreement that hypotension follows a sudden fall of an elevated P_{CO_2}. Together with the fall of plasma catecholamine level, this is believed to account for the hypotension which follows cyclopropane anaesthesia (which is frequently accompanied by hypercapnia if respiration is spontaneous). Hypercapnia causes a rise in pulmonary arterial pressure and pulmonary vascular resistance (Barer, Howard and McCurrie, 1967).

Regional blood flow appears to be influenced by the P_{CO_2} in different ways for different organs (Tenney and Lamb, 1965). Brain (Kety and Schmidt, 1948; Lassen, 1959), heart and skin blood flow increases with rising P_{CO_2}, while skeletal muscle blood flow is reduced by hypercapnia although this effect is much diminished by general anaesthesia (McArdle and Roddie, 1958). Vance, Brown and Smith (1973) showed that hypocapnia (P_{CO_2}, 3·3 kPa or 25 mm Hg) in anaesthetized dogs caused a highly significant reduction in myocardial blood flow. However, oxygen extraction was increased and myocardial oxygen consumption was unchanged.

Effect upon the kidney

Renal blood flow and glomerular filtration rate are little influenced by minor changes of P_{CO_2}. However, at high levels of P_{CO_2} there is constriction of the glomerular afferent arterioles, leading to anuria. This effect is abolished in the denervated kidney (Irwin, Draper and Whitehead, 1957).

Chronic hypercapnia results in increased resorption of bicarbonate by the kidneys, further raising the plasma bicarbonate level, and constituting a secondary or compensatory 'metabolic alkalosis'. Chronic hypocapnia decreases renal bicarbonate resorption, resulting in a further fall of plasma bicarbonate and producing a secondary or compensatory 'metabolic acidosis'. In each case the arterial pH returns towards the normal value but the bicarbonate ion concentration departs even further from normality.

Although acute changes of P_{CO_2} do not produce a true metabolic acid–base change, conventional techniques of acid–base measurement indicate an apparent base deficit of about 2 mmol/l when the P_{CO_2} of a normal patient is acutely raised from 5·3 to 10·7 kPa (40 to 80 mm Hg). Similarly, a base excess of about 2 mmol/l appears when the P_{CO_2} is actually lowered to 2·7 kPa (20 mm Hg). Both abnormalities disappear immediately when the P_{CO_2} is restored to normal. These changes arise from the fact that the *in vivo* CO_2 equilibration curve of a patient is flatter than the *in vitro* curve of sampled blood (*Figures 113 and 114*). This interesting artefact is too small to be of practical consequence unless the P_{CO_2} is outside the limits 2·7–10·7 kPa (20–80 mm Hg). Such cases are comparatively rare and correction can be applied if this is required (Prys-Roberts, Kelman and Nunn, 1966).

Effect on blood electrolyte levels

Hypercapnia is accompanied by a leakage of potassium from the cells into the plasma (Clowes, Hopkins and Simeone, 1955). Hepatectomy has demonstrated that most of the potassium comes from the liver, probably in association with glucose which is mobilized in response to the rise in plasma catecholamine levels (Fenn and Asano, 1956). Since the plasma potassium level takes an appreciable time to return to normal, repeated bouts of hypercapnia at short intervals result in a stepwise rise in plasma potassium.

A reduction in the ionized fraction of the total calcium has, in the past, been thought to be the cause of the tetany which accompanies severe hypocapnia. However, the changes which occur are too small to account for tetany, which only occurs in parathyroid disease when there has been a fairly gross reduction of ionized calcium (Tenney and Lamb, 1965). Hyperexcitability affects all nerves and spontaneous activity ultimately occurs. The spasms probably result from activity in proprioceptive fibres causing reflex muscle contraction.

Effect upon drug action

Changes in P_{CO_2} may affect drug action as a result of a great number of different mechanisms. Firstly, the distribution of the drug may be influenced by changes in perfusion of organs. Secondly, the ionization of drugs may be altered by the change in blood pH. Thirdly, the solubility of the drug in body fluids and the protein binding may be influenced. The effect of changes in Pco_2 and pH on the older neuromuscular blockers have been studied by Hughes (1970), who also reviewed the earlier literature. Dann (1971) reported no effect of changes in Pco_2 on the duration of action of the steroid neuromuscular blocker, pancuronium. Wyke (1957) reviewed the effect of changes in pH on the action of barbiturates.

Therapeutic uses of carbon dioxide

The varied and powerful effects of increased Pco_2 suggest that the inhalation of carbon dioxide gas mixtures would have a clear place in therapy. In fact this is not so and some believe that carbon dioxide has no place in the fields of anaesthesia, resuscitation and intensive therapy. Fear of accidental administration of high concentrations of carbon dioxide has caused many to omit cylinders of the gas from anaesthetic and other inhalational apparatus.

The main therapeutic indication for the administration of carbon dioxide is to stimulate respiration. This is useful to expedite the uptake and elimination of inhalational anaesthetic agents, and reference has already been made to the administration of carbon dioxide to raise the arterial Pco_2 above the apnoeic threshold in order to encourage the resumption of spontaneous breathing after passive hyperventilation of unconscious patients (page 366). Although carbon dioxide may be used to stimulate breathing in these situations, its use in the treatment of ventilatory failure is very limited. Many patients in respiratory failure have a diminished or absent response to exogenous carbon dioxide and in such patients carbon dioxide will be ineffective in raising the minute volume, and may actually cause a decrease, possibly leading to carbon dioxide narcosis. Carbon dioxide is also likely to be ineffective or harmful if ventilation is limited by malfunction of the efferent motor pathway, the respiratory muscles or by raised airway resistance. Such patients will already have a raised Pco_2 and show a flattened Pco_2/ventilation response curve which is very similar to that produced by depression of the central chemoreceptors (*Figure 17*).

Carbon monoxide poisoning remains one of the clearest indications for the administration of carbon dioxide gas mixtures. Not only will stimulation of respiration hasten the elimination of carbon monoxide, but the venous Po_2 will be substantially increased by the shift of the dissociation curve of the remaining normal haemoglobin (page 410). Elevation of venous (and tissue) Po_2 by displacement of the dissociation curve of normal haemoglobin seems to be a rational therapeutic use for carbon dioxide but its clinical role for this purpose has not been fully explored. There is also clear evidence that elevation of Pco_2 will usually improve both cardiac output and regional perfusion of certain organs, particularly the brain. However, there has been surprisingly little interest in this potentially important therapeutic use for carbon dioxide.

If carbon dioxide is used clinically, careful attention must be paid to dosimetry. Thus, maximal effectiveness in its use as a respiratory stimulant requires control of the concentration in the inspired gas. Therapy based on an elevation of arterial Pco_2 would clearly be ineffective if the patient's ventilatory response prevented any appreciable increase in ventilation. Ivanov and Nunn (1969) have examined quantitative aspects of some of the simpler methods of administration of exogenous and endogenous carbon dioxide (*see* above, page 357).

CLINICAL RECOGNITION OF HYPERCAPNIA

There are no infallible diagnostic signs of hypercapnia. The patient's skin is usually flushed and the pulse is generally full and bounding, with occasional extrasystoles and possibly other forms of arrhythmia. The blood pressure is often raised but this is not always the case. However, hypercapnia should always be considered when there is an unexplained hypertension during anaesthesia. Hyperventilation will obviously be absent if hypercapnia is caused by hypo-ventilation. However, it may be noticed during accidental elevation of the concentration of carbon dioxide in the inspired gas. Muscle twitchings and a characteristic flap of the hands are seen when the P_{CO_2} approaches the level at which coma occurs. Convulsions occur at high levels. It must be stressed that coma and depressed breathing may be the only signs of severe hypercapnia and the diagnosis may not be at all obvious. Respiratory depression occurs at high levels of P_{CO_2} and the mortality of the condition is very high unless the attendants are aware of the importance of prompt and vigorous treatment.

Tests for hypercapnia

In all cases of undiagnosed coma, the arterial P_{CO_2} should be measured. If this is not practicable, the mixed venous P_{CO_2} may be measured by the rebreathing technique (*see* later). If it is found that the minute volume is substantially below the normal value (particularly if there is likely to be an increase in physiological dead space), hypercapnia is inevitable unless there is a reduction in metabolic rate (e.g. in hypothermia). A useful therapeutic test for hypercapnia is to ventilate the patient vigorously with a CO_2-free gas. In true cases of hypercapnia, there is a dramatic return of consciousness (Scurr, 1954). This may result in hypotension.

OUTLINE OF METHODS OF MEASUREMENT OF CARBON DIOXIDE

Fractional concentration in gas mixtures

The reference method is chemical absorption. In medical circles the most accurate method usually employed is Lloyd's modification of the Haldane apparatus (Cormack, 1972). A simpler version of Haldane's apparatus which is sufficiently accurate for clinical work has been described by Campbell (1960). The popularity of the Scholander apparatus has declined in Great Britain in recent years, but it may still be required for the analysis of very small samples (Scholander, 1947). All these methods are markedly influenced by the presence of nitrous oxide in gas samples and modifications of technique are required (Nunn, 1958b; Glossop, 1963; Meade and Owen-Thomas, 1975).

Infrared absorption can be used to compare the concentration of carbon dioxide in an unknown sample with the concentration in a known sample (DuBois et al., 1952). Unfortunately, the presence of other gases has an appreciable effect upon the response of the instrument to a particular concentration of carbon dioxide (Cooper, 1957). This effect, known as collision broadening, is best overcome by calibrating with a known concentration of carbon dioxide in a diluent gas mixture which is similar to the gas sample for analysis. The particular virtue of infrared analysers is that they can be made to respond within less than a quarter of a second and will thus show the changes in carbon dioxide concentration during a single respiratory cycle. Cormack and Powell (1972) have described refinements of technique which permit greater accuracy. The broken line in *Figure 115* shows a typical capnogram from which the following information may be derived.

1. The end-expiratory carbon dioxide concentration.
2. The inspiratory carbon dioxide concentration.
3. In conjunction with a record of the patient's tidal exchange, it is possible to see how much gas is exhaled before the carbon dioxide concentration at the lips rises to the alveolar plateau. This is the anatomical dead space.
4. The slope of the alveolar P_{CO_2} plateau indicates the rate of rise of the alveolar P_{CO_2} during the course of expiration. This is increased by maldistribution of inspired gas or by an increase in the mixed venous/arterial P_{CO_2} difference.

Rapid analysis of gas mixtures for carbon dioxide can also be carried out with a mass spectrometer.

Blood carbon dioxide concentration

For many years the concentration of carbon dioxide in blood or plasma has been measured by vacuum extraction followed by chemical absorption in the manometric apparatus of Van Slyke and Neill (1924). The microapparatus of Natelson (1951) is considerably easier to handle. A convenient alternative technique is dissociation of bicarbonate by adding a large volume of acid to the blood followed by measurement of P_{CO_2} of the blood-plus-acid (Linden, Ledsome and Norman, 1965). By suitable calibration with solutions of known concentrations of sodium bicarbonate, the method is capable of satisfactory accuracy. P_{CO_2} is measured by means of the P_{CO_2}-sensitive electrode (*see* below).

Blood P_{CO_2}

Four methods of measurement are available.

1. A tiny bubble of gas may be equilibrated with blood at the patient's body temperature and then analysed quantitatively for carbon dioxide (Riley, Campbell and Shephard, 1957). P_{CO_2} is derived from the carbon dioxide concentration of the bubble and is close to that of the blood. The technique is difficult, and unsuitable for use in the presence of nitrous oxide.

2. For many years P_{CO_2} was derived from the form of the Henderson–
Hasselbalch equation given earlier in this Chapter (equation 8, page 337).
This method is no longer popular since measurements of pH and CO_2
content are required and there is always uncertainty of the value which
should be taken for pK'. Nevertheless, tolerable accuracy is attainable
(Thornton and Nunn, 1960).

3. P_{CO_2} of blood may be conveniently measured by interpolating the actual
pH in a plot of P_{CO_2} against pH derived from aliquots of the same blood
sample. The plot is linear (*Figure 114*) and the whole operation became a
practical proposition following the introduction of the microapparatus
described by Siggaard-Andersen et al. (1960). A small error is introduced
if the sample is desaturated. Minor refinements of technique and the level
of accuracy have been described by Kelman, Coleman and Nunn (1966).
Accuracy is uninfluenced by the presence of anaesthetic gases.

4. P_{CO_2} of any gas or liquid may be determined directly by the use of the
P_{CO_2}-sensitive electrode (Severinghaus and Bradley, 1958; Severinghaus,
1965). The P_{CO_2} of a film of bicarbonate solution is allowed to come into
equilibrium with the P_{CO_2} of a sample across a membrane permeable to
carbon dioxide. The pH of the bicarbonate solution is constantly
monitored with a glass electrode and the log of the P_{CO_2} is inversely
proportional to the recorded pH. The pH scale may therefore be engraved
to read P_{CO_2} directly. The accuracy obtainable is comparable to that of
other techniques and is uninfluenced by the presence of anaesthetic gases.
Recent advances in design have resulted in the production of equipment of
high reliability, and the P_{CO_2}-sensitive electrode is now the commonest
technique in routine use, with a 95 per cent limit of error of the order of
±0·5 kPa (3·8 mm Hg) when correctly operated.

Indirect measurement of arterial P_{CO_2}

Measurement of end-expiratory P_{CO_2} is of limited value due to the variable
arterial/end-expiratory P_{CO_2} gradient caused by anaesthesia or lung disease
(page 226). However, the method is useful for recording changes. If a rapid
carbon dioxide analyser is not available, end-expiratory samples may be
collected (Rahn et al., 1946a; Nunn and Pincock, 1957).

Measurement of mixed venous P_{CO_2} is of greater value than measurement of
end-expiratory P_{CO_2} and it may be estimated indirectly with very simple
apparatus, using the rebreathing technique of Campbell and Howell (1960). Its
modified use in children has been described by Sykes (1960). The collection of
the gas sample which has been equilibrated with mixed venous blood is perfectly
feasible in the unconscious patient and the technique should be available in
hospitals where there are no facilities for measurement of P_{CO_2} of blood
samples.

It was originally recommended that 0·8 kPa (6 mm Hg) should be subtracted
from the mixed venous (rebreathing) P_{CO_2} to give the arterial P_{CO_2} since this is
the normally accepted difference between mixed venous and arterial P_{CO_2} (*see
Table 26*). However, many workers have found that the mixed venous P_{CO_2}
measured by the rebreathing technique seems to give a higher value than would

be expected. McEvoy, Jones and Campbell (1974) have reconsidered the theoretical background of the method and drawn attention to a number of factors which raise the rebreathing P_{CO_2}. Most important is the fact that the rebreathing method measures the P_{CO_2} of venous blood as it would be if fully oxygenated. The Haldane effect (*Figure 111*) then raises the P_{CO_2} 0·5–1 kPa (3·8–7·5 mm Hg) higher than the true mixed venous P_{CO_2}. Furthermore, the mixed venous/arterial P_{CO_2} gradient will be increased in hypercapnia (due to the curvature of the carbon dioxide dissociation curve), in arterial hypoxaemia, reduced cardiac output and anaemia. An additional factor is the finite time required for the physicochemical equilibration of carbon dioxide in the blood, the rate-limiting step being equation (2) on page 334. P_{CO_2} of arterial blood when sampled and analysed may be different from the value when the blood leaves the pulmonary capillary where it is in equilibrium with alveolar gas. In general, the observed mixed venous P_{CO_2} (as measured by the rebreathing technique) is likely to exceed the arterial P_{CO_2} by 1–2 kPa (7·5–15 mm Hg) in the normal resting subject and certainly does so in the author. Since this difference rises with increasing P_{CO_2}, McEvoy and his co-workers now suggest that the indirect arterial P_{CO_2} should be calculated as 0·8 times the mixed venous P_{CO_2} measured by the rebreathing technique. Denison et al. (1971) and Godfrey and Wolf (1972) have described the use of the method in exercise.

Measurement of P_{CO_2} *of venous blood draining from skin* has been advanced as an alternative, to avoid arterial puncture. The results are quite acceptable for clinical purposes (Forster et al., 1972). However, it is surprisingly difficult to collect a good sample of blood anaerobically from the veins on the back of the hand. As a rough rule, if the sample is very difficult to collect, the circulation is unlikely to be good enough for the arterial and venous P_{CO_2} to be acceptably close. Cooper and Smith (1961) found that agreement between arterial and cutaneous venous P_{CO_2} was good in the majority of a series of anaesthetized patients, but considerable discrepancies appeared in a minority of patients, thought to have circulatory disturbances. Blood from veins draining muscles (e.g. the median cubital vein) has a P_{CO_2} much higher than the arterial level.

Measurement of capillary P_{CO_2} on blood obtained from a skin prick suffers from the same uncertainties which surround cutaneous venous P_{CO_2}. However, the technique is clearly useful in neonates. It is perhaps important to remember that an error of 0·6 kPa (4·5 mm Hg) is seldom of much consequence in the management of a patient.

Handling of blood samples

It is important that samples be preserved from contact with air or oil, to which they may lose carbon dioxide. Analysis should be undertaken quickly as the P_{CO_2} of blood *in vitro* rises by about 0·013 kPa/min (0·1 mm Hg/min) at 37°C. If analysis is not carried out at the patient's body temperature, a correction factor should be applied, as the P_{CO_2} of an anaerobic blood sample falls by about 4 per cent of each degree celsius cooling. Nomograms for correction for both these errors have been presented by Kelman and Nunn (1966b) and are to be found in Appendix D (*Figures 145 and 146*).

Chapter 12   Oxygen

THE ROLE OF OXYGEN IN THE CELL

Dissolved molecular oxygen enters into many metabolic processes in the mammalian body. From the point of view of respiratory physiology, much the most important is the *electron-transfer oxidase system* which is responsible for about 90 per cent of the total oxygen consumption and is concerned with the production of high-energy compounds which are the general source of biological energy. High-energy phosphate bonds are used for the short-term storage of energy and the process is described below under the heading of oxidative phosphorylation. Other electron-transfer oxidase systems are responsible for the dehydrogenation of flavoproteins. These are important in intermediary metabolism and account for an appreciable part of the total body oxygen consumption. However, flavoprotein dehydrogenation is not directly relevant to respiratory physiology and is not considered further in the present volume.

A second group of oxidative reactions is characterized by one atom of an oxygen molecule entering a substrate to form a hydroxyl group, while the other is reduced to water. The enzymes concerned are known as *mixed function oxidases*, hydroxylases or monoxygenases; they include the cytochrome P-450 enzymes which are of considerable importance in the biotransformation of drugs and are considered briefly below.

A third group of oxidative reactions involves the introduction of both atoms of a molecule of oxygen into substrates such as catechol, homogentisate, l-tryptophan and myoinositol. The enzymes are known as *oxygenases*, oxygen-transferases or dioxygenases. These oxidations are also important steps in intermediary metabolic pathways but are not directly relevant to respiratory physiology and will not be discussed further.

375

Oxidative phosphorylation

Most of the energy deployed in the mammalian body is derived from the oxidation of food-fuels, of which the most important is glucose:

$$C_6H_{12}O_6 + 6\,O_2 = 6\,CO_2 + 6\,H_2O + energy$$

The equation accurately describes the combustion of glucose *in vitro*, but is only a crude, over-all representation of the oxidation of glucose in the body. The direct reaction does not produce energy in a form in which it can be utilized for the various activities of the living body. The biological oxidation proceeds by a large number of stages, with phased production of energy. This energy is not all immediately released but is partly stored by means of the reaction of adenosine diphosphate (ADP) with inorganic phosphate ion to form adenosine tri-phosphate (ATP):

$$ADP + inorganic\ phosphate\ ion + energy \rightleftharpoons ATP$$

The third phosphate radical in ATP is held by a high energy bond which releases its energy when ATP is split back into ADP and inorganic phosphate ion. ADP is thus recycled indefinitely with ATP acting as a short-term store of energy available in a form which may be used directly for work such as muscle contraction, ion pumping, protein synthesis and secretion. ATP is commonly transported short distances between the sites of synthesis and utilization. For example, in voluntary muscles, it is formed in the mitochondria and used in the myofibrils.

There is no large store of ATP in the body and it must be synthesized continuously as it is being used. The ATP/ADP ratio is an indication of the level of energy which is currently carried in the ADP/ATP system and the ratio is normally related to the state of oxidation of the cell. The ADP/ATP system is not the only short-term energy store in the body but it is the most important.

The uses of ATP in the body lie outside the scope of this book, but its production from ADP is highly relevant to this chapter since the most efficient methods of production of ATP require the consumption of oxygen. However, the anaerobic methods are of great biological importance and were universal in the Pre-Cambrian era before the atmospheric P_{O_2} was sufficiently high for aerobic pathways of metabolism. Anaerobic metabolism is still the rule in certain organisms and in the mammalian body when energy requirements outstrip oxygen supply as, for example, during severe exercise and in hypoxia.

The aerobic pathway permits the release of far greater quantities of energy from the same amount of substrate and is therefore used whenever possible. In simplified form, the contrasting pathways can be shown as follows.

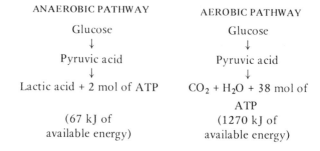

ANAEROBIC PATHWAY	AEROBIC PATHWAY
Glucose	Glucose
↓	↓
Pyruvic acid	Pyruvic acid
↓	↓
Lactic acid + 2 mol of ATP	$CO_2 + H_2O$ + 38 mol of ATP
(67 kJ of available energy)	(1270 kJ of available energy)

In vitro combustion of glucose liberates 2820 kJ/mol. Thus, under conditions of oxidative metabolism, 45 per cent of the total energy is made available for biological work and this compares favourably with most man-made machines.

Localization of oxidative phosphorylation in the cell. The oxygen consumption occurs in the mitochondria, where it combines with hydrogen to form water. The hydrogen has previously been removed from a variety of substrates by nicotinamide adenine dinucleotide (NAD), and then passed along a chain of hydrogen carriers to combine with oxygen at cytochrome a_3 which is the end of the chain. *Figure 124* shows the transport of hydrogen along the chain, which

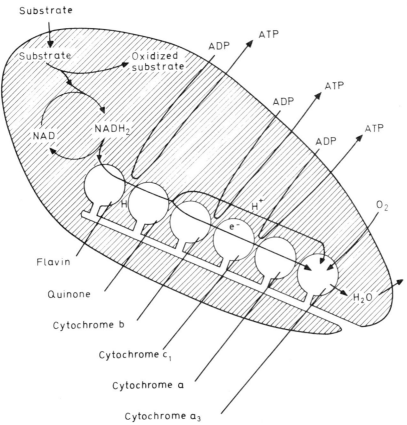

Figure 124. Diagrammatic representation of oxidation within the mitochondrion. The substrate diffuses from the cytoplasm into the mitochondrion where hydrogen is removed under the influence of the appropriate dehydrogenase enzyme. The hydrogen is carried by intramitochondrial NAD to the first of the chain of hydrogen carriers which are attached to the cristae of the mitochondria. When the hydrogen reaches the cytochromes, ionization occurs: the proton passes into the lumen of the mitochondrion while the electron is passed along the cytochromes where it converts ferric iron to the ferrous form. The final stage is at cytochrome a_3 where the proton and the electron combine with oxygen to form water. Three molecules of ADP are converted to ATP at the stages shown in the diagram. ADP and ATP can cross the mitochondrial membrane freely while there are separate pools of intra- and extramitochondrial NAD which cannot interchange

consists of structural entities just visible under the electron microscope and arranged in rows along the cristae of the mitochondria. Three molecules of ATP are formed at various stages of the chain during the transfer of two atoms of hydrogen. The process is not associated directly with the production of carbon dioxide which is formed elsewhere in the metabolic pathways. Oxidative phosphorylation can only take place when the Po_2 within the mitochondrion is above a critical level, thought to be of the order of 0·1 kPa. When the Po_2 falls below this level, metabolism reverts to anaerobic pathways.

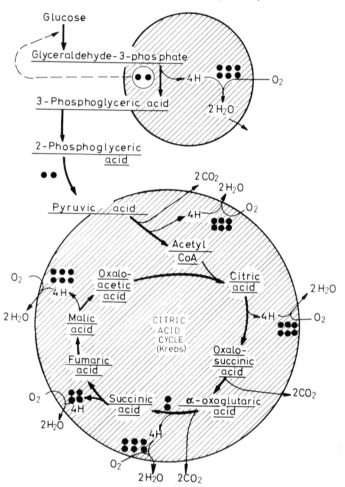

Figure 125. Successive stages in the principal oxidative metabolic pathway of glucose by the citric acid cycle. Many stages have been omitted for clarity. The two shaded circles represent mitochondria and indicate the reactions which can only take place within them. The names of substances which cross the membranes show those which are capable of diffusion into and out of the mitochondria. Underlining indicates that two molecules are formed from one of glucose. Black dots show where ATP is formed (the first two to be produced are offset by two which are required for the conversion of glucose to glyceraldehyde-3-phosphate). Note the dissociation between O_2 and CO_2 production. The conversion of glyceraldehyde-3-phosphate to 3-phosphoglyceric acid can also take place in the cytoplasm as shown in Figure 126 but, in that case, it is not possible for the liberated hydrogen to be oxidized to water, since the NADH$_2$ cannot diffuse into the mitochondria

The role of oxidative phosphorylation in the aerobic degradation of glucose is illustrated in *Figure 125*. One molecule of glucose is converted into two molecules of glyceraldehyde-3-phosphate in the cytoplasm of the cell. The latter substance then diffuses into the mitochondria where it is converted into 3-phosphoglyceric acid when hydrogen is removed by NAD and oxidized after transport along the chain shown in *Figure 124*. The next reactions can take place in the cytoplasm down to the point where pyruvic acid is formed. The oxidation of pyruvic acid, however, can only take place in the mitochondria where hydrogen is removed and oxidized at successive stages of the familiar citric acid cycle. It will be seen that the production of carbon dioxide also occurs within the mitochondria but that it is not directly associated with oxygen consumption. The scheme shown in *Figure 125* also accounts for the consumption of oxygen in the metabolism of fat. After hydrolysis, glycerol is converted into pyruvic acid while the fatty acids shed a series of 2-carbon molecules in the form of acetyl CoA. Pyruvic acid and acetyl CoA enter the citric acid cycle and are then degraded in the same manner as though they were derived from glucose. Amino acids are dealt with in similar manner after deamination. Oxidative phosphorylation has been reviewed by Lardy and Ferguson (1969) and Cohen (1972).

Figure 126 illustrates the anaerobic metabolism of glucose, a pathway which is followed either when there is a shortage of oxygen or, in the case of erythrocytes, when there is an absence of the respiratory enzymes located in the mitochondria. The conversion of glyceraldehyde-3-phosphate to 3-phospho-

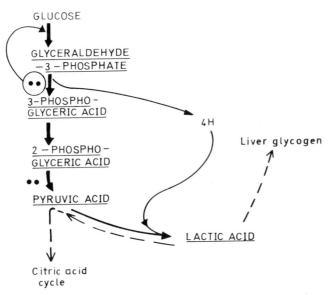

Figure 126. *The Embden–Meyerhof pathway for anerobic metabolism of glucose. Underlining indicates that two molecules are formed from one molecule of glucose. ATP production is shown by black dots, those produced in the second reaction being set against the two which are required to energize the first reaction. There is thus a net production of only two molecules of ATP per molecule of glucose. The hydrogen released at the second reaction is carried by extramitochondrial NAD and used in the reduction of pyruvic acid to lactic acid. No mitochondrial enzymes are used and no oxygen is required. The pathway has been greatly simplified in this diagram and many intermediate compounds have been omitted for clarity*

glyceric acid can take place in the plasma with hydrogen released as in the aerobic pathway but, in this case, to extramitochondrial NAD. This hydrogen cannot be oxidized but it is taken up lower down the pathway by the reduction of pyruvic acid to lactic acid. This series of changes is associated with the formation of only two molecules of ATP in contrast to the 38 produced in the course of aerobic metabolism. However, considerable chemical energy remains in the lactic acid which, in the presence of oxygen, can be reconverted to pyruvic acid and then oxidized in the citric acid cycle, producing the balance of 36 molecules of ATP. Alternatively, lactic acid may be converted into liver glycogen to await more favourable conditions for oxidation.

Significance of oxidative phosphorylation.   The production of a high yield of ATP requires oxygen. The alternative anaerobic pathways must either consume very much larger quantities of glucose or, alternatively, yield less ATP. In high-energy-consuming organs such as brain, kidney and liver it is not, in fact, possible to transfer the increased quantities of glucose and therefore these organs suffer ATP depletion under hypoxic conditions. In contrast, voluntary muscle is able to function satisfactorily on aerobic metabolism during short periods of time and this is normal in the diving mammals.

Anaerobic metabolism carries not only the penalty of ATP depletion but also the serious disadvantage of production of two moles of lactic acid from one of glucose (*Figure 126*). At normal intracellular pH, the lactic acid so formed is almost entirely ionized. In most organs both hydrogen and lactate ions escape into the circulation, producing 'lactacidosis'. However, the situation in the brain is quite different. The blood-brain barrier is relatively impermeable to charged ions and both hydrogen and lactate ions are largely retained within the neurone, lowering the intracellular pH. The biochemical and physiological consequences of hypoxia are discussed below (page 414 et seq.).

The critical oxygen tension of aerobic metabolism.   When the mitochondrial Po_2 is reduced, oxidative phosphorylation continues normally down to a level of about 0·3 kPa (2 mm Hg). Below this level oxygen consumption falls and the various members of the electron transport chain revert to the reduced state. $NADH/NAD^+$ and lactate/pyruvate ratios rise and the ATP/ADP ratio falls. The critical oxygen tension varies between different organs and different species but, as an approximation, a mitochondrial Po_2 of about 0·13 kPa (1 mm Hg) may be taken as the level below which there is serious impairment of oxidative phosphorylation and a switch to anaerobic metabolism. This level is, of course, far below the critical arterial Po_2 because there normally exists a large gradient of Po_2 between arterial blood and the site of utilization of oxygen in the mitochondria. This gradient is discussed as the oxygen cascade, below.

The critical Po_2 for oxidative phosphorylation is also known as the Pasteur point and has applications beyond the pathophysiology of hypoxia in man. In particular, it has a powerful bearing on putrefaction, many forms of which are the results of anaerobic metabolism resulting from a fall of Po_2 below the Pasteur point in, for example, polluted rivers.

Cytochrome P-450

The cytochrome P-450 enzymes are the terminal oxidases for many mixed function oxidase systems, the typical over-all reaction being:

$$RH + NADPH + H^+ + O_2 \rightarrow ROH + NADP^+ + H_2O$$

One atom of the oxygen molecule enters the substrate to form the hydroxyl radical while the other is reduced to water.

Cytochrome P-450 enzymes occupy a position at the end of an electron transport chain in a position rather similar to cytochrome a_3 (*Figure 124*) but there are very important differences. Firstly, these enzymes are bound to the membrane of the smooth endoplasmic reticulum (microsomes in homogenized and centrifuged preparations). Secondly, they are not concerned with synthesis of ATP but with hydroxylation of a wide range of substrates, including many drugs. They are thus very important not only in detoxification but also in the formation of biotransformation products which may be more toxic than the original drug. These functions are largely carried out in the liver. It is generally possible to demonstrate that the substrate for hydroxylation is bound to cytochrome P-450 *in vitro* with characteristic changes of its spectral properties.

The cytochrome P-450 enzymes derive their name from the difference spectrum between preparations treated with nitrogen and carbon monoxide. The difference spectrum shows a strong band at a wavelength of 450 nm. It is likely that a number of mixed function oxidases share this property and they are known collectively as cytochrome P-450.

The hepatic smooth endoplasmic reticulum hypertrophies as a result of *in vivo* treatment with enzyme inducers such as phenobarbitone. There is also an increased level of cytochrome P-450 with enhanced activity towards a wide variety of substrates. Induction with 3-methylcholanthrene causes synthesis of different structural form of cytochrome with the peak of the difference spectrum at 448 nm (cytochrome P-448).

The likely scheme of action of cytochrome P-450 is shown in *Figure 127*.

Oxygenase-catalysed biological hydroxylations have been reviewed by Gunsalus, Pederson and Sligar (1975). Halothane, methoxyflurane and enflurane (but not diethyl ether) cause spectral changes *in vitro* indicative of binding to cytochrome P-450 (Takahashi, Shigematsu and Furukawa, 1974). Bio-transformation by P-450 system is an essential feature of the toxicity of fluroxene; enzyme induction with phenobarbitone increases conversion to trifluoroethanol and thereby the toxicity of fluroxene in animals but not man (Cascorbi and Singh-Amaranath, 1972).

An entirely different role of cytochrome P-450 is its suggested function in the facilitated transport of oxygen and carbon monoxide, a role which is perhaps analogous to that of myoglobin as an oxygen carrier in skeletal muscle (Whittenberg, 1970). It has been observed that, in the sheep, placental transfer of oxygen is about 100 times that of argon for an equal partial pressure gradient. Since the physical properties of oxygen and argon are similar, this suggests the

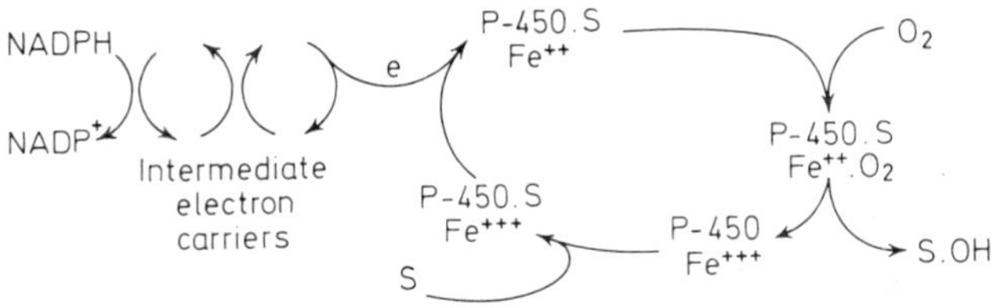

Figure 127. The likely scheme of action of cytochrome P-450. S indicates the substrate: both C- and N- oxygenations can occur.

existence of a carrier system. Cytochrome P-450 is abundant in the placenta, and treatment with agents known to inactivate cytochrome P-450 (e.g. SKF 525-A) cause a marked reduction in oxygen transfer across the placenta (Gurtner and Burns, 1972, 1973). Reference has been made in Chapter 10 to the reduction in pulmonary diffusing capacity for carbon monoxide on treatment with diphenhydramine which is known to bind to cytochrome P-450 (page 327). A more recent paper by Gurtner and Burns (1975) provides convincing evidence that oxygen transport across the placenta is perfusion-limited to contrast to argon transport which is diffusion-limited. This provides further evidence in support of their theory that there is active transport of oxygen in the placenta.

THE OXYGEN CASCADE

The P_{O_2} of dry air at sea level is 21·2 kPa (159 mm Hg). Oxygen moves down a partial pressure gradient from air, through the respiratory tract, the alveolar gas, the arterial blood, the systemic capillaries, the cell and finally reaches its lowest level within the mitochondria where it is consumed (*Figure 128*). At this point, the P_{O_2} is probably within the range 0·5–3 kPa (3·8–22·5 mm Hg) varying from one tissue to another, from one cell to another, and from one part of a cell to another.

The steps by which the P_{O_2} decreases from air to the mitochondria are known as the oxygen cascade and are of great practical importance. Any one step in the cascade may be increased under pathological circumstances and this may result in hypoxia. The steps will now be considered *seriatim*.

Dilution of inspired oxygen by water vapour

Analysis with the Haldane apparatus indicates the true fractional concentration of oxygen in a dry gas mixture. If the gas sample is humidified, the added water vapour is ignored and the indicated fractional concentration of oxygen is still that of the dry part of the gas mixture. Thus the normal value for atmospheric oxygen (20·94 per cent) indicates the concentration of oxygen in the dry gas phase regardless of whether the gas is humidified or not. However, humidification such as occurs when dry air is inhaled through the upper respiratory tract, dilutes air with water vapour and so reduces the P_{O_2}. The process is similar to the reduction in P_{O_2} which occurs when ether vapour is added to air (Scott, 1847).

When dry gas kept at normal barometric pressure is humidified with water vaporized at 37° C, 100 volumes of the dry gas take up about 6 volumes of water vapour, giving a total gas volume of 106 units but containing the same number of molecules of oxygen. The P_{O_2} is thus reduced by the fraction $\frac{6}{106}$. It follows from Boyle's law that P_{O_2} after humidification is indicated by the following expression:

$$\begin{matrix} \text{fractional concentration of oxygen} \\ \text{in the dry gas phase} \\ \text{(Haldane value)} \end{matrix} \times \left(\begin{matrix} \text{barometric} \\ \text{pressure} \end{matrix} - \begin{matrix} \text{saturated water} \\ \text{vapour pressure} \end{matrix} \right)^*$$

Therefore the effective Po_2 of inspired air at a body temperature of $37^\circ C$ is:

$$\frac{20 \cdot 94}{100} \times (101 \cdot 3 - 6 \cdot 3)^* = \frac{20 \cdot 94}{100} \times 95$$

$$= 19 \cdot 9 \text{ kPa}$$

or, in old units:

$$\frac{20 \cdot 94}{100} \times (760 - 47)^* = \frac{20 \cdot 94}{100} \times 713$$

$$= 149 \text{ mm Hg}$$

As a rough approximation, the partial pressure in kPa is close to the percentage concentration at normal barometric pressure. Partial pressure in mm Hg may be

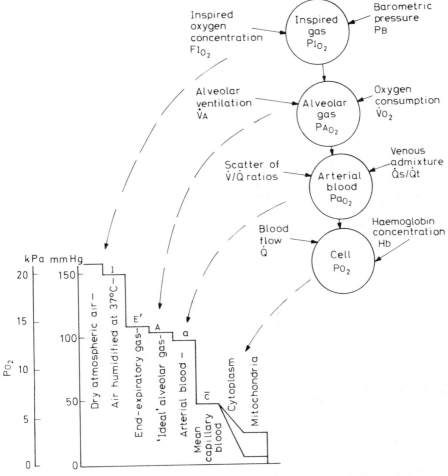

Figure 128. On the left is shown the oxygen cascade with PO_2 falling from the level in the ambient air down to the level in mitochondria, which is the site of utilization. On the right is shown a summary of the factors influencing oxygenation at different levels in the cascade

* The quantity in parentheses is known as the 'dry barometric pressure'.

approximately derived by multiplying the percentage concentration by 7; e.g. Po_2 of air is approximately $21 \times 7 = 147$ mm Hg, tension of 2 per cent halothane is approximately $2 \times 7 = 14$ mm Hg, and the tension of 5 per cent carbon dioxide is approximately $5 \times 7 = 35$ mm Hg.

In respiratory physiology, gas tensions are almost always considered as being exerted by gas humidified at body temperature. This applies to inspired gas because it cannot participate in gas exchange until after it has been humidified in the upper respiratory tract. Therefore calculations almost always employ the *dry* barometric pressure whether considering inspired, alveolar or expired gas.

Factors influencing alveolar tension of oxygen

The general equation for the calculation of the alveolar tension of a gas has been stated on pages 186 et seq. In the case of oxygen:

$$\text{alveolar } Po_2 \doteq \begin{matrix} \text{dry} \\ \text{barometric} \\ \text{pressure} \end{matrix} \left(\begin{matrix} \text{inspired} \\ \text{oxygen} \\ \text{concentration} \end{matrix} - \frac{\text{oxygen uptake}}{\text{alveolar ventilation}} \right) \quad \ldots (1)$$

This equation is only approximate and does not include the second order correction factor due to the small difference in volume between the inspired and expired gas. Normally this factor is small but, during the exchange of a soluble gas such as nitrous oxide, the difference may be quite large.

Various forms of the alveolar air equation may be used to correct for this difference. The commonest forms assume that the number of molecules of nitrogen inhaled equals the number exhaled. This, of course, is very seldom true during and after anaesthesia, and in the intensive therapy unit. Therefore, under these circumstances it is necessary to use a special form of the equation introduced by Filley, MacIntosh and Wright (1954), which makes no assumptions of inert gas equilibrium and is appropriate to most of the varied conditions encountered by the anaesthetist and intensive therapist:

$$PA_{O2} = PI_{O2} - PA_{CO2} \left(\frac{PI_{O2} - P\bar{E}_{O2}}{P\bar{E}_{CO2}} \right) \quad \ldots (2)$$

Applications of the equation have been discussed by Nunn (1963). A further modification has been described by Kelman and Prys-Roberts (1967) which allows for the addition of carbon dioxide to the inspired gas of the patient.

In its more accurate forms (e.g. equation 2), the alveolar air equation is used principally for calculation of the 'ideal' alveolar Po_2, a theoretical entity which was introduced on page 214 and explained in greater detail on pages 307 et seq. 'Ideal' alveolar gas approximates in composition to the mixed gas which is exhaled at the end of expiration from the perfused alveoli. In practice it is defined as having a Pco_2 equal to that of arterial blood, and a respiratory exchange ratio equal to that of mixed expired gas. Comparison of 'ideal' alveolar Po_2 with arterial Po_2 is the standard method of measurement of 'venous admixture' (pages 306 et seq.).

In its simplified form (equation 1), the alveolar air equation is useful for consideration of the important quantitative relationships between barometric pressure, inspired oxygen concentration, oxygen uptake and alveolar ventilation. *Figure 129* shows the relationship for normal barometric pressure and basal oxygen consumption. The quantitative basis of the relationship was considered on pages 186 et seq. It suffices here to stress the following points.

Dry barometric pressure. Other factors remaining constant, the alveolar P_{O_2} will be directly proportional to the dry barometric pressure which falls with increasing altitude to become zero at 19 kilometres where the actual barometric pressure equals the saturated vapour pressure of water at body temperature. A pressure of two atmospheres (absolute) approximately doubles the alveolar P_{O_2} if other factors remain constant.

Ventilation. There is a hyperbolic relationship between alveolar P_{O_2} and alveolar ventilation. As ventilation is increased, the alveolar P_{O_2} rises asymptotically towards (but never reaches) the P_{O_2} of the inspired gas (*Figure 129*). It will be seen from the shape of the curves that changes in

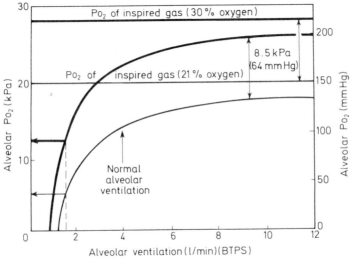

Figure 129. *The effect on alveolar P_{O_2} of increasing the inspired oxygen concentration from 21 per cent (thin curve) to 30 per cent (heavy curve). The patient is assumed to have an oxygen consumption of 200 ml/min (STPD). In this example, the alveolar P_{O_2} is reduced to a dangerously low level when breathing air at an alveolar ventilation of 1·5 l/min. At this point, oxygen enrichment of the inspired gas to 30 per cent is sufficient to raise the alveolar P_{O_2} almost to within the normal range. All points on the heavy curve are 8·5 kPa (64 mm Hg) above the corresponding points on the thin curve at the same ventilation*

ventilation *above* the normal level have comparatively little effect upon alveolar P_{O_2}. In contrast, changes in ventilation *below* the normal level may have a very marked effect on alveolar P_{O_2}. At very low levels of ventilation, the alveolar ventilation is quite critical and small changes may precipitate gross hypoxia. The critical zone may be deduced from a study of *Figure 129*.

Oxygen consumption. The role of oxygen consumption has received insufficient attention and there is an unfortunate tendency to consider that all patients consume 250 ml of oxygen per minute under all circumstances. Oxygen consumption must, of course be raised by exercise but is often above basal in a patient 'at rest'. It tends to be just those patients in whom there is a respiratory problem who have oxygen consumptions significantly different from basal. For example, a patient with chronic obstructive airway disease tends to become trapped between the pincers of a falling ventilatory capacity and a rising ventilatory requirement until, in due course, his ventilatory capacity can no longer sustain his resting ventilatory requirement. We have mentioned above (page 229) that his ventilatory requirement is raised by a high physiological dead space and, in the case of oxygen, by an increased alveolar/arterial P_{O_2} difference. To these troubles there is usually added a raised oxygen consumption, due perhaps to pyrexia, laboured breathing or merely to agitation in response to dyspnoea. The raised oxygen consumption may well be the final straw which precipitates the onset of ventilatory failure. Weaning from artificial ventilation may be made unexpectedly difficult by an unsuspected high oxygen consumption. This may be measured directly but is admittedly difficult in the circumstances of the intensive therapy unit. Thyrotoxicosis, convulsions and, to a lesser extent, shivering (Bay, Nunn and Prys-Roberts, 1968) cause a very marked rise in oxygen consumption and should, of course, be controlled. The value of measurement of oxygen consumption in the management of tetanus has recently been stressed by Femi-Pearse et al. (1976).

No less important is the reduction in oxygen consumption which occurs during anaesthesia, hypothermia and myxoedema. Oxygen consumption during anaesthesia tends to be about 15 per cent below basal on the usual standards (*see Table 15*) but approximates to the basal values proposed by Robertson and Reid (1952) for patients who were either well rested or sedated. This factor tends to reduce the ventilatory requirement during anaesthesia but is more than offset by the increase in dead space and alveolar/arterial P_{O_2} gradient. Hypothermia

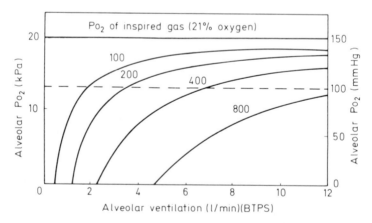

Figure 130. The relationship between alveolar ventilation and alveolar P_{O_2} for different values of oxygen consumption for a patient breathing air at normal barometric pressure. The figures on the curves indicate the oxygen consumption in ml/min (STPD). Alveolar ventilation is in l/min (BTPS). A typical value for oxygen consumption by an anaesthetized patient is 200 ml/min; 100 ml/min would be an average figure during hypothermia at 30° C. Higher values may be brought about by restlessness, struggling, pyrexia or shivering. Note that the alveolar ventilation required to maintain any particular alveolar P_{O_2} is directly proportional to the oxygen consumption. (In calculations of this type it is important to make the correction required by the fact that oxygen consumption and alveolar ventilation values are commonly expressed at different temperatures and pressures—see Appendix B)

causes marked reductions in oxygen consumption with values of about 50 per cent of basal at 31°C. Artificial ventilation of hypothermic patients very commonly results in hypocapnia unless a conscious effort is made to reduce the minute volume or increase the apparatus dead space. *Figure 130* shows the effect of different values for oxygen consumption on the relationship between alveolar ventilation and alveolar P_{O_2} for a patient breathing air.

The oxygen consumption of a patient is the sum of the oxygen consumptions of the individual organ systems. Approximately 20 per cent of the total is accounted for by the brain. This rises during convulsions and is markedly depressed by barbiturates though to a lesser extent by inhalational anaesthetics (*see Table 27*). Myocardial oxygen consumption is of the same order and it has been shown that this declines progressively with deepening halothane anaesthesia (Theye, 1972).

Cardiac output.   In the short term, cardiac output can influence the alveolar P_{O_2}. For example, if other factors remain constant, a sudden reduction in cardiac output will temporarily raise the alveolar P_{O_2} since less blood passes through the lungs to remove oxygen from the alveolar gas. However, the reduced cardiac output also causes increased oxygen extraction in the tissues supplied by the systemic circulation and before long the mixed venous oxygen level is decreased. When that has happened, the removal of oxygen from the alveolar gas returns to its original level as the reduction in blood flow rate is compensated by the greater amount of oxygen which is taken up per unit volume of blood flowing through the lungs. Thus, in the long term cardiac output does not directly influence the alveolar P_{O_2} and only the oxygen consumption appears in equation (1).

Inspired oxygen concentration.   The alveolar P_{O_2} will be raised or lowered by an amount equal to the change in the inspired gas P_{O_2}, provided that other factors remain constant. Since the concentration of oxygen in the inspired gas should always be under control, it is a most important therapeutic tool which may be used to counteract a number of different factors which may impair oxygenation.

The effect of an increase in the inspired oxygen concentration from 21 to 30 per cent is shown in *Figure 129*. For any alveolar ventilation, the improvement of alveolar P_{O_2} will be 8·5 kPa or 64 mm Hg. This will be of great importance if hypoventilation while breathing air has reduced the alveolar P_{O_2} to 4 kPa (30 mm Hg), a value which is close to the lowest level compatible with life. Oxygen enrichment of inspired gas to 30 per cent will then increase the alveolar P_{O_2} to 12·5 kPa (94 mm Hg), which is almost within the normal range. However, at this level of hypoventilation, P_{CO_2} would have been 13 kPa (98 mm Hg) and might well have risen further on withdrawal of the hypoxic drive to ventilation. Thus 30 per cent is the maximum concentration of oxygen in the inspired gas which will be required to correct the alveolar P_{O_2} of a patient breathing air, who has become hypoxaemic as a result of hypoventilation. If higher concentrations are required, the patient could not survive while breathing air and the elevation of P_{CO_2} (uninfluenced directly by changes in inspired oxygen) will be dangerously high. Such cases require treatment by increase of alveolar ventilation such as, for example, by artificial ventilation or tracheostomy. In *Figure 65*, ventilation/alveolar P_{O_2} curves were constructed for a wide range of inspired oxygen concentrations. This figure indicates the protection against hypoxaemia (due to hypoventilation) which is afforded by different concentrations of oxygen in the inspired gas.

An entirely different problem is hypoxaemia due to venous admixture, which can be alleviated partially or fully by increasing the inspired oxygen concentration to a level which is determined by the degree of venous admixture and various other factors. This may require concentrations as high as 100 per cent or even hyperbaric oxygen. Quantitative aspects are shown in *Figure 102* and are also considered below (page 431). It should be noted that these high concentrations of oxygen are not without danger (page 426).

For completeness, it should be mentioned that high concentrations of oxygen may be used for clearing gas loculi (page 422) and also to provide an increase in the body stores of oxygen (page 412).

The 'concentration', third gas or Fink effect. The above diagrams and equations have ignored a factor which influences alveolar P_{O_2} during exchanges of large quantities of soluble gases such as nitrous oxide. This effect was mentioned briefly in connection with carbon dioxide on page 350. Its effect on oxygen is probably more important.

During the administration of nitrous oxide, large quantities of the more soluble gas replace smaller quantities of the less soluble nitrogen previously dissolved in body fluids. There is thus a net uptake of 'inert' gas into the body from the alveoli, causing a *temporary* increase in the concentration of both oxygen and carbon dioxide, which will thus *temporarily* exert a higher tension than would otherwise be expected. Conversely, during recovery from nitrous oxide anaesthesia, large quantities of nitrous oxide leave the body to be replaced with smaller quantities of nitrogen. There is thus a net loss of 'inert' gas from the body into the alveoli causing dilution of oxygen and carbon dioxide, both of which will *temporarily* exert a lower tension than would otherwise be expected.

The alveolar/arterial P_{O_2} difference

The next step in the oxygen cascade is of great clinical relevance. In the healthy young adult breathing air, the alveolar/arterial P_{O_2} difference does not exceed 2 kPa (15 mm Hg) but rises to about 5 kPa (37·5 mm Hg) in aged but healthy subjects. These values may be exceeded in any lung disease which causes shunting or mismatching of ventilation and perfusion. Typical examples are pulmonary collapse, consolidation, neoplasm or infection. Uncomplicated anaesthesia increases the alveolar/arterial P_{O_2} difference, probably because of a decrease in lung volume. Extrapulmonary shunting (e.g. Fallot's tetralogy) will also increase the difference. It is a fact of life that the alveolar/arterial P_{O_2} difference is substantially raised in all patients undergoing intensive therapy regardless of their diagnosis! Without doubt, an increased alveolar/arterial P_{O_2} difference is the commonest cause of arterial hypoxaemia in clinical practice and is a very important step in the oxygen cascade.

Unlike the alveolar P_{O_2}, the alveolar/arterial P_{O_2} difference cannot be predicted from other more easily measured quantities, and there is no simple means of knowing the magnitude of the alveolar/arterial P_{O_2} difference in a particular patient other than by measurement of the arterial blood gases. It is, therefore, important to understand the factors which influence the difference and the principles of restoration of arterial Po_2 by increasing the inspired oxygen concentration.

Factors influencing the magnitude of the alveolar/arterial Po_2 difference

In Chapter 9 it was explained how the alveolar/arterial Po_2 difference results from venous admixture (or physiological shunt) which consists of two components: (1) shunted venous blood which mingles with the oxygenated blood leaving the pulmonary capillaries; (2) a component due to scatter of ventilation/perfusion ratios in different parts of the lungs. In the present state of knowledge, any component due to impaired diffusion across the alveolar/capillary membrane can probably be ignored (page 320).

Figure 97 shows the derivation of the following axiomatic relationship for the first component:

$$\frac{\dot{Q}s}{\dot{Q}t} = \frac{Cc'_{o_2} - Ca_{o_2}}{Cc'_{o_2} - C\bar{v}_{o_2}}$$

Two points should be noted.

1. The equation gives a slightly false impression of precision since it assumes that all the shunted blood is *mixed* venous. This is not the case, Thebesian and bronchial venous blood being obvious exceptions.
2. Oxygen content of pulmonary end-capillary blood (Cc'_{o_2}) is, in practice, calculated on the basis of the end-capillary oxygen tension (Pc'_{o_2}) being equal to the 'ideal' alveolar Po_2 (*see* page 307).

The equation may be cleared and solved for the pulmonary end-capillary/arterial oxygen content difference as follows:

$$Cc'_{o_2} - Ca_{o_2} = \frac{\dfrac{\dot{Q}s}{\dot{Q}t}(Ca_{o_2} - C\bar{v}_{o_2})^*}{1 - \dfrac{\dot{Q}s}{\dot{Q}t}} \qquad \ldots (3)$$

$Ca_{o_2} - C\bar{v}_{o_2}$ is the arterial/mixed venous oxygen content difference and is a function of the oxygen consumption and the cardiac output thus:

$$\dot{Q}t\,(Ca_{o_2} - C\bar{v}_{o_2}) = \dot{V}o_2 \text{ (Fick equation)}^* \qquad \ldots (4)$$

Substituting for $(Ca_{o_2} - C\bar{v}_{o_2})$ in equation (3), we have:

$$Cc'_{o_2} - Ca_{o_2} = \frac{\dot{V}o_2\,\dfrac{\dot{Q}s}{\dot{Q}t}}{\dot{Q}t\left(1 - \dfrac{\dot{Q}s}{\dot{Q}t}\right)}^* \qquad \ldots (5)$$

This equation shows the content difference in terms of oxygen consumption $(\dot{V}o_2)$, the venous admixture $(\dot{Q}s/\dot{Q}t)$ and the cardiac output $(\dot{Q}t)$.

The significance of cardiac output has not received due attention until recent

---

* Scaling factors are required to correct for the inconsistency of the units which are customarily used for the quantities in this equation.

years. However, it will be clear that this factor must be of considerable importance, since a reduced cardiac output results in an increased arterial/mixed venous oxygen content difference. This means that the shunted blood will be more desaturated and will therefore cause a greater fall of the arterial oxygen level than would less desaturated blood flowing through a shunt of the same magnitude.

The final stage in the calculation is to convert the end-capillary/arterial oxygen *content* difference to the *tension* difference. The oxygen content of blood is the sum of the oxygen in physical solution and that which is combined with haemoglobin:

$$\text{oxygen content of blood} = \alpha P_{O_2} + S_{O_2} \times Hb \times 1\cdot39^*$$

where: α is the solubility coefficient of oxygen in blood (not plasma!); S_{O_2} is the saturation, and varies with P_{O_2} according to the oxygen dissociation curve, which itself is influenced by temperature, pH and base excess (Bohr effect); Hb is the haemoglobin concentration (g/100 ml); $1\cdot39$ is the volume of oxygen (ml) which can combine with 1 g of haemoglobin.*

Carriage of oxygen in the blood is discussed in detail on pages 399 et seq.

Derivation of the oxygen content from the P_{O_2} is excessively laborious if due account is taken of pH, base excess, temperature and haemoglobin concentration. Derivation of P_{O_2} from content is even more laborious as an iterative approach is required. Tables of tension/content relationships are particularly useful, and *Table 29* is an extract from Kelman and Nunn (1968) to show the format and general influence of the several variables.

The principal factors influencing the magnitude of the alveolar/arterial P_{O_2} difference caused by venous admixture may be summarized as follows.

The magnitude of the venous admixture increases the alveolar/arterial P_{O_2} difference with direct proportionality for small shunts, although this is lost with larger shunts (*Figure 131*). The resultant effect on arterial P_{O_2} is shown in *Figure 102*. Different forms of venous admixture are considered on pages 291 et seq.

$\dot{V}/\dot{Q}$ scatter.   It was explained in Chapter 9 that scatter in ventilation/perfusion ratios produces an alveolar/arterial P_{O_2} difference for the following reasons.

1. More blood flows through the underventilated overperfused alveoli, and the mixed arterial blood is therefore heavily weighted in the direction of the suboxygenated blood from areas of low $\dot{V}/\dot{Q}$ ratio. The smaller amount of blood flowing through areas of high $\dot{V}/\dot{Q}$ ratio cannot compensate for this (*see Figure 98*).
2. Due to the bend in the upper part of the dissociation curve, the fall in saturation in blood from areas of low $\dot{V}/\dot{Q}$ ratio tends to be greater than the rise in saturation in blood from areas of high $\dot{V}/\dot{Q}$ (*see Figure 99*). This provides a second reason why blood from alveoli with a high $\dot{V}/\dot{Q}$ cannot compensate for blood from alveoli with a high $\dot{V}/\dot{Q}$ ratio.

---

* $1\cdot39$ is the theoretical value based on the molecular weight of haemoglobin. This value is not obtained in practice (*see page 401*).

Table 29 OXYGEN CONTENT OF HUMAN BLOOD (ml/100 ml) AS A FUNCTION OF PO_2 AND OTHER VARIABLES (VALUES FROM THE COMPUTER-WRITTEN TABLES OF KELMAN AND NUNN, 1968)

	Haemoglobin concentration (g/100 ml)		
	10	*14*	*18*
PO_2 at pH 7·4, 37°C, base excess zero			
50	11·99	16·72	21·45
70	13·29	18·53	23·76
100	13·85	19·27	24·69
150	14·20	19·70	25·20
200	14·41	19·94	25·47
PO_2 at pH 7·2, 37°C, base excess zero			
50	10·45	14·57	18·69
70	12·60	17·56	22·52
100	13·62	18·94	24·27
150	14·11	19·58	25·04
200	14·37	19·87	25·38
PO_2 at pH 7·4, 34°C, base excess zero			
50	12·81	17·87	22·93
70	13·59	18·94	24·30
100	13·96	19·43	24·89
150	14·24	19·76	25·28
200	14·44	19·98	25·51

The fourth significant figure is not of clinical importance but is useful for interpolation.

The actual alveolar PO_2 has a profound but non-linear effect on the alveolar/arterial PO_2 gradient (*Figure 131*). The alveolar/arterial oxygen *content* is uninfluenced by the alveolar PO_2 (equation 5), and the effect on the *tension* difference arises entirely in conversion of *content* to *tension*: it is thus a function of the slope of the dissociation curve at the PO_2 of the alveolar gas. For example, a loss of 1 vol. per cent of oxygen from blood with a PO_2 of 93 kPa (700 mm Hg) causes a fall of PO_2 of about 43 kPa (325 mm Hg), most of the oxygen being lost from physical solution. However, if the initial PO_2 were 13 kPa (100 mm Hg), a loss of 1 vol. per cent would only cause a fall of PO_2 of 4·6 kPa (35 mm Hg), most of the oxygen being lost from combination with haemo-globin. Should the initial PO_2 be only 6·7 kPa (50 mm Hg), a loss of 1 vol. per cent would cause a very small change in PO_2 of the order of 0·7 kPa (5 mm Hg), drawn almost entirely from combination with haemoglobin at a point where the dissociation curve is steep.* This effect is clearly shown in *Figure 131*. The clinical implication of this is that the alveolar/arterial PO_2 difference will be greatest when the alveolar PO_2 is highest (other factors being the same). If the alveolar PO_2 be reduced (e.g. by underventilation), then the alveolar/arterial PO_2 gradient will be diminished if other factors remain the same. The arterial PO_2 thus falls less than the alveolar PO_2. This is fortunate and may be considered as

* These figures only apply to certain specified conditions—haemoglobin concentration 14 g/100 ml, 37° C, pH 7·40, base excess zero. A change in any of these factors will alter the figures.

one of the many benefits deriving from the shape of the oxygen dissociation curve. With a 50 per cent venous admixture, the arterial P_{O_2} is almost independent of changes in alveolar P_{O_2} (*Figure 102*).

Cardiac output changes produce inverse changes of the arterial/mixed venous oxygen content difference if the patient's oxygen consumption remains the same (Fick equation 4). Equation (5) shows that there is also an inverse relationship between the cardiac output and the alveolar/arterial oxygen *content* difference if the venous admixture is constant (*Figure 132b*). However, when the *content* difference is converted to *tension* difference, the relationship to cardiac output is no longer truly inverse, but assumes a complex non-linear form in consequence of the shape of the oxygen dissociation curve. The relationship between cardiac

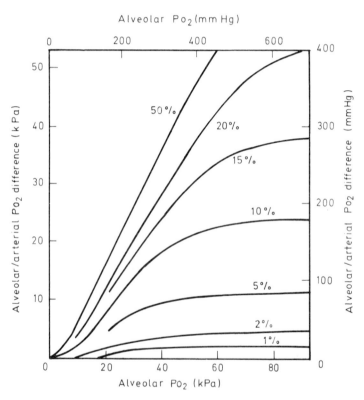

Figure 131. Influence of shunt on alveolar/arterial P_{O_2} *difference at different levels of alveolar* P_{O_2}. *For small shunts, the difference (at constant alveolar* P_{O_2}*) is roughly proportional to the magnitude of the shunt. For a given shunt, the alveolar/arterial* P_{O_2} *difference increases with alveolar* P_{O_2} *in non-linear manner governed by the oxygen dissociation curve. At high alveolar* P_{O_2}*, a plateau of alveolar/arterial* P_{O_2} *difference is reached but the alveolar* P_{O_2} *at which the plateau is reached is higher with larger shunts. Note that, with a 50 per cent shunt, an increase in alveolar* P_{O_2} *produces an almost equal increase in alveolar/arterial* P_{O_2} *difference. Therefore, the arterial* P_{O_2} *is virtually independent of changes in alveolar* P_{O_2}*, if other factors remain constant. Constants incorporated in this diagram: arterial/venous oxygen content difference, 5 ml/100 ml; Hb concentration, 14 g/100 ml; temperature of blood, 37°C; pH of blood, 7·40; base excess, zero. Figures in the graph indicate shunt as percentage of total pulmonary blood flow*

output and alveolar/arterial Po₂ difference shown in *Figure 132a* applies only to the conditions specified, particularly the alveolar Po₂, which was assumed to be 24 kPa (180 mm Hg) in the preparation of this diagram. The combination of a moderate degree of venous admixture and a low cardiac output can clearly lead to severe arterial hypoxaemia in a patient breathing air.

The temperature, pH and base excess of the patient's blood influence the dissociation curve (page 404). In addition, temperature affects the solubility coefficient of oxygen in blood. All three factors influence the relationship between tension and content (*see Table 29*).

Therefore, the effect of venous admixture on the alveolar/arterial Po₂ difference is influenced by these factors although the effect is not usually important except in extreme deviations from normal.

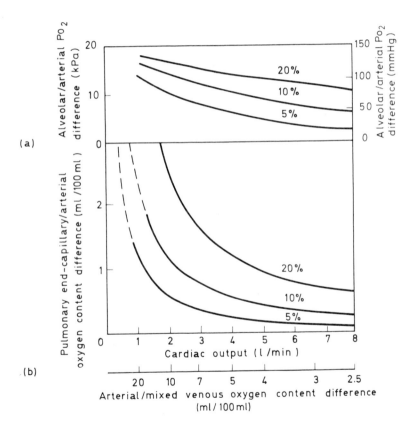

Figure 132. Influence of cardiac output on the alveolar/arterial Po₂ difference. In this example it is assumed that the patient has an oxygen consumption of 200 ml/min and an alveolar Po₂ of 24 kPa (180 mm Hg). Changes in cardiac output produce an inverse change in the pulmonary end-capillary/arterial oxygen content difference (graph b). When converted to tension differences, the inverse relationship is distorted by the effect of the oxygen dissociation curve in a manner which is applicable only to the particular alveolar Po₂ of the patient (graph a). (Alveolar Po₂ is assumed equal to pulmonary end-capillary Po₂)

The haemoglobin concentration influences the partition of oxygen between physical solution and chemical combination. While the heamoglobin concentration does not influence the pulmonary end-capillary/arterial oxygen *content* difference (equation 5), it exerts an effect on the *tension* difference. For example, at a cardiac output of 5 l/min and oxygen consumption of 200 ml/min, venous admixture of 20 per cent results in a pulmonary end-capillary/arterial oxygen content difference of 0·5 vol. per cent. Assuming an alveolar Po_2 of 24 kPa (180 mm Hg), the alveolar/arterial Po_2 difference is influenced by haemoglobin concentration as shown in *Table 30*. (Different figures would be obtained by selection of a different value for alveolar Po_2.)

Table 30 EFFECT OF DIFFERENT HAEMOGLOBIN CONCENTRATIONS ON THE ARTERIAL PO_2 UNDER VENOUS ADMIXTURE CONDITIONS DEFINED IN TEXT

Haemoglobin concentration	*Alveolar/arterial PO_2 difference*		*Arterial PO_2*	
(g/100 ml)	*kPa*	*mm Hg*	*kPa*	*mm Hg*
8	15·0	113	9·0	67
10	14·5	109	9·5	71
12	14·0	105	10·0	75
14	13·5	101	10·5	79
16	13·0	98	11·0	82

Alveolar ventilation.   The over-all effect of changes in alveolar ventilation on the arterial Po_2 presents an interesting problem, and serves to illustrate the integration of the separate aspects of the factors discussed above. An increase in the alveolar ventilation may be expected to have the following results.

1. *The alveolar* Po_2 must be raised provided the barometric pressure, inspired oxygen concentration and oxygen consumption remain the same (equation 1 and *Figure 129*).
2. *The alveolar/arterial* Po_2 *difference* is increased for the following reasons.
    a. The increase in the alveolar Po_2 will increase the alveolar/arterial Po_2 difference if other factors remain the same (*Figure 131*).
    b. Under many conditions it has been demonstrated that a fall of Pco_2 (resulting from an increase in alveolar ventilation) reduces the cardiac output, which will increase the alveolar/arterial Po_2 difference if other factors remain the same (equation 5 and *Figure 132*).
    c. The change in arterial pH resulting from the reduction in Pco_2 causes a small, unimportant increase in alveolar/arterial Po_2 difference.

Thus an increase in alveolar ventilation may be expected to raise the alveolar Po_2 *and* the alveolar/arterial Po_2 difference. The resultant change in arterial Po_2 will depend upon the relative magnitude of the two changes. *Figure 133* shows the changes in arterial Po_2 caused by variations of alveolar ventilation at an inspired oxygen concentration of 30 per cent in the presence of varying degrees of venous admixture, assuming that cardiac output is influenced by Pco_2 as described in the legend. Up to an alveolar ventilation of 1·5 l/min, an increase in ventilation will always raise the arterial Po_2. Beyond that, in the example cited, further increases in alveolar ventilation will only increase the arterial Po_2 if the

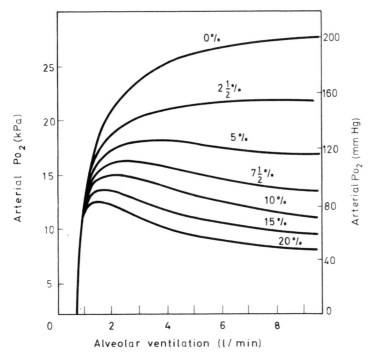

Figure 133. *The effect of alveolar ventilation on arterial* PO_2 *is the algebraic sum of the effect upon the alveolar* PO_2 *(Figure 129) and the alveolar/arterial* PO_2 *difference. When the increase in the latter exceeds the increase in the former, the arterial* PO_2 *will be diminished. The figures in the diagram indicate the percentage venous admixture. The curve corresponding to zero per cent venous admixture will indicate the alveolar* PO_2. *Constants incorporated in the design of this figure: inspired* O_2 *concentration, 30 per cent;* O_2 *consumption, 200 ml/min; respiratory exchange ratio, 0·8. It has been assumed that the cardiac output is influenced by the* PCO_2 *according to the equation:* $\dot{Q} = 0·039 \times PCO_2$ *(mm Hg) + 2·23. (Reproduced from Kelman and his colleagues, 1967, by courtesy of the Editor of the* British Journal of Anaesthesia)

venous admixture is less than 3 per cent. For larger values of venous admixture, the increase in the alveolar/arterial PO_2 difference exceeds the increase in the alveolar PO_2 and the arterial PO_2 is thus decreased.

Compensation for increased alveolar/arterial PO_2 *difference by raising the inspired oxygen concentration*

Hypoxaemia is to be expected in patients with most forms of severe cardiac or respiratory dysfunction. In the type of patient presenting for intensive therapy, hypoxaemia while breathing air is almost always present. As a broad classification, hypoxaemia may be due to hypoventilation or to venous admixture or to a combination of the two. The first line of treatment is clearly to remove the cause of the hypoxaemia but, when this is not immediately possible, it is necessary to raise the inspired oxygen concentration of the inspired gas to the level required to restore a normal arterial PO_2 (the normal range of arterial PO_2 is considered on page 411).

When hypoxaemia is primarily due to hypoventilation and when it is not appropriate or possible to restore the normal ventilation, then the arterial P_{O_2} may be restored by elevation of the inspired oxygen within the range 21–30 per cent, as explained above (page 387). When hypoxaemia is primarily due to venous admixture, it is possible to restore the arterial P_{O_2} by oxygen enrichment of the inspired gas provided the venous admixture does not exceed the equivalent of a shunt of 30 per cent of the cardiac output. The quantitative aspects of the relationship are best considered in relation to the iso-shunt diagram described by Benatar, Hewlett and Nunn in 1973 (*see Figure 102*). This diagram, introduced on page 290, makes the assumption that the haemoglobin concentration and arterial P_{CO_2} lie within the limits shown and that the arterial/mixed venous oxygen content difference is 5 ml/100 ml. The bands indicate the value of arterial P_{O_2} which can be expected for different values of inspired oxygen concentration for a range of shunt values. It will be seen that the relationships are non-linear and not intuitively obvious.

At the practical level, the iso-shunt diagram may be used in several different ways. Firstly, from simultaneous values of arterial P_{O_2} and inspired oxygen concentration, it is possible to read off the virtual shunt value for a patient. The virtual shunt is defined as the shunt which would account for the arterial P_{O_2} if the arterial/mixed venous oxygen content difference were 5 ml/100 ml. It thus includes a factor related to the ratio of cardiac output to oxygen consumption. The virtual shunt line may than be used to indicate the arterial P_{O_2} which may be expected for any inspired oxygen concentration or, alternatively, to indicate the inspired oxygen concentration which will be necessary to give any particular arterial P_{O_2}. For example, if the arterial P_{O_2} is 30 kPa (225 mm Hg) during the inhalation of 90 per cent oxygen, the patient has a virtual shunt of 20 per cent. If we consider that an arterial P_{O_2} of 10 kPa (75 mm Hg) will be sufficient, then we can reduce the inspired oxygen concentration to about 45 per cent. The virtual shunt can be seen to fall during resolution of pulmonary pathology and thus has some prognostic value. Caution is necessary in its use. If the venous admixture is due mainly to ventilation/perfusion mismatch without a major shunt, then arterial P_{O_2} will rise above iso-shunt lines as the inspired oxygen is increased (King et al., 1974). Also, cardiac output may well change with the arterial P_{O_2} and therefore the virtual shunt may alter even if the true shunt remains the same. In practice, however, the iso-shunt diagram has proved useful although it is prudent to check the new arterial P_{O_2} after a major change of inspired oxygen concentration.

During routine anaesthesia, there is usually a virtual shunt of 10 per cent, probably due to the reduction in lung volume (*see Figure 106*). Maintenance of a satisfactory arterial P_{O_2} requires an inspired oxygen concentration of 30–40 per cent, which is normal practice.

Figure 102 shows that elevation of the inspired oxygen concentration will only restore the arterial P_{O_2} if the virtual shunt is less than about 35 per cent. For larger shunts, even 100 per cent oxygen will not restore normal arterial oxygenation and this is a well known observation in patients with massive shunts such as are seen in Fallot's tetralogy. In fact, it is possible to restore the arterial P_{O_2} under these circumstances if 100 per cent oxygen is administered at greater than normal atmospheric pressure.

The purpose of this concern about selection of the optimal arterial P_{O_2} is to avoid hypoxia on one side and pulmonary oxygen toxicity on the other side (*see* page 426). In general, one is reluctant to use concentrations higher than 60 to 70 per cent for more than a short period and every means should be employed for so doing. It is thus important to ensure that pulmonary function is as good as is possible by careful attention to control of secretions, infection and expansion of areas of collapse. Positive end-expiratory pressure is a particularly valuable method of decreasing the virtual shunt (*see* page 128).

There is little point in deciding what is the optimal inspired oxygen concentration unless the means are available for delivery of the selected oxygen concentration to the patient. This important topic is considered below (page 431).

Transport of oxygen from the lungs to the cell

We may regard the most important function of the respiratory and circulatory systems to be the supply of oxygen to the cells of the body. The quantity of oxygen transferred in one minute has been termed the 'oxygen flux' (Nunn and Freeman, 1964), and is equal to the following:

$$\text{cardiac output} \times \text{arterial oxygen content}$$

$$= \quad \frac{5000}{\text{ml/min}} \quad \times \quad \frac{20}{100} \quad = 1000 \text{ ml/min}$$

$$\text{ml } O_2/\text{ml blood}$$

Of this 1000 ml/min, approximately 250 is utilized by the conscious resting subject. The circulating blood thus loses 25 per cent of its oxygen and the mixed venous blood is approximately 75 per cent saturated. The 75 per cent of unextracted oxygen forms an important reserve which may be drawn upon under the stress of such conditions as exercise, to which additional extraction forms one of the integrated adaptations (Barcroft, 1934).

The arterial oxygen content consists predominantly of oxygen in combination with haemoglobin and this fraction is given by the following expression:

$$\text{saturation} \times \text{haemoglobin concentration} \times 1 \cdot 39^*$$

Ignoring the oxygen in physical solution, the full expression for the oxygen flux is as follows:

$$\frac{\text{cardiac}}{\text{output}} \times \frac{\text{arterial } O_2}{\text{saturation}} \times \frac{\text{haemoglobin}}{\text{concentration}} \times 1 \cdot 39 = \text{oxygen flux}$$

$$\frac{5000}{\text{ml(min}} \times \frac{95}{100} \times \frac{15}{100} \times 1 \cdot 39 = \frac{1000}{\text{ml/min}}$$

$$\text{g/ml}$$

Note that three variable factors determine the oxygen flux.

1. *Cardiac output* or, for a particular organ, the regional blood flow. Failure of this factor has been termed 'stagnant anoxia' (Barcroft, 1920).
2. *Arterial oxygen saturation.* Failure of this (for whatever reason) has been termed 'anoxic anoxia'.

---

* 1·39 is the theoretical volume of oxygen (ml) which will combine with 1 g of haemoglobin (*see* page 401).

3. *Haemoglobin concentration* deficiency, as a cause of tissue hypoxia, has been termed 'anaemic anoxia'.

The three types of 'anoxia' may be conveniently displayed on a Venn diagram (*Figure 134*) which clearly displays the possibility of combinations of any two types of anoxia or all three together. For example, the combination of anaemia and low cardiac output, which occurs in untreated haemorrhage, would be indicated by the overlapping area of the stagnant and anaemic circles. If the patient also suffered from 'shock lung' he might then move into the central area, indicating the addition of anoxic anoxia. On a more cheerful note, compensations are more usual. Patients with anaemia normally have a high cardiac output; subjects resident at altitude have polycythaemia, and so on. Such considerations provide a classic example of the importance of viewing a patient as a whole. The question of the lowest permissible haemoglobin concentration for major surgery can only be answered after consideration of the actual and projected cardiac output during surgery, the pulmonary function and so on. No general answer is possible.

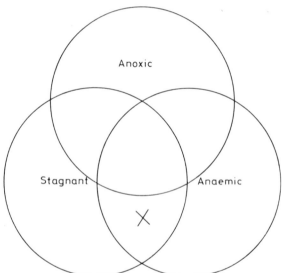

Figure 134. Barcroft's classification of causes of hypoxia displayed on a Venn diagram to illustrate the possibility of combinations of more than one type of hypoxia. The lowest area of overlap, marked with a cross, shows co-existent anaemia and low cardiac output. The central area illustrates a combination of all three types of hypoxia (e.g. a patient with haemorrhage and 'shock lung')

It is important to note that the oxygen flux equals the product of the three variables and one constant. If one variable is halved, the oxygen flux is halved, but if all three variables are halved, the oxygen flux is reduced to one-eighth of the original value. One-eighth of 1000 is 125 ml/min, and this is a value which, if maintained for any length of time, is incompatible with life, although the reductions of the individual variables are not in themselves lethal.

The quantitative implications of the oxygen flux have been explored by Nunn and Freeman (1964) who stressed the conclusion that criteria for the adequacy of each variable must be considered in relation to the other variables. Thus a degree of arterial hypoxaemia which may be tolerated in the otherwise healthy patient may be dangerous in patients with impaired circulation or anaemia.

Tissue P_{O_2}. It is often useful to refer to the tissue P_{O_2} and much of intensive therapy is directed towards increasing tissue P_{O_2}. However, it is almost impossible to quantify tissue P_{O_2}. It is evident that there are differences between different organs, with the tissue P_{O_2} influenced not only by arterial P_{O_2} and tissue perfusion but also by oxygen uptake of the organ. However, even greater difficulties arise from the regional variations in tissue P_{O_2} in different parts of the same organ. They are presumably caused by regional variations in tissue perfusion and oxygen consumption. Nor is this the whole story. An advancing P_{O_2}-sensitive microelectrode detects variations in P_{O_2} which can be interpreted in relation to the proximity of the electrode to small vessels (*see Figure 109*). Very large variations have been demonstrated with exploring electrodes in the brain (Cater et al., 1961). 'Tissue P_{O_2}' is thus an unsatisfactory quantitative index of the state of oxygenation of an organ.

THE CARRIAGE OF OXYGEN IN THE BLOOD

Oxygen is carried in the blood in two forms. Much the greater part is in reversible chemical combination with haemoglobin, while a smaller part is in physical solution in plasma and intracellular fluid. The ability to carry large quantities of oxygen in the blood is of great importance to the organism, since without haemoglobin the amount carried would be so small that the cardiac output would need to be increased by a factor of about 20 to give an adequate oxygen flux. This would require a considerable increase in blood volume and, under such handicaps, animals could not have developed to their present extent. The biological significance of the haemoglobin-like compounds is thus immense and they may be compared with chlorophyll, which closely resembles haemoglobin although containing magnesium in place of iron.

Haemoglobin

The haemoglobin molecule has been the subject of many years of detailed X-ray crystallographic analysis by the team led by Perutz in Cambridge. We now know a great deal about its structure and can postulate a structural basis for some of its remarkable properties (Roughton, 1964; Lehmann and Huntsman, 1966; Perutz, 1969).

The haemoglobin molecule consists of four protein chains, each of which carries a haem group (*Figure 135*), the total molecular weight being 64 458·5 (Braunitzer, 1963). The amino acids comprising the chains have now been identified and it is known that, in the commonest type of adult human haemoglobin (Hb A), there are two types of chain, two of each occurring in each molecule. The two α chains each have 141 amino-acid residues, with the haem attached to a histidine* residue occupying position 87. The two β chains each have 146 amino-acid residues, with the haem attached to a histidine residue occupying position 92. *Figure 135b* shows details of the point of attachment of the haem in the α chain. Similar information for the β chain is given on page 340.

The four chains of the haemoglobin molecule lie in a ball like a crumpled necklace. However, the form is not random and the actual shape (the quaternary structure) is of critical importance and governs the reaction with oxygen. The shape is maintained by loose bonds between certain amino acids on different chains and also between some amino acids on the same chain. One consequence of these bonds is that the haem groups lie in crevices formed by weak bonds between the haem groups and histidine residues, other than those to which they are attached by normal valency linkages. For example, *Figure 135c* shows a section of an α chain with the haem group attached to the iron atom which is bound to the histidine residue in position 87. However, the haem group is also attached by a loose bond to the histidine residue in position 58 and also by non-polar bonds to many other amino acids. This forms a loop and places the haem group in a crevice which limits and controls the ease of access for oxygen molecules.

Structural basis of the Bohr effect

The precise shape of the haemoglobin molecule is altered by factors which influence the strength of the loose bonds and such factors include temperature, pH, ionic strength and carbon dioxide binding to the N-terminal amino acid residues as carbamate (Kilmartin and Rossi-Bernardi, 1973). This alters the accessibility of the haem groups to oxygen and is believed to be the basis of the mechanism by which the affinity of haemoglobin for oxygen is altered by these factors, an effect which is generally considered in terms of its influence upon the dissociation curve (*see Figure 138*).

Structural basis of the Haldane effect (page 338)

The quaternary structure of the haemoglobin molecule is altered by the uptake of oxygen to form oxyheamoglobin. It is believed that this increases the ionization of certain $-NH_2$ or $=NH$ groups and so reduces their ability to undertake carbamino carriage of carbon dioxide (*Figure 110*).

* Histidine is an amino acid with the following formula (*see* page 340).

$$
\begin{array}{c}
\text{H} \\
\text{C} \\
\diagup \diagdown \\
\text{N} \quad \text{NH} \\
| \quad | \\
\text{HC}=\text{C} \\
| \\
\text{CH}_2 \\
| \\
\text{NH}_2-\text{C}-\text{COOH} \\
| \\
\text{H}
\end{array}
$$

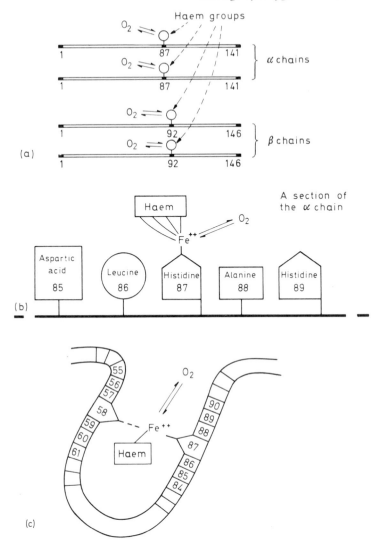

Figure 135. The haemoglobin molecule consists of four amino-acid chains, each carrying a haem group. (a) Two chains are identical, each with 141 amino-acid residues (α chains). The other two are also identical and have 146 amino-acid residues (β chains). (b) shows the attachment of the haem group to the α chain. (c) depicts the crevice which contains the haem group

Oxygen combining capacity of haemoglobin

There has been some confusion over the oxygen combining capacity of haemoglobin. Until recently the value was taken to be 1·34 ml/g. Following the determination of the molecular weight of haemoglobin, the theoretical value of 1·39 ml/g was derived and passed into general use. However, it gradually became clear that this value was not obtained when direct measurements of haemoglobin concentration and oxygen capacity were compared. After an exhaustive study of the subject, Gregory (1974) proposed the values of 1·306 ml/g for human adult blood and 1·312 ml/g for fetal blood. Haemoglobin concentrations are ultimately compared with the International Cyanmethaemoglobin Standard, which is based on iron content and not on oxygen combining capacity. Since some of the iron is likely to be in the form of haemochromagens, it is not altogether surprising that the observed oxygen combining capacity is less than the theoretical value of 1·39.

Abnormal forms of haemoglobin

There are a great number of abnormal forms of haemoglobin. Many changes in the molecule alter the reaction with oxygen, even though they concern a part of the amino-acid chain remote from the attachment of the haem group. Apart from the α and β chains already mentioned, γ and δ chains occur normally in combination with α chains. γ and δ chains have different amino-acid sequences. The combination of two γ chains with two α chains constitutes fetal haemoglobin (Hb F) and the combination of two δ chains with two α chains constitutes A_2 haemoglobin (Hb A_2) which forms 2 per cent of the total haemoglobin in normal adults. Other variations in the amino-acid chains can be considered abnormal, and many are associated with disordered oxygen carriage or impaired solubility.

Sickle cell anaemia is caused by the presence of Hb S in which valine replaces glutamic acid in position 6 on the two β chains. This apparently trivial substitution is sufficient to cause critical loss of solubility in the reduced state. It is a hereditary condition and in the homozygous state is a grave abnormality. The heterozygous form (sickle cell trait) is much less serious and there is no convincing evidence that it presents an increased hazard in anaesthesia (Gilbertson; Ball; and Watson-Williams, 1967).

Thalassaemia is another hereditary disorder of haemoglobin. It consists of a suppression of formation of Hb A with a compensatory production of fetal haemoglobin (Hb F) which persists throughout life instead of falling to low levels after birth. the functional disorder thus includes a shift of the dissociation curve to the left (*Figure 136*).

Abnormal ligands. The iron in haemoglobin is able to combine with other inorganic molecules apart from oxygen. The compounds so formed are, in general, more stable than oxyhaemoglobin and therefore block the combination of haemoglobin with oxygen. The most important of these abnormal compounds is carboxyhaemoglobin but ligands may also be formed with nitric oxide, cyanide, ammonia and a number of other substances. Apart from the loss of oxygen-carrying power, there is often a shift of the dissociation curve to the left (*see* later), so that the remaining oxygen is only released at lower tensions of oxygen. This may cause tissue hypoxia when the arterial P_{O_2} and oxygen content would otherwise appear to be at a safe level.

Methaemoglobin consists of haemoglobin in which the iron has assumed the trivalent ferric form. Methaemoglobin is unable to combine with oxygen but is slowly reconverted to haemoglobin in the normal subject by the action of enzymes which are deficient in familial methaemoglobinaemia (Lehmann and Huntsman, 1966). Alternatively, conversion may be brought about by reducing agents such as ascorbic acid or methylene blue. The nitrite ion is a potent cause of methaemoglobin formation and is a major factor in poisoning by higher oxides of nitrogen (see symposium in May 1967 issue of *British Journal of Anaesthesia*). Methaemoglobin and sulphaemoglobin are a brownish colour and produce a slate-grey colouring of the patient which may be confused with cyanosis.

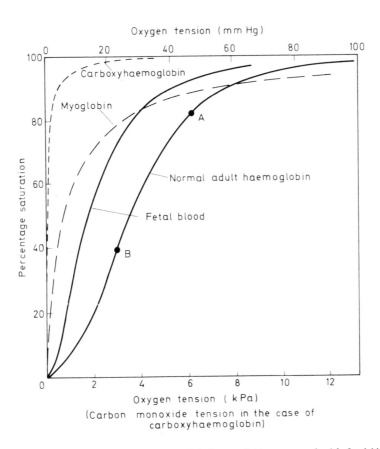

Figure 136. Dissociation curves of normal adult haemoglobin compared with fetal blood. Curves for myoglobin and carboxyhaemoglobin are shown for comparison. Note: (1) Fetal blood is adapted to operate at a lower PO_2 than adult blood. (2) Myoglobin approaches full saturation at PO_2 levels pertaining in voluntary muscle 2–4 kPa (15–30 mm Hg); the bulk of its oxygen can only be released at very low oxygen tension. (3) Carboxyhaemoglobin can only be dissociated by the maintenance of very low levels of PCO_2. After birth, fetal haemoglobin is progressively replaced with adult haemoglobin and the dissociation curve gradually moves across to the position of the adult curve. In a patient with a normal circulation and haemoglobin concentration, point A represents the greatest deterioration of arterial oxygenation which should pass untreated. Arterial blood corresponding to point B is at the threshold of loss of consciousness from hypoxia

Kinetics of the reaction of oxygen with haemoglobin

There is now ample experimental proof of Adair's intermediate compound hypothesis (1925) which proposed that the oxidation of haemoglobin proceeds in four separate stages. If the whole haemoglobin molecule, with its four haem groups, is designated as 'Hb$_4$', the reactions may be presented as follows:

$$Hb_4 + O_2 \underset{k_1}{\overset{k_1'}{\rightleftharpoons}} Hb_4O_2 \qquad K_1 = \frac{k_1'}{k_1}$$

$$Hb_4O_2 + O_2 \underset{k_2}{\overset{k_2'}{\rightleftharpoons}} Hb_4O_4 \qquad K_2 = \frac{k_2'}{k_2}$$

$$Hb_4O_4 + O_2 \underset{k_3}{\overset{k_3'}{\rightleftharpoons}} Hb_4O_6 \qquad K_3 = \frac{k_3'}{k_3}$$

$$Hb_4O_6 + O_2 \underset{k_4}{\overset{k_4'}{\rightleftharpoons}} Hb_4O_8 \qquad K_4 = \frac{k_4'}{k_4}$$

The velocity constant of each dissociation is indicated by a small k, while the addition of a prime ($'$) indicates the velocity constant of the corresponding forward reaction. k_3' is thus the velocity constant of the reaction of Hb_4O_4 with O_2 to yield Hb_4O_6. The ratio of the forward velocity constant to the reverse velocity constant equals the equilibrium constant of each reaction in the series (represented by capital K).

The separate velocity constants have been measured and it is now known that the last reaction has a forward velocity constant (k_4') which is much higher than that of the other reactions. During the saturation of the last 75 per cent of reduced haemoglobin, the last reaction will predominate and the high velocity counteracts the effect of the ever-diminishing number of oxygen-receptors which would otherwise slow the reaction rate by the law of mass action (Staub, Bishop and Forster, 1961). In fact, the reaction proceeds at much the same rate until saturation is completed. The significance of this to oxygen transfer in the lung has been presented by Staub (1963a), and its importance in the matter of 'diffusing capacity' is discussed on page 317.

The velocity of the dissociation of oxyhaemoglobin is somewhat slower than its formation. The velocity constant of the combination of carbon monoxide with haemoglobin is of the same order, but the rate of dissociation of carboxyhaemoglobin is extremely slow by comparison.

The oxyhaemoglobin dissociation curve

Under standard conditions, the relationship between Po_2 and percentage saturation of haemoglobin with oxygen is fixed but non-linear. The relationship is shown in graphical form for adult and fetal haemoglobin and also for myoglobin and carboxyheamoglobin in *Figure 136*. It is displayed as a line chart in *Figure 137*.

Displacement of the dissociation curve and the P_{50}.   Various factors displace the dissociation curve sideways, and the familiar effect of pH (the Bohr effect) is shown in *Figure 138*. Shifts may be defined as the ratio of the Po_2 which

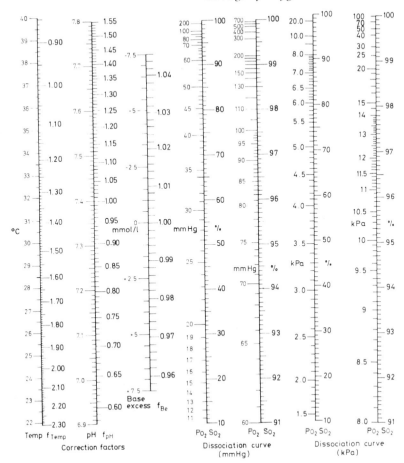

Figure 137. The standard oxyhaemoglobin dissociation curve with factors which displace it. The two right-hand line charts give corresponding values of PO₂ and saturation for standard conditions (temperature, 37° C; pH, 7·40; base excess, zero). The remaining lines indicate the factors by which the actual measured PO₂ should be multiplied before entering the standard dissociation curve to determine the saturation. When more than one factor is required, they should be multiplied together as in the example given in the text. (Reproduced from Kelman and Nunn (1966b) by courtesy of the Editor of the Journal of Applied Physiology, *modified in accord with data of Roughton and Severinghaus (1973) and with the addition of kPa scales)*

produces a particular saturation under standard conditions to the P_{O_2} which produces the same saturation under special conditions. Standard conditions include pH 7·400, temperature 37° C and zero base excess. In *Figure 138*, a saturation of 80 per cent is produced by P_{O_2} 6 kPa (45 mm Hg) at pH 7·4 (standard). At pH 7·0 the P_{O_2} required for 80 per cent saturation is 9·4 kPa (70·3 mm Hg). The ratio is 0·64 and this applies to all saturation at pH 7·0. The ratio is indicated on the line chart in *Figure 137*, which also shows the ratios (or correction factors) for different values of temperature and base excess.

Since the effects of temperature, pH and base excess are all similar, their influence on the dissociation curve may be considered simultaneously. The usual practice is to derive a factor for the influence of each and then to multiply them

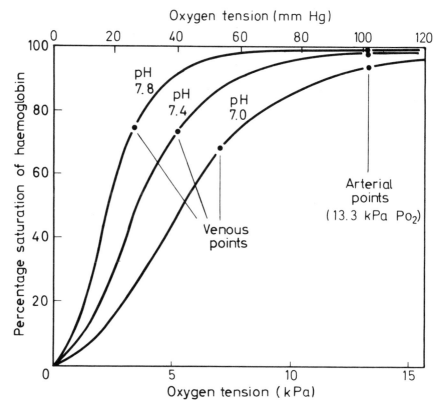

Figure 138. The Bohr effect and its effect upon oxygen tension. The centre curve is the normal curve under standard conditions; the other two curves show the displacement caused by the indicated changes in pH, other factors remaining constant. The venous points have been determined on the basis of a fixed arterial/venous oxygen saturation difference of 25 per cent in each case. They are thus 25 per cent saturation less than the corresponding arterial saturation which is equivalent to a PO₂ of 13·3 kPa (100 mm Hg) in each case. Under the conditions shown, alkalosis lowers venous PO₂ and acidosis raises venous PO₂. This effect is reversed in severe arterial hypoxaemia. Tissue PO₂ is related to venous PO₂. Temperature, 37° C; base excess, zero

together. This combined factor is then multiplied by the observed P_{O_2} to give the apparent P_{O_2} which may be entered into the standard dissociation curve to indicate the saturation. The factors may be determined from the line charts in *Figure 137*; its use is illustrated by the following example.

	Factor
Blood temperature 33·7 °C	1·20
Blood pH 7·08	0·70
Blood base excess — 7 mmol/l	1·04

Combined factor = 1·20 × 0·70 × 1·02 = 0·87
Observed P_{O_2} = 9·3 kPa (70 mm Hg);
    apparent P_{O_2} = observed P_{O_2} × 0·86 = 8·1 kPa (61 mm Hg)
Calculated saturation (from line chart) = 91·3 per cent

This calculation may be expeditiously performed on the slide rule described by Severinghaus (1966). The factors are also incorporated in the digital computer subroutine described by Kelman (1966a) and feature in the tables produced by Kelman and Nunn (1968).

An alternative approach to quantifying a shift of the dissociation curve is to indicate the P_{O_2} required for 50 per cent saturation. This is known as the P_{50} and, under the standard conditions shown in *Figure 137*, is 3·5 kPa (26·5 mm Hg).

Clinical significance of the Bohr effect. There is a good deal of confusion about the clinical significance of the Bohr effect. It is generally appreciated that a shift to the right (caused by low pH) impairs oxygenation in the lungs but aids release of oxygen in the tissue. However, there is often a failure to appreciate the over-all significance of these two effects in combination. It is essential to think in quantitative terms and an illustrative example is set out in *Figure 138*. The arterial P_{O_2} is assumed to be 13·3 kPa (100 mm Hg) and arterial saturation is clearly decreased by a reduction of pH. However, the effect is small except when the arterial P_{O_2} is very low (less than about 8 kPa or 60 mm Hg) or when the pH falls to extremely low values at normal P_{O_2} (Prys-Roberts, Smith and Nunn, 1967).

At the venous point the position is quite different, and the examples in *Figure 138* show the venous oxygen tensions to be very markedly affected. Assuming that the arterial/venous oxygen saturation difference is constant at 25 per cent it will be seen that at low pH the venous P_{O_2} is raised to 6·9 kPa (52 mm Hg), while at high pH the venous P_{O_2} is reduced to 3·5 kPa (26 mm Hg). This is important as the tissue P_{O_2} is influenced directly by the venous P_{O_2}. Over a wide range of conditions it will be found that a shift of the curve to the right will always raise the venous P_{O_2} provided other factors remain constant. In fact other factors are unlikely to remain constant, and both cerebral blood flow and cardiac output are likely to be increased by a moderate respiratory acidosis which would further tend to raise the venous and tissue P_{O_2}. Thus, far from being universally harmful as is so often assumed, there seems no doubt that respiratory acidosis raises tissue P_{O_2}, particularly in the brain. Of course, this is not the whole story and it would be equally wrong to believe that respiratory acidosis is universally beneficial. Considerable judgement and a good deal more research are necessary to indicate in what circumstances the condition of a patient may be improved by shifting the curve to the right as, for example, by the deliberate induction of an acidosis or the avoidance of an alkalosis.

Factors which shift the dissociation curve. It is well known that the curve is shifted to the right (P_{50} raised) by an increase of hydrogen ion concentration, P_{CO_2}, temperature, ionic strength or haemoglobin concentration. Certain abnormal haemoglobins (such as San Diego and Chesapeake) have a high P_{50} while others (such as sickle and Kansas) have a low P_{50}.

In 1967 it was found independently by Benesch and Benesch and by Chanutin and Curnish that the presence of certain organic phosphates in the erythrocyte has a pronounced effect on the P_{50}. The most important of these compounds is 2,3-diphosphoglycerate (2,3-DPG), one molecule of which is able to bind preferentially to the β chains of one tetramer of deoxyhaemoglobin, resulting in a conformational change which reduces oxygen affinity (Arnone,

1972). The percentage occupancy of the 2,3-DPG-binding sites governs the over-all P_{50} of a blood sample within the range 2–4·5 kPa (15–34 mm Hg).

2,3-DPG is formed in the Rapoport–Luebering shunt off the glycolytic pathway (*see Figure 126*) and its level is determined by the balance between synthesis and degradation (*Figure 139*).

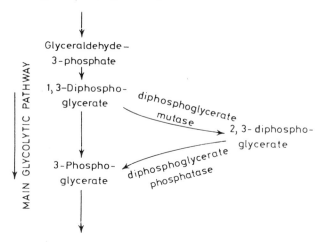

Figure 139. Rapoport–Luebering shunt for synthesis of 2,3-diphosphoglycerate

Activity of the DPG mutase is enhanced and the DPG phosphatase diminished at high pH, which thus increases the level of 2,3-DPG.

The relationship between 2,3-DPG levels and P_{50} suggested that 2,3-DPG levels would have a most important bearing on clinical practice and therefore much research effort was devoted to determining those conditions which might result in substantial changes in 2,3-DPG levels.

Storage of bank blood with acid-citrate-dextrose (ACD) preservative results in depletion of all 2,3-DPG within the usual period of three weeks' storage, P_{50} being reduced to about 2 kPa (15 mm Hg) (McConn and Derrick, 1972). A massive transfusion of old blood shifts the patient's dissociation curve to the left but restoration is usually well advanced within a few hours (see review by Valeri, 1975). Changes in P_{50} of a patient do not usually exceed 0·5 kPa (3·8 mm Hg). Storage in citrate-phosphate-dextrose (CDP) substantially reduces the rate of 2,3-DPG depletion (Shafer et al., 1971).

Anaemia results in a raised 2,3-DPG level with P_{50} of the order of 0·5 kPa (3·7 mm Hg) higher than control levels (Torrance et al., 1970). This must raise the partial pressure of oxygen delivery to the tissues, and supplements the effect of increased tissue perfusion.

Altitude is reported to cause a 2,3-DPG-mediated shift to the right (Lenfant et al., 1968) with an increase in P_{50} of the order of 0·5 kPa (3·8 mm Hg). This has not been confirmed by Weiskopf and Severinghaus (1972) and it should also be noted that, at an altitude of 4000 metres, the arterial P_{CO_2} is of the order of 7 kPa (52·5 mm Hg), below which a rightward shift of the dissociation curve is not advantageous since oxygenation in the lung is impaired to a degree which is not outweighed by improved off-loading in the tissues.

Ventilatory failure does not appear to cause any significant change in either 2,3-DPG levels or the P_{50}. Fairweather, Walker and Flenley (1974) and Flenley et al. (1975) studied a total of 71 patients with arterial PCO_2 ranging from 6·7 to 10·7 kPa (50 to 80 mm Hg) and PO_2 4·3–8·7 kPa (32–65 mm Hg). P_{50} values (at pH 7·4) ranged from 3–4 kPa (22·5–30 mm Hg) and did not appear to differ from the normal value by more than the experimental error of determination. 2,3-DPG levels were widely scattered about the normal value.

Haemorrhagic and endotoxic shock do not appear to be associated with any significant changes of 2,3-DPG or 2,3-DPG-mediated changes in P_{50} (Naylor et al., 1972).

In general it may be said that subsequent research has failed to substantiate the earlier suggestions that 2,3-DPG was of fundamental importance in clinical problems of oxygen delivery. In fact, the likely effects of changes in P_{50} mediated by 2,3-DPG seem to be of marginal significance in comparison with changes in arterial PO_2 and tissue perfusion. Similarly, there has been little application of the suggestions that drug-induced shifts of the dissociation curve would have a major therapeutic role. A valuable review of the subject has been presented by Shappell and Lenfant (1972).

Effect of anaesthetics. It has long been known that anaesthetics bind to haemoglobin and this accounts for a substantial part of their carriage in blood (Featherstone et al, 1961). More recently, Barker et al. (1975) have identified specific changes in the nuclear magnetic resonance spectrum for haemoglobin in equilibrium with halothane, methoxyflurane and diethyl ether, suggesting different binding sites for each agent. It was clearly a possibility that hydrophobic binding of anaesthetics to haemoglobin might result in a conformational change which would alter the P_{50}, and certain preliminary reports suggested this possibility. However, a series of carefully controlled studies have now established that even with high concentrations of methoxy-flurane, halothane and cyclopropane, there is no measurable change in P_{50} (Cohen and Behar, 1970; Millar, Beard and Hulands, 1971; Weiskopf, Nishimura and Severinghaus, 1971).

Physical solution of oxygen in blood

In addition to combination with haemoglobin, oxygen is carried in physical solution in both erythrocytes and plasma. The total amount carried in normal blood in solution at 37°C is about 0·0225 ml/100 ml per kPa or 0·003/100 ml per mm Hg. At normal arterial PO_2, the oxygen in physical solution is thus about 0·25 ml/100 ml or rather more than 1 per cent of the total oxygen carried in all forms. However, when breathing 100 per cent oxygen, the level rises to about 2 ml/100 ml. Breathing 100 per cent oxygen at 3 atmospheres pressure absolute (303 kPa), the amount of oxygen in physical solution rises to about 6 ml/100 ml, which is sufficient for the arteriovenous extraction. The amount of oxygen in physical solution rises with decreasing temperature for the same PO_2.

Carbon monoxide in combination with haemoglobin

Carbon monoxide is well known to displace oxygen from combination with haemoglobin, the affinity being approximately 300 times greater than the affinity for oxygen. The presence of carboxyhaemoglobin also causes a leftward shift of the dissociation curve of the remaining oxyhaemoglobin (Roughton and Darling, 1944), partly mediated by a reduction in 2,3-DPG levels. This is conveniently shown on a plot of oxygen content against P_{O_2} (*Figure 140*), the values on the ordinate being the sum of dissolved and combined oxygen. The upper curve is for the normal concentration of haemoglobin without carbon monoxide. The lowest of the three curves applies to a patient with haemoglobin at half the normal concentration. At each P_{O_2}, the oxygen concentration is approximately half that of the patient with a normal concentration of

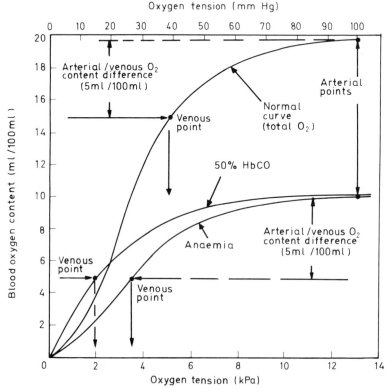

Figure 140. Influences of anaemia and carbon monoxide poisoning on the relationship between oxygen tension and content. The normal curve is constructed for a haemoglobin concentration of 14·4g/100 ml. Assuming an arterial/venous oxygen content difference of 5 ml/100 ml, the venous P_{O_2} is about 5·3 kPa (40 mm Hg). The curve of anaemic blood is constructed for a haemoglobin concentration of 7·2 g/100 ml. If the arterial/venous oxygen content difference remains unchanged, the venous P_{O_2} will fall to 3·6 kPa (27 mm Hg), a level which is low but not dangerously so. The curve of 50 per cent carboxyhaemoglobin is based on a total haemoglobin (incl. carboxyhaemoglobin) of 14·4 g/100 ml. The curve is interpolated from Roughton (1964). Assuming an arterial/venous oxygen content difference of 5 ml/100 ml, the venous P_{O_2} is only 1·9 kPa (14 mm Hg), a level which is dangerously low as it must be associated with a greatly reduced tissue P_{O_2}. Arterial P_{O_2} is assumed to be 13·3 kPa (100 mm Hg) in all cases

haemoglobin. The intermediate curve applies to blood with normal haemoglobin concentration but with half of the haemoglobin bound to carbon monoxide, resulting in a displacement of the dissociation curve of the remaining haemoglobin. It will be seen that, in comparison with the anaemic blood, this displacement has little effect on the oxygen content of the arterial blood provided that it is in excess of about 8 kPa (60 mm Hg). However, the effect on the venous Po_2, after unloading of oxygen in the tissues, is very great. Assuming an arterial Po_2 of 13·3 kPa (100 mm Hg) and an arterial venous oxygen content difference of 5 ml/100 ml, the venous points are as follows:

Normal haemoglobin concentration	5·3 kPa (40 mm Hg)
Half normal haemoglobin concentration	3·6 kPa (27 mm Hg)
50 per cent carboxyhaemoglobin	1·9 kPa (14 mm Hg)

The disappearance of coal gas for domestic use in many countries has decreased the popularity of carbon monoxide for attempted suicide. However, carbon monoxide is still to be found in the blood of patients, in trace concentrations as a result of its production in the body but mainly as a result of the internal combustion engine and smoking. Jones, Commins and Cernik (1972) reported levels of 0·4–9·7 per cent in London taxi drivers but the highest level in a non-smoking driver was 3·0 per cent. Levels up to 10 per cent of carboxyhaemoglobin were also found in smokers by Castleden and Cole (1974). Maternal smoking results in appreciable levels of carboxyhaemoglobin in fetal blood (Longo, 1970), and smoking prior to blood donation may result in levels of carboxyhaemoglobin up to 10 per cent in the blood. This level appears to persist throughout the usual three weeks of storage (Millar and Gregory, 1972).

THE 'NORMAL' ARTERIAL OXYGEN TENSION

In contrast to the arterial Pco_2, the arterial Po_2 shows a progressive decline with age. Marshall and Whyche (1972) have analysed 12 studies of healthy subjects and from the pooled results have suggested the following relationship in subjects breathing air:

$$\text{mean arterial } Po_2 = 13·6 \quad - 0·044 \text{ (age in years)} \qquad kPa$$
$$\text{or } 102 - 0·33 \text{ (age of years)} \qquad mm\ Hg$$

About this regression line there are 95 per cent confidence limits (2 s.d.) of ±1·33 kPa (10 mm Hg) (*Table 31*). Five per cent of normal patients will lie outside these limits and it is therefore preferable to refer to this as the reference range rather than the normal range.

It seems likely that some of the scatter of values for Po_2 is due to transient changes in ventilation, perhaps associated with arterial puncture. Because of the

Table 31

Age (years)	Arterial Po_2	
	mean and range (kPa)	*mean and range (mm Hg)*
20–29	12·5 (11·2–13·9)	94 (84–104)
30–39	12·1 (10·8–13·5)	91 (81–101)
40–49	11·7 (10·4–13·1)	88 (78–98)
50–59	11·2 (9·9–12·5)	84 (74–94)
60–69	10·8 (9·5–12·1)	81 (71–91)

ARP—14*

small body oxygen stores, such changes have a greater effect on PO_2 than on PCO_2.

When breathing oxygen the most important factor causing scatter of values for arterial PO_2 is failure to exclude air from the breathing system. Provided that great care is taken to prevent dilution with air, very high values of arterial PO_2 may be obtained. A number of studies of normal conscious subjects have been reviewed by Raine and Bishop (1963) and by Laver and Seifen (1965). Mean values for arterial PO_2 in these studies range from 80 to 86·7 kPa (600 to 650 mm Hg), but individual values range from 73·3 kPa (550 mm Hg) to values which are (no doubt erroneously) in excess of the alveolar PO_2.

Reports of 'abnormalities' of oxygenation must be interpreted against the high degree of scatter in normal subjects under normal conditions.

OXYGEN STORES AND THE STEADY STATE

It is a fact of the utmost importance that the body oxygen stores are meagre and, if replenishment ceases, are normally insufficient to sustain life for more than a few minutes. The principal stores are shown in *Table 32*.

Table 32

	While breathing air		While breathing 100% oxygen
In the lungs (FRC)		450 ml	3 000 ml
In the blood		850 ml	950 ml
Dissolved in tissue fluids		50 ml	? 100 ml
In combination with myoglobin	?	200 ml	? 200 ml
Total		1 550 ml	4 250 ml

While breathing air the total oxygen stores are small. To make matters worse, very little of this small store of oxygen can be released without an unacceptable reduction in PO_2. Reference to the dissociation curves in *Figure 136* shows that blood will not release substantial quantities of oxygen until the PO_2 falls below 5·3 kPa (40 mm Hg). Myoglobin is even more reluctant to part with its oxygen and very little can be released above a PO_2 2·7 kPa (20 mm Hg).

Breathing oxygen causes a substantial increase in total oxygen stores. Most of the additional oxygen is accommodated in the alveolar gas where 80 per cent of it may be withdrawn without causing the PO_2 to fall below the normal value. With 2400 ml of easily available oxygen, there is no difficulty in breath holding, after breathing oxygen for as long as eight minutes without becoming hypoxic.

The small size of the oxygen stores means that changes in factors affecting the alveolar or arterial PO_2 will produce their full effects very quickly after the change. This is in contrast to carbon dioxide where the size of the stores buffers the body against rapid changes. *Figure 141* shows the time course of changes in

PO_2 produced by the same changes in ventilation. *Figure 120* showed how the time course of changes of PCO_2 was different for falling and rising PCO_2.

Factors which reduce the PO_2 always act rapidly, but the following is the order of rapidity of changes which produce anoxia.

1. *Circulatory arrest.* When the circulation is arrested, hypoxia supervenes as soon as the oxygen in the tissues and stagnant capillaries has been exhausted. In the case of the brain, with its high rate of oxygen consumption, there is a mere 10 seconds before consciousness is lost. If the eyeball is compressed to occlude its vessels, vision commences to be lost at the periphery within about six seconds (a convincing experiment which was suggested by Rahn, 1964). Circulatory arrest also differs from other forms of hypoxia in the failure of clearance of products of anaerobic metabolism (e.g. lactic acid) which, with the exception of the brain, is not a factor in simple arterial hypoxaemia.

2. *Exposure to a barometric pressure of less than 6·3 kPa (47 mm Hg).* At a pressure of less than 6·3 kPa (47 mm Hg), body fluids boil and alveolar gas is replaced with 100 per cent steam. The PO_2 rapidly falls to zero and consciousness is lost within one circulation time, which is of the order of 15 seconds (Ernsting and McHardy, 1960).

3. *Inhalation of nitrogen.* Washing out the alveolar oxygen by hyperventilation with nitrogen results in a very rapid fall of arterial PO_2, which reached 4 kPa (30 mm Hg) in 30 seconds in a series of dogs (Cater et al., 1963). Even more rapid changes were obtained in human volunteers by Ernsting (1963).

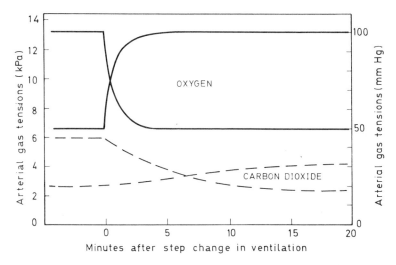

Figure 141. The upper pair of curves indicates the rate of change of arterial PO_2 following step changes in ventilation. Half of the total change occurs in about 30 seconds. The rising curve could be produced by an increase of alveolar ventilation from 2 to 4 l/min while breathing air (see Figure 129). The falling curve could result from the corresponding reduction of alveolar ventilation from 4 to 2 l/min. The lower pair of curves indicates the time course of changes in PCO_2 which are very much slower than for oxygen. These changes are shown in greater detail in Figure 120

4. *Inhalation of nitrous oxide.* Alveolar wash-out with a soluble gas such as nitrous oxide would be expected to cause a slower fall of Po_2 because of the loss of the flushing gas into the tissues. This is, however, difficult to demonstrate as many variables are hard to control. Heller and Watson (1962) showed a precipitous descent of arterial Po_2 in one patient breathing 100 per cent nitrous oxide. A level of $3 \cdot 2$ kPa (24 mm Hg) was reached after 30 seconds.

5. *Apnoea.* The rate of onset of anoxia is dependent upon the initial alveolar Po_2 and the rate of oxygen consumption. It is, for example, more rapid while swimming underwater than while breath holding in the laboratory. Generally speaking, after breathing air, 90 seconds of apnoea results in a substantial fall of Po_2 to a level which threatens the subject with loss of consciousness. If a patient has previously inhaled oxygen, the arterial Po_2 should remain above $13 \cdot 3$ kPa (100 mm Hg) for at least three minutes of apnoea (Heller and Watson, 1961), and this is the basis of the usual method of protection against hypoxia during the interference with ventilation which accompanies tracheal intubation. (If the patient is pre-oxygenated and then connected to a supply of oxygen while apnoeic, the arterial Po_2 is well maintained for a long time by the process of 'apnoeic mass-movement oxygenation'—*see* page 358.)

Since a steady state for oxygen is very rapidly attained, it follows that oxygen uptake is seldom appreciably different from oxygen consumption. Therefore, measurement of oxygen uptake usually gives a satisfactory estimate of the oxygen consumption. In contrast, measured values of carbon dioxide output may be very different from the simultaneous level of carbon dioxide production if the ventilation is unsteady. During the irregular breathing of anaesthesia with spontaneous respiration, values for carbon dioxide output may range widely, while values for oxygen consumption are reasonably steady (Nunn and Matthews, 1959; Nunn, 1964).

For a fuller discussion of oxygen stores, the reader is referred to Farhi and Rahn (1955a), Farhi (1964), Rahn (1964) and Cherniack and Longobardo (1970).

HYPOXIA

Biochemical changes in hypoxia

The essential feature of hypoxia is the cessation of oxidative phosphorylation when the mitochondrial Po_2 falls below the critical level. Anaerobic pathways, in particular the glycolytic pathway (*see Figure 126*), then come into play. Glycosis is switched on under hypoxic conditions by the accumulation of ADP which acts on rate-limiting steps in the metabolic pathway (see review by Cohen, 1972).

Anaerobic metabolism cannot produce the yield of ATP which is possible during aerobic metabolism and, therefore, during hypoxia the ATP/ADP ratio of the brain falls and there is a decline in the level of high energy compounds, including phosphocreatine (*Figure 142*). The changes are very rapid in an organ with a high metabolic rate and, in the rat brain, respiratory arrest results in a precipitous fall of all high energy compounds within a few minutes. Very similar changes occur in response to arterial hypotension (Kaasick, Nilsson and Siesjö, 1970b). These changes will rapidly block cerebral function but organs with a lower energy requirement will continue to function for a longer time. Relative resistance to hypoxia is discussed below in relation to survival times.

The end-products of aerobic metabolism are carbon dioxide and water, both of which are easily diffusible and lost from the body. The main anaerobic pathway produces hydrogen and lactate ions which are retained within the brain since the blood-brain barrier is relatively impermeable to charged ions. In the rest of the body hydrogen and lactate ions escape into the circulation where they may be conveniently quantified in terms of the base deficit and the lactate/pyruvate ratio.

In severe cerebral hypoxia, it seems likely that the intracellular acidosis is more harmful than the depletion of high energy compounds. In particular, pH falls below the optimum for certain enzymes and the acidosis may be the main cause of the development of post-anoxic cerebral oedema. When anoxia follows

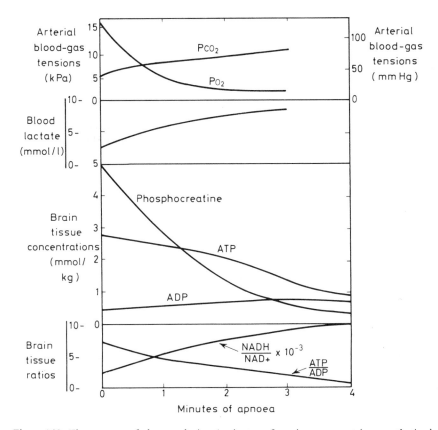

Figure 142. Time course of changes during 4 minutes of respiratory arrest in anaesthetized and curarized rats previously breathing 30 per cent oxygen. Recovery of all values, except blood lactate, was complete within 5 minutes of restarting pulmonary ventilation after 3 minutes' apnoea. Effects of sustained levels of hypoxaemia have been reported by Siesjö and Nilsson (1971). (Drawn from the data of Kaasik, Nilsson and Siesjö, 1970a)

chronic hypoxia, there is, surprisingly, less evidence of cell damage than in acute anoxia. It is thought that this is due to the reduction in lactic acid formation, owing to glucose depletion during the period of chronic hypoxaemia (Lindenberg, 1963; Geddes, 1967). A comparison of available energy (page 376) shows that a nineteenfold increase in glucose consumption is required during anoxia. This quantity of glucose is beyond the capacity of the transport mechanism of the neurones which therefore suffer both energy depletion and reduction of intracellular glucose concentration during anoxia.

Quantification of cerebral hypoxia presents considerable difficulty since the usual indicators (hydrogen and lactate ions) are not released into the jugular venous blood. It is possible to detect rapid changes of CSF pH and lactate during arterial hypotension (Kaasik, Nilsson and Siesjö, 1970a) since the CSF is on the same side of the blood-brain barrier as the neurones. However, an index of hypoxia available from the jugular venous blood is more elusive. Venous P_{O_2} is perhaps the best of the simple measurements. Arterial/venous differences offer further possibilities but, again, lactate and base deficit are not helpful. A more sophisticated measurement is the ratio of arterial/venous differences of oxygen and glucose. With full aerobic metabolism the theoretical ratio is 6 : 1 (moles). A decrease indicates anaerobic consumption of glucose (usually in increased quantity) and the validity of this index is not affected by the blood-brain barrier.

P_{O_2} *levels and hypoxia*

Cellular P_{O_2} is the starting point for quantitative consideration of hypoxia. Oxidative phosphorylation to form ATP occurs in the mitochondria and will continue down to a P_{O_2} of about 0·13 kPa, or 1 mm Hg (page 380). P_{O_2} gradients within the cell are considered on page 399, and there is reason to believe that neurones will no longer function when the P_{O_2} at their surface is reduced below about 2·7 kPa (20 mm Hg). P_{O_2} varies from one cell to another and is also different in different parts of the same cell. There are therefore insuperable difficulties in defining or measuring 'the tissue P_{O_2}'.

Venous P_{O_2} is a more feasible measurement than cellular P_{O_2}, and the venous P_{O_2} approximates to the mean P_{O_2} at the surface of the cells in the region drained by the venous blood.* Some cells close to the arterial end of the capillaries will have a higher P_{O_2} while others lying between the venous end of two or more capillaries will have a lower P_{O_2} (*Figure 109*). Nevertheless, the venous P_{O_2} is a useful practicable measure of the state of oxygenation of an organ, and conciousness is lost when the internal jugular venous P_{O_2} falls below about 2·7 kPa, or 20 mm Hg (McDowell, personal communication).

Lowest tolerable level of arterial P_{O_2}. It is now interesting to extend this argument and consider in what circumstances the venous P_{O_2} may fall below the

---

* The significance of the venous P_{O_2} is lost when there are shunts which permit arterial blood to mix with blood draining the tissue. However, significant shunts do not occur in the organs which are most vulnerable to hypoxia.

critical level of 2·7 kPa (20 mm Hg), which in normal blood corresponds to 32 per cent saturation and about 6·4 ml/100 ml oxygen content. If the brain has an oxygen consumption of 46 ml/min and a blood flow of 620 ml/min, it follows that the arterial/venous oxygen content difference is about 7·4 ml/100 ml. We may then say that, *under these conditions and so far as the brain is concerned,* an arterial oxygen content of 13·8 ml/100 ml is the minimum which will avoid cerebral hypoxia. It is a simple matter to show that with normal haemoglobin concentration, pH, etc., this would correspond to a saturation of 68 per cent and an arterial P_{O_2} of 4·8 kPa (36 mm Hg). This calculation and others under various different conditions are set out in *Table 33.*

The calculation which has just been made leads to the conclusion that an arterial P_{O_2} of less than 4·8 kPa (36 mm Hg) would result in cerebral hypoxia, *if all other factors remained normal.* The major difficulties arise from the last clause. Other factors may not be normal but may be unfavourable as a result of multiple disability in the patient (e.g. anaemia combined with a low cerebral blood flow). Alternatively, other factors may be favourably influenced by the powerful homeostatic mechanisms which exist to protect the brain from hypoxia. These include the polycythaemia of chronic arterial hypoxaemia, increased cerebral blood flow in anaemia and the vasopressor response to cerebral hypoxia. Cerebral vascular resistance is diminished by reduced arterial blood pressure and arterial hypoxaemia. Cerebral oxygen requirements are reduced by hypothermia or anaesthesia (*see Table 27*). Myocardial oxygen consumption is reduced by deep anaesthesia (Theye, 1972).

The possible combinations of conditions are so great that it is not feasible to discuss every possible situation. Instead, certain important examples have been selected which illustrate the fundamentals of the problem, and these have been set out in *Table 33.* Further consideration of *arterial hypoxaemia* shows that a twofold increase of cerebral blood flow would permit a further fall of arterial P_{O_2} from 4·8 to 3·6 kPa (36 to 27 mm Hg) before the cerebral venous P_{O_2} reached 2·7 kPa (20 mm Hg). This is important as an increase in cerebral blood flow may be expected to follow severe hypoxia. Polycythaemia (haemoglobin concentration of about 18 g/100 ml) does not confer the same degree of benefit and the lower limit of arterial P_{O_2} would then be 4·3 kPa (32 mm Hg). Alkalosis, which may be expected to result from the hypoxic drive to respiration, confers no advantage at all. Considerable advantage derives from hypothermia but this is all due to the reduction in cerebral metabolism, and not at all to the shift of the dissociation curve.

Uncompensated *ischaemia* is seen to be dangerous, and a 45 per cent reduction in cerebral blood flow means that the arterial P_{O_2} cannot fall below the normal value without exposing the brain to risk of hypoxia. Uncompensated *anaemia* is almost equally dangerous, although an increase in cerebral blood flow restores a satisfactory safety margin. In the example in *Table 33*, a 40 per cent reduction of blood oxygen capacity and a 40 per cent increase of cerebral blood flow permits the arterial P_{O_2} to fall to 5·3 kPa (40 mm Hg) without the cerebral venous P_{O_2} falling below 2·7 kPa (20 mm Hg), a situation which is close to that which applies in uncomplicated arterial hypoxaemia. The last line in *Table 33* shows the very dangerous combination of anaemia and ischaemia. In this example the haemoglobin concentration is reduced to about 11 g/100 ml and the cerebral blood flow to three-quarters of the normal value. Neither abnormality is very serious considered separately, but in combination the arterial

Table 33 LOWEST ARTERIAL OXYGEN LEVELS COMPATIBLE WITH A CEREBRAL VENOUS PO$_2$ OF 2·7 kPa (20 mm Hg) UNDER VARIOUS CONDITIONS

	Blood O$_2$ capacity (ml/100 ml)	Brain O$_2$ consump. (ml/min)	Cerebral blood flow (ml/min)	Cerebral venous blood				A.-v. O$_2$ content difference (ml/100 ml)	Arterial blood			
				PO$_2$ (kPa)	PO$_2$ (mm Hg)	Sat. (%)	O$_2$ content (ml/100 ml)		O$_2$ content (ml/100 ml)	Sat. (%)	PO$_2$ (kPa)	PO$_2$ (mm Hg)
Normal values	20	46	620	4·4	33	63	12·6	7·4	20·0	97·5	13·3	100
Uncompensated arterial hypoxaemia	20	46	620	2·7	20	32	6·4	7·4	13·8	68	4·8	36
Arterial hypoxaemia with increased cer. blood flow	20	46	1 240	2·7	20	32	6·4	3·7	10·1	50	3·6	27
Arterial hypoxaemia with polycythaemia	25	46	620	2·7	20	32	8·0	7·4	15·4	61	4·3	32
Arterial hypoxaemia with alkalosis*	20	46	620	2·7	20	46	9·2	7·4	16·6	82	4·9	37
Arterial hypoxaemia with hypothermia†	20	23	620	2·7	20	57	11·4	3·7	15·1	75	3·6	27
Uncompensated cerebral ischaemia	20	46	340	2·7	20	32	6·4	13·5	19·9	98	14·9	112
Uncompensated anaemia	12	46	620	2·7	20	32	3·8	7·4	11·2	93	8·9	67
Anaemia with increased cer. blood flow	12	46	870	2·7	20	32	3·8	5·3	9·1	75	5·3	40
Combined anaemia and ischae·.ia	15	46	460	2·7	20	32	4·8	10·0	18·8	97	12·3	92

* pH 7·6   † temp. 30°C; cerebral O$_2$ consumption reduced to half normal

Po$_2$ cannot be reduced below 12·3 kPa (92 mm Hg) without the cerebral venous Po$_2$ falling below 2·7 kPa (20 mm Hg).

This Table must not be taken too literally. There are many minor factors which have not been considered and it appears that maximal cerebral vasodilatation may be expected to occur in any condition which threatens cerebral oxygenation. We must also bear in mind that there may be circumstances in which the critical organ is not the brain but the heart, liver or kidney. However the message of *Table 33* is that there is no simple answer to the question 'What is the safe lower limit of arterial Po$_2$?'. We may say that, in an otherwise normal patient who is able to respond with cerebral vasodilatation, the lowest tolerable arterial Po$_2$ would appear to be about 3·6 kPa (27 mm Hg). This figure accords with the fact than men have remained conscious while breathing air on the summit of Everest where the alveolar Po$_2$ may be calculated to be about 3·7 kPa (28 mm Hg) with the arterial Po$_2$ only a little lower. Patients presenting with severe respiratory disease who are still conscious while breathing air tend to have a lower limit of arterial Po$_2$ of about 2·7 kPa (20 mm Hg) (Refsum, 1963; McNicol and Campbell, 1965). Such patients would have compensatory polycythaemia and maximal cerebral vasodilatation.

Questions of fitness for surgery and anaesthesia in the presence of disorders of factors influencing oxygen flux cannot be decided in isolation but must be answered after considering the patient as a whole, and in the light of the additional disturbances which may be expected to result from operation and anaesthesia.

Compensatory mechanisms in hypoxia

Hypoxia presents a serious threat to the body and vigorous compensatory mechanisms come into play. These mechanisms are usually robust and not easily impaired by drugs or disease. Where they conflict with other mechanisms acting in the opposite direction, the compensation for hypoxia is usually dominant. Thus, for example, in hypoxia with concomitant hypocapnia, hyperventilation and increase of cerebral blood flow occur in spite of the lowered Pco$_2$ (Turner et al., 1957). Certain compensatory mechanisms will come into play whatever the reason for the hypoxia, although their effectiveness will depend to a large extent upon its actual cause. For example hyperventilation will be largely ineffective in stagnant hypoxia since hyperventilation while breathing air can do little to increase the oxygen content of the arterial blood, and usually nothing to increase perfusion.

Hyperventilation results from a fall of arterial Po$_2$ but the response is non-linear (page 44). Moderate falls of arterial Po$_2$ below the normal level have little effect, but falls below 6·7 kPa (50 mm Hg) cause a marked increase which becomes maximal at about 3·3 kPa (25 mm Hg). The interrelationship between hypoxia and other factors in the control of breathing is discussed in Chapter 2.

Pulmonary distribution of blood flow is improved by hypoxia as a result of the increase in pulmonary artery pressure (page 254).

Cardiac output is increased by hypoxia together with the regional blood flow to almost every major organ, particularly the brain (Cohen et al., 1967).

Haemoglobin concentration is not increased by acute hypoxia in man, although it is elevated by chronic hypoxia due to residence at altitude, chronic respiratory disease, etc.

Dissociation curve may be displaced to the right by an increase in 2,3-diphosphoglycerate or as a result of acidosis (page 408). This tends to raise tissue P_{O_2} (*see Figure 138*).

Autonomic system is concerned in many of the responses to hypoxia. The immediate response to cardiac output is reflex and is initiated by the chemoreceptors: it occurs before there has been any measurable rise in circulating catecholamines. The reduction of cerebral and probably the myocardial vascular resistance is not dependent upon circulating catecholamines or on autonomic innervation. The effect appears to be due to a local response within the vessels themselves. Nevertheless, catecholamine levels are raised in due course.

Anaerobic metabolism is increased in severe hypoxia in an attempt to maintain the production of ATP. This may be detected by an increase in arterial/venous excess lactate difference. Attempts have been made to use this as an index of hypoxia but results have been disappointing (Price et al., 1966). In the case of the brain, lactate may be retained within the neurones, causing a delay in the rise of the venous lactate level.

Organ survival times

Lack of oxygen stops the machine and, if prolonged, wrecks the machinery. The time of circulatory arrest up to the first event (survival time) must be distinguished from the duration of anoxia which results in the second event (the revival time), the latter being defined as the time beyond which no recovery of function is possible. Anoxia lasting more than the survival time but less than the revival time may result in prolonged impairment of function during recovery (Graham, 1961).

Survival times depend upon many factors. There is a pronounced difference between different organs, ranging from less than a minute for the cerebral cortex to about two hours for skeletal muscle. Heart is intermediate with a survival time of about five minutes, liver and kidney probably being about ten minutes. Revival times tend to be about four times as long as survival times but the ratio is greater in the case of the brain which has a revival time of the order of five minutes.

Apart from the inherent differences in sensitivity of organs, survival time is influenced by oxygen consumption and oxygen stores in the tissue. An inactive organ (such as a heart in asystole or an anaesthetized brain) has increased resistance to hypoxia (Wilhjelm, 1966) and there is a small but definite increase in survival time after hyperbaric oxygenation. Hypothermia decreases oxygen demand and increases oxygen storage in physical solution. Both factors, particularly the former, increase resistance to hypoxia.

Survival of an organ after anoxia depends on many secondary factors which influence oxygen transport during the recovery phase. If the heart has been severely affected in generalized hypoxaemia, there may be a depression of function during recovery which will diminish oxygen transport to other organs. Tissue oedema, particularly in the brain, may decrease the local perfusion and oxygen transport for a considerable time during recovery.

HYPEROXIA

Extreme hyperventilation, while breathing air, may raise the arterial Po_2 to about 16 kPa (120 mm Hg). Higher levels can only be obtained by oxygen-enrichment of the inspired gas, or by elevation of the ambient pressure. Although by this means the arterial Po_2 can be raised to very high levels, the increase in arterial oxygen *content* is, in the normal subject, quite small since the additional oxygen is mainly confined to the fraction in physical solution (*Table 34*). Provided that the arterial/venous oxygen content difference remains constant, it follows that the increase in venous oxygen content is the same as that of the arterial blood. This means that, with a normal arterial/venous oxygen content difference, the venous blood will not become fully saturated during the inhalation of 100 per cent oxygen until the pressure is elevated to more than 2 atmospheres absolute. Unless the venous blood is more than about 95 per cent saturated, the rise in venous Po_2 is not at all spectacular (*Table 34*). Since the tissue Po_2 is related to the venous Po_2, it follows that the tissue Po_2 is not raised to anything like the level of the arterial Po_2 during oxygen therapy at normal and raised barometric pressure.

Table 34 OXYGEN LEVELS ATTAINED IN THE NORMAL SUBJECT BY CHANGES IN THE OXYGEN TENSION OF THE INSPIRED GAS

	At normal barometric pressure		*At 2 atm. absolute*	*At 3 atm. absolute*
Inspired gas	Air	Oxygen	Oxygen	Oxygen
Inspired gas Po_2 (humidified				
(kPa)	20	95	190	285
(mm Hg)	150	713	1 426	2 139
Arterial Po_2*				
(kPa)	13	80	175	270
(mm Hg)	100	600	1 313	2 026
Arterial oxygen content†				
(ml/100 ml)	19·3	21·3	23·4	25·5
Arterial/venous oxygen content				
difference (ml/100 ml)	5·0	5·0	5·0	5·0
Venous oxygen content				
(ml/100 ml)	14·3	16·3	18·4	20·5
Venous Po_2				
(kPa)	5·2	6·4	9·1	48·0
(mmHg)	39	48	68	360

(Tissue perfusion may be reduced by elevation of Po_2. This tends to increase the arterial/venous oxygen content difference which will limit the rise in venous Po_2. The increases in venous Po_2 shown in this Table will therefore be too great in certain circumstances.)

* Reasonable values have been assumed for Pco_2 and alveolar/arterial Po_2 difference.

† Normal values are assumed for Hb, pH, etc.

It is convenient to consider two degrees of hyperoxia. The first ranges from normal levels up to a Po_2 of inspired gas of one atmosphere. This may be attained either by the inhalation of 100 per cent oxygen at normal barometric pressure or by the inhalation of air at 5 atmospheres absolute pressure. The second degree ranges above an inspired gas Po_2 of 1 atmosphere and may be attained by the inhalation of 100 per cent oxygen at pressure in excess of 1 atmosphere. This is still being evaluated for therapeutic purposes under the term 'hyperbaric oxygenation'. Comparable values of Po_2 may be obtained by breathing air at pressures in excess of 5 atmospheres absolute.

Hyperoxia produced by oxygen-enrichment of inspired gas at normal barometric pressure

Indications

The commonest indications for oxygen-enrichment of inspired gas are the prevention of arterial hypoxaemia caused either by hypoventilation or by venous admixture. These applications have been discussed in detail elsewhere (pages 194 and 395). In addition, oxygen-enrichment may also be used to mitigate the effects of ischaemia or anaemia (stagnant and anaemic hypoxia). Further specific indications are clearance of gas loculi and the treatment of carbon monoxide poisoning.

Stagnant anoxia can be marginally relieved by the inhalation of oxygen, which will elevate the oxygen content of the arterial blood to the extent shown in *Table 34.* The Po_2 increase is impressive but the content change is small and therefore the improvement in oxygen flux can only be marginal unless tissue perfusion is improved. However, before dismissing oxygen therapy for stagnant hypoxia, it should be remembered that the improvement in oxygen flux may be critical and may result in significant improvement of myocardial function. Freeman (1962) has demonstrated reduction of mortality in critically bled dogs following the administration of oxygen. Possible modes of action were explored by Freeman and Nunn (1963). Definitive treatment should, of course, be aimed at improving the circulation.

Anaemic hypoxia can be relieved by oxygen therapy for the reasons outlined above. However, since the combined oxygen is less than in the normal subject, the effect of the additional oxygen carried in solution will be relatively more important.

Clearance of gas loculi in the body may be greatly accelerated by inhalation of 100 per cent oxygen which may also be considered as denitrogenation. The principle of this form of therapy depends upon the reduction of the total tension of the dissolved gases in the venous blood. This results in the blood draining the tissues having surplus capacity to carry away gas dissolved from the loculi within the area of venous drainage. In the normal subject breathing air, the total gas tensions in venous blood are always about 7 kPa (53 mm Hg) less than in the arterial blood since the arterial/venous Po_2 fall is about ten times greater than the corresponding Pco_2 rise (*Table 35*). It is of the utmost

Table 35 NORMAL ARTERIAL AND MIXED VENOUS BLOOD-GAS TENSIONS
BREATHING AIR

	kPa		*mm Hg*	
	arterial blood	*venous blood*	*arterial blood*	*venous blood*
PO_2	13·3	5·3	100	40
PCO_2	5·3	6·1	40	46
PN_2	76·0	76·0	570	570
Total gas tensions	94·6	87·4	710	656

importance that the venous blood should have a total gas tension which is subatmospheric. This means that there is always capacity to dissolve away a gas loculus and ensures that all potential spaces in the body remain empty and can even sustain a pressure below atmospheric. The importance of this in the pleural 'cavity' has already been stressed (page 64).

When a subject breathes 100 per cent oxygen, the difference between the total gas tensions of arterial and venous blood becomes even greater (*Table 36*).

Table 36 NORMAL ARTERIAL AND MIXED VENOUS BLOOD-GAS TENSIONS
BREATHING OXYGEN

	kPa		*mm Hg*	
	arterial blood	*venous blood*	*arterial blood*	*venous blood*
PO_2	80·0	6·7	600	50*
PCO_2	5·3	6·1	40	46
PN_2	0	0	0	0
Total gas tensions	85·3	12·8	640	96

* *See Table 34.*

The total gas tension of the venous blood is now very markedly subatmospheric and the venous blood has a greatly increased capacity to dissolve gas which is lying in loculi.

The use of oxygen to remove gas is indicated after air embolus. It may also be used to ease intestinal gas pressure in patients with intestinal obstruction or pneumatosis coli (Down and Castleden, 1975), to hasten recovery from pneumoencephalography and to aid absorption of pneumoperitoneum and pneumothorax.

Carbon monoxide poisoning has long been recognized as a most important indication for oxygen therapy. Not only is the oxygen content of the arterial blood improved, but the clearance rate of carboxyhaemoglobin is accelerated (Sharp, Ledingham and Norman, 1962).

Oxygen toxicity

It is an extraordinary fact that oxygen, which is essential for the efficient synthesis of ATP required by all higher organisms, should be universally toxic to all forms of life. The possibility was recognized by Priestley in 1776 and demonstrated by Paul Bert in 1878. The P_{O_2} at which toxic effects become manifest varies widely, being low in anaerobic bacteria and high in aerobic organisms which are equipped with a range of protective systems against the harmful effects of oxygen. Oxygen toxicity is markedly dose-dependent. One range of toxic effects become evident when the P_{O_2} is raised from that of room air to that of 100 per cent oxygen, and another range is encountered when the pressure of 100 per cent is raised above 1 atmosphere (hyperbaric).

The mode of action of toxicity of oxygen is complex and not fully understood. At the molecular level it is not clear to what extent toxicity is due to oxygen itself and how far free radicals are involved. Molecular oxygen contains two unpaired orbital electrons and therefore may be considered as a free radical itself although conventionally it is not normally displayed as a free radical. Molecular oxygen undergoes a progressive reduction to water but with formation of a series of free radicals and molecules as short-lived intermediates (Gerschman, 1964; Menzel, 1970; Fridovich, 1975). Changes which have been suggested include those shown in *Figure 143*. All intermediates in this scheme are highly toxic. Fortunately, they have very short half-lives in the body and some were not detected until recently. The two enzymes, superoxide dismutase and catalase, play an important role in reducing the half-lives of the superoxide ion radical and hydrogen peroxide respectively.

Oxygen-dependent radiosensitivity

In the presence of oxygen and water, ionizing radiations produce a somewhat similar range of intermediates to those shown in *Figure 143* but with the addition of H_2O^+ and H_3O^+ (Gerschman, 1964). These intermediates are responsible for a part of the total tissue damage produced by radiation in the presence of oxygen. As tissue P_{O_2} is reduced below about 2 kPa (15 mm Hg), there is a progressively increased resistance to radiation damage until, at zero

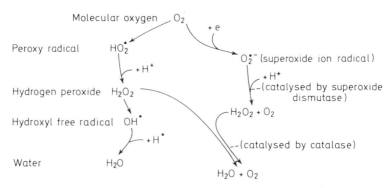

Figure 143. Suggested stages in the in vivo reduction of oxygen. (The small black circle indicates the unpaired electron of a free radical)

Po$_2$, resistance is increased threefold (Gray et al., 1953). The oxygen-dependent component of radiosensitivity is of great practical importance in radiotherapy because hypoxic areas of tumours have greater resistance, and cells near the necrotic centre of tumours tend to survive.

Hyperbaric oxygenation has been used as an adjunct to radiotherapy in an attempt to raise the Po$_2$ in hypoxic areas of tumours and so increase their radiosensitivity (Foster, 1965). An alternative approach was nitrogen inhalation with the hope of reducing the sensitivity of the host tissues to the level of the hypoxic areas of the tumour, thereby permitting an increased dosage of irradiation (Cater et al., 1963). Perhaps more encouraging have been the reports that oxygen-dependent radiosensitivity is reduced by anaesthetics (Ebert and Hornsey, 1958).

There are, in fact, many features in common between oxygen toxicity and the effects of irradiation (Swartz, 1973). It is tempting to believe that certain free radicals play a part in both processes.

Biochemical changes of oxygen toxicity

Although it is not possible to be certain whether the responsible agent is oxygen or free radicals, it has nevertheless been possible to identify certain biochemical lesions which follow exposure to high partial pressures of oxygen. These have been reviewed by Haugaard (1968), Menzel (1970), Swartz (1973) and Wolfe and deVries (1975), and include the following.

1. Enzyme inhibition, particularly the flavoproteins (page 375) and those which contain sulphydryl groups. Such enzymes are important in metabolism. There may be interference with oxidative phosphorylation and metabolism of glutamate and γ-aminobutyric acid (GABA), brain levels of which are reduced in the intact animal exposed to high pressures of oxygen.
2. Lipid peroxidation is common to both oxygen toxicity and irradiation damage. Vulnerable sites include the unsaturated fatty acids of the cell membrane, and membrane damage is an important feature of pulmonary oxygen toxicity (*see* below).
3. Apart from enzymes, other compounds containing sulphydryl groups may be oxidized. They include glutathione, lipoic acid and coenzyme A.

There is considerable difficulty in relating the histopathological effects of oxygen toxicity described below to the biochemical effects outlined above.

Substances which modify oxygen toxicity. There has been much interest in the possibility of chemical protection against the effects of high Po$_2$. Suggested protective agents have included glutathione, which scavenges free radicals, the reducing agent ascorbic acid, vitamin E and γ-aminobutyric acid. An alternative approach is to raise the levels of enzymes which destroy the active intermediate radicals and compounds. Although there are considerable practical difficulties, protection might be conferred by raised levels of superoxide dismutase, catalase and peroxidases. Superoxide dismutase has, in fact, been effective in the treatment of paraquat poisoning which produces pulmonary changes similar to those of oxygen toxicity (Autor, 1974). Various forms of symptomatic treatment are effective, particularly the use of anticonvulsants to prevent convulsions during exposure to hyperbaric oxygen. Anaesthetics are reputed to reduce oxygen-dependent radiosensitivity (*see* above) and it is tempting to hope that they might modify the biochemical effects of oxygen toxicity.

Pulmonary oxygen toxicity (the Lorrain–Smith effect)

This subject is of great practical importance in intensive therapy. Recent reviews have included those by Clark and Lambertsen (1971) and Winter and Smith (1972). Pulmonary tissue has the highest Po_2 in the body and therefore the lung is the most vulnerable organ.

Cellular changes.   Weibel (1971) has contributed a valuable summary of the work of his group. Electron microscopy has shown that, in rats exposed to 1 atmosphere of oxygen, the primary change is in the capillary endothelium, which becomes vacuolated and thinned. Permeability is increased and fluid accumulates in the interstitial space. At a later stage, in monkeys, the epithelial lining is lost over large areas of the alveoli. This process affects the type I epithelial cell (page 18) and is accompanied by a proliferation of the type II cells which appear to be attempting to make good the loss of type I cells. Weibel postulates that the cytological differentiation of the type I cell decreases its resistance to oxygen-induced damage. The cytoplasm of the type I cells consists mainly of the very thin sheets of alveolar membrane which is poor in organelles which are required for repair of biochemical damage. Over-all the alveolar-capillary membrane is thickened as a result of fluid accumulation in the interstitial space.

Limits of survival.   Pulmonary effects of oxygen vary greatly between different species. Most strains of rats will not survive for much more than three days in 1 atmosphere of oxygen. Monkeys survive oxygen breathing for about two weeks and man is probably even more resistant. Pulmonary oxygen-tolerance curves for normal man, based on reduction in vital capacity, have been prepared by Clarke and Lambertsen (1971). In general, there is an approximately inverse relationship between Po_2 and duration of tolerable exposure. Thus 20 hours of 1 atmosphere produces an effect similar to 10 hours of 2 atmospheres or 5 hours of 4 atmospheres.

American space craft contain 100 per cent oxygen at a pressure of one-third of an atmosphere. There is abundant evidence that prolonged exposure to this environment does not cause pulmonary changes. This establishes a safe limit of environmental Po_2 of 34 kPa (252 mm Hg) and, furthermore, shows that it is partial pressure rather than concentration which is dangerous, at least in healthy subjects. It will be clear that there are formidable practical difficulties in the experimental determination of man's ability to withstand higher partial pressures of oxygen. There is general agreement that 10 hours' exposure to 1 atmosphere of oxygen produces substernal distress and the first measurable reduction in vital capacity in fit subjects. Beyond these early symptoms, study of healthy man is not feasible.

Oxygen toxicity in the presence of pre-existing pulmonary pathology.   The other source of evidence for pulmonary oxygen toxicity in man is from therapeutic administration of oxygen, particularly in the intensive therapy situation. There is very great difficulty in separating the effects of the pulmonary disease which required oxygen administration from effects which may be attributed to the oxygen. Nash, Blennerhassett and Pontoppidan (1967) reviewed 70 patients who died after prolonged artificial ventilation. Pulmonary abnormalities (particularly fibrin membranes, oedema and fibrosis) were greater in those patients who had received more than 90 per cent oxygen. However, it must be remembered that very high concentrations of oxygen are only employed in patients with grossly defective gas exchange who cannot maintain a safe arterial Po_2 in any other way. Therefore, a study of patients who died after receiving 100 per cent oxygen for long periods will necessarily comprise patients with gross lung pathology not attributable to oxygen.

In an attempt to exclude the factor of lung pathology antedating the administration of 100 per cent oxygen, Singer et al. (1970) ventilated a group of patients with 100 per cent oxygen for 24 hours following heart operations with cardiopulmonary bypass. In addition, two patients received 100 per cent oxygen for 5 and 7 days respectively. Various pulmonary parameters (VD/VT ratio, shunt and compliance) were not significantly different from a control group breathing less than 42 per cent oxygen. A second study mounted by Barber, Lee and Hamilton (1970) showed a significant increase in VD/VT ratio and shunt of patients with irreversible head injuries ventilated with 100 per cent oxygen for 31–72 hours when compared with a control group ventilated with air. There were no differences in the lung histology between the two groups.

Available information on pulmonary oxygen toxicity in man is incomplete. It seems likely that pre-existing lung pathology may play a major role in determining sensitivity to oxygen and it is impossible to predict the outcome of administration of 100 per cent oxygen. Unfortunately, this may be required for survival in spite of meticulous attention to clearance of secretions, expansions, expansion of collapsed areas of lung, the use of positive end-expiratory pressure (PEEP) and other measures to improve gas exchange. Many intensive therapy units regard 70 per cent oxygen as the safe upper limit.

Pulmonary absorption collapse.   Whatever the uncertainties about pulmonary oxygen toxicity in man, there is no doubt that high concentrations of oxygen in areas of the lung with a low ventilation/perfusion ratio will result in collapse (*see Figure 105*). This may easily be demonstrated in the healthy volunteer. A few minutes' breathing 100 per cent oxygen at residual volume results in radiological evidence of collapse, a reduced arterial Po_2 and substernal pain on attempting a maximal inspiration (Nunn et al., 1965b).

Ventilatory depression.   Perhaps the greatest danger of oxygen therapy is the production of ventilatory depression in patients who have lost their sensitivity to carbon dioxide and rely upon the hypoxic drive to breathing (page 194). This is particularly dangerous in the patient with chronic bronchitis (the blue bloater). The administration of 100 per cent oxygen may cause respiratory arrest within minutes, and even modest increases of inspired oxygen within the range 25–35 per cent may cause substantial increases in arterial Pco_2. Great caution is necessary in such patients and the inspired oxygen must always be under control. Venturi masks are the best method of controlled oxygen administration (*see* below).

Balancing the risks.   In the face of the various respiratory hazards associated with the use of oxygen, it remains necessary to stress that severe hypoxia is dangerous and must be treated as a first priority. Nevertheless, it is pointless and often dangerous to administer a needlessly high concentration of oxygen. A reasonable safe working arterial P_{O_2} is 10 kPa (75 mm Hg) but, if this cannot be maintained without using very high concentrations of oxygen or precipitating ventilatory failure, it may be necessary to settle for a lower arterial P_{O_2} and 6·7 kPa (50 mm Hg) has been suggested by Hutchison, Flenley and Donald (1964). Levels of the order of 3 kPa (23 mm Hg) have been tolerated by Himalayan mountaineers. It is, however, important to appreciate that oxygen delivery to the tissues is an integrated process and all aspects of the problem must be considered for an individual patient before pronouncing a value for his safe minimal arterial P_{O_2} (page 416).

Other hazards of oxygen

Retrolental fibroplasia consists of vascular obliteration and fibroblastic infiltration in the retina, and only occurs in neonates who have been hyperoxygenated (Patz, 1958). The condition does not contraindicate the use of oxygen in the neonate but care must be exercised to prevent the P_{O_2} rising higher than is necessary.

Fire risk is enormously increased when inflammable material is exposed to an atmosphere of oxygen (Denison, Ernsting and Cresswell, 1966).

The dangers of oxygen which have been described above apply to patients who are anaesthetized with inhalational agents, such as halothane and/or cyclopropane, carried in very high concentrations of oxygen. An additional disadvantage of such techniques is that it excludes the use of nitrous oxide which many regard as a useful anaesthetic agent. These are the prices which must be paid for the virtual guarantee of oxygenation afforded by the use of near-100 per cent concentrations of oxygen.

Special hazards of hyperbaric oxygenation

The most important toxic effect of oxygen in man is the convulsive effect which occurs during exposure to pressures in excess of 2 atmospheres absolute. This effect is named after Paul Bert who first described it. Its cause is still unknown although it is thought to result from interference with enzyme systems, and convulsions are encountered under conditions in which the tissue P_{O_2} rises steeply. The fact that more than 2 atmospheres of oxygen is required accords with the relationship to tissue P_{O_2} shown in *Table 34*. Further evidence is the effect of an elevation of P_{CO_2} which diminishes the arterial P_{O_2} at which convulsions occur (Lambertsen, 1965). This, no doubt, results from the increase in cerebral blood flow which would reduce the difference between arterial and cerebral tissue P_{O_2}.

The possibility of oxygen convulsions may be reduced by general anaesthesia and by hyperventilation. The onset of convulsions is variable ranging from 2 to

30 minutes at 3 atmospheres absolute. When a patient with normal arterial blood oxygenation is exposed to high pressures of oxygen (in excess of 3 atmospheres) it is usual to employ general anaesthesia. Others, however, have relied on curtailing the duration of exposure.

Many of the untoward effects associated with the use of hyperbaric oxygenation are due to the elevation of ambient pressure and are not related to oxygen at all. These effects are common to the circumstances of compressed-air working and include bends, ruptured air cysts (Walder, 1965) and avascular necrosis of bone (Davidson, 1965). Oxygen bends are very rare but have been described in goats (Donald, 1955). It should also be remembered that patients in caissons are, to a greater or lesser extent, isolated from the normal facilities of a hospital. This reaches its greatest extent in one-man tanks which prevent the possibility of nursing or emergency medical attention. Access may depend on emergency decompressions but there are certain patients who cannot be safely subjected to this procedure.

Hyperoxia with P_{O_2} in excess of one atmosphere absolute

Oxygen tensions in excess of 1 atmosphere may be obtained by the use of 100 per cent oxygen at pressures in excess of 1 atmosphere. Alternatively, lower concentrations of oxygen may be employed at proportionately higher pressures. The special features of hyperbaric oxygenation are as follows.

1. Arterial P_{O_2} values reach very high values in excess of 130 kPa (975 mm Hg).
2. Pulmonary tissue P_{O_2} presumably reaches levels of the same order as those of the alveolar gas.
3. In contrast to the inhalation of oxygen at 1 atmosphere, hyperbaric oxygenation results in a steep rise of venous and tissue P_{O_2} (*Table 34*).

In any consideration of hyperbaric oxygenation it is important to think in terms of the P_{O_2} of the tissues. It is easy to think that, because a patient has an arterial P_{O_2} of, say, 200 kPa (1500 mm Hg), the tissue P_{O_2} must also be very high. In fact, the simple calculations shown in *Table 34*, supported by experimental observations, show that large rises of venous (and presumably tissue) P_{O_2} do not occur until the P_{O_2} of the arterial blood is of the order of 300 kPa (2250 mm Hg), and the whole of the tissue oxygen requirement can be met from dissolved oxygen. The situation varies from one tissue to another depending upon their oxygen extraction.

An interesting effect of hyperbaric oxygenation is the effect upon carriage of carbon dioxide in the blood. If the dissolved oxygen in the arterial blood is sufficient for the tissue requirements, it follows that the venous blood will contain a negligible quantity of reduced haemoglobin (Gessell, 1923). This causes a marked reduction of buffering power and carbamino carriage. It seems likely that this will result in some tissue retention of carbon dioxide although the elevation of P_{CO_2} is not likely to exceed about 1 kPa (7·5 mm Hg). In the brain this may increase cerebral blood flow and lead to secondary rise of tissue P_{O_2}.

Clinical applications of hyperbaric oxygenation which are under evaluation

Space does not permit a full discussion of the difficult problem of the role of hyperbaric oxygenation in clinical medicine. Many of the factors have been presented in the last few pages but theory can only point the way to controlled clinical trials from which clear answers have been slow to emerge.

Prolongation of safe period of circulatory arrest would appear at first sight to be an obvious benefit to be expected from hyperbaric oxygenation. In fact, results have been very disappointing at normal temperature although somewhat better during hypothermia (Ledingham and Norman, 1965). *Table 34* shows that tissue Po_2 is not likely to be greatly increased by pressures up to 2 atmospheres absolute and therefore there is little additional stored oxygen dissolved in tissue fluids. However, during hypothermia, not only is the oxygen consumption decreased but also the solubility of oxygen in tissue fluids is increased.

Symptomatic treatment of patients with gross shunts is not possible at atmospheric pressure when the shunt exceeds about 40 per cent of cardiac output. *Figure 102* shows that the administration of 100 per cent oxygen does very little to raise the arterial Po_2 in such cases. However, administration of high pressures of oxygen will restore normal arterial Po_2 up to a shunt of 50 per cent, as shown in *Table 37*.

Hypoxia due to hypoperfusion can be relieved by hyperbaric oxygenation provided that the perfusion is only marginally inadequate, since the small amount of additional oxygen carried in blood cannot compensate for a gross inadequacy of circulation. In an organ suffering from partial ischaemia, the zone of surviving tissue may be enlarged. Satisfactory results have been obtained in experimental ligation of the left circumflex coronary artery in dogs (Smith and Lawson, 1958). Satisfactory protection has also been obtained during diffuse embolization of the coronary arteries of dogs at 3 atmospheres of oxygen (Jacobson et al., 1965). However, evidence of satisfactory results in clinical myocardial infarction has remained elusive (Cameron et al., 1965).

Table 37 OXYGEN LEVELS WITH 50 PER CENT SHUNT

Oxygen at:	Pulmonary end-capillary blood			Arterial blood			Mixed venous blood		
	PO_2		O_2 content	PO_2		O_2 content	PO_2		O_2 content
	(kPa)	(mm Hg)	(ml/100 ml)	(kPa)	(mm Hg)	(ml/100 ml)	(kPa)	(mm Hg)	(ml/100 ml)
1 atm. abs*	80	600	21	6·3	47	16	4·0	30	11
2 atm. abs*	173	1 300	23	8·3	62	18	4·7	35	13
3 atm. abs.*	267	2 000	25	26·7	200	20	5·6	42	15

* The pressure in atmospheres absolute is equal to the sum of the barometric pressure and the gauge pressure (which shows the difference between the chamber pressure and the atmosphere). It is very important to distinguish clearly between absolute and gauge pressure since both scales are in routine use in different laboratories.

Isolated case histories have been reported of patients with cerebral ischaemia who have recovered consciousness during hyperbaric oxygenation. Improvement has been temporary and sustained recovery has not been reported (Ingvar, 1965).

There is a clinical impression that partially severed limbs have been saved with hyperbaric oxygenation at 2 atmospheres absolute, the remaining blood flow presumably being just insufficient to maintain life with conventional oxygen therapy. Such cases are rare but have been described (Smith et al., 1961). The value of such therapy would be lost if perfusion were to be reduced by the elevated P_{O_2}. Mortality from haemorrhagic shock is reduced by hyperbaric oxygenation (Attar, Scanlan and Cowley, 1966). There is also a strong clinical impression that varicose and senile ulcers heal more rapidly with intermittent exposure to hyperbaric oxygen.

Infection offers a promising field for the application of hyperbaric oxygenation. Good results have been claimed with anaerobic infections (Brummelkamp, 1965). Pulmonary infections also appear suitable for investigation since very high tissue P_{O_2} can be attained in the lung (Ross and McAllister, 1965). Hyperbaric oxygen is cidal not only to anaerobes but also to most aerobes.

Radiotherapy has been employed under conditions of hyperbaric oxygenation since 1955, the rationale being based on the influence of P_{O_2} on tissue radiosensitivity (*see* above). Technique has been reviewed by Foster (1965). There is evidence of improved results in certain conditions but full results of controlled trials are still awaited.

Carbon monoxide poisoning may be treated more effectively with oxygen at high pressure (Sharp, Ledingham and Norman, 1962). However, its clinical value will be maximal at an early stage when hyperbaric facilities are unlikely to be available. This consideration has led to interest in the possibility of mounting small chambers in ambulances (Williams and Hopkins, 1965).

CONTROL OF THE INSPIRED OXYGEN CONCENTRATION

Much of this chapter has been devoted to the problem of selection of the optimal inspired oxygen concentration for a particular pathophysiological state. It now remains to be considered how this should be put into effect.

Interface with the patient's airway

A crucial factor in oxygen therapy is the nature of the seal between the patient's airway and the external breathing apparatus. Airtight seals may be obtained with cuffed endotracheal or tracheostomy tubes and these give complete control over the composition of the inspired gas. An anaesthetic facemask will usually provide an airtight seal with the face, but it must be held by a trained person (preferably an anaesthetist) and is at best a temporary measure. Physiological mouthpieces with a nose clip are satisfactory for short-term use with co-operative subjects but cannot be tolerated for long periods. There is no mask available for clinical use which can be guaranteed to provide an airtight fit to a patient's face unless it is actually held on to the face by trained staff. Most disposable oxygen masks do not attempt to provide an airtight fit.

Gas mixing

The most satisfactory technique for the control of the inspired oxygen concentration is to mix the required proportions of air and oxygen. Gas mixtures are conveniently obtained from air and oxygen pipeline installations with appropriate humidification. A pair of rotameters may be used, and *Figure 150* shows a simple wall chart to facilitate the calculation of flow rates. A far more satisfactory arrangement is to employ a mixing device with separate controls for total flow rate and oxygen concentration. It is important that such devices should have a visible indication of oxygen flow (Richardson, Chinn and Nunn, 1976).

Air/oxygen mixtures can be delivered to ventilators, passed over a T-piece for patients breathing spontaneously with a cuffed endotracheal tube or passed to the patient by means of a valvular non-rebreathing system. They can also be passed to loose-fitting disposable masks but, under these circumstances, high flow rates are required, preferably in excess of the peak inspiratory flow rate (page 121).

Use of venturi devices

Oxygen may be passed through the jet of a venturi to entrain air. This is a convenient and highly economical method of preparing oxygen mixtures in the range 25–40 per cent concentration. For example, 1 l/min of oxygen with an entrainment ratio of 8 : 1 will deliver 9 l/min of 30 per cent oxygen. Higher oxygen concentrations require a lower entrainment ratio and therefore a higher oxygen flow in order to maintain an adequate total delivered flow rate. The familiar venturi mask was introduced by Campbell (1960b) on the suggestion of the author who had used a venturi to provide the oxygen-enriched carrier gas for an anaesthetic apparatus designed for use in the Antarctic (Nunn, 1961b).

With the availability of an ample flow rate of the air/oxygen mixture, the venturi mask need not fit the face with an airtight junction. The high flow rate escapes round the cheeks and room air is effectively excluded. Numerous studies have indicated that the venturi mask gives excellent control over the inspired oxygen concentration with an accuracy of ±1 per cent, unaffected by variations in the ventilation of the patient (Leigh, 1973). There is no doubt that this is the most satisfactory method of controlling the inspired oxygen concentration of a patient who is breathing spontaneously and is not intubated.

Control of the patient's gaseous environment

Oxygen tents have been in use for many years but suffer from the disadvantage of the large volume and high rate of leakage which makes it difficult to attain and maintain a high oxygen concentration, unless the volume is reduced and a high gas flow rate is used (Wayne and Chamney, 1969). In addition, the fire hazard cannot be ignored. These problems are minimized when the patient is an infant, and oxygen control within an incubator is a highly satisfactory method of administering a precise oxygen concentration under these circumstances. Largely because of the danger of retrolental fibroplasia (page 428), it is mandatory to monitor the oxygen concentration in the incubator.

Spectacles, nasal catheters, simple disposable oxygen masks, etc.

A wide range of simple devices aim to blow oxygen at or into the air passages. This oxygen is mixed with inspired air to give an inspired oxygen concentration which is a complex function of the geometry of the device, the oxygen flow rate, the patient's ventilation and whether the patient is breathing through his mouth or nose. The effective inspired oxygen concentration is impossible to predict and may vary within very wide limits (Leigh, 1973). These devices cannot be used for oxygen therapy when the exact inspired oxygen concentration is critical (e.g. ventilatory failure), but may be useful in less critical situations such as recovery from routine anaesthesia. Fairly high oxygen concentrations may be obtained with a combination of two techniques such as nasal catheters used under an MC mask, an arrangement with which Down and Castleden (1975) obtained an arterial Po_2 of 52 kPa (388 mm Hg).

Hyperbaric oxygenation

Two systems are in use. One-man chambers are filled with 100 per cent oxygen and the patient is entirely exposed to high pressure 100 per cent oxygen: no mask is required. Larger chambers are pressurized with air which is breathed by staff; 100 per cent oxygen is made available to the patient by means of a well fitting facemask. The quality of the airtight fit is obviously crucial and has caused considerable difficulties in the past.

Monitoring oxygen concentrations

When the inspired gas has a fixed composition (e.g. in oxygen tents, with venturi masks and with delivery of air/oxygen mixtures), there is no problem in sampling inspired gas and determining the oxygen concentration with devices such as paramagnetic analysers (*see* below). With variable performance devices (e.g. oxygen spectacles, nasal catheters, MC mask, etc.), it is extremely difficult to determine the inspired oxygen which may not be constant throughout the duration of inspiration, and the measured oxygen concentration may be highly dependent on the point from which the sample was taken. In the face of these difficulties it may be preferable to measure the end-expiratory oxygen concentration or even the arterial blood Po_2. However, if such measures are necessary it would be wiser to use a device with a fixed performance.

OXYGEN LEVELS DURING ANAESTHESIA

There has been evidence of interest in oxygenation of patients under the effect of anaesthetic agents since the birth of the speciality. In Davy's *Researches* (1800) there is comment by Beddoes on the colour of blood flowing from leech bites, and in Robinson's book of 1847 there is the remark that arterial blood presents its normal appearance during etherization.

Until about 1960, studies of oxygenation generally related to the saturation rather than the Po_2 of the arterial blood, and were of limited value since considerable reduction of Po_2 can occur without much change in saturation due to the shape of the oxygen dissociation curve. However, since 1960, the introduction of the polarograph has led to many studies of arterial Po_2 which have shed a great deal of light on factors governing the oxygenation of the arterial blood during anaesthesia. The contributions of most of these studies to the fundamental understanding of the problems have already been discussed in the appropriate parts of this book, and all that now remains is to summarize the principal factors in relation to anaesthesia.

Inspired oxygen concentration probably exceeds all other factors in importance. When the inspired oxygen concentration exceeds 80 per cent the arterial Po_2 of apparently healthy anaesthetized patients is almost never found to be below 30 kPa (225 mm Hg). When the inspired oxygen concentration is below 21 per cent the arterial Po_2 is usually below 13·3 kPa (100 mm Hg). Inspired oxygen concentrations within the range 30–40 per cent usually result in an arterial Po_2 between 10 and 20 kPa (75 and 150 mm Hg) (*Figure 144*) but surprisingly low

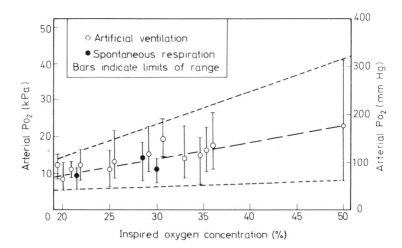

Figure 144. Pooled data on arterial Po_2 levels during anaesthesia reported by the following authors as a function of the inspired oxygen concentration: Campbell, Nunn and Peckett (1958); Theye and Tuohy (1964a, b); Nunn (1964); Salter et al. (1965); Sykes, Young and Robinson (1965); Nunn, Bergman and Coleman (1965); Webb and Nunn (1967); Roberts et al. (1974); Hewlett et al. (1974c). Note the high correlation between mean arterial Po_2 and inspired oxygen concentration. Mean arterial Po_2 is about half the inspired gas Po_2. Factors varying between the different studies seem to have surprisingly little effect and most studies contain one or more patients whose Po_2 is unexpectedly low. The middle broken line corresponds closely to the 10 per cent iso-shunt line (Figure 102)

values are occasionally found in patients who show no signs of respiratory or circulatory disease.

An increase in inspired oxygen concentration will usually produce a corresponding increase in alveolar PO_2 (page 387). However, other factors remaining constant, the alveolar/arterial PO_2 difference is increased (page 391) and improvement in arterial PO_2 is thus less than might be expected. *Figure 144* shows this as a disappointingly flat response curve.

There is a school of thought which believes that oxygenation is of such importance that all anaesthetized patients should receive an inspired gas containing at least 80 per cent oxygen. This virtually guarantees adequate arterial oxygenation under almost all exigencies of anaesthesia, including gross hypoventilation (*Table 38*). However, it obliges the anaesthetist to forgo the use of nitrous oxide and seems to engender an attitude which tolerates elevation of PCO_2 to levels which many would regard as dangerous (Birt and Cole, 1965).

Table 38 VALUES FOR ARTERIAL PO_2 REPORTED DURING ANAESTHESIA WITH AN INSPIRED GAS CONCENTRATION CLOSE TO 100%

Year	Authors	Type of respiration	Arterial PO_2					
			minimum		mean		maximum	
			kPa	mm Hg	kPa	mm Hg	kPa	mm Hg
1960	Stark and Smith	Spontaneous	36·3	272	44·3	332	51·7	388
		Artificial	28·1	211	45·7	343	59·3	445
1963	Bendixen, Hedley-Whyte and Laver	Artificial	20·0	150	58·7	440	81·1	608
1964	Nunn	Spontaneous	34·5	259	63·5	476	75·9	569
1964	Bendixen and his colleagues	Spontaneous	—	—	53·6	402	—	—
		Artificial	—	—	73·7	553	—	—
1965	Nunn, Bergman and Coleman	Artificial	56·1	421	68·9	517	84·8	636
1968	Panday and Nunn	Spontaneous	44·3	332	60·0	450	70·7	530

A number of studies have been omitted where there was inadequate evidence of nitrogen elimination. These studies included those in which the patients were allowed to breathe from closed circuits with an inflow of a few hundred millilitres of oxygen per minute. Measurements have shown that there is still about 20% nitrogen circulating after 1 hour of such conditions, sufficient to reduce the arterial PO_2 by about 19 kPa (140 mm Hg).

Ventilation is of critical importance below the normal value of alveolar ventilation (*Figure 129*). At high levels of ventilation and when breathing 100 per cent oxygen, changes of ventilation have relatively little effect upon the alveolar PO_2, although an increased tidal ventilation may re-expand collapsed lung.

The alveolar/arterial PO_2 difference is a major factor influencing the arterial PO_2 during anaesthesia and has been accorded considerable attention in this chapter (page 388). Its magnitude is influenced by the following factors: (1) shunt; (2) scatter of ventilation/perfusion ratios; (3) cardiac output; (4) the alveolar PO_2; and (5) haemoglobin, pH, temperature and other minor factors.

There is no doubt that the alveolar/arterial PO_2 difference is increased in all anaesthetized patients except perhaps for children and young adults undergoing brief operations. There is also little doubt that the increase is largely due to the increased pulmonary venous admixture which has been found to be of the order of 10 per cent of cardiac output during uncomplicated anaesthesia (*Table 21* and *Figure 106*). The pulmonary venous admixture is not consistently reduced by the inhalation of 100 per cent oxygen and thus is probably caused by shunting, although the contribution of areas of low ventilation/perfusion ratio is not known at the time of writing. Increased alveolar/arterial Po_2 difference correlates with reduction of lung volume (page 69) and airway closure seems the most likely cause of the shunt. Reduction of cardiac output and mixed venous oxygen content also plays a part. Reduction of oxygen consumption helps to minimize the fall in arterial Po_2 but the effect is too small to offset other factors and oxygen-enrichment of the inspired gas within the range 30–50 per cent oxygen is normal practice.

Thoracic surgery.   Problems of the lateral position and open pneumothorax have been discussed on pages 235 and 276. The problems of oxygenation during one-lung anaesthesia have been extensively investigated (see, for example, Khanam and Branthwaite, 1973; Kerr et al., 1974). As might be expected, cessation of ventilation of the exposed lung results in a fall of arterial Po_2 but this may be reversed by occluding the vessels of the exposed lung. No support has been found for the theory that perfusion ceases spontaneously during the first few minutes after collapse of a lung. Kerr's group recommend that 100 per cent oxygen should be used to prevent hypoxaemia during one-lung ventilation, particularly if circulation continues through the non-ventilated lung. With either two-lung ventilation or else one-lung ventilation with vessels occluded, arterial Po_2 can usually be maintained within normal limits when the inspired oxygen concentration is in the range 40–50 per cent. However, unexpectedly low values of arterial Po_2 are not infrequently encountered in thoracic surgery and are often related to pulmonary pathology resulting in shunting. Hypoxaemia in relation to anaesthesia has been reviewed by Marshall and Wyche (1972).

In the post-operative period, there are many possible causes of arterial hypoxaemia. Withdrawal of nitrous oxide at the end of an anaesthetic causes dilution of alveolar gas with nitrous oxide. Alveolar and arterial Po_2 are reduced by this mechanism originally known as 'diffusion anoxia' (page 388). Marshall and Millar (1965) considered this to be the principal cause of early post-operative hypoxaemia but reductions of arterial Po_2 commonly occur in patients who have not received nitrous oxide and, in patients who have received nitrous oxide, the hypoxaemia usually outlasts the period of nitrous oxide wash-out (Nunn and Payne, 1962). Alexander et al (1973) showed that reduction of lung volume continued into the post-operative period and correlated with hypoxaemia. It therefore seems that airway closure is an important factor, as it is during operation. A study by Bay, Nunn and Prys-Roberts (1968) showed that there was no universal cause for early post-operative hypoxaemia. In some patients there was a large venous admixture, while in others the main abnormality was excessive desaturation of mixed venous blood caused by a high oxygen consumption which was not matched by the cardiac output. Substantial increases in oxygen consumption were found in shivering patients. Surprisingly, hypoventilation was not a major cause of arterial hypoxaemia in the patients studied, and minute volumes as high as 25 l/min were recorded in shivering patients. Clearly the ventilation might be limited in other patients by pulmonary disease or faulty anaesthetic technique with, for example, residual neuromuscular block.

The severity of early post-operative hypoxaemia has no obvious connection with the nature of the operation except that there is a relation to duration of anaesthesia (Marshall and Millar, 1965). Hypoxaemia is more marked in older patients and there is a negative correlation between arterial P_{O_2} and the age of the patient (Nunn, 1965), the regression line lying below and parallel to that observed in conscious patients. There is a great deal of scatter in individual observations but mean results of pooled data from many sources yield the following regression equation:

$$\text{early post-operative arterial } P_{O_2} = \frac{12 \cdot 6 - 0 \cdot 061 \text{ (age) in kPa}}{94 \cdot 3 - 0 \cdot 455 \text{ (age) in mm Hg}}$$

(Nunn, 1965)

(patient breathing air)

Early post-operative arterial hypoxaemia does not last beyond the day of operation and persistent hypoxaemia, when it persists, is usually due to overt pulmonary collapse (Palmer and Gardiner, 1964; Palmer, Gardiner and McGregor, 1965).

In the pre-operative period it has been shown that patients awaiting surgery (without premedication) have a normal arterial P_{O_2} for their age (Conway, Payne and Tomlin, 1965). Atropine was found to have no effect on arterial P_{O_2} of volunteers (Daly, Roll and Behnke, 1963; Nunn and Bergman, 1964) but Tomlin, Conway and Payne (1964) reported a fall of arterial P_{O_2} of 2 kPa (15 mm Hg) after intramuscular administration of atropine to patients awaiting surgery. Papaveretum and hyoscine administered together were found to result in a fall of arterial P_{O_2} of about 1·3 kPa (10 mm Hg), patients acting as their own control (Prys-Roberts, 1966).

CYANOSIS

The commonest method of detection of hypoxia is by the appearance of cyanosis, and the change in colour of haemoglobin on desaturation affords the patient a safeguard of immense value. Indeed, it is interesting to speculate on the additional hazards of anaesthesia if gross hypoxia could occur without overt changes in the colour of the blood. There must have been countless occasions in which the appearance of cyanosis has given warning of hypoventilation, pulmonary shunting, stagnant circulation or decreased oxygen concentration of inspired gas.

Central and peripheral cyanosis

If shed arterial blood is seen to be purple, this indicates arterial desaturation. However, when skin or mucous membrane is inspected, most of the blood which colours the tissue is lying in veins and its oxygen content is related to the arterial oxygen content as follows:

$$
\begin{matrix}
\text{venous} & & \text{arterial} & & \text{arterial/venous} \\
\text{oxygen} & = & \text{oxygen} & - & \text{oxygen content} \\
\text{content} & & \text{content} & & \text{difference}
\end{matrix}
$$

The last term may be expanded in terms of the tissue metabolism and perfusion:

$$
\begin{matrix}
\text{venous} & & \text{arterial} \\
\text{oxygen} & = & \text{oxygen} \\
\text{content} & & \text{content}
\end{matrix}
- \left(\frac{\text{tissue oxygen consumption}}{\text{tissue blood flow}} \right)
$$

The oxygen consumption by the skin is usually very low in relation to its circulation so that the quantity in the bracket is generally small. Therefore the venous oxygen content is close to that of the arterial blood and inspection of the skin gives a reasonable indication of arterial oxygen content. However when circulation is reduced in relation to skin oxygen consumption, cyanosis may occur in the presence of normal arterial oxygen levels. This occurs typically in cold weather and in the face of a patient in the Trendelenburg position, but may occur in a wide range of circulatory disorders.

The influence of anaemia

Lundsgaard and Van Slyke (1923) stressed the importance of anaemia in appearance of cyanosis. There is general acceptance of their statement that cyanosis is apparent when there are 5 g of reduced haemoglobin per 100 ml of capillary blood. They defined capillary blood as having a reduced haemoglobin concentration which was the mean of the levels in arterial and venous blood. If, for example, the arterial blood contained 3 g/100 ml of reduced haemoglobin (80 per cent saturation at normal haemoglobin concentration) and the arterial/venous difference for the skin were 4 ml/100 ml of oxygen (corresponding to the reduction of a further 3 g/100 ml of haemoglobin), the 'capillary' blood would contain 4·5 g/100 ml of reduced haemoglobin and the degree fo hypoxaemia would be just below the threshold at which cyanosis should be evident. In cases of severe anaemia, the reduced haemoglobin concentration of the capillary blood is unlikely to attain the level of 5 g/100 ml, which is said to be required for the appearance of cyanosis and, clearly, cyanosis could never occur if the haemoglobin concentration were only 5 g/100 ml.

There seems little doubt that qualitatively the views of Lundsgaard and Van Slyke are sound. There has been little quantitative confirmation of their theory but it is generally found that cyanosis can be detected at an arterial oxygen saturation of about 85 per cent although there is much variation (Comroe and Botelho, 1947). Such a level would probably correspond to a 'capillary' saturation of more than 80 per cent and a reduced haemoglobin of about 3 g/100 ml.

Sites for detection of cyanosis

Kelman and Nunn (1966a) carried out a comparison of the appearance of cyanosis in different sites with various biochemical indices of hypoxaemia of arterial blood. Best correlations were obtained with cyanosis observed in the buccal mucosa and lips, but there was no significant correlation between the oxygenation of the arterial blood and the appearance of cyanosis in the ear lobes, nail bed or conjunctivae.

The importance of colour-rending properties of source of illumination

Kelman and Nunn also compared the use of five types of fluorescent lighting in use in hospitals. There was no significant difference in the correlation between hypoxaemia and cyanosis for the different lights. None was therefore more *reliable* than the others for the detection of hypoxaemia. However, there was a striking difference in the *degree* of cyanosis with the different lights, some tending to make the patient pinker and others imparting a bluer tinge to the patients. The former gave false negatives (no cyanosis in the presence of hypoxaemia) while the latter gave false positives (cyanosis in the absence of hypoxaemia), the total number of false results being approximately the same with all tubes.

It is potentially dangerous for patients to be inspected under lamps of different colour-rendering properties, particularly if the medical and nursing staff do not know the characteristics of each type of lamp. It would be too much to suggest that the staff should calibrate their impressions of cyanosis for a particular lamp by relation to arterial oxygen levels, but it is not too much to expect that hospitals will standardize their lighting and acquaint staff with the colour-rendering properties of the type which is finally chosen.

Sensitivity of cyanosis as an indication of hypoxaemia

It has been stressed above that the appearance of cyanosis is considerably influenced by the circulation, haemoglobin concentration and lighting conditions. Even when all these are optimal, cyanosis is by no means a precise indication of the arterial oxygen level and should be regarded as a warning sign rather than a measurement. Kelman and Nunn (1966a) detected cyanosis in about 50 per cent of patients who had a saturation of 93 per cent. Cyanosis was detected in about 95 per cent of patients with a saturation of 89 per cent. It should be remembered that 89 per cent saturation corresponds to about 7·7 kPa (58 mm Hg) Po_2, a level which many would consider unacceptable. Absence of cyanosis does not necessarily mean normal arterial oxygen levels.

PRINCIPLES OF MEASUREMENT OF OXYGEN LEVELS
(see review by Wilson and Laver, 1972)

Oxygen concentration in gas samples

For many years the use of the Haldane apparatus, or its modification by Lloyd (Cormack, 1972), has been the standard method of measurement of oxygen concentrations in physiological gas samples. Recently, analysers working on the paramagnetic properties of oxygen (Pauling, Wood and Sturdivant, 1946) have attained a degree of accuracy and reliability which has enabled them to supplant the older chemical methods of analysis (Nunn et al., 1964; Ellis and Nunn, 1968). A particularly attractive feature of the method is that interference by other gases likely to be present in anaesthetized patients does not cause major inaccuracies and, if particularly high accuracy is required, correction factors may be employed. The apparatus manufactured by Servomex Controls Ltd. has proved to be reliable and is based on a robust measuring cell developed by the Distillers Company. Fuel cells have recently been introduced for analysis of oxygen in gas mixtures (Weil, Sodal and Speck, 1967).

Measurement of breath-to-breath changes in oxygen concentrations of respired gases requires an instrument with a response time of less than about 300 ms. Formerly the only suitable technique for oxygen measurement was the mass spectrometer (Fowler and Hugh-Jones, 1957). However, a number of alternative methods have now been described although their use has remained limited at the time of writing. The first of these was a modification of the polarograph (Severinghaus, 1963), followed by a fast-response version of the Servomex DCL 83 paramagnetic oxygen analyser (Cunningham, Kay and Young, 1965). A hitherto unapplied principle was employed in the oxygen-sensitive solid electrochemical cell described by Elliot, Segger and Osborn (1966). All of these instruments are capable of giving a continuous indication of the oxygen concentration of respired gases from which it is possible to observe the end-expiratory concentration.

Oxygen content of blood samples

The older chemical methods are those of Van Slyke and Neill (1924) and Haldane (1920). Gregory (1973) has described a technique for assessment of the accuracy of the Van Slyke apparatus against hydrogen peroxide. There was no significant systematic error, but random error was in the range of ±0.3 ml/100 ml. More recently, the Natelson apparatus (1951) appears a simpler alternative to the Van Slyke manometric apparatus but many have found it unexpectedly difficult to obtain reliable results for oxygen content.

Still more recently, the polarographic method of measurement of Po_2 (*see* page 422) has been utilized to measure oxygen content. Chemically combined oxygen is liberated from blood by saponin-ferricyanide solution and the Po_2 of the resultant solution is proportional to the oxygen content of the blood sample (Linden, Ledsome and Norman, 1965). This method is uninfluenced by the presence of inhalational anaesthetic agents, and has proved to be simple, accurate and reliable.

The latest technique for determination of content uses a fuel cell for measurement of evolved oxygen. Satisfactory results have been reported by Kusumi, Butts and Ruff (1973), but Selman, White and Tait (1975) obtained 95 per cent confidence limits of ±2 ml/100 ml in comparison with the Van Slyke.

Blood oxygen saturation

The classical method of measurement of saturation is in the form of the ratio of content to capacity (with dissolved oxygen subtracted from each):

$$\text{saturation} = \frac{HbO_2}{Hb + HbO_2} = \frac{\text{oxygen content} - \text{dissolved oxygen}}{\text{oxygen capacity} - \text{dissolved oxygen}}$$

Oxygen capacity is determined as the content after saturation of the blood by exposure to oxygen.

Nowadays, it is more usual to measure saturation photoelectrically. Methods are based on the fact that the absorption of monochromatic light of wavelength 805 nm is the same for reduced and oxygenated haemoglobin. At other wavelengths (particularly 650 nm) there is a marked difference between the absorption of transmitted or reflected light by the two forms of haemoglobin (Zijlstra, 1958). Various devices are marketed which depend upon the simultaneous absorption of light at these two wavelengths and so indicate the saturation directly. Unfortunately, these instruments tend to be used uncritically and their calibration is seldom checked for the simple reason that such a check is a difficult and time-consuming operation.

Saturation may be derived from PO_2. This is reasonably accurate above a PO_2 of about 7·3 kPa (55 mm Hg) where the dissociation curve is flat. However, it is inaccurate at lower tensions since, on the steep part of the curve, the saturation changes by 3 per cent for a tension change of 0·13 kPa (1 mm Hg).

At a superficial glance the concept of saturation appears simple enough. However, on further consideration there are seen to be difficulties which cannot easily be overcome. They arise chiefly from the presence of abnormal forms and compounds of haemoglobin. Methaemoglobin is usually present as about 5 per cent of total haemoglobin, and carboxyhaemoglobin may be as high as 10 per cent of total haemoglobin in smokers.

Blood PO_2

Four methods of measurement are available.

1. A tiny bubble of gas may be equilibrated with blood at the patient's body temperature and then analysed quantitatively for oxygen (Riley, Campbell and Shepard, 1957). PO_2 is derived from the oxygen concentration of the bubble. The technique is difficult and inaccurate when the PO_2 is more than 12·7 kPa (95 mm Hg). It cannot be used in the presence of anaesthetic gases.

2. If the dissociation curve is known, the PO_2 may be derived from the saturation (*see* above). This method is quite accurate on the steep part of the dissociation curve, but is of limited value when the PO_2 is more than 7·3 kPa (55 mm Hg) and quite inaccurate when the PO_2 is over about 11·3 kPa (85 mm Hg).

3. PO_2 of blood is directly proportional to the oxygen content of the plasma. This relationship may be used for deriving PO_2 from content, provided that blood can be separated anaerobically without change in the distribution of oxygen between plasma and erythrocytes. The solubility of oxygen in the patient's plasma must be accurately known. The method is difficult because of the small quantities of oxygen dissolved in plasma. However, Stark and Smith (1960) successfully used the method of Smith

and Pask (1959) for measuring plasma oxygen content and derived values for blood Po₂ in a pioneer study.

4. Since 1960, polarography has virtually displaced all other methods of measurement of blood Po_2. This technique has been of immense value in anaesthesia since it is uninfluenced by the presence of anaesthetic agents. It has been used both for research and for the management of patients who present difficult problems of oxygenation. The apparatus consists essentially of a cell formed by a silver anode and a platinum cathode, both in contact with an electrolyte in dilute solution. If a potential difference of about 700 millivolts is applied to the cell, a current is passed which is directly proportional to the Po_2 of the electrolyte in the region of the cathode. In use, the electrolyte is separated from the sample by a thin membrane which is permeable to oxygen. The electrolyte thus attains the same Po_2 as the sample and the current passed by the cell is proportional to the Po_2 of the sample, which may be gas, blood or other liquids. A disturbing source of error in the polarographic measurement of blood Po_2 is the difference in reading between blood and gas of the same Po_2. Estimates of the ratio vary between 1·0 and 1·17 but it may change unexpectedly due to changes in the position of the membrane. This error may be avoided by calibration with tonometer-equilibrated blood, but some workers prefer to calibrate on gas and then use a correction factor. A third approach is to calibrate with a solution of 30 per cent glycerol in water. This solution gives the same reading as blood of the same Po_2. Studies of the performance of polarographs for the measurement of blood Po_2 include those by Polgar and Forster (1960), Staub (1961) and Bishop et al. (1966). The subject has been reviewed with special reference to anaesthesia by Laver and Seifen (1965) and Adams, Morgan-Hughes and Sykes (1967).

The major errors in the measurement of blood oxygen levels usually arise from faulty sampling and handling of the sample (Nunn, 1962b) and from failure to correct for differences in temperature between the patient and the measurement system. The following points require attention.

1. The blood sample must be collected without exposure to air.
2. Oxygen is consumed by blood (Greenbaum et al., 1967), and avoidance of error due to the consequent fall in Po_2 after sampling requires one of the following actions:
   a. immediate analysis after sampling;
   b. storage of sampled blood at $0°C$;
   c. application of a correction factor for oxygen consumed during the interval between sampling and analysis (*see Figure 145*).
   (The first is the most satisfactory method.)
3. If blood Po_2 is measured at a lower temperature than the patient, the measured Po_2 will be less than the Po_2 of the blood while it was in the patient. It is often difficult to maintain the measuring apparatus at the patient's body temperature, and significant error results from a temperature difference of more than about 1 degree C. Correction is possible but the factor is variable depending upon the saturation (Nunn et al., 1965a). A convenient nomogram has been described by Kelman and Nunn (1966b) and is included in Appendix D as *Figure 146.*

Cutaneous oximetry

On superficial acquaintance, cutaneous oximetry appears an attractive alternative to direct measurement of arterial oxygen levels. The blood which is visualized by the apparatus is venous or capillary rather than arterial and the method is, therefore, dependent upon a brisk blood flow being maintained through the skin. Perhaps the most serious objection is that the apparatus is usually standardized according to a routine provided by the manufacturers and few users calibrate the apparatus against measurements on arterial blood. An indirect method of calibration suggested by Campbell (unpublished) has been described by Nunn et al. (1965b). Generally speaking arterial puncture and direct measurement of oxygen levels is no more difficult and a great deal more reliable.

Measurement of mixed venous Po_2

The usual method of measurement of mixed venous Po_2 (or oxygen content) is to sample blood from the right ventricle or pulmonary artery and analyse it according to the methods described above. It has, however, been suggested that a rebreathing technique might be used to derive mixed venous Po_2 indirectly along the same lines as the Campbell and Howell technique for measurement of mixed venous Pco_2 (page 373). The technique for oxygen was described by Cerretelli et al. (1966) and requires the rebreathing of a mixture of carbon dioxide in nitrogen. This procedure causes a reduction of the arterial Po_2 which, although of short duration, may be unacceptable for some patients. There is, however, a more serious objection to the method. Calculations show that the cardiac output in most patients will not be sufficiently high for the alveolar Po_2 to be brought into equilibrium with the mixed venous Po_2 in one circulation time (Spence and Ellis, 1971). Furthermore, the change in alveolar Po_2 is likely to be so slow that there may be a false impression that equilibrium has been attained.

Indirect methods of measurement of arterial Po_2

Unfortunately, indirect methods of measurement of arterial Po_2 are of limited value in the healthy subject, and of no value in the anaesthetized patient or in patients with respiratory disease. The arterial/venous Po_2 difference is so large that the rebreathing method of measurement of mixed venous Po_2 (*see* above) is valueless for indirect assessment of the arterial Po_2. The end-expiratory Po_2 differs from the arterial Po_2 in patients with increased alveolar dead space, for reasons identical to those producing a difference in the Pco_2 (page 226); End-expiratory Po_2 will not therefore indicate the actual level of arterial Po_2 during anaesthesia, although it may give some indication of changes. Cutaneous venous or capillary blood Po_2 may, under ideal conditions, be close to the arterial Po_2, but a modest reduction in skin perfusion will cause a substantial fall in Po_2 since the oxygen is consumed at a point on the dissociation curve where small changes in content correspond to large changes in tension. Unsatisfactory correlation between arterial and 'arterialized' venous Po_2 has been reported by Forster et al. (1972). For these reasons, if a reliable indication of the arterial Po_2

is required, there appears to be no alternative to arterial puncture and direct measurement.

Tissue Po_2

Clearly the tissue Po_2 is of greater significance than the Po_2 at various intermediate stages higher in the oxygen cascade. It would therefore appear to be logical to attempt the measurement of Po_2 in the tissues, but this has proved difficult both in technique and in interpretation. Difficulties of measurement arise from the extremely small size of the polarographic electrode which is needed to avoid excessive damage to the tissues. Difficulties of interpretation arise from the fact that Po_2 varies from one cell to another and from one part of a cell to another, the most important factor being the relation of the electrode to the capillaries (*Figure 109*). The significance of measurements of tissue Po_2 depends upon the precise location of the electrode and the degree of damage caused by its insertion: this requires meticulous attention to detail. Cater et al. (1961) have inserted electrodes by a stereotaxic technique, fixed the tissues before removal and then examined serial sections cut along the track of the electrode to determine its position in relation to blood vessels and to exclude the possibility of a haematoma around the tip of the electrode.

Such are the difficulties of measurement of tissue Po_2 that many prefer to measure the venous Po_2 of blood draining a particular tissue. Even the significance of this measurement is not entirely clear, but the venous Po_2 is roughly related to the mean pressure head of oxygen for diffusion into the cells of the area drained by the blood.

Oxygen consumption

Oxygen consumption may be measured either as the loss of oxygen from a closed rebreathing system or, more accurately, by the subtraction of the quantity of oxygen exhaled from the quantity inhaled. Measurement of the minute volume and the concentration of oxygen in the inspired and expired gas presents no great difficulty and the main problem centres on the measurement of the difference between the inspired and expired minute volumes. This is easy enough when a patient is in equilibrium with the nitrogen in ambient air but, when he is breathing an artificial gas mixture, the difficulties increase (Nunn and Pouliot, 1962).

Appendix A

PHYSICAL QUANTITIES AND UNITS OF MEASUREMENT

SI units

At the time of going to press we are in a state of transition from old to new metric units. The old system was based on the centimetre-gram-second (CGS) and was supplemented with many non-coherent derived units such as the millimetre of mercury for pressure and the calorie for work which could not be related to the basic units by factors which were powers of ten. The new system, the Système Internationale or SI, is based on the metre-kilogram-second (MKS) and comprises base and derived units which are obtained simply by multiplication or division without the introduction of numbers, not even powers of ten.

Base units are metre (length), kilogram (mass), second (time), ampere (electric current), kelvin (thermodynamic temperature), mole (amount of substance) and candela (luminous intensity).

Derived units include newton (force—kilograms metre second^{-1}), pascal (pressure—newton metre^{-2}), joule (work—newton metre) and hertz (periodic frequency—second^{-1}).

Special non-SI units are recognized as having sufficient practical importance to warrant retention for general or specialized use. These include litre, day, hour, minute and the standard atmosphere.

Non-recommended units include the dyne, bar and calorie and gravity-dependent units such as the kilogram-force, centimetre of water and millimetre of mercury, which are expected to disappear within a few years.

The introduction of SI units into anaesthesia and respiratory physiology has been reviewed by Padmore and Nunn (1974). While it is still too early to define the full extent of the change of units, it is clear that the kilopascal will replace the millimetre of mercury for blood-gas tensions. Its introduction for fluid pressures in the medical field is being delayed for, what appears to the author, an entirely specious attachment to the mercury or water manometer. The scale on a sphygmomanometer or central venous pressure manometer can easily be engraved to read kilopascals and we appear to be condemned to a further period during which we record arterial pressure in mm Hg, venous pressure in cm H_2O, cerebrospinal fluid pressure in mm H_2O and, in the author's intensive therapy unit, a suction pump calibrated in cm Hg. The existing situation would be less dangerous if all staff knew the relationship between a millimetre of mercury and a centimetre of water.

The replacement of the calorie by the joule should end the confusion between the calorie and the Calorie. It is not yet clear whether the 'amount of substance' (mol) will replace the gas volume in expressions of, for example, oxygen consumption. This transition would be fairly inconvenient. It is likely that the litre will replace the '100 ml' as the reference quantity of a liquid.

In this book, both SI and old units are given in situations in which the change is likely to be made in the life of this edition. It is hoped that text and figures can be read with equal facility by those accustomed to each system. Conversion factors are listed below (*Table 39*). For the physical quantities listed below, the

Table 39 CONVERSION FACTORS FOR UNITS OF MEASUREMENT

Force	
1 N (newton)	$= 10^5$ dyn
Pressure	
1 kPa (kilopascal)	$= 7\cdot50$ mm Hg
	$= 10\cdot2$ cm H_2O
	$= 0\cdot009\ 87$ standard atmospheres
	$= 10\ 000$ dyn/sq. cm (microbars)
1 standard atmosphere	$= 101\cdot3$ kPa
	$= 760$ mm Hg
	$= 1\ 033$ cm H_2O
1 mm Hg (almost equal to the torr)	$= 1\cdot36$ cm H_2O
Compliance	
1 l kPa^{-1} s	$= 0\cdot098$ l/cm H_2O
Flow resistance	
1 kPa l^{-1} s	$= 10\cdot2$ cm H_2O/l/s
Work	
1 J (joule)	$= 0\cdot102$ kilopond metres
	$= 0\cdot239$ calories
Power	
1 W (watt)	$= 1$ J s^{-1}
Surface tension	
1 N m^{-1} (newton/metre or pascal metre)	$= 1\ 000$ dyn/cm
Note: 1 mN m^{-1}	$= 1$ dyn/cm
Amount of substance	
1 mmol of oxygen	$= 22\cdot39$ ml (STPD)
1 mmol of carbon dioxide	$= 22\cdot26$ ml (STPD)

In the figures and text of this book 1 kPa has been taken to equal $7\cdot5$ mm Hg or 10 cm H_2O

dimensions are given in mass/length/time (MLT) units. These units provide a most useful check of the validity of equations and other expressions which are derived in the course of studies of respiratory function. Only quantities with identical MLT units can be added or subtracted and the units must be the same on the two sides of an equation.

Volume (dimensions: L^3)

In this book we are concerned with volumes of blood and gas. Strict SI units would be cubic metres and submultiples. However, the litre (l) and millilitre (ml) are recognized as special non-SI units and will remain in use. For practical purposes, we may ignore changes in the volume of liquids which are caused by changes of temperature. However, the changes in volume of gases caused by changes of temperature or pressure are by no means negligible and constitute an important source of error if they are ignored. Gas volumes are usually measured at ambient (or environmental) temperature and pressure, either dry (as from a cylinder passing through a rotameter) or saturated with water vapour at ambient temperature (e.g. an expired gas sample). Customary abbreviations are ATPD (ambient temperature and pressure, dry) and ATPS (ambient temperature and pressure, saturated).

It is not good practice to report gas volumes under the conditions prevailing during their measurement. In the case of oxygen uptake, carbon dioxide output and the exchange of 'inert' gases, we need to know the actual quantity (i.e. number of molecules) of gas exchanged and this is most conveniently expressed by stating the gas volume as it would be under standard conditions; i.e. $0°C$, 101.3 kPa (760 mm Hg) pressure and dry (STPD). Conversion from ATPS to STPD is by application of Charles' and Boyle's law (*see* page 1). A table of conversion factors is given in Appendix B. In the case of volumes which relate to anatomical measurements (e.g. vital capacity, tidal volume and dead space) it is necessary to express gas volumes as they would be at body temperature and pressure, saturated with water vapour (BTPS). Conversion from ATPS to BTPS is also based on Charles' and Boyle's law and factors are listed in Appendix B.

Amount of substance (dimensionless)

In clinical chemistry there is a progressive move towards reporting concentrations in terms of 'amount of substance' concentration (mmol l^{-1}) in place of mass concentration (mg/100 ml). In the respiratory field this may be extended to gases and vapours. For an ideal gas, 1 mmol corresponds to 22.4 ml and this figure applies to oxygen and nitrogen. For non-ideal gases such as nitrous oxide and carbon dioxide the figure is reduced to 22.25.

Gas concentrations may be expressed as mmol/l and for a mixture of ideal gases the sum of the concentrations of the components would be 44.6 mmol/l at standard temperature and pressure (dry). The advantages and disadvantages of expressing gas concentrations in terms of millimoles have been reviewed by Piiper et al. (1971). If haemoglobin is expressed as millimoles of the monomer, then 1 mmol of haemoglobin combines with 1 mmol of oxygen.

Fluid flow rate (dimensions: L^3/T, i.e. L^3T^{-1})

In the case of liquids, flow rate is the physical quantity of cardiac output, regional blood flow, etc. The strict SI units would be metre^3 second^{-1}, but litres per minute (l/min) and millilitres per minute (ml/min) are special non-SI units which may be retained. For gases, the dimension is applied to the delivery rate of fresh gases in anaesthetic gas circuits, minute volume of respiration, oxygen consumption, etc. The units are the same as those for liquids except that litres per second are used for the high instantaneous flow rates which occur during the course of inspiration and expiration.

In the case of gas flow rates, just as much attention should be paid to the matter of temperature and pressure as when volumes are being measured. Measurement is usually made at ambient temperature, but gas exchange rates are reported after correction to STPD, while ventilatory gas flow rates should be corrected to BTPS. As a very rough rule, gas volumes at STPD are about 10 per cent less than at ATPS, while volumes at BTPS are about 10 per cent more.

Force (dimensions: MLT^{-2}) (LT^{-2} or L/T^2 are the units of acceleration)

In respiratory physiology we are chiefly concerned with force in relation to pressure, which is force per unit area. An understanding of the units of force is essential to an understanding of the units of pressure. Force, when applied to a free body, causes it to change either the magnitude or the direction of its velocity.

The units of force are of two types. The first is the force resulting from the action of gravity on a mass and is synonymous with weight. It includes the kilogram-force and the pound-force (as in the pound per square inch). All such units are non-recommended under the SI and will disappear. The second type of unit of force is absolute and does not depend on the magnitude of the gravitational field. In the CGS system, the absolute unit of force was the dyne and this has been replaced under the MKS system and the SI by the newton (N) which is defined as the force which will give a mass of 1 kilogram an acceleration 1 metre per second per second.

$$1 \text{ N} = 1 \text{ kg m s}^{-2}$$

Pressure (dimensions: MLT^{-2}/L^2, i.e. $ML^{-1}T^{-2}$)

Pressure is defined as force per unit area. The SI unit is the pascal (Pa) which is 1 newton per square metre.

$$1 \text{ Pa} = 1 \text{ N m}^{-2}$$

The pascal is inconveniently small (one ten-thousandth of an atmosphere) and the kilopascal (kPa) has been adopted for general use in the medical field. Its introduction is simplified by the fact that the kPa is very close to 1 per cent of an atmosphere. Thus a standard atmosphere is 101·3 kPa and the Po_2 in dry air is very close to 21 kPa; 1 kPa is also approximately equal to 10 cm water. The kilopascal will replace the millimetre of mercury and the centimetre of water, both of which are gravity-based. The centimetre of water can be considered as the pressure at the bottom of a centimetre cube of water which would be one gram-force acting on a square centimetre.

The standard atmosphere may continue to be used under SI. It is defined as $1·013\ 25 \times 10^5$ pascals.

The torr came into use only shortly before the move towards SI units. This is unfortunate, for the memory of Torricelli as the torr will disappear from use. The torr is defined as exactly equal to 1/760 of a standard atmosphere and it is therefore very close to the millimetre of mercury, the two units being considered identical for practical purposes. The only distinction is that the torr is absolute, while the millimetre of mercury is gravity-based.

The bar is the absolute unit of pressure in the old CGS system and is defined as 10^6 dyn/sq cm. The unit was convenient because the bar is close to 1 atmosphere (1·013 bars) and a millibar is close to 1 centimetre of water (0·9806 millibars).

Compliance (dimensions: $M^{-1}L^4T^2$)

The term 'compliance' is used in respiratory physiology to denote the volume change of the lungs in response to a change of pressure. The dimensions are therefore volume divided by pressure and the commonest units have been litres (or millilitres) per centimetre of water. It is likely that this will change to litres per kilopascal (l/kPa). Elastance is the reciprocal of compliance.

Resistance to fluid flow (dimensions: $ML^{-4}T^{-1}$)

Under conditions of laminar flow (Chapter 4) it is possible to express resistance to gas flow as the ratio of pressure difference to gas flow rate. This is analogous to electrical resistance which is expressed as the ratio of potential difference to current flow. The dimensions of resistance to gas flow are pressure difference divided by gas flow rate, and typical units in the respiratory field have been cm H_2O/litre/second or dynes sec cm^{-5} in absolute units. Appropriate SI units will probably be kilopascals $litre^{-1}$ second (kPa l^{-1} s).

Work (dimensions: ML^2T^{-2}, derived from MLT^{-2} x L or $ML^{-1}T^{-2}$ x L^3)

Work is done when a force moves its point of application or gas is moved in response to a pressure gradient. The dimensions are therefore either force times distance or pressure times volume, in each case simplifying to ML^2T^{-2}. The multiplicity of units of work has caused confusion in the past. Under SI, the erg, calorie and kilopond-metre will disappear in favour of the joule, which is defined as the work done when a force of 1 newton moves its point of application 1 metre. It is also the work done when a litre of gas moves in response to a pressure gradient of 1 kilopascal. This represents a welcome simplification.

$$1 J = 1 N m = 1 l kPa$$

The kilojoule will replace the kilocalorie in metabolism.

Power (dimensions: ML^2T^{-2}/T, i.e. ML^2T^{-3})

Power is the rate at which work is done and so has the dimensions of work divided by time. The SI unit is the watt, which equals 1 joule per second. Power is the correct dimension for the rate of continuous expenditure of biological energy, although one talks loosely about the 'work of breathing', for example (Chapter 6). This is incorrect and 'power of breathing' is the correct term.

Surface tension (dimensions: MLT^{-2}/L, i.e. MT^{-2})

Surface tension has become important to the respiratory physiologist since the realization of the part it plays in the 'elastic' recoil of the lungs (page 72). The CGS units of surface tension are dynes per centimetre (of interface). The appropriate SI unit would be the newton per metre. This has the following rather curious relationships:

$$1 \text{ N/m} = 1 \text{ Pa m} = 1 \text{ kg/s}^2$$

The unit for surface tension is likely to be called the pascal metre (Pa m) which is identical to the newton per metre. A millinewton per metre (or a millipascal metre) is identical in value to the familiar CGS unit, the dyn/cm.

General notes

The symbol for second is now changed from sec to s. In the case of temperature, the symbol $^{\circ}C$ now represents degrees Celsius and not degrees Centigrade. The values are identical.

Division may be indicated by a solidus (/) provided that only one is used. For example, m/s and m s^{-1} are equally correct for metres per second. In expressions with more than two terms, confusion may be avoided by the exclusive use of negative indices (*see* Padmore and Nunn, 1974).

Appendix B

CONVERSION FACTORS FOR GAS VOLUMES

Conversion factors for gas volumes—ATPS to BTPS

Gas volumes measured by spirometry and other methods usually indicate the volume at ambient temperature and pressure, saturated (ATPS). Tidal volume, minute volume, dead space, lung volumes, etc., should be converted to the volumes as they would be in the lungs of the patient at body temperature and pressure, saturated (BTPS).

Table 40 FACTORS FOR CONVERSION OF GAS VOLUMES MEASURED UNDER CONDITIONS OF AMBIENT TEMPERATURE AND PRESSURE, SATURATED (ATPS) TO THE VOLUMES WHICH WOULD BE OCCUPIED UNDER CONDITIONS OF BODY TEMPERATURE AND PRESSURE, SATURATED (BTPS)

Ambient temperature (°C)	Conversion factor	Saturated water vapour pressure	
		kPa	mm Hg
15	1·129	1·71	12·8
16	1·124	1·81	13·6
17	1·119	1·93	14·5
18	1·113	2·07	15·5
19	1·108	2·20	16·5
20	1·103	2·33	17·5
21	1·097	2·48	18·6
22	1·092	2·64	19·8
23	1·086	2·80	21·0
24	1·081	2·99	22·4
25	1·075	3·16	23·7
26	1·069	3·66	25·2

Derivation of correction factors:

$$\text{volume }_{\text{(BTPS)}} = \text{volume }_{\text{(ATPS)}} \left(\frac{273 + 37}{273 + t}\right) \left(\frac{P_B - P_{H_2O}}{P_B - 6\cdot3}\right)$$

P_B is barometric pressure and the table has been prepared for a barometric pressure of 100 kPa (750 mm Hg): variations within the range 99–101 kPa (740–760 mm Hg) gave a negligible effect upon the factors.

t is ambient temperature (°C). The table has been prepared for a body temperature of 37°C: variations within the range 35–39°C are of small importance.

P_{H_2O} is the water vapour pressure of the sample (kPa).

451

Conversion factors for gas volumes—ATPS to STPD

Measurement of absolute amounts of gases (e.g. oxygen consumption) requires conversion of measured gas volumes to standard conditions (0°C, 101·3 kPa (760 mm Hg), dry). Under these conditions, one mole of an ideal gas occupies 22·4 litres.

Table 41 FACTORS FOR CONVERSION OF GAS VOLUMES MEASURED UNDER CONDITIONS OF AMBIENT TEMPERATURE AND PRESSURE, SATURATED (ATPS) TO THE VOLUMES WHICH WOULD BE OCCUPIED UNDER CONDITIONS OF STANDARD TEMPERATURE AND PRESSURE, DRY (STPD)–0°C, 101·3 kPa (760 mm Hg)

Ambient temperature ($^\circ$C)	Barometric pressure, kPa (mm Hg)			
	97·3 (730)	98·7 (740)	100 (750)	101·3 (760)
15	0·895	0·907	0·919	0·932
16	0·890	0·903	0·915	0·928
17	0·886	0·899	0·911	0·923
18	0·882	0·894	0·907	0·919
19	0·878	0·890	0·902	0·915
20	0·873	0·886	0·898	0·910
21	0·869	0·881	0·893	0·906
22	0·865	0·877	0·889	0·901
23	0·860	0·872	0·885	0·897
24	0·856	0·868	0·880	0·892
25	0·851	0·863	0·875	0·887
26	0·847	0·859	0·871	0·883

Derivation of correction factors:

$$\text{volume}_{(STPD)} = \text{volume}_{(ATPS)} \left(\frac{273}{273+t}\right)\left(\frac{P_B - P_{H_2O}}{101}\right)$$

P is barometric pressure (kPa).
t is ambient temperature.
P_{H_2O} is the saturated vapour pressure of water at ambient temperature (*see Table 40*).

Appendix C

Symbols

Symbols used in this book are in accord with the recommendations of the committee for standardization of definitions and symbols in respiratory physiology (Pappenheimer et al., 1950). The use of these symbols is very helpful for an understanding of the quantitative relationships which are so important in respiratory physiology.

Primary symbols (large capitals) denoting physical quantities.

>F   fractional concentration of gas
>P   pressure, tension or partial pressure of a gas
>V   volume of a gas
>Q   volume of blood
>C   content of a gas in blood
>S   saturation of haemoglobin with oxygen
>R   respiratory exchange ratio (RQ)
>D   diffusing capacity

denotes a time derivative; e.g. $\dot{V}$ ventilation
$$\dot{Q} \text{ blood flow}$$

Secondary symbols denoting location of quantity.

in gas phase (small capitals)	*in blood* (lower case)
I inspired gas	a arterial blood
E expired gas	v venous blood
A alveolar gas	c capillary
D dead space	t total
T tidal	s shunt
B barometric (usually pressure)	

¯ denotes mixed or mean; e.g. $\bar{v}$ mixed venous blood
$$\bar{E} \text{ mixed expired gas}$$
′ denotes end; e.g. E′ end-expiratory gas
$$c' \text{ end-capillary blood}$$

Tertiary symbols indicating particular gases.

O_2 oxygen
CO_2 carbon dioxide
N_2O nitrous oxide
etc.

f denotes the respiratory frequency

BTPS, ATPS and STPD, *see Appendix B*

Examples of respiratory symbols

PA_{O_2} alveolar oxygen tension
$C\bar{v}_{O_2}$ oxygen content of mixed venous blood
$\dot{V}_{O_2}$ oxygen consumption

The system is well adapted to the expression of quantitative relationships.

$$\dot{Q}\,(Ca_{O_2} - C\bar{v}_{O_2}) = \dot{V}_{O_2} \qquad \text{(Fick equation)}$$

$$VD = VE \left(\frac{Pa_{CO_2} - P\bar{E}_{CO_2}}{Pa_{CO_2}} \right) \qquad \text{(Bohr equation)}$$

$$R = \frac{\dot{V}_{CO_2}}{\dot{V}_{O_2}}$$

Definitions of words used in a special sense or which have little general use

Ambient: surrounding or environmental (e.g. room air)

Parameter: a quantity which is a constant in a particular relationship, but which varies from one relationship to another; e.g. a and b in the equation $y = a + bx$ (x and y are variables).

Variable: any quantity of which the value is likely to change; e.g. haemoglobin concentration might be considered as a variable over a number of days but as a parameter when a series of blood samples are drawn in rapid succession without there being a change of haemoglobin concentration. P_{O_2} would probably be a variable in both situations.

Phase: a continuous fluid medium. The lungs contain a gas phase and a blood phase, separated by the alveolar-capillary membrane.

Appendix D

NOMOGRAMS AND CORRECTION CHARTS

Blood-gas correction nomograms for time

This nomogram is designed for the application of corrections for metabolism occurring between sampling and analysis when blood at $37°C$ is drawn into a 5 ml glass or 2 ml plastic syringe at room temperature, followed by storage at room temperature. Elapsed time between sampling and analysis is shown on the ordinate. Line charts indicate the change in PCO_2 (which rises), pH (which falls) and base excess (which falls). A graph is required for the change in PO_2 (which falls) because the rate of fall depends upon the PO_2. For details, see Kelman and Nunn (1966b).

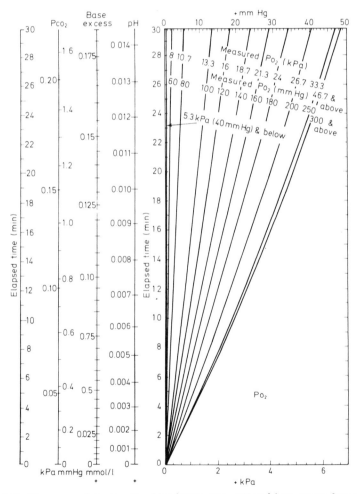

Figure 145. Nomogram for correcting blood PCO_2, PO_2, pH and base excess for metabolic changes occurring between sampling and analysis. (Reproduced from Kelman and Nunn (1966b) by courtesy of the Editors of the Journal of Applied Physiology)

Blood-gas correction nomogram for temperature

Enter with the patient's temperature on the abscissa. *Multiply* the measured gas tension by the factor shown on the ordinate, using the appropriate curve for Po_2 based on the saturation of the sample. The broken line should be used for Pco_2, whatever the level of Pco_2. The line chart at the top of the graph may be used for the pH correction which should be *added*. For details, see Kelman and Nunn (1966b).

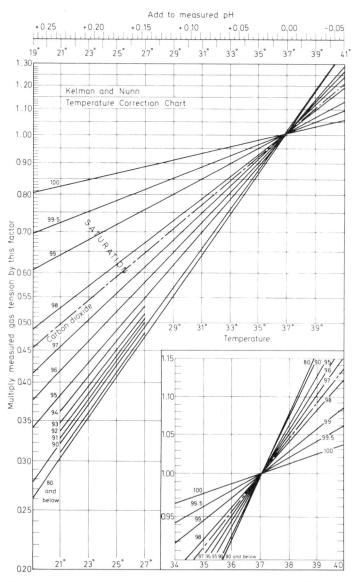

Figure 146. Nomogram for correction of blood PCO_2, PO_2 and pH for differences between temperature of patient and electrode system (assumed to be 37°C). (Reproduced from Kelman and Nunn (1966b) by courtesy of the Editors of the Journal of Applied Physiology)

Nomogram for haemoglobin dissociation curve

The right-hand line charts give corresponding values for Po_2 and saturation under standard conditions (temperature, 37° C; pH, 7·40; base excess, zero). The remaining lines indicate the factors by which the actual measured Po_2 should be multiplied to give the 'virtual Po_2' with which to enter the standard dissociation curve for determination of saturation. When more than one factor is required, they should be multiplied together (page 405).

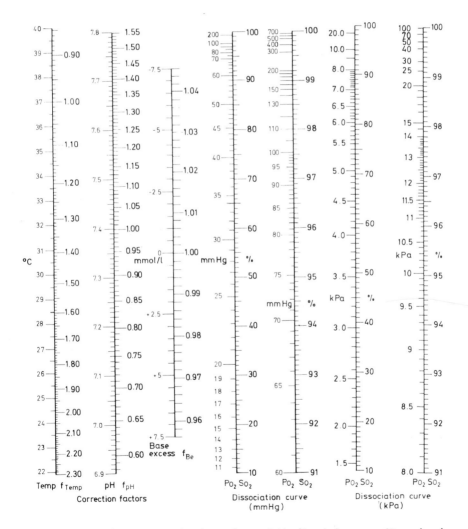

Figure 147. Line charts representing the oxyhaemoglobin dissociation curve. (Reproduced after Kelman and Nunn (1966b) by courtesy of the Editors of the Journal of Applied Physiology*)*

Nomogram for R.Q. and oxygen consumption

The respiratory exchange ratio of a patient breathing air may be determined from the concentrations of oxygen and carbon dioxide in the expired gas by using the left-hand section of the chart. Oxygen consumption may be determined from the mixed expired oxygen concentration and the volume of gas expired in 2 or 3 minutes, by using the right-hand section of the chart. The nomogram for calculation of the respiratory exchange ratio has only a very small error. The nomogram for calculating the oxygen consumption has an error of less than 10 ml/min if the respiratory exchange ratio is within the limits 0·7–0·9. For details, see Nunn (1972).

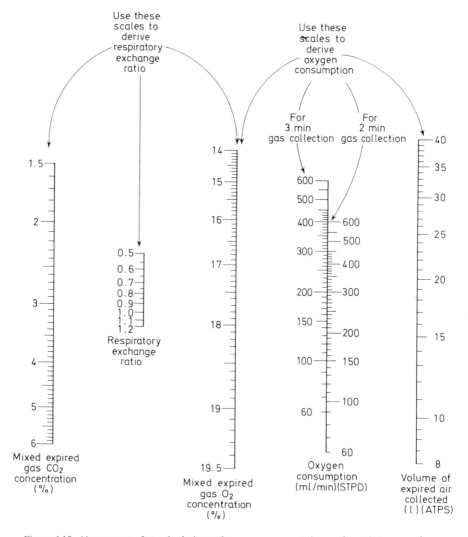

Figure 148. Nomograms for calculation of oxygen consumption and respiratory exchange ratio of a patient breathing air. (Reproduced from Nunn (1972) by courtesy of the Editor of the British Medical Journal)

The iso-shunt chart

Diagram of the theoretical relationship between arterial P_{O_2} and inspired oxygen concentration for different values of virtual shunt. The shaded areas enclose all relationships within the limits of haemoglobin concentration 10–14 g/100 ml and arterial P_{CO_2} 3·3–5·3 kPa (25–40 mm Hg). Virtual shunt is defined as the shunt which gives the relationships depicted when the arterial/mixed venous oxygen content difference is 5 ml/100 ml. For further details, *see* text (page 290) and Benatar, Hewlett and Nunn (1973).

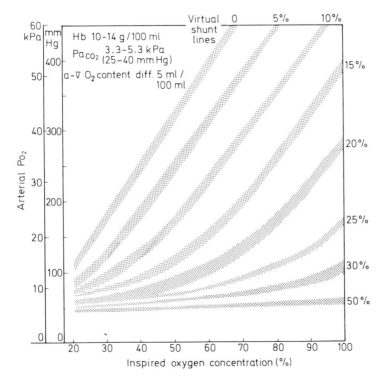

Figure 149. Iso-shunt lines for control of oxygen therapy. (Reproduced from Benatar, Hewlett and Nunn (1973) by courtesy of the Editor of the British Journal of Anaesthesia)

Air-oxygen mixing chart

This chart is used for determining air and oxygen flow rates required to give various total gas flow rates at various oxygen concentrations. Chart prepared by Dr A. M. Hewlett.

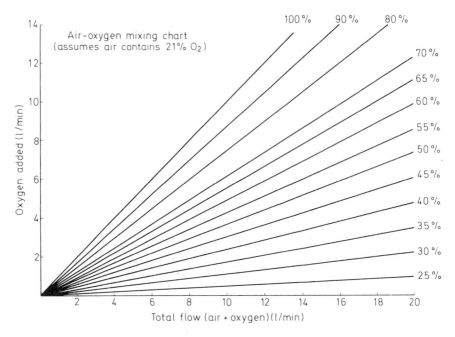

Figure 150. Air-oxygen mixing chart for oxygen therapy. (Reproduced from Richardson, Chinn and Nunn (1977) by courtesy of the Editor of British Journal of Anaesthesia*)*

Appendix E

THE EXPONENTIAL FUNCTION*

Examples of exponential functions recur throughout this book. They are, in fact, so common in biological systems that the exponential function is sometimes referred to as the law of organic growth.

The anaesthetist is deeply implicated in practical applications of exponential functions. The examples quoted below will show that much of this work is devoted to guiding certain variables of his patients along exponential curves. The success which attends his work depends to a large extent upon his skill in performing this task.

Many anaesthetists have had no formal instruction in exponential functions and lack much of the background knowledge which is needed for their comprehension. This is unfortunate since orthodox mathematical texts tend to proceed in an orderly manner with the assumption that the student has understood all that has gone before. It is, therefore, difficult for the anaesthetist to pick up a textbook of mathematics and 'read up exponential functions'. The best approach is without doubt a friendly mathematician. Failing that, the less orthodox books such as *Mathematics for the Million*, by Lancelot Hogben (1967), and *Calculus Made Easy*, by Silvanus P. Thompson (1965), will be found helpful.

General statement

An exponential function describes a change in which the rate of change of one variable, in relation to the other, is proportional to the magnitude of the first variable. Thus, if y varies with respect to x, the rate of change of y with respect to x (i.e. dy/dx)† varies in proportion to the value of y at that instant. That is to say;

$$\frac{dy}{dx} = ky$$

where k is a constant.

This general equation appears with minor modifications in three main forms. To the biological worker they may be conveniently described as the tear-away, the wash-out and the wash-in.

_____

* *See also* Waters and Mapleson (1964).

† dy/dx is the mathematical shorthand for rate of change of y with respect to x. The 'd' means 'a very small bit of'; dy/dx thus means a very small bit of y divided by a very small bit of x. This is equal to the slope of the graph of y against x at that point. In the case of a curve, it is the slope of a tangent drawn to the curve at that point.

THE TEAR-AWAY EXPONENTIAL FUNCTION

This must be described first as it is the simplest form of the exponential function. It is, however, the least important of the three to the anaesthetist.

Simple statement

In a tear-away exponential function, the quantity under consideration increases at a rate which is in direct proportion to its actual value—the richer one is, the faster one makes money.

Examples

Classical examples are compound interest, and the mythical water-lily which doubles its diameter every day (*Figure 151*). A typical biological example is the free spread of a bacterial colony in which (for example) each bacterium divides every 20 minutes. The doubling time of this example would be 20 minutes.

Mathematical statement

By convention we consider y as the quantity which is changing in relation to x. However, for the anaesthetist, x almost invariably represents time and so we shall take the liberty of replacing x with t throughout. The tear-away function may thus be represented as follows:

$$\frac{dy}{dt} = ky$$

A little mathematical processing will convert this equation into a more useful form, which will indicate the instantaneous value of y at any time, t.

First multiply both sides by dt/y:

$$\frac{1}{y} dy = k \, dt$$

Next integrate both sides with respect to t:

$$\log_e y^* + C_1 = kt + C_2$$

(C_1 and C_2 are constants of integration and may be collected on the right-hand side.)

$$\log_e y = (C_2 - C_1) + kt$$

Finally, take antilogs of each side to the base e:

$$y = e^{(C_2 - C_1)} \times e^{kt}$$

At zero time, $t = 0$ and $e^{kt} = 1$. Therefore the constant $e^{(C_2 - C_1)}$ equals the initial value of y which we may call y_0. Our final equation is thus:

$$y = y_0 \, e^{kt}$$

* This is a difficult step for most of us. See Thompson (1965).

y_0 is the initial value of the variable y at zero time.

e is the base of natural or Napierian logarithms (discovered in 1619 before the circulation of the blood was known). This constant (2·718 28...) possesses many remarkable properties which are lucidly expounded by Hogben (1967).

k is a constant which defines the speed of the particular function. For example, it will differ by a factor of two if our mythical water-lily doubles its size every 12 hours instead of every day. In the case of the wash-out and wash-in, we shall see that k is directly related to certain important physiological

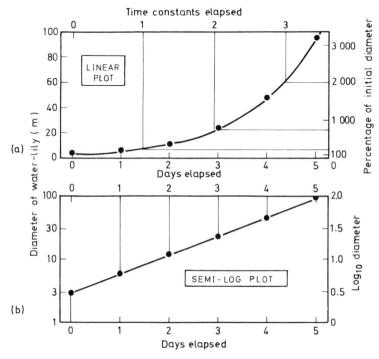

Figure 151. The growth of a water-lily which doubles its diameter every day—a typical tear-away exponential function. Initial diameter, 3 metres; size doubled every day (i.e. doubling time = 1 day). Compare the figures in the table below with those in Table 42

	Elapsed time (days)	Diameter of water-lily	
		metres	percentage of initial diameter
Diameter of water-lily = $3e^{t/1·44}$	0	3	100
(t is measured in days, diameter in metres)	1	6	200
	1·44	6·5	217
	2	12	400
	2·88	22·2	739
	3	24	800
	4	48	1 600
	4·32	60·3	2 009
	5	96	3 200

quantities, from which we may predict the speed of certain biological changes.

To many of us, e is unfamiliar and fairly alarming. We may, if we wish avoid it by using the more familiar base 10:

$$y = y_0 10^{k_1 t}$$

This is a perfectly valid way of expressing a tear-away exponential function, but you will notice that the constant k has changed to k_1. This new constant does *not* have the simple relationships of physiological variables mentioned above. It does, however, bear a constant relationship to k, as follows:

$$k_1 = 0.4343k \quad \text{(approx.)}$$

When an exponential function is considered to proceed by steps of whole numbers, it is known as a geometrical progression.

Graphical representation

On linear graph paper, a tear-away exponential functional rapidly disappears off the top of the paper (*Figure 151*). If plotted on semi-logarithmic paper (time on a linear axis and y on a logarithmic axis), the plot becomes a straight line and this is a most convenient method of presenting such a function. The logarithmic plots in *Figures 151–153* are all plotted on semi-log paper.

THE WASH-OUT OR DIE-AWAY EXPONENTIAL FUNCTION

The account of the tear-away exponential function has really been a curtain-raiser for the wash-out or die-away exponential function, which is of great importance to the biologist in general, and the anaesthetist in particular.

Simple statement

In a wash-out exponential function, the quantity under consideration falls at a rate which decreases progressively in proportion to the distance it still has to fall. It approaches but, in theory, never reaches zero.

Examples

Classical examples are cooling curves, radioactive decay and (nearer home) water running out of the bath. In the latter example the rate of flow down the plug-hole is proportional to the pressure of water, which is proportional to the depth of water in the bath, which in turn is proportional to the quantity of water in the bath (assuming that the sides are vertical). Therefore, the flow rate of water down the plug-hole is proportional to the amount of water left in the bath, and decreases as the bath empties. The last molecule of bath water takes an infinitely long time to drain away. A similar example is the mountaineer who each day ate half of the food which he carried. In this way he made his food last indefinitely.

Biological examples include:

1. Passive expiration (*Figure 152*)
2. The elimination of inhalational anaesthetics
3. The fall of arterial Pco_2 to its new level after a step increase in ventilation
4. The fall of arterial Po_2 to its new level after a step decrease in ventilation
5. The fall of blood Pco_2 towards the alveolar level as it progresses along the pulmonary capillary
6. The fall of blood Po_2 towards the tissue level as blood progresses through the tissue capillaries

Mathematical statement

When a quantity *decreases* with any time, the rate of change is *negative*. Therefore, the wash-out exponential function is written thus:

$$\frac{dy}{dt} = -ky$$

from which we may derive the following equations, which give the value of y at any time t.

$$y = y_0 \, e^{-kt}$$

which is simply another way of saying:

$$y = \frac{y_0}{e^{kt}}$$

y_0 is again the initial value of y at zero time. In *Figure 152* y_0 is the initial value of (lung volume−FRC) at the start of expiration; that is to say, the tidal volume inspired.

e is again the base of natural logarithms (2·718 28...).

k is the constant which defines the rate of decay, and really comes into its own in the wash-out exponential function. It is the reciprocal of a most important quantity known as the *time constant*. There are three things which should be known about the time constant.

1. *Figure 152* shows a tangent drawn to the first part of the curve. This shows the course events would take if the initial rate were maintained instead of slowing down in the manner characteristic of the wash-out curve. The time which would then be required for completion would be $1/k$ which is called the *time constant* and designated by the Greek letter *tau* (τ). The wash-out exponential function may thus be written:

$$y = y_0 \, e^{-t/\tau}$$

2. After one time constant, y will have fallen to $1/e$ of its original value. After two time constants, y will have fallen to $1/e^2$ of its initial value, and so on.
   After 1 time constant, y will have fallen to approximately 37 per cent of its initial value.
   After 2 time constants, y will have fallen to approximately $13\frac{1}{2}$ per cent of its initial value.

After 3 time constants, y will have fallen to approximately 5 per cent of
its initial value.

After 5 time constants, y will have fallen to approximately 1 per cent of
its initial value.

(More precise values are indicated in *Table 42*).

3. The time constant is often determined by physiological factors. When air

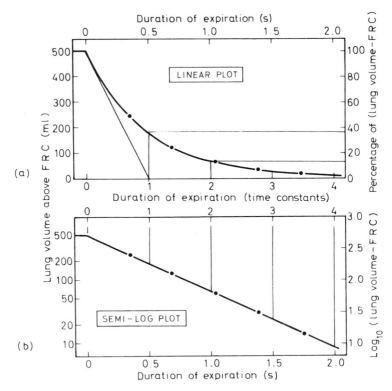

*Figure 152. Passive expiration—a typical wash-out exponential function. Tidal volume,
500 ml; compliance, 0·5 l/kPa (50 ml/cm H₂O); airway resistance 1 kPa l⁻¹ s (10 cm
H₂O/1000 ml/sec; time constant, 0·5 s; half-life, 0·35 s. The points on the curves indicate
the passage of successive half lives*

	Elapsed time (constants)	Lung volume remaining above FRC	
		ml	percentage of tidal volume
Lung volume above FRC $= 500e^{-(t/0\cdot5)}$	0	500	100
	0·69	250	50
	1	184	36·8
	2	67·5	13·5
	3	25	5·0
	4	9	1·8

*Note that the logarithmic co-ordinate has no zero. This accords with the lung volume
approaching, but never actually equalling, the FRC*

escapes passively from a distended lung, the time constant is governed by two variables, compliance and resistance (Chapters 3, 4 and 5).

Let V represent the lung volume (above FRC), then $-(dV/dt)$ is the instantaneous expiratory gas flow rate. Assuming Poiseuille's law is obeyed (page 96):

$$-\frac{dV}{dt} = \frac{P}{R}$$

when P is the instantaneous alveolar-to-mouth pressure gradient and R is the airway resistance.

But

$$\text{compliance } C = \frac{V}{P} \text{ (page 71)}$$

therefore

$$-\frac{dV}{dt} = \frac{1}{CR} V$$

or

$$\frac{dV}{dt} = -\frac{1}{CR} V$$

Then by integration and the taking of antilogs as described above:

$$V = V_0 e^{-(t/CR)}$$

By analogy with the general equation of the wash-out exponential function, it is clear that $CR = 1/k = \tau$ (the time constant). Thus the *time constant equals the product of compliance and resistance.*[*] This is analogous to the discharge of an electrical capacitor through a resistance, when the time constant of discharge equals the product of the capacitance and the resistance. Analysis of the passive expiration has been considered in greater detail on page 150 and by Bergman (1969).

Rather similar is the wash-out of anaesthetic from a body or organ. Here the 'capacitance' equals the product of the mass of the body or organ and the solubility in it of the agent. The agent's 'resistance' to escape is inversely related to ventilation, diffusion, blood flow, renal function, etc. In the more complex situations, wash-out curves remain exponential in form, but are compounded of a number of individual wash-out curves. Each has its own time constant which equals the product of capacitance (for the anaesthetic) and resistance (to wash-out) for each part. An example of the technique for separation of individual components from an over-all wash-out curve is the analysis of nitrogen clearance curves (Comroe et al., 1962).

Wash-out of a substance from an organ by perfusion with blood which is free of the substance is another example of a wash-out exponential function where the time constant may be stated in terms of certain physiological factors.

Let Q represent the volume of an organ and C be the concentration in the organ of a substance whose solubility in the organ equals its solubility in blood.

---

[*] It is strange at first sight that two quantities as complex as compliance and resistance should have a product which boils down to anything as simple as time. In fact the mass/length/time units check perfectly well (*see* Appendix A).

$$\text{compliance} \times \text{resistance} = \text{time}$$
$$M^{-1}L^4T^2 \times ML^{-4}T^{-1} = T$$

Imagine a small quantity of blood (dQ) to enter the organ. The concentration is then reduced by dC:

$$\frac{C - dC}{C} = \frac{Q + dQ}{Q}$$

Subtracting 1 from each side:

$$-\frac{dC}{C} = \frac{dQ}{Q}$$

If blood enters the organ at a constant rate, dQ/dt may be represented by $\dot{Q}$ (the usual symbol for blood flow rate). It then follows that:

$$-\frac{dC}{C} = \frac{\dot{Q}.dt}{Q}$$

and so

$$-\frac{dC}{dt} = \frac{\dot{Q}}{Q}C$$

from which if follows that:

$$C = C_o e^{-(\dot{Q}/Q)t}$$

Again, by analogy, it is clear that $Q/\dot{Q} = 1/k = \tau$ (the time constant). Thus the *time constant equals the tissue volume divided by its blood flow.*

Similarly, the time constant of wash-out of a substance from the alveolar gas equals the FRC divided by the alveolar ventilation (assuming that none of the substance crosses the alveolar-capillary membrane during the process, as is nearly true with helium, for example).

This important relationship is used in the nitrogen wash-out test of uniformity of intrapulmonary gas mixing, in which gas is considered as being washed out of two compartments, one fast and one slow. A compound wash-out curve is obtained and is subsequently analysed for different components (Comroe et al., 1962). It is also the basis of the Lassen and Ingvar (1961) technique for measurement of organ blood flow. The theory is delightfully simple. The time constant is determined for the wash-out of a freely diffusible radioactive substance from the organ. Since the reciprocal of the time constant equals the organ blood flow divided by the organ volume, the answer is immediately available in blood flow per unit volume of tissue (usually expressed as ml min^{-1} 100 ml of tissue). This again makes the assumption that the solubility of the substance is the same for blood and tissue. If it is not, a correction factor can easily be applied.

Half-life.   It is often convenient to use the half-life instead of the time constant. This is the time required for y to change by a factor of two (or a half). The special attraction of the half-life is its ease of measurement. The half-life of a radioactive element may be determined quite simply. First of all the degree of activity is measured and the time noted. Its activity is then followed and the time noted at which its activity is exactly half the initial value. The difference between the two times is the half-life and is constant at all levels of activity. Half-lives are shown in *Figures 151–153* as dots on the curves. For a particular exponential function there is a constant relationship between the time constant and the half-life.

Half-life = 0·69 times the *time constant*
Time constant = 1·44 times the *half-life*

(For practical purposes, the time constant is 1·5 times the half-life.)

Graphical representation

Plotting a wash-out exponential function is similar to the tear-away function (*Figure 152*). Semi-log paper may be used in the same way and is of considerable practical importance as the curve (being straight) may then be defined by far fewer observations. It is also easy to extrapolate backwards to zero time if the initial value is required but could not be measured directly for some reason. It is, for example, an essential step in the measurement of cardiac output with a dye which is rapidly lost from the circulation (page 271).

THE WASH-IN EXPONENTIAL FUNCTION

The wash-in function is of special importance to the anaesthetist and is the mirror image of the wash-out function.

Simple statement

In a wash-in exponential function, the quantity under consideration rises towards a limiting value, at a rate which decreases progressively in proportion to the distance it still has to rise.

Examples

A typical example would be a mountaineer who each day manages to climb half the remaining distance between his overnight camp and the summit of the mountain. His rate of ascent declines exponentially and he will never reach the summit. A graph of his altitude plotted against time would resemble a 'wash-in' curve.

Biological examples include the reverse of those listed for the wash-out function.

1. Inflation of the lungs of a paralysed patient by a sustained increase of mouth pressure (*Figure 153*).
2. The uptake of inhalational anaesthetics.
3. The rise of arterial P_{CO_2} to its new level after a step decrease of ventilation.
4. The rise or arterial P_{O_2} to its new level after a step increase of ventilation.

5. The rise of blood P_{O_2} to the alveolar level as it progresses along the pulmonary capillary.
6. The rise of blood P_{CO_2} to the venous level as blood progresses through the tissue capillaries.

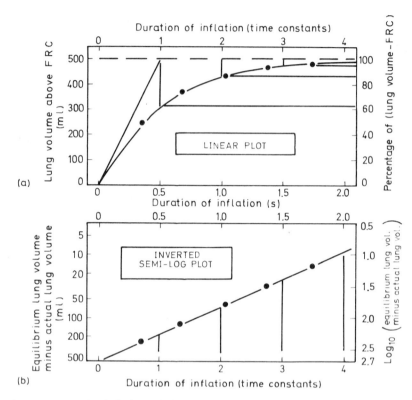

Figure 153. Passive inflation of the lungs with a sustained mouth pressure—a typical wash-in exponential function. Eventual tidal volume, 500 ml; compliance, 0·5 l/kPa (50 ml/cm H_2O); airway resistance, 1 kPa l^{-1} s (10 cm H_2O/1000 ml/sec; time constant, 0·5 s; half-life, 0·35 s. The points on the curves indicate the passage of successive half-lives.

	Elapsed time (constants)	Lung volume attained above FRC	
		ml	percentage of tidal volume
Lung volume above FRC $= 500 (1 - e^{-(t/0·5)})$	0	0	0
	0·69	250	50
	1	316	63·2
	2	433	86·5
	3	475	95·0
	4	491	98·2

Note that, for the semi-log plot, the log scale (ordinate) is from above downwards and indicates the difference between the equilibrium lung volume (inflation pressure maintained indefinitely) and the actual lung volume

Mathematical statement

With a wash-in exponential function, y increases with time and therefore the rate of change is positive. As time advances, the rate of change falls towards zero. The initial value of y is often zero but y approaches a final limiting value which may designate y_∞, that is the value of y when time is infinity (∞). A change of this type is indicated thus:

$$\frac{dy}{dt} = k(y_\infty - y)$$

As y approaches y_∞ so the quantity within the bracket approaches zero, and the rate of change slows down. The corresponding equation which indicates the instantaneous value of y is:

$$y = y_\infty (1 - e^{-kt})$$

y_∞ is the limiting value of y (attained only at infinite time).

e is again the base of natural logarithms.

k is a constant defining the rate of build-up and, as is the case of the wash-out function, it is the reciprocal of the *time constant* the significance of which is described above. It is the time which would be required to reach completion, if the initial rate were maintained without slowing down.

After 1 time constant, y will have risen to approximately $100 - 37 = 63$ per cent of its final value.

After 2 time constants, y will have risen to approximately $100 - 13\frac{1}{2} = 86\frac{1}{2}$ per cent of its final value.

After 3 time constants, y will have risen to approximately $100 - 5 = 95$ per cent of its final value.

After 5 time constants, y will have risen to approximately $100 - 1 = 99$ per cent of its final value.

(More precise values are indicated in *Table 42*.)

Table 42 PERCENTAGE CHANGE OF y AFTER LAPSE OF DIFFERENT NUMBERS OF TIME CONSTANTS

Time elapsed in time constants	*Tear-away function* $y = y_0 e^{kt}$ *(expressed as % of y_0)*	*Wash-out function* $y = y_0 e^{-kt}$ *(expressed as % of y_0)*	*Wash-in function* $y = y_\infty(1 - e^{-kt})$ *(expressed as % of y_∞)*
0	100	100	0
0·693*	200	50	50
1	272	36·8	63·2
2	739	13·5	86·5
3	2 009	4·98	95·02
4	5 460	1·83	98·17
5	14 841	0·67	99·33
10	2 202 650	0·004 5	99·995 5
∞	∞	0	100

* Half-life or doubling time.

Note: $272 = 100 \times e$
    $739 = 100 \times e^2$
    $2\ 009 = 100 \times e^3$
    etc.

Finally, the time constant for a wash-in exponential function equals the product of compliance and resistance, tissue volume divided by blood flow, or FRC divided by alveolar ventilation as the case may be. As above, the time constant is approximately 1·5 times the half-life.

There are many examples of both a wash-in and a wash-out in a single system with fixed parameters. The time constant for each function will then be the same. A classical example is the charging of an electrical capacitor through a resistance, and then allowing to discharge to earth through the same resistor. The time constant is the same for each process and equals the product of capacitance and resistance. *Figure 153* shows inflation of the lung by a sustained pressure applied to the mouth. Assuming that compliance and airway resistance are the same for inflation and expiration, the inflation curve in *Figure 153* will be the mirror image of the expiration curve in *Figure 152*, and each will have the same time constant (equal to compliance times resistance).

Graphical representation

The wash-in function may be represented on linear paper as for the other types of exponential function. However, for the semi-log plot, the paper must be turned upside down and the plot made as indicated in *Figure 153*. The curve will then be a straight line.

Bibliography and References

Adair, G. S. (1925). 'The hemoglobin system. VI. The oxygen dissociation curve of hemoglobin.' *J. biol. Chem.*, **63**, 529.

Adams, A. P., Morgan-Hughes, J. O. and Sykes, M. K. (1967). 'pH and blood-gas analysis.' *Anaesthesia*, **22**, 575.

Adams, A. P., Morgan, M., Jones, B. C. and McCormick, P. W. (1969). 'A case of massive aspiration of gastric contents during obstetric anaesthesia.' *Br. J. Anaesth.*, **41**, 176.

Adams, A. P., Economides, A. P., Finlay, W. E. I. and Sykes, M. K. (1970). 'The effects of variations of inspiratory flow waveform on cardiorespiratory function during controlled ventilation in normo-, hypo- and hypervolaemic dogs.' *Br. J. Anaesth.*, **42**, 818.

Adams, R. W., Gronert, G. A., Sundt, T. M. and Michenfelder, J. D. (1972). 'Halothane, hypocapnia, and cerebrospinal fluid pressure in neurosurgery.' *Anesthesiology*, **37**, 510.

Agostoni, E. (1962). 'Diaphragm activity and thoraco-abdominal mechanics during positive pressure breathing.' *J. appl. Physiol.*, **17**, 215.

Agostoni, E. (1963). 'Diaphragm activity during breath-holding: factors related to its onset.' *J. appl. Physiol.*, **18**, 30.

Agostoni, E. (1965). 'Mechanical significance of the changes in chest wall shape.' In *Breathlessness*. Ed. by J. B. L. Howell and E. J. M. Campbell. Oxford; Blackwell.

Agostoni, E., Sant'Ambrogio, G. and Carrasco, H. D. P. (1960). 'Electromyography of the diaphragm in man and transdiaphragmatic pressure.' *J. appl. Physiol.*, **15**, 1093.

Alexander, J. I., Spence, A. A., Parikh, R. K. and Stuart, B. (1973). 'The role of airway closure in postoperative hypoxaemia.' *Br. J. Anaesth.*, **45**, 34.

Alexander, S. C., James, F. M., Colton, E. T., Gleaton, H. R. and Wollman, H. (1968). 'Effects of cyclopropane on cerebral blood flow and carbohydrate metabolism in man.' *Anesthesiology*, **29**, 170.

de Almeida, A. J. de M. P. (1975). 'Some effects of inspiratory flow patterns on blood gas exchange in artificial ventilation during anaesthesia.' *PhD Thesis*, University of Birmingham.

Angus, G. E. and Thurlbeck, W. M. (1972). 'Number of alveoli in the human lung.' *J. appl. Physiol.*, **32**, 483.

Anthonisen, N. R., Danson, J., Robertson, P. C. and Ross, W. R. D. (1969). 'Airway closure as a function of age.' *Resp. Physiol.*, **8**, 58.

Armitage, G. H. and Taylor, A. B. (1956). 'Non-bronchospirometric measurement of differential lung function.' *Thorax*, **11**, 281.

Arndt, H., King, T. K. C. and Briscoe, W. A. (1970). 'Diffusing capacities and ventilation: perfusion ratios in patients with the clinical syndrome of alveolar capillary block.' *J. clin. Invest.*, **49**, 408.

Arnone, A. (1972). 'X-ray diffraction study of binding of 2, 3-diphosphoglycerate to human deoxyhaemoglobin.' *Nature, Lond.*, **237**, 146.

Ashbaugh, D. G., Bigelow, D. B., Petty, T. L. and Levine, B. E. (1967). 'Acute respiratory distress in adults.' *Lancet*, **2**, 319.

Askrog, V. F., Pender, J. W., Smith, T. C. and Eckenhoff, J. E. (1964). 'Changes in respiratory dead space during halothane, cyclopropane and nitrous oxide anesthesia.' *Anesthesiology*, **25**, 342.

Asmussen, E. and Nielsen, M. (1960). 'Alveolar–arterial gas exchange at rest and during work at different oxygen tensions.' *Acta physiol. scand.*, **50**, 153.

Åstrand, P., Cuddy, T. E., Saltin, B. and Stenberg, J. (1964). 'Cardiac output during submaximal and maximal work.' *J. appl. Physiol.*, **19**, 268.

Attar, S., Scanlan, E. and Cowley, R. A. (1966). 'Further evaluation of hyperbaric oxygen in haemorrhagic shock.' In *Proceedings of the Third International Conference on Hyperbaric Medicine*. Ed. by I. W. Brown and B. G. Cox. Washington DC; Nat. Acad. Sci.

Aub, J. C. and DuBois, E. F. (1917). 'The basal metabolism of old men.' *Archs intern. Med.*, **19**, 823.

Austrian, R., McClement, J. H., Renzetti, A. D., Donald, K. W., Riley, R. L. and Cournand, A. (1951). 'Clinical and physiological features of some types of pulmonary diseases with impairment of alveolar–capillary diffusion.' *Am. J. Med.*, **11**, 667.

Autor, A. P. (1974). 'Reduction of paraquat toxicity by superoxide dismutase.' *Life Sci.*, **14**, 1309.

Avery, M. E. and Mead, J. (1959). 'Surface properties in relation to atelectasis and hyaline membrane disease.' *Archs Dis. Childh.*, **97**, 517.

Aviado, D. M. (1960). 'Effects of acute atelectasis on lobar blood flow.' *Am. J. Physiol.*, **198**, 349.

Aviado, D. M. (1965). *The Lung Circulation.* Oxford; Pergamon.

Aviado, D. M. (1975). 'Regulation of bronchomotor tone during anaesthesia.' *Anesthesiology*, **42**, 68.

Bainton, C. R. and Mitchell, R. A. (1965). 'Posthyperventilation apnea in awake man.' *Fedn Proc.*, **24**, 273.

Bake, B., Wood, L., Murphy, B., Macklem, P. T. and Milic-Emili, J. (1974). 'Effect of inspiratory flow rate on regional distribution of inspired gas.' *J. appl. Physiol.*, **37**, 8.

Bakhle, Y. S. and Block, A. J. (1976). 'Effects of halothane on pulmonary inactivation of noradrenalin and prostaglandin E_2 in anaesthetized dogs.' *Clin. Sci.*, **50**, 87.

Bakhle, Y. S. and Vane, J. R. (1974). 'Pharmacokinetic function of the pulmonary circulation.' *Physiol. Rev.*, **54**, 1007.

Ball, I. M., Dundee, J. W. and Stevenson, H. M. (1973). 'Ventilation during bronchoscopy with an injector.' *Br. J. Anaesth.*, **45**, 1063.

Banchero, N., Schwartz, P. E., Tsakiris, A. G. and Wood, E. H. (1967). 'Pleural and esophageal pressures in the upright body position.' *J. appl. Physiol.*, **23**, 228.

Banister, J. and Torrance, R. W. (1960). 'The effects of the tracheal pressure on flow: pressure relations in the vascular bed of isolated lungs.' *Q. Jl exp. Physiol.*, **45**, 352.

Bannister, R. G., Cunningham, D. J. C. and Douglas, C. G. (1954). 'The carbon dioxide stimulus to breathing in severe exercise.' *J. Physiol.*, **125**, 90.

Barber, R. E., Lee, J. and Hamilton, W. K. (1970). 'Oxygen toxicity in man. A prospective study in patients with irreversible brain damage.' *New Engl. J. Med.*, **283**, 1478.

Barcroft, J. (1920). 'Physiological effects of insufficient oxygen supply.' *Nature, Lond.*, **106**, 125.

Barcroft, J. (1934). *Features in the Architecture of Physiological Function.* Cambridge; University Press. (Reissued, 1972, Hafner.)

Barer, G. R., Howard, P. and McCurrie, J. R. (1967). 'The effect of carbon dioxide and changes in blood pH on pulmonary vascular resistance in cats.' *Clin. Sci.*, **32**, 361.

Barker, R. W., Brown, F. F., Drake, R., Halsey, M. J. and Richards, R. E. (1975). 'Nuclear magnetic resonance studies of anaesthetic interactions with haemoglobin.' *Br. J. Anaesth.*, **47**, 25.

Bartels, J., Severinghaus, J. W., Forster, R. E., Briscoe, W. A. and Bates, D. V. (1954). 'The respiratory dead space measured by single breath analysis of oxygen, carbon dioxide, nitrogen or helium.' *J. clin. Invest.*, **33**, 41.

Barth, L. (1954). 'Untersuchungen über die Diffusionsatmung des Menschen.' In *Anaesthesieprobleme. Abh. dt. Akad. Wiss. Berl., Klasse für med.*

Barton, F. and Nunn, J. F. (1975). 'Totally closed circuit nitrous oxide/oxygen anaesthesia.' *Br. J. Anaesth.*, **47**, 350.

Bates, D. V., Macklem, P. T. and Christie, R. V. (1971). *Respiratory Function in Disease,* 2nd edn. Philadelphia, Pa. and London; W. B. Saunders.

Bay, J., Nunn, J. F. and Prys-Roberts, C. (1968). 'Factors influencing arterial Po_2 during recovery from anaesthesia.' *Br. J. Anaesth.*, **40**, 398.

Bellville, J. W. and Seed, J. C. (1960). 'The effect of drugs on the respiratory response to carbon dioxide.' *Anesthesiology*, **21**, 727.

Benatar, S. R., Hewlett, A. M. and Nunn, J. F. (1973). 'The use of iso-shunt lines for control of oxygen therapy.' *Br. J. Anaesth.*, **45**, 711.

Bendixen, H. H. and Bunker, J. P. (1962). 'Measurement of inspiratory force in anesthetized dogs.' *Anesthesiology*, **23**, 315.

Bendixen, H. H., Hedley-Whyte, J. and Laver, M. B. (1963). 'Impaired oxygenation in surgical patients during general anesthesia with controlled ventilation.' *New. Engl. J. Med.*, **269**, 991.

Bendixen, H. H., Smith, G. M. and Mead, J. (1964). 'Pattern of ventilation in young adults.' *J. appl. Physiol.*, **19**, 195.

Bendixen, H. H., Bullwinkel, B., Hedley-Whyte, J. and Laver, M. B. (1964). 'Atelectasis and shunting during spontaneous ventilation in anesthetized patients.' *Anesthesiology*, **25**, 297.

Bendixen, H. H., Egbert, L. D., Hedley-Whyte, J., Laver, M. B. and Pontoppidan, H. (1965). *Respiratory Care*. St. Louis, Mo.; C. V. Mosby London; Kimpton.

Benesch, R. and Benesch, R. E. (1967). 'Effects of organic phosphates from human erythrocytes on the allosteric properties of haemoglobin.' *Biochem. Biophys. Res. Commun.*, **26**, 162.

Bennett, E. D., Jayson, M. I. V., Rubinstein, D. and Campbell, E. J. M. (1962). 'The ability of man to detect added non-elastic loads to breathing.' *Clin. Sci.*, **23**, 155.

Benzinger, T. (1937). 'Untersuchungen über die Atmung und den Gasstoffwechsel insbesondere bei Sauerstoffmangel und Unterdruck, mit fortlaufend unmittelbar aufzeichnenden Methoden.' *Ergebn. Physiol.*, **40**, 1.

Bergman, N. A. (1963a). 'Effect of different pressure breathing patterns on alveolar–arterial gradients in dogs.' *J. appl. Physiol.*, **18**, 1049.

Bergman, N. A. (1963b). 'Distribution of inspired gas during anesthesia and artificial ventilation.' *J. appl. Physiol.*, **18**, 1085.

Bergman, N. A. (1966). 'Measurement of respiratory resistance in anesthetized subjects.' *J. appl. Physiol.*, **21**, 1913.

Bergman, N. A. (1967). 'Effects of varying waveforms on gas exchange.' *Anesthesiology*, **28**, 390.

Bergman, N. A. (1969). 'Properties of passive exhalations in anesthetized subjects.' *Anesthesiology*, **30**, 379.

Bergman, N. A. (1970). 'Pulmonary diffusing capacity and gas exchange during halothane anesthesia.' *Anesthesiology*, **32**, 317.

Bergman, N. A. (1972). 'Intrapulmonary gas trapping during mechanical ventilation at rapid frequencies.' *Anesthesiology*, **37**, 626.

Bergman, N. A. and Waltemath, C. L. (1974). 'A comparison of some methods for measuring total respiratory resistance.' *J. appl. Physiol.*, **36**, 131.

Bernstein, L. and Mendel, D. (1951). 'Accuracy of spirographic tracings at high rates.' *Thorax*, **6**, 297.

Bernstein, L., D'Silva, J. L. and Mendel, D. (1952). 'The effect of rate on M.B.C. determination with a new spirometer.' *Thorax*, **7**, 225.

Berry, E. M., Edmonds, J. F. and Wyllie, J. H. (1971). 'Release of prostaglandin E_2 and unidentified factors from ventilated lungs.' *Br. J. Surg.*, **58**, 189.

Bert, P. (1878). *La Pression Barometrique*. Paris; Masson. (English translation by M. A. Hitchcock and F. A. Hitchcock, 1943. Columbus, Ohio; College Book Co.)

Bertrand, F., Hugelin, A. and Vibert, J. F. (1974). 'A stereologic model of pneumotaxic oscillator based on spatial and temporal distributions of neuronal bursts.' *J. Neurophysiol.*, **37**, 91.

Birt, C. and Cole, P. V. (1965). 'Some physiological effects of closed circuit halothane anaesthesia.' *Anaesthesia*, **20**, 258.

Biscoe, T. J. (1971). 'Carotid body structure and function.' *Physiol. Rev.*, **5**, 437.

Biscoe, T. J. and Millar, R. A. (1964). 'The effect of halothane on carotid sinus baroreceptor activity.' *J. Physiol.*, **173**, 24.

Bishop, J. M., Pincock, A. C., Hollyhock, A., Raine, J. and Cole, R. B. (1966). 'Factors affecting the measurement of the partial pressure of oxygen in blood using a covered electrode system.' *Resp. Physiol.*, **1**, 225.

Bitter, H. S. and Rahn, H. (1956). 'Redistribution of alveolar blood flow with passive lung distension.' *Wright Air Dev. Ctr. Tech. Rep.* 56–466, 1.

Björk, V. O. (1953). 'Circulation through an atelectatic lung in man.' *J. thorac. Surg.*, **26**, 533.

Black, A. M. S. and Torrance, R. W. (1971). 'Respiratory oscillations in chemoreceptor discharge in the control of breathing.' *Resp. Physiol.*, **13**, 221.

Black, G. W., Linde, H. W., Dripps, R. D. and Price, H. L. (1959). 'Circulatory changes accompanying respiratory acidosis during halothane (Fluothane) anaesthesia in man.' *Br. J. Anaesth.*, **31**, 238.

Blackburn, J. P., Conway, C. M., Leigh, J. M., Lindop, M. J. and Reitan, J. A. (1972). '$PaCO_2$ and the pre-ejection period.' *Anesthesiology*, **37**, 268.

Blackburn, J. P., Conway, C. M., Davies, R. M., Enderby, G. E. H., Edridge, A. W., Leigh, J. M., Lindop, M. J., Phillips, G. D. and Strickland, D. A. P. (1973). 'Valsalva responses and systolic time intervals during anaesthesia and induced hypotension.' *Br. J. Anaesth.*, **45**, 704.

Bodman, R. I. (1963). 'Clinical applications of pulmonary function tests.' *Anaesthesia*, **18**, 355.

Bodman, R. I. and Latimer, R. D. (1975). 'Arterial oxygen tensions during the induction of ether and air anaesthesia with spontaneous respiration.' *Anaesthesia*, **30**, 539.

Bohr, C. (1891). 'Über die Lungenathmung.' *Skand. Arch. Physiol.*, **2**, 236.

Bohr, C. (1909). 'Über die spezifische Tätigkeit der Lungen bei der respiratorischen Gasaufnahme.' *Skand. Arch. Physiol.*, **22**, 221.

Bookallil, M. and Smith, W. D. A. (1964). 'A proportional respiratory sampling apparatus.' *Br. J. Anaesth.*, **36**, 527.

Boothby, W. M. and Sandiford, I. (1924). 'Basal metabolism.' *Physiol. Rev.*, **18**, 1085.

Bradley, R. D. and Semple, S. J. G. (1962). 'A comparison of certain acid–base characteristics of arterial blood, jugular venous blood, and cerebrospinal fluid in man, and the effect on them of some acute and chronic acid–base disturbances.' *J. Physiol.*, **160**, 381.

Braunitzer, G. (1963). 'Molekulare struktur der Hämoglobine.' *Nova Acta Acad. Caesar. Leop. Carol.*, **26**, 471.

Braunwald, E., Binion, J. T. and Morgan, W. L. (1957). 'Alterations in central blood volume and cardiac output induced by positive pressure breathing and counteracted by metaraminol (Aramine). *Circulation Res.*, **5**, 670.

Brendstrup, A. (1966). 'The effect of artificial respiration on the regional distribution of ventilation examined with xenon-133.' *Acta anaesth. scand.*, suppl. **23**, 1, 180.

Breuer, J. (1868). 'Die Selbsteuerung der Athmung durch den Nervus Vagus.' *Sber. Akad. Wiss. Wien*, **58**, 909.

Briscoe, W. A. and Cournand, A. (1962). 'The degree of variation of blood perfusion and of ventilation within the emphysematous lung.' In: Ciba Symposium on *Pulmonary Structure and Function*, p. 304. Ed. by A. V. S. de Rueck and M. O'Connor. Edinburgh and London; Churchill Livingstone.

Briscoe, W. A., Forster, R. E. and Comroe, J. H. (1954). 'Alveolar ventilation at very low tidal volumes.' *J. appl. Physiol.*, **7**, 27.

Brown, E. B. (1953). 'Physiological effects of hyperventilation.' *Physiol. Rev.*, **33**, 445.

Brown, E. B. and Miller, F. (1952). 'Ventricular fibrillation following a rapid fall in alveolar carbon dioxide concentration.' *Am. J. Physiol.*, **169**, 56.

Brown, E. S., Johnson, R. P. and Clements, J. A. (1959). 'Pulmonary surface tension.' *J. appl. Physiol.*, **14**, 717.

Brownlee, W. E. and Allbritten, F. F. (1956). 'The significance of the lung–thorax compliance in ventilation during thoracic surgery.' *J. thorac. Surg.*, **32**, 454.

Brummelkamp, W. H. (1965). 'Reflections on hyperbaric oxygen therapy at 2 atmospheres absolute for *Clostridium welchii* infections.' In; *Hyperbaric Oxygenation*. Ed. by I. Ledingham. Edinburgh and London; Churchill Livingstone.

Burton, A. C. (1951). 'On the physical equilibrium of small blood vessels.' *Am. J. Physiol.*, **164**, 319.

Burton, A. C. and Patel, D. J. (1958). 'Effect on pulmonary vascular resistance of inflation of the rabbit lungs.' *J. appl. Physiol.*, **12**, 239.

Butler, J. (1960). 'The work of breathing through the nose.' *Clin. Sci.*, **19**, 55.

Butler, J. and Smith, B. H. (1957). 'Pressure–volume relationships of the chest in the completely relaxed anaesthetised patient.' *Clin. Sci.*, **16**, 125.

Butler, J., White, H. C. and Arnott, W. M. (1957). 'The pulmonary compliance in normal subjects.' *Clin. Sci.*, **16**, 709.

Byles, P. H. (1960). 'Observations on some continuously-acting spirometers.' *Br. J. Anaesth.*, **32**, 470.

Cain, C. C. and Otis, A. B. (1949). 'Some physiological effects resulting from added resistance to respiration.' *J. Aviat. Med.*, **20**, 149.

Cain, S. M. and Otis, A. B. (1961). 'Carbon dioxide transport in anesthetized dogs during inhibition of carbonic anhydrase.' *J. appl. Physiol.*, **16**, 1023.

Cameron, A. J. V., Gibb, B. H., Ledingham, I. McA. and McGuiness, J. B. (1965). 'A controlled clinical trial of hyperbaric oxygen in the treatment of acute myocardial infarction.' In *Hyperbaric Oxygenation*. Ed. by I. Ledingham. Edinburgh and London; Churchill Livingstone.

Campbell, E. J. M. (1952). 'An electromyographic study of the role of the abdominal muscles in breathing.' *J. Physiol.,* 117, 222.

Campbell, E. J. M. (1955). 'An electromyographic examination of the role of the intercostal muscles in breathing in man.' *J. Physiol.,* 129, 12.

Campbell, E. J. M. (1957). 'The effects of increased resistance to expiration on the respiratory behaviour of the abdominal muscles and intra-abdominal pressure.' *J. Physiol.* 136, 556.

Campbell, E. J. M. (1958). *The Respiratory Muscles and the Mechanics of Breathing.* London; Lloyd-Luke.

Campbell, E. J. M. (1960a). 'Simplification of Haldane's apparatus for measuring CO_2 concentration in respired gases in clinical practice.' *Br. med. J.,* 1, 457.

Campbell, E. J. M. (1960b). 'A method of controlled oxygen administration which reduces the risk of carbon-dioxide retention.' *Lancet,* 2, 12.

Campbell, E. J. M. (1962). 'RIpH'. *Lancet,* 1, 681.

Campbell, E. J. M. and Dickinson, C. J. (1960). *Clinical Physiology.* Oxford; Blackwell.

Campbell, E. J. M. and Howell, J. B. L. (1960). 'Simple rapid methods of estimating arterial and mixed venous PCO_2.' *Br. med J.* 1, 458.

Campbell, E. J. M. and Howell, J. B. L. (1962). 'Proprioceptive control of breathing.' In Ciba Foundation Symposium on *Pulmonary Structure and Function.* Ed. by A. V. S. de Rueck and M. O'Connor. Edinburgh and London; Churchill Livingstone.

Campbell, E. J. M. and Howell, J. B. L. (1963). 'The sensation of breathlessness.' *Br. med. Bull.,* 19, 36.

Campbell, E. J. M., Howell, J. B. L. and Peckett, B. W. (1957). 'The pressure-volume relationships of the thorax of anaesthetized human subjects.' *J. Physiol.,* 136, 563.

Campbell, E. J. M., Nunn, J. F. and Peckett, B. W. (1958). 'A comparison of artificial ventilation and spontaneous respiration with particular reference to ventilation–blood-flow relationships.' *Br. J. Anaesth.,* 30, 166.

Campbell, E. J. M. Westlake, E. K. and Cherniack, R. M. (1957). 'Simple methods of estimating oxygen consumption and efficiency of the muscles of breathing.' *J. appl. Physiol.,* 11, 303.

Campbell, E. J. M., Freedman, S., Smith, P. S. and Taylor, M. E. (1961). 'The ability of man to detect added elastic loads to breathing.' *Clin. Sci.,* 20, 223.

Campbell, E. J. M., Freedman, S., Clark, T. J. H., Robson, J. G. and Norman, J. (1967). 'The effect of muscular paralysis induced by tubocurarine on the duration and sensation of breath-holding.' *Clin. Sci.,* 32, 425.

Campbell, E. J. M., Godfrey, S., Clark, T. H. J., Freedman, S. and Norman, J. (1969). 'The effect of muscular paralysis induced by tubocurarine on the duration and sensation of breath holding during hypercapnia.' *Clin. Sci.,* 36, 323.

Carlens, E., Hanson, H. E. and Nordenström, B. (1951). 'Temporary occlusion of the pulmonary artery.' *J. thorac. Surg.,* 22, 527.

Caro, C. G., Butler, J. and DuBois, A. B. (1960). 'Some effects of restriction of chest cage expansion on pulmonary function in man.' *J. clin. Invest.,* 39, 573.

Cascorbi, H. F. and Singh-Amaranath, A. V. (1972). 'Fluroxene toxicity in mice.' *Anesthesiology,* 37, 480.

Castleden, C. M. and Cole, P. V. (1974). 'Variations in carboxyhaemoglobin levels in smokers.' *Br. med. J.* 4, 736.

de Castro, F. (1926). 'Sur la structure et l'innervation de la glande intercarotidienne.' *Trab. Lab. Invest. biol. Univ. Madrid,* 24, 365.

Cater, D. B., Garatini, S. Marina, F. and Silver, I. A. (1961). 'Changes of oxygen tension in brain and somatic tissues induced by vasodilator and vasoconstrictor drugs.' *Proc. R. Soc. B,* 155, 136.

Cater, D. B., Hill, D. W., Lindop, P. J., Nunn, J. F. and Silver, I. A. (1963). 'Oxygen washout studies in the anesthetized dog.' *J. appl. Physiol.,* 18, 888.

Cerretelli, P., Cruz, J. C., Farhi, L. E. and Rahn, H. (1966). 'Determination of mixed venous O_2 and CO_2 tensions and cardiac output by a rebreathing method.' *Resp. Physiol.,* 1, 258.

Channin, E. and Tyler, J. (1962). 'Effect of increased breathing frequency on inspiratory resistance in emphysema.' *J. appl. Physiol.,* 17, 605.

Chanutin, A. and Curnish, R. (1967). 'Effect of organic and inorganic phosphates on the oxygen equilibrium of human erythrocytes.' *Arch. Biochem. Biophys.,* 121, 96.

Cherniack, N. S. and Longobardo, G. S. (1970). 'Oxygen and carbon dioxide gas stores of the body.' *Physiol. Rev.*, 50, 196.

Christensen, M. S. (1974). 'Acid–base changes in cerebrospinal fluid and blood, and blood volume changes following prolonged hyperventilation in man.' *Br. J. Anaesth.*, 46, 348.

Christensen, M. S., Hoedt-Rasmussen, K. and Lassen, N. A. (1967). 'Cerebral vasodilatation by halothane anaesthesia in man and its potentiation by hypotension and hypercapnia.' *Br. J. Anaesth.*, 39, 927.

Christiansen, J., Douglas, C. G. and Haldane, J. S. (1914). 'The adsorption and dissociation of carbon dioxide by human blood.' *J. Physiol.*, 48, 244.

Clark, J. M. and Lambertsen, C. J. (1971). 'Pulmonary toxicity—a review.' *Pharmac. Rev.*, 23, 37.

Clark, T. J. H. (1968). 'The ventilatory response to CO_2 in chronic airways obstruction measured by a rebreathing method.' *Clin. Sci.*, 34, 559.

Clark, T. J. H., Clarke, B. G. and Hughes, J. M. B. (1966). 'A simple technique for measuring changes in ventilatory response to carbon dioxide.' *Lancet* 2, 368.

Clarke, S. W., Jones, J. G. and Oliver, D. R. (1970). 'Resistance to two-phase gas–liquid flow in airways.' *J. appl. Physiol.*, 29, 464.

Clements, J. A. (1970). 'Pulmonary surfactant.' *Am. Rev. resp. Dis.*, 101, 984.

Clowes, G. H. A., Hopkins, A. L. and Simeone, F. A. (1955). 'A comparison of physiological effects of hypercapnia and hypoxia in the production of cardiac arrest.' *Ann. Surg.*, 142, 446.

Clutton-Brock, J. (1957). 'The cerebral effects of overventilation.' *Br. J. Anaesth.*, 29, 111.

Cockett, F. B. and Vass, C. C. N. (1951). 'A comparison of the role of the bronchial arteries in the bronchiectasis.' *Thorax*, 6, 268.

Cohen, J. J., Brackett, N. C. and Schwartz, W. B. (1964). 'The nature of the carbon dioxide titration curve in the normal dog.' *J. clin. Invest.*, 43, 777.

Cohen, P. J. (1972). 'The metabolic function of oxygen and biochemical lesions of hypoxia.' *Anesthesiology*, 37, 148.

Cohen, P. J. and Behar, M. G. (1970). 'The in vitro effect of anesthesia on the oxyhemoglobin dissociation curve.' *Fedn Proc.*, 29, 329.

Cohen, P. J., Alexander, S. C., Smith, T. C., Reivich, M. and Wollman, H. (1967). 'Effects of hypoxia and normocarbia on cerebral blood flow and metabolism in conscious man.' *J. appl. Physiol.*, 23, 183.

Cole, R. B. and Bishop, J. M. (1963). 'Effects of varying inspired oxygen tension on alveolar–arterial O_2 tension difference in man.' *J. appl. Physiol.*, 18, 1043.

Cole, R. B. and Bishop, J. M. (1967). 'Variation in alveolar–arterial O_2 tension difference at high levels of alveolar O_2 tension.' *J. appl. Physiol.*, 22, 685.

Colgan, F. J., Barrow, R. E. and Fanning, G. (1971). 'Constant positive-pressure breathing and cardiorespiratory function.' *Anesthesiology*, 34, 145.

Colville, P., Shugg, C. and Ferris B. G. (1956). 'Effects of body tilting on respiratory mechanics.' *J. appl. Physiol.*, 9, 19.

Comroe, J. H. (1939). 'The location and function of the chemoreceptors of the aorta.' *Am. J. Physiol.*, 127, 176.

Comroe, J. H. and Botelho, S. (1947). 'The unreliability of cyanosis in the recognition of arterial anoxemia.' *Am. J. med. Sci.*, 214, 1.

Comroe, J. H. and Dripps, R. D. (1946). 'Artificial respiration'. *J. Am. med. Ass.*, 130, 381.

Comroe, J. H. and Schmidt, C. F. (1938). 'The part played by reflexes from the carotid body in the chemical regulation of respiration in the dog.' *Am. J. Physiol.*, 121, 75.

Comroe, J. H., Nisell, O. I. and Nims, R. G. (1954). 'A simple method of concurrent measurement of compliance and resistance to breathing in anesthetized animals and man.' *J. appl. Physiol.*, 7, 225.

Comroe, J. H., Forster, R. E. DuBois, A. B., Briscoe, W. A. and Carlsen, E. (1962). *The Lung*, 2nd edn. Chicago; Year Book Medical Publ. London; Lloyd-Luke.

Conway, C. M., Payne, J. P. and Tomlin, P. (1965). 'Arterial oxygen tensions of patients awaiting surgery.' *Br. J. Anaesth.*, 37, 405.

Cooper, E. A. (1957). 'Infra-red analysis for the estimation of carbon dioxide in the presence of nitrous oxide.' *Br. J. Anaesth.*, 30, 486.

Cooper, E. A. (1959). 'The estimation of minute volume.' *Anaesthesia*, 14, 373.

Cooper, E. A. (1961). 'Behaviour of respiratory apparatus.' *Med. Res. Memo. natn. Coal Bd med. Serv.*, 2.

Cooper, E. A. (1967). 'Physiological dead space in passive ventilation.' *Anaesthesia*, 22, 199.

Cooper, E. A. and Smith, H. (1961). 'Indirect estimation of arterial pCO_2.' *Anaesthesia*, 16, 445.

Corda, M., von Euler, C. and Lennerstrand, G. (1965). 'Proprioceptive innervation of the diaphragm.' *J. Physiol.*, 178, 161.

Cormack, R. S. (1972). 'Eliminating two sources of error in the Lloyd–Haldane apparatus.' *Resp. Physiol.*, 14, 382.

Cormack, R. S. and Powell, J. N. (1972). 'Improving the performance of the infra-red carbon dioxide meter.' *Br. J. Anaesth.*, 44, 131.

Cormack, R. S. Cunningham, D. J. C. and Gee, J. B. L. (1957). 'The effect of carbon dioxide on the respiratory response to want of oxygen in man.' *Q. Jl exp. Physiol.*, 42, 303.

Cotes, J. E. (1975). *Lung Function*, 3rd edn. Oxford; Blackwell.

Cottrell, T. S., Levine, O. R., Senior, R. M., Wiener, J., Spiro, D. and Fishman, A. P. (1967). 'Electron microscopic alterations at the alveolar level in pulmonary edema.' *Circulation Res.*, 21, 783.

Cournand, A., Motley, H. L., Werko, L. and Richards, D. W. (1948). 'Physiological studies of the effects of intermittent positive pressure breathing on cardiac output in man.' *Am. J. Physiol.*, 152, 162.

Cox, J., Woolmer, R. W. and Thomas, V. (1960). 'Expired air resuscitation.' *Lancet*, 1, 727.

Cozine, R. A. and Ngai, S. H. (1967). 'Medullary surface chemoreceptors and regulation of respiration in the cat.' *J. appl. Physiol.*, 22, 117.

Craig, D. B., Wahba, W. M. and Don, H. (1971). 'Airway closure and lung volumes in surgical positions.' *Can. Anaesth. Soc. J.*, 18, 92.

Craig, D. B., Wahba, W. M. Don, H. F., Couture, J. G. and Becklake, M. R. (1971). ' "Closing volume" and its relationship to gas exchange in seated and supine positions.' *J. appl. Physiol.*, 31, 717.

Cross, K. W., Klaus, M., Tooley, W. H. and Weisser, K. (1960). 'The response of the new-born baby to inflation of the lungs. *J. Physiol.*, 151, 551.

Crul, J. F. (1962). 'Measurement of arterial pressure.' *Acta anaesth. scand.*, suppl. 11, 135.

Cullen, D. J. and Eger, E. I. (1974). 'Cardiovascular effects of carbon dioxide in man.' *Anesthesiology*, 41, 345.

Cunningham, D. J. C. (1974). 'The control system regulating breathing in man.' *Q. Rev. Biophys.* 6, 433.

Cunningham, D. J. C. and Lloyd, B. B., Eds. (1963). *The Regulation of Human Respiration.* Oxford; Blackwell.

Cunningham, D. J. C. and Ward, S. A. (1975a). 'The form of the respiratory interaction between an alternate-breath oscillation of $PACO_2$ and hypoxia in man.' *J. Physiol.*, 251, 37P.

Cunningham, D. J. C. and Ward, S. A. (1975b). 'The separate effects of alternate-breath oscillations of $PACO_2$ during hypoxia on inspiration and expiration.' *J. Physiol.*, 252, 33P.

Cunningham, D. J. C., Howson, M. G. and Pearson, S. B. (1973). 'The respiratory effects in man of altering the time profile of alveolar CO_2 and O_2 within each respiratory cycle.' *J. Physiol.* 234, 1.

Cunningham, D. J. C. Kay, R. H. and Young, J. M. (1965). 'A fast response paramagnetic oxygen analyser.' *J. Physiol.*, 181, 15P.

Cunningham, D. J. C., Hey, E. N., Patrick, J. M. and Lloyd, B. B. (1963). 'The effect of noradrenalin infusion on the relation between pulmonary ventilation and the alveolar PO_2 and PCO_2 in man.' *Ann. N.Y. Acad. Sci.*, 109, 756.

Dail, C. W., Affeldt, J. E. and Collier, C. R. (1955). 'Clinical aspects of glossopharyngeal breathing.' *J. Am. med. Ass.*, 158, 445.

Daly, N. J., Ross, J. C. and Behnke, R. H. (1963). 'The effect of changes in the pulmonary vascular bed produced by atropine, pulmonary engorgement and positive pressure breathing on diffusing and mechanical capacity of the lung.' *J. clin. Invest.*, 42, 1083.

Dann, W. L. (1971). 'The effects of different levels of ventilation in the action of pancuronium in man.' *Br. J. Anaesth.*, 43, 959.

Dantzker, D. R., Wagner, P. D. and West, J. B. (1975). 'Instability of lung units with low $V\dot{A}/\dot{Q}$ ratios during O_2 breathing.' *J. appl. Physiol.*, 38, 886.

Davenport, H. W. (1958). *The ABC of Acid–Base Chemistry*, 4th edn. Chicago and London; University of Chicago Press. (6th edn., published 1974.)

Davidson, J. K. (1965). 'Avascular necrosis of bone.' In: *Hyperbaric Oxygenation*. Ed. by I. Ledingham. Edinburgh and London; Churchill Livingstone.

Davidson, J. T., Whipp, B. J., Wasserman, K., Koyal, S. N. and Lugliani, R. (1974). 'Role of carotid bodies in breath-holding.' *New Engl. J. Med.*, 290, 819.

Davies, H. W., Haldane, J. S. and Priestley, J. G. (1919). 'Response to respiratory resistance.' *J. Physiol.*, 53, 60.

Davy, H. (1800). *Researches, Chemical and Philosophical; chiefly concerning nitrous oxide or dephlogisticated nitrous air, and its respiration*. London; J. Johnson.

Defares, J. G., Lundin, G., Arborelius, M., Stromblad, R. and Svanberg, L. (1960). 'Effect of "unilateral hypoxia" on pulmonary blood flow distribution in normal subjects.' *J. appl. Physiol.*, 15, 169.

Dejours, P. (1964). 'Control of respiration in muscular exercise.' *Handbk Physiol. section 3*, 1, 631.

Dejours, P. (1966). *Respiration*. (Translated by L. E. Farhi.) New York and Oxford; Oxford University Press.

Dempsey, J. A., Forster, H. V. and doPico, G. A. (1974). 'Ventilatory acclimatization to moderate hypoxemia in man.' *J. clin. Invest.*, 53, 1091.

Denison, D. M., Ernsting, J. and Cresswell, A. W. (1966). 'Fire and hyperbaric oxygen.' *Lancet*, 2, 1404.

Denison, D., Edwards, R. H. T., Jones, G. and Pope, H. (1971). 'Estimates of the CO_2 pressures in systemic arterial blood during rebreathing on exercise.' *Resp. Physiol.*, 11, 186.

Déry, R., Pelletier, J., Jacques, A., Clavet, M. and Houde, J. (1965). 'Alveolar collapse induced by denitrogenation.' *Can. Anaesth. Soc. J.*, 12, 531.

Dexter, L., Whittenberger, J. L., Haynes, F. W., Goodale, W. T., Gorlin, R. and Sawyer, C. G. (1951). 'Effect of exercise on circulatory dynamics of normal individuals.' *J. appl. Physiol.*, 3, 439.

Dollfuss, R. E., Milic-Emili, J. and Bates, D. V. (1967). 'Regional ventilation of the lung studied with boluses of [133]xenon.' *Resp. Physiol.*, 2, 234.

Don, H. F. and Robson, J. G. (1965). 'The mechanics of the respiratory system during anesthesia.' *Anesthesiology*, 26, 168.

Don, H. F., Wahba, W. M. and Craig, D. B. (1972). 'Airway closure, gas trapping, and the functional residual capacity during anesthesia.' *Anesthesiology*, 36, 533.

Don, H. F., Wahba, M. Cuadrado, L. and Kelkar, K. (1970). 'The effects of anesthesia and 100 per cent oxygen on the functional residual capacity of the lungs.' *Anesthesiology*, 32, 521.

Donald, K. W. (1955). 'Oxygen bends.' *J. appl. Physiol.*, 7, 639.

Donald, K. W. and Christie, R. V. (1949). 'A new method of clinical spirometry.' *Clin. Sci.*, 8, 21.

Donald, K. W., Renzetti, A., Riley, R. L. and Cournand, A. (1952). 'Analysis of factors affecting the concentrations of oxygen and carbon dioxide in gas and blood of lungs: results.' *J. appl. Physiol.*, 4, 497.

Donald, K. W., Bishop, J. M., Cumming, G. and Wade, O. L. (1953). 'Effect of nursing positions on cardiac output in man.' *Clin. Sci.*, 12, 199.

Douglas, C. G. and Haldane, J. S. (1909). 'The causes of periodic or Cheyne–Stokes breathing.' *J. Physiol.*, 38, 401.

Dowman, C. E. (1927). 'Relief of diaphragmatic tic, following encephalitis, by section of phrenic nerves,' *J. Am. med. Ass.*, 88, 95.

Down, R. H. L. and Castleden, W. M. (1975). 'Oxygen therapy for pneumatosis coli.' *Br. med. J.*, 1, 493.

Downes, J. J. (1976). 'CPAP and PEEP—a perspective.' *Anesthesiology*, 44, 1.

Downes, J. J. and Raphaely, R. C. (1975). 'Pediatric intensive care.' *Anesthesiology*, 43, 238.

Downs, J. B., Klein, E. F. and Modell, J. H. (1973). 'The effect of incremental PEEP on PaO_2 in patients with respiratory failure.' *Anesth. Analg.*, 52, 210.

Downs, J. B., Klein, E. F., Desautels, D., Modell, J. H. and Kirby, R. R. (1973). 'Intermittent mandatory ventilation: a new approach to weaning patients from mechanical ventilators.' *Chest*, 64, 331.

Draper, W. B. and Whitehead, R. W. (1944). 'Diffusion respiration in the dog anesthetized by pentothal sodium.' *Anesthesiology*, 5, 262.

DuBois, A. B., Botelho, S. Y. and Comroe, J. H. (1956). 'A new method of measuring airway resistance in man using a body plethysmograph.' *J. clin. Invest.*, 35, 327.

DuBois, A. B., Fowler, R. C., Soffer, A. and Fenn, W. O. (1952). 'Aveolar CO_2 measured by expiration into the rapid infra-red gas analyzer.' *J. appl. Physiol.*, 4, 526.

DuBois, A. B., Botelho, S. Y., Bedell, G. N., Marshall, R. and Comroe, J. H. (1956). 'A rapid plethysmographic method for measuring thoracic gas volume.' *J. clin. Invest.*, 35, 322.

Duke, H. N. (1954). 'The site of action of anoxia on the pulmonary blood vessels of the cat.' *J. Physiol.*, 125, 373.

Dunbar, B. S., Ovassapian, A. and Smith, T. C. (1967). 'The effects of methoxyflurane on ventilation in man.' *Anesthesiology*, 28, 1020.

Dundee, J. W. (1952). 'Influence of controlled respiration on dosage of thiopentone and *d*-tubocurarine chloride required for abdominal surgery.' *Br. med. J.*, 2, 893.

Dutton, R. E., Fitzgerald, R. S. and Gross, N. (1968). 'Ventilatory response to square-wave forcing of carbon dioxide at the carotid bodies.' *Resp. Physiol.*, 4, 101.

Dymond, J. H. and Smith, E. B. (1969). *The Virial Coefficients of Gases: a critical compilation.* Oxford; Oxford University Press.

Ebert, M. and Hornsey, S. (1958). 'Effect of nitrous oxide on the radiosensitivity of mouse Ehrlich ascites tumour.' *Nature, Lond.*, 182, 1240.

Eckenhoff, J. E., Enderby, G. E. H., Larson, A., Edridge, A. and Judevine, D. E. (1963). 'Pulmonary gas exchange during deliberate hypotension. *Br. J. Anaesth.*, 35, 750.

Egbert, L. D. and Bisno, D. (1967). 'The educated hand of the anesthesiologist.' *Anesth. Analg.*, 46, 195.

Eger, E. I. (1974). *Anesthetic Uptake and Action.* Baltimore, Md.; Williams & Wilkins.

Eger, E. I. and Bahlman, S. H. (1971). 'Is the end-tidal anesthetic partial pressure an accurate measure of the arterial anesthetic partial pressure?' *Anesthesiology*, 35, 301.

Eger, E. I., Dolan, W. M., Stevens, W. C., Miller, R. D. and Way, W. L. (1972). 'Surgical stimulation antagonizes the respiratory depression produced by forane.' *Anesthesiology*, 36, 544.

Eisele, J. H., Eger, E. I. and Muallem, M. (1967). 'Narcotic properties of carbon dioxide in the dog.' *Anesthesiology*, 28, 856.

Eisele, J. H., Trenchard, D., Burki, N. and Guz, A. (1968). 'The effect of chest wall block on respiratory sensation and control in man.' *Clin. Sci.*, 35, 23.

Eisele, J. H., Noble, M. I. M., Katz, J., Fung, D. L. and Hickey, R. F. (1972). 'Bilateral phrenic-nerve block in man.' *Anesthesiology*, 37, 64.

Elam, J. O. (1962). In: *Artificial Respiration.* Ed. by J. L. Whittenberger. New York and London; Harper and Row.

Elam, J. O. and Greene, D. G. (1962). In: *Artificial Respiration.* Ed. by J. L. Whittenberger. New York and London; Harper and Row.

Elliott, S. E., Segger, F. J. and Osborn, J. J. (1966). 'A modified oxygen gauge for the rapid measurement of Po_2 in respiratory gases.' *J. appl. Physiol.*, 21, 1672.

Ellis, F. R. and Nunn, J. F. (1968). 'The measurement of gaseous oxygen tension utilising paramagnetism: an evaluation of the Servomex OA 150 analyser.' *Br. J. Anaesth.*, 40, 569.

Ellison, R. G., Ellison, L. T. and Hamilton, W. F. (1955). 'Analysis of respiratory acidosis during anaesthesia.' *Ann. Surg.*, 141, 375.

Enghoff, H. (1931). 'Zur Frage des schädlichen Raumes bei der Atmung.' *Skand. Arch. Physiol.*, 63, 15.

Enghoff, H. (1938). 'Volumen inefficax. Bemerkungen zur Frage des schädlichen Raumes.' *Uppsala LäkFör Förh.*, 44, 191.

Enghoff, H., Holmdahl, M. H:son and Risholm, L. (1951). 'Diffusion respiration in man.' *Nature, Lond.*, 168, 830.

Engineer, S. and Jennett, S. (1972). 'Respiratory depression following single and repeated doses of pentazocine and pethidine.' *Br. J. Anaesth.*, 44, 795.

Ernsting, J. (1963). 'The effect of brief profound hypoxia upon the arterial and venous oxygen tensions in man.' *J. Physiol.*, 169, 292.

Ernsting, J. and McHardy, G. J. R. (1960). 'Brief anoxia following rapid decompression from 560 to 150 mm Hg.' *J. Physiol.*, 153, 73P.

Evans, J. M., Hogg, M. I. J., Lunn, J. N. and Rosen, M. (1974). 'Degree and duration of reversal by naloxone of effects of morphine in conscious subjects.' *Br. med. J.*, 2, 589.

Eve, F. C. (1932). 'Actuation of the inert diaphragm by a gravity method.' *Lancet*, 2, 995.

Fairley, H. B. and Blenkarn, G. D. (1966). 'Effect on pulmonary gas exchange of variations in inspiratory flow rate during intermittent positive pressure ventilation.' *Br. J. Anaesth.,* 38, 320.

Fairweather, L. J., Walker, J. and Flenley, D. C. (1974). '2,3-Diphosphoglycerate concentrations and the dissociation of oxyhaemoglobin in ventilatory failure.' *Clin. Sci.,* 47, 577.

Farhi, L. E. (1964). 'Gas stores of the body.' *Handbk Physiol., section 3,* 1, 873.

Farhi, L. E. and Rahn, H. (1955a). 'Gas stores of the body and the unsteady state.' *J. appl. Physiol.,* 7, 472.

Farhi, L. E. and Rahn, H. (1955b). 'A theoretical analysis of the alveolar–arterial O_2 difference with special reference to the distribution effect.' *J. appl. Physiol.,* 7, 699.

Farhi, L. E., Otis, A. B. and Proctor, D. F. (1957). 'Measurement of intrapleural pressure at different points in the chest of the dog.' *J. appl. Physiol.,* 10, 15.

Faulconer, A., Gaines, T. R. and Grove, J. S. (1946). 'Atelectasis during operations on the upper urinary tract.' *Anesthesiology,* 7, 637.

Featherstone, R. M., Muehlbaecher, C. A., DeBon, F. L. and Forsaith, J. A. (1961). 'Interactions of inert gases with proteins.' *Anesthesiology,* 22, 6.

Femi-Pearse, D., Afonja, A. O., Elegbeleye, O. O. and Odusote, K. A. (1976). 'Value of determination of oxygen consumption in tetanus.' *Br. med. J.,* 1, 74.

Fencl, V., Miller, T. B. and Pappenheimer, J. R. (1966). 'Studies of the respiratory response to disturbances of acid–base balance, with deductions concerning the ionic composition of cerebral interstitial fluid. *Am. J. Physiol.,* 210, 459.

Fenn, W. O. and Asano, T. (1956). 'Effects of carbon dioxide inhalation on potassium liberation from the liver.' *Am. J. Physiol.,* 185, 567.

Fenn, W. O., Otis, A. B. Rahn, H., Chadwick, L. E. and Hegnauer, A. H. (1947). 'Displacement of blood from the lungs by pressure breathing.' *Am. J. Physiol.,* 151, 258.

Ferguson, J. K. W. (1936). 'Carbamino compounds of CO_2 with human haemoglobin and their role in the transport of CO_2.' *J. Physiol.,* 88, 40.

Ferguson, J. K. W. and Roughton, F. J. W. (1934). 'The direct chemical estimation of carbamino compounds of CO_2 with haemoglobin.' *J. Physiol.,* 83, 68.

Ferris, B. G., Mead, J. and Frank, N. R. (1959). 'Effect of body position on esophageal pressure and measurement of pulmonary compliance.' *J. appl. Physiol.,* 14, 521.

Ferris, B. G., Mead, J. Whittenberger, J. L. and Saxton, G. A. (1952). 'Pulmonary function in convalescent poliomyelitis patients. 3. Compliance of the lungs and thorax. *New Engl. J. Med.,* 40, 664.

Ferris, E. B., Engel, G. L., Stevens, C. D. and Webb, J. (1946). 'Voluntary breath holding.' *J. clin. Invest.,* 25, 734.

Filley, G. F. MacIntosh, D. J. and Wright, G. W. (1954). Carbon monoxide uptake and pulmonary diffusing capacity in normal subject at rest and during exercise.' *J. clin. Invest.,* 33, 530.

Fink, B. R. (1961). 'Influence of cerebral activity in wakefulness on regulation of breathing.' *J. appl. Physiol.,* 16, 15.

Fink, B. R., Carpenter, S. L. and Holaday, D. A. (1954). 'Diffusion anoxia during recovery from nitrous oxide/oxygen anesthesia.' *Fedn Proc.,* 13, 354.

Fink, B. R., Ngai, S. H. and Holaday, D. A. (1958). 'Effect of air flow resistance on ventilation and respiratory muscle activity.' *J. Am. med. Ass.,* 168, 2245.

Finlay, W. E. I. Wightman, A. E., Adams, A. P. and Sykes, M. K. (1970). 'The effects of variations in inspiratory : expiratory ratio on cardiorespiratory function during controlled ventilation in normo-, hypo- and hypervolaemic dogs.' *Br. J. Anaesth.,* 42, 935.

Finley, T. N., Swenson, E. W. and Comroe, J. H. (1962). 'The cause of arterial hypoxemia at rest in patients with "alveolar–capillary block syndrome".' *J. clin. Invest.,* 41, 618.

Finucane, K. E. and Colebatch, H. J. H. (1969). 'Elastic behavior of the lung in patients with airway obstruction.' *J. appl. Physiol.,* 26, 330.

Fishman, A. P. (1972). 'Pulmonary oedema. The water exchanging function of the lung.' *Circulation,* 46, 390.

Flenley, D. C., Fairweather, L. J., Cooke, N. J. and Kirby, B. J. (1975). 'Changes in haemoglobin binding curve and oxygen transport in chronic hypoxic lung disease.' *Br. med. J.,* 1, 602.

Folkow, B. and Pappenheimer, J. R. (1955). 'Components of the respiratory dead space and their variation with pressure breathing and with broncho-active drugs.' *J. appl. Physiol.,* 8, 102.

Forrest, J. B. (1972). 'The effect of hyperventilation on pulmonary surface activity.' *Br. J. Anaesth.* **44**, 313.

Forster, H. V., Dempsey, J. A. and Chosy, L. W. (1975). 'Incomplete compensation of CSF [H$^+$] in man during acclimatization to high altitude (4,300 m).' *J. appl. Physiol.,* **38**, 1067.

Forster, H. V. Dempsey, J. A., Thomson, J., Vidruk, E. and doPico, G. A. (1972). 'Estimation of arterial PO$_2$, PCO$_2$, pH and lactate from arterialized venous blood.' *J. appl. Physiol.,* **32**, 134.

Forster, R. E. (1964a). 'Rate of gas uptake by red cells.' *Handbk Physiol., section 3,* **1**, 827.

Forster, R. E. (1964b). 'Diffusion of gases.' *Handbk Physiol., section 3,* **1**, 839.

Foster, C. A. (1965). 'Hyperbaric oxygen and radiotherapy.' In: *Hyperbaric Oxygenation.* Ed. by I. Ledingham. Edinburgh and London; Churchill Livingstone.

Fourcade, H. E., Larson, C. P., Hickey, R. F., Bahlman, S. H. and Eger, E. I. (1972). 'Effects of time on ventilation during halothane and cyclopropane anesthesia.' *Anesthesiology,* **36**, 83.

Fowler, K. T. and Hugh-Jones, P. (1957). 'Mass spectrometry applied to clinical practice and research.' *Br. med. J.,* **1**, 1205.

Fowler, W. S. (1948). 'Lung function studies: II. The respiratory dead space.' *Am. J. Physiol.,* **154**, 405.

Fowler, W. S. (1950a). 'Lung function studies. IV. Postural changes in respiratory dead space and functional residual capacity.' *J. clin. Invest.,* **29**, 1437.

Fowler, W. S. (1950b). 'Lung function studies. V. Respiratory dead space in old age and in pulmonary emphysema.' *J. clin Invest.,* **29**, 1439.

Fowler, W. S. (1954). 'Breaking point of breath-holding.' *J. appl. Physiol.,* **6**, 539.

Fowler, W. S., and Blakemore, W. S. (1951). 'Lung function studies: VII. The effect of pneumonectomy on respiratory dead space.' *J. thorac. Surg.,* **21**, 433.

Freeman, J. (1962). 'Survival of bled dogs after halothane and ether anaesthesia.' *Br. J. Anaesth.,* **34**, 832.

Freeman, J. and Nunn, J. F. (1963). 'Ventilation–perfusion relationships after haemorrhage.' *Clin. Sci.* **24**, 135.

Freund, F., Roos, A. and Dodd, R. B. (1964). 'Expiratory activity of the abdominal muscles in man during general anesthesia.' *J. appl. Physiol.,* **19**, 693.

Freund, F. K. Martin, W. E., Wong, K. C. and Hornbein, T. F. (1973). 'Abdominal-muscle rigidity induced by morphine and nitrous oxide.' *Anesthesiology,* **38**, 358.

Fridovich, I. (1975). 'Superoxide dismutases.' *A. Rev. Biochem.,* **44**, 147.

Fritts, H. W., Odell, J. E., Harris, P., Braunwald, E. W. and Fishman, A. P. (1960). 'Effects of acute hypoxia on the volume of blood in the thorax.' *Circulation,* **22**, 216.

Froese, A. B. and Bryan, A. C. (1974). 'Effects of anesthesia and paralysis on diaphragmatic mechanics in man.' *Anesthesiology* **41**, 242.

Froman, C. (1966). 'Correction of cerebrospinal fluid metabolic acidosis by intrathecal injection of bicarbonate.' *Br. J. Anaesth.,* **39**, 90.

Froman, C. and Crampton-Smith, A. (1966). 'Hyperventilation associated with low pH of cerebrospinal fluid after intracranial haemorrhage.' *Lancet,* **1**, 780.

Frumin, M. J. Epstein, R. M. and Cohen, G. (1959). 'Apneic oxygenation in man.' *Anesthesiology,* **20**, 789.

Fry, D. L., Ebert, R. V. Stead, W. W. and Brown, C. C. (1954). 'The mechanics of pulmonary ventilation in normal subjects and in patients with emphysema.' *Am. J. Med.,* **16**, 80.

Geddes, I. C. (1967). 'Recent studies in metabolic aspects of anaesthesia.' In: *Modern Trends in Anaesthesia,* 3. Ed. by F. T. Evans and T. C. Gray. London; Butterworths.

Geddes, I. C. and Gray, T. C. (1959). 'Hyperventilation for the maintenance of anaesthesia.' *Lancet,* **2**, 4.

Georg, G., Lassen, N. A., Mellemgaard, K. and Vinther, A. (1965). 'Diffusion in the gas phase of the lungs in normal and emphysematous subjects.' *Clin. Sci.,* **29**, 525.

Gerbershagen, H. U. and Bergman, N. A. (1967). 'The effect of *d*-tubocurarine on respiratory resistance in anesthetized man.' *Anesthesiology,* **28**, 981.

Gerschman, R. (1964). 'Biological effects of oxygen.' In: *Oxygen in the Animal Organism.* Ed. by F. Dickens and E. Neil. Oxford; Pergamon.

Gerst, P. H., Rattenborg, C. and Holaday, D. A. (1959). 'The effects of hemorrhage on pulmonary circulation and respiratory gas exchange.' *J. clin. Invest.,* **38**, 524.

Gessell, R. (1923). 'On the chemical regulation of respiration.' *Am. J. Physiol.,* **66**, 5.

Giesecke, A. H. Gerbershagen, H. U., Dortman, C. and Lee, D. (1973). 'Comparison of the ventilating and injection bronchoscopes.' *Anesthesiology,* 38, 298.

Gilbertson, A. A., Ball, P. A. J. and Watson-Williams, E. J. (1967). 'The management of anaesthesia in sickle cell states.' *Proc. R. Soc. Med.,* 60, 631.

Gillis, C. N. (1973). 'Metabolism of vasoactive hormones by lung.' *Anesthesiology,* 39, 626.

Gilmour, I., Burnham, M. and Craig, D. B. (1976). 'Closing capacity measurement during general anesthesia.' *Anesthesiology,* 45, 477.

Ginn, R. and Vane, J. R. (1968). 'Disappearance of catecholamines from the circulation. *Nature, Lond.* 219, 740.

Glazier, J. B., Hughes, J. M. B., Maloney, J. E. and West, J. B. (1967). 'Vertical gradient of alveolar size in lungs of dogs frozen intact.' *J. appl. Physiol.,* 23, 694.

Glazier, J. B., Hughes, J. M. B. Maloney, J. E. and West, J. B. (1969). 'Measurements of capillary dimensions and blood volume in rapidly frozen lungs.' *J. appl. Physiol.,* 26, 65.

Glossop, M. W. (1963). 'A simple method for the estimation of carbon dioxide concentration in the presence of nitrous oxide. *Br. J. Anaesth.,* 35, 17.

Gluck, L. (1971). 'Biochemical development of the lung.' *Clin. Obstet. Gynec.,* 14, 710.

Gluck, L., Kulovich, M. V. Borer, R. C., Brenner, P. H., Anderson, G. G. and Spellacy, W. N. (1971). 'Diagnosis of the respiratory distress syndrome by amniocentesis.' *Am. J. Obstet. Gynec.,* 109, 440.

Godfrey, S. and Wolf, E. (1972). 'An evaluation of rebreathing methods for measuring mixed venous PCO_2 during exercise.' *Clin. Sci.,* 42, 345.

Gold, M. I. and Helrich, H. (1965). 'Pulmonary compliance during anesthesia.' *Anesthesiology,* 26, 281.

Gold, M. I. and Helrich, M. (1967). 'Ventilation and blood gases in anaesthetized patients.' *Can. Anaesth. Soc. J.* 14, 424.

Gordon, A. S., Sadove, M. S., Raymon, F. and Ivy, A. C. (1951a). 'Critical survey of manual artificial respiration.' *J. Am. med. Ass.,* 147, 1444.

Gordon, A. S., Affeldt, J. E. Sadove, M. S., Raymon, F., Whittenberger, J. L. and Ivy, A. C. (1951b). 'Air-flow patterns and pulmonary ventilation during manual artificial respiration on apneic normal adults. *J. appl. Physiol.,* 4, 408.

Gordon, A. S., Prec, L., Wedell, H., Sadove, M. S., Raymon, F., Nelson, J. T. and Ivy, A. C. (1951c). 'Circulatory studies during artificial respiration on apneic normal adults.' *J. appl. Physiol.,* 4, 421.

Gracey, D. R. Divertie, M. B. and Brown, A. L. (1968). 'Alveolar–capillary membrane in idiopathic interstitial pulmonary fibrosis.' *Am. Rev. resp. Dis.,* 98, 16.

Graham, G. R. (1961). 'Physiological aspects of circulatory arrest and resuscitation.' *Br. J. Anaesth.* 33, 480.

Graham, G. R., Hill, D. W. and Nunn, J. F. (1960). 'Die Wirkung hoher CO_2-Konzentrationen auf Kreislauf und Atmung.' *Anaesthetist,* 9, 70.

Granit, R. (1955). *Receptors and Sensory Perception.* New Haven, Conn. and London ; Yale University Press.

Gray, L. H., Conger, A. D. Ebert, M., Hornsey, S. and Scott, O. C. A. (1953). 'The concentration of oxygen dissolved in tissues at the time of irradiation as a factor in radiotherapy.' *Br. J. Radiol.,* 26, 638.

Gray, T. C. and Rees, G. J. (1952). 'The role of apnoea in anaesthesia for major surgery.' *Br. med. J.* 2, 891.

Greenbaum, R., Nunn, J. F. Prys-Roberts, C., Kelman, G. R. and Silk, F. F. (1965). 'Cardio-pulmonary function after fat embolism. *Br. J. Anaesth.,* 37, 554.

Greenbaum, R. Bay, J., Hargreaves, M. D., Kain, M. L., Kelman, G. R., Nunn, J. F., Prys-Roberts, C. and Siebold, K. (1967a). 'Effects of higher oxides of nitrogen on the anaesthetized dog.' *Br. J. Anaesth,* 39, 393.

Greenbaum, R. Nunn, J. F., Prys-Roberts, C. and Kelman, G. R. (1967b). 'Metabolic changes in whole human blood (*in vitro*) at 37° C.' *Resp. Physiol.,* 2, 274.

Greene, D. G., Dameron, J. T. and Bush, E. T. (1952). 'Treatment of pulmonary edema with different types of portable mechanical respirators.' *Surg. Forum.,* 389.

Green, D. G., Bauer, R. O. Janney, C. D. and Elam, J. O. (1957). 'Oxygen and carbon dioxide exchange and energy cost of expired air resuscitation.' *J. Am. med. Ass.,* 167, 328.

Gregory, G. A. Kitterman, J. A., Phibbs, R. H., Tooley, W. H. and Hamilton, W. K. (1971). 'Treatment of idiopathic respiratory-distress syndrome with continuous positive airway pressure.' *New Engl. J. Med.,* 284, 1333.

Gregory, G. A., Eger, E. I., Smith, N. T. and Cullen, B. F. (1974). 'The cardiovascular effects of carbon dioxide in man awake and during diethyl ether anesthesia.' *Anesthesiology*, **40**, 301.

Gregory, I. C. (1973). 'Assessment of Van Slyke manometric measurements of oxygen content.' *J. appl. Physiol.*, **34**, 715.

Gregory, I. C. (1974). 'The oxygen and carbon monoxide capacities of foetal and adult blood.' *J. Physiol.*, **236**, 625.

Grollman, A. (1929). 'The determination of the cardiac output of man by the use of acetylene.' *Am. J. Physiol.*, **88**, 285.

Gunsalus, I. C. Pederson, T. C. and Sligar, S. G. (1975). 'Oxygenase-catalyzed biological hydroxylations.' *A. Rev. Biochem.*, **44**, 377.

Gurtner, G. H. and Burns, B. (1972). 'Possible facilitated transport of oxygen across the placenta.' *Nature, Lond.*, **240**, 473.

Gurtner, G. H. and Burns, B. (1973). 'The role of cytochrome P-450 of placenta in facilitated oxygen diffusion ' *Drug Metab. Disposit.*, **1**, 368.

Gurtner, G. and Burns, B. (1975). 'Physiological evidence consistent with the presence of a specific O_2 carrier in the placenta.' *J. appl. Physiol.*, **39**, 728.

Gurtner, G. H. and Fowler, W. S. (1971). 'Interrelationships of factors affecting the pulmonary diffusing capacity.' *J. appl. Physiol.*, **30**, 619.

Guyton, A. C. and Lindsey A. W. (1959). 'Effect of elevated left atrial pressure and decreased plasma protein concentration on the development of pulmonary edema.' *Circulation Res.*, **7**, 649.

Guz, A. (1975). 'Regulation of respiration in man. *A. Rev. Physiol.*, **37**, 303.

Guz, A., Noble, M. I. M. Trenchard, D., Cochrane, H. L. and Makey, A. R. (1964). 'Studies on the vagus nerves in man: their role in respiratory and circulatory control.' *Clin. Sci.*, **27**, 293.

Guz, A., Noble, M. I. M. Widdicombe, J. G., Trenchard, D. and Mushin, W. W. (1966a). 'Peripheral chemoreceptor block in man.' *Resp. Physiol.*, **1**, 38.

Guz, A., Noble, M. I. M. Widdicombe, J. G., Trenchard, D., Mushin, W. W. and Makey, A. R. (1966b). 'The role of the vagal and glossopharyngeal afferent nerves in respiratory sensation, control of breathing and arterial pressure regulation in conscious man.' *Clin. Sci.*, **30**, 161.

Guz, A., Noble, M. I. M. Eisele, J. H. and Trenchard, D. (1971). 'The effect of lung deflation on breathing in man.' *Clin. Sci.*, **40**, 451.

Haldane, J. S. (1920). 'A new apparatus for accurate blood-gas analysis.' *J. Path. Bact.*, **23**, 443.

Haldane, J. S. and Priestley, J. G. (1905). 'The regulation of the lung ventilation.' *J. Physiol.*, **32**, 225.

Hales, S. (1731). *Vegetable Staticks: analysis of the air* p. 240. London.

Hamburger, H. J. (1918). 'Anionenwanderungen in serum und Blut unter dem Einfluss von CO_2, Säure und Alkali. *Biochem, Z.*, **86**, 309.

Hamilton, W. K., McDonald, J. S. Fischer, H. W. and Bethards, R. (1964). 'Postoperative respiratory complications.' *Anesthesiology*, **25**, 607.

Hanks, E. C., Ngai, S. H. and Fink, B. R. (1961). 'The respiratory threshold for carbon dioxide in anesthetized man.' *Anesthesiology*, **22**, 393.

Harlan, W. R. and Said, S. I. (1969). 'Selected aspects of lung metabolism.' Chapter 12 in: *The Biological Basis of Medicine.* Ed. by E. E. Bittar and N. Bittar. New York and London; Academic Press.

Harris, E. A., Hunter, M. E., Seelye E. R., Vedder, M. and Whitlock, R. M. L. (1973). 'Prediction of the physiological dead-space in resting normal subjects.' *Clin. Sci.*, **45**, 375.

Harris, E. A., Kenyon, A. M. Nisbet, H. D., Seelye, E. R. and Whitlock, R. M. L. (1974). 'The normal alveolar–arterial oxygen-tension difference in man. *Clin. Sci.*, **46**, 89.

Harris, P. and Heath, D. (1962). *The Human Pulmonary Circulation.* Edinburgh and London; Churchill Livingstone.

Hasselbalch, K. A. (1916). 'Berechnung der Wasserstoffzahl des Blutes usw.' *Biochem. Z.*, **78**, 112.

Haugaard, N. (1968). 'Cellular mechanisms of oxygen toxicity.' *Physiol. Rev.*, **48**, 311.

von Hayek, H. (1960). *The Human Lung.* Translated from *Die Menschliche Lunge* by V. E. Krahl. New York and London; Hafner.

Head, H. (1889). 'On the regulation of respiration.' *J. Physiol.*, **10**, 1.

Hedenstierna, G. and McCarthy, G. (1975). 'Mechanics of breathing, gas distribution and functional residual capacity at different frequencies of respiration during spontaneous and artifical ventilations.' *Br. J. Anaesth.*, 47, 706.

Hedenstierna, G., McCarthy, G. and Bergström, M. (1976). 'Airway closure during mechanical ventilation.' *Anesthesiology*, 44, 114.

Heinemann, H. O. and Fishman, A. P. (1969). 'Non-respiratory functions of mammalian lung.' *Physiol. Rev.*, 49, 1.

Heller, M. L. and Watson, T. R. (1961). 'Polarographic study of arterial oxygenation during apnea in man.' *New Engl. J. Med.*, 264, 326.

Heller, M. L. and Watson, T. R. (1962). 'The role of preliminary oxygenation prior to induction with high nitrous oxide mixtures.' *Anesthesiology*, 23, 219.

Hemmingsen, A. and Scholander, P. E. (1960). 'Specific transport of oxygen through haemoglobin solutions.' *Science* 132, 1379.

Henderson, L. J. (1909). 'Das Gleichgewicht zwischen Basen und Säuren im tierischen Organismus.' *Ergebn. Physiol.*, 8, 254.

Henderson, Y. Chillingworth, F. P. and Whitney, J. L. (1915). 'The respiratory dead space.' *Am. J. Physiol.*, 38, 1.

Henry, J. M., McArdle, A. H., Bounous, G., Hampson, L. G., Scott, H. J. and Gurd, F. N. (1967). 'The effect of experimental hemorrhagic shock on pulmonary alveolar surfactant.' *J. Trauma*, 7, 691.

Herholdt, J. D. and Rafn, C. G. (1796). *Life-saving Methods for Drowning Persons.* Copenhagen; H. Tikiob. Reprinted in 1960, Aarhuus, Denmark; Stiftsbogtrykkerie.

Hering, E. (1868). 'Die Selbsteuerung der Athmung durch den Nervus Vagus.' *Sber. Akad. Wiss. Wien*, 57, 672.

Hewlett, A. M., Hulands, G. H., Nunn, J. F. and Minty, K. B. (1974a). 'Functional residual capacity during anaesthesia. I: Methodology.' *Br. J. Anaesth.*, 46, 479.

Hewlett, A. M., Hulands, G. H., Nunn, J. F. and Heath, J. R. (1974b). 'Functional residual capacity. II: Spontaneous respiration.' *Br. J. Anaesth.*, 46, 486.

Hewlett, A. M., Hulands, G. H., Nunn, J. F. and Milledge, J. S. (1974c). 'Functional residual capacity during anaesthesia. III: Artificial ventilation. *Br. J. Anaesth.*, 46, 495.

Heymans, C. and Neil, E. (1958). *Reflexogenic Areas of the Cardiovascular System.* Boston, Mass.; Little/London; Churchill.

Heymans, C., Bouckaert, J. J. and Dautrebande, L. (1930). 'Sinus carotidien et réflexes respiratoire.' *Archs int. Pharmacodyn. Thér.*, 39, 400.

Heymans, J. F. and Heymans, C. (1927). 'Sur les modifications directes et sur la régulation reflexe de l'activité du centre respiratoire de la tête isolée du chien.' *Archs int. Pharmacodyn. Thér.*, 33, 272.

Hickey, R. F., Visick, W., Fairley, H. B. and Fourcade, H. E. (1973). 'Effects of halothane anesthesia on functional residual capacity and alveolar–arterial oxygen tension difference.' *Anesthesiology*, 38, 20.

Hickman, H. H. (1824). A letter on suspended animation. Ironbridge, W. Smith (addressed to T. A. Knight of Downton Castle).

Higgins, H. L. and Means, J. H. (1915). 'The effect of certain drugs on the respiration and gaseous metabolism in normal human subjects.' *J. Pharmac. exp. Ther.*, 7, 1.

Hill, D. W. (1972). *Physics Applied to Anaesthesia*, 2nd edn. London and Boston, Mass.; Butterworths.

Hill, J. D., Main, F. B., Osborn, J. J. and Gerbode, F. (1965). 'Correct use of respirator on cardiac patient after operation.' *Archs. Surg.*, 91, 775.

Hirshman, C. A., McCullough, R. E., Cohen, P. J. and Weil, J. V. (1975). 'Effect of pentobarbitone on hypoxic ventilatory drive in man.' *Br. J. Anaesth.*, 47, 963.

Hoedt-Rasmussen, K., Skinhoj, E., Paulson, O., Ewald, J., Bjerrum, J. K., Fahrenkrug, A. and Lassen, N. A. (1967). 'Regional cerebral blood flow in acute apoplexy. The "luxury perfusion syndrome" of brain tissue.' *Archs Neurol.*, 17, 271.

Hoff, H. E. and Breckenridge, C. G. (1949). 'The medullary origin of respiratory periodicity in the dog.' *Am. J. Physiol.*, 158, 157.

Hogben, L. (1951). *Mathematics for the Million*, 3rd edn. London; Allen and Unwin.

Hogg, M. I. J., Davies, J. M., Mapleson, W. W. and Rosen, M. (1974). 'Proposed upper limit of respiratory resistance for inhalational apparatus used in labour.' *Br. J. Anaesth.*, 46, 149.

Holdcroft, A., Lumley, J. and Gaya, H. (1973). 'Why disinfect ventilators?' *Lancet*, 1, 240.

Holmdahl, M. H:son. (1953). 'Apnoeic diffusion oxygenation in electroconvulsion therapy.' *Acta Soc. Med. upsal.*, 58, 269.

Holmdahl, M. H:son (1956). 'Pulmonary uptake of oxygen, acid-base metabolism and circulation during prolonged apnoea.' *Acta chir. scand.*, suppl. 212.

Hornbein, T. F. and Pavlin, E. G. (1975). 'Distribution of H^+ and HCO_3^- between CSF and blood during respiratory alkalosis in dogs.' *J. Physiol.*, 228, 1149.

Hornbein, T. F. and Roos, A. (1963). 'Specificity of H ion concentration as a carotid chemoreceptor stimulus.' *J. appl. Physiol.*, 18, 580.

Hornbein, T. F., Griffo, Z. J. and Roos, A. (1961). 'Quantitation of chemoreceptor activity: interrelation of hypoxia and hypercapnia.' *J. Neurophysiol.*, 24, 561.

Howell, J. B. L. and Peckett, B. W. (1957). 'Studies of the elastic properties of the thorax of supine anaesthetized paralysed human subjects.' *J. Physiol.*, 136, 1.

Howell, J. B. L., Permutt, S., Proctor, D. F. and Riley, R. L. (1961). 'Effect of inflation of the lung on different parts of pulmonary vascular bed.' *J. appl. Physiol.*, 16, 71.

Huckabee, W. E. (1961). 'Henderson vs Hasselbalch.' *Clin. Res.*, 9, 116.

Hughes, J. M. B., Glazier, J. B., Maloney, J. E. and West, J. B. (1968). 'Effect of lung volume on the distribution of pulmonary blood flow in man.' *Resp. Physiol.*, 4, 58.

Hughes, J. M. B., Grant, B. J. B., Greene, R. E., Iliff, L. D. and Milic-Emili, J. (1972). 'Inspiratory flow rate and ventilation distribution in normal subjects and in patients with simple chronic bronchitis.' *Clin. Sci.*, 43, 583.

Hughes, R. (1970). 'The influence of changes in acid–base balance on neuromuscular blockade in cats.' *Br. J. Anaesth.*, 42, 658.

Hugh-Jones, P. and West, J. B. (1960). 'Detection of bronchial and arterial obstruction by continuous gas analysis from individual lobes and segments of the lung.' *Thorax*, 15, 154.

Hulands, G. H., Green, R., Iliff, L. D. and Nunn, J. F. (1970). 'Influence of anaesthesia on the regional distribution of perfusion and ventilation in the lung.' *Clin. Sci.*, 38, 451.

Hultgren, H. N. and Grover, R. F. (1968). 'Circulatory adaptation to high altitude.' *A. Rev. Med.*, 19, 119.

Hutchison, D. C. S., Flenley, D. C. and Donald, K. W. (1964). 'Controlled oxygen therapy in respiratory failure.' *Br. med. J.*, 2, 1159.

Hutchison, D. C. S., Cook, P. J. L., Barter, C. E., Harris, H. and Hugh-Jones, P. (1971). 'Pulmonary emphysema and α_1-antitrypsin deficiency.' *Br. med. J.*, 1, 689.

Ingvar, D. H. (1965). In: *Hyperbaric Oxygenation*, discussion page 199. Ed. by I. Ledingham. Edinburgh and London; Churchill Livingstone.

Ingvar, D. H. and Bulow, K. B. (1963). 'Respiratory regulation in sleep.' *Ann. N. Y. Acad. Sci.*, 109, 870.

Inkster, J. S. and Pearson, D. T. (1967). 'Some infant ventilator systems.' *Br. J. Anaesth.*, 39, 667.

Irwin, R. L., Draper, W. B. and Whitehead, R. W. (1957). 'Urine secretion during diffusion respiration after apnea from neuromuscular block.' *Anesthesiology*, 18, 594.

Ivanov, S. D. and Nunn, J. F. (1968). 'Influence of duration of hyperventilation on rise time of PCO_2 after step reduction of ventilation.' *Resp. Physiol.*, 4, 243.

Ivanov, S. D. and Nunn, J. F. (1969). 'Methods of elevation of PCO_2 for restoration of spontaneous breathing after artificial ventilation of anaesthetised patients.' *Br. J. Anaesth.*, 41, 28.

Jacobson, J. H., Wang, M. C. H., Yamaki, T., Kline, H. J., Kark, A. E. and Kuhn, L. A. (1965). 'Hyperbaric oxygenation in diffuse myocardial infarction.' In: *Hyperbaric Oxygenation.* Ed. by I. Ledingham. Edinburgh and London; Churchill Livingstone.

Jain, S. K., Trenchard, D., Reynolds, F., Noble, M. I. M. and Guz, A. (1973). 'The effect of local anaesthesia of the airway on respiratory reflexes in the rabbit.' *Clin. Sci.*, 44, 519.

Janney, C. D. (1959). 'Super-syringe.' *Anesthesiology*, 20, 709.

Jaques, E. (1957). 'The use of the modified Beaver respirator.' *Br. J. Anaesth.*, 29, 181.

Jennett, W. B., McDowall, D. G. and Barker, J. (1967). 'The effect of halothane on intracranial pressure in cerebral tumours: report of two cases.' *J. Neurosurg.*, 26, 270.

Jerusalem, E. and Starling, E. H. (1910). 'On the significance of carbon dioxide for the heart beat.' *J. Physiol.*, 40, 279.

Johnson, S. R. (1951). 'The effect of some anesthetic agents on the circulation in man. *Acta chir. scand.*, 102, suppl. 158.

Johnstone, R. E. Jobes, D. R., Kennell, E. M., Behar, M. G. and Smith, T. C. (1974). 'Reversal of morphine anesthesia with naloxone.' *Anesthesiology*, 41, 361.

Jones, J. G., Faithfull, D. and Minty, B. D. (1976). 'The relative contribution to tidal volume of the chest wall and the abdomen in awake and anaesthetised subjects.' *Br. J. Anaesth.*, 48, (in the press).

Jones, J. G., Fraser, V. B. and Nadel, J. A. (1975). 'Prediction of maximum expiratory flow rate from area-transmural pressure curve of compressed airway.' *J. appl. Physiol.*, **38**, 1002.

Jones, R. D., Commins, B. T. and Cernik, A. A. (1972). Blood lead and carboxyhaemoglobin levels in London taxi drivers.' *Lancet*, **2**, 302.

Julian, D. G., Travis, D. M., Robin, E. D. and Crump, C. H. (1960). 'Effect of pulmonary artery occlusion upon end-tidal CO_2 tension.' *J. appl. Physiol.*, **15**, 87.

Kaasik, A. E., Nilsson, L. and Siesjö, B. K. (1970a). 'The effect of asphyxia upon the lactate, pyruvate and bicarbonate concentrations of brain tissue and cisternal CSF, and upon the tissue concentrations of phosphocreatine and adenine nucleotides in anesthetized rats.' *Acta physiol. scand.*, **78**, 433.

Kaasik, A. E., Nilsson, L. and Siesjö, B. K. (1970b). 'The effect of arterial hypotension upon the lactate, pyruvate and bicarbonate concentrations of brain tissue and cisternal CSF, and upon the tissue concentrations of phosphocreatine and adenine nucleotides in anesthetized rats.' *Acta physiol. scand.*, **78**, 448.

Kain, M. L., Panday, J. and Nunn, J. F. (1969). 'The effect of intubation on the dead space during halothane anaesthesia.' *Br. J. Anaesth.*, **41**, 94.

Kalia, M., Senapati, J. M., Parida, B. and Panda, A. (1972). 'Reflex increase in ventilation by muscle receptors with nonmedullated fibers (C fibers).' *J. appl. Physiol.*, **32**, 189.

Kaneko, K., Milic-Emili, M. E., Dolovich, M. B., Dawson, A. and Bates, D. V. (1966). 'Regional distribution of ventilation and perfusion as a function of body position.' *J. appl. Physiol.*, **21**, 767.

Kao, F. F. (1963). 'An experimental study of the pathways involved in exercise hyperpnoea employing cross-circulation techniques.' In: *The Regulation of Human Respiration.* Ed. by D. J. C. Cunningham and B. B. Lloyd. Oxford; Blackwell.

Karpovich, P. V. (1962). In: *Artificial Respiration.* Ed. by J. L. Whittenberger. New York and London; Harper and Row.

Karpovich, P. V., Hale, C. J. and Bailey, T. L. (1951). 'Pulmonary ventilation in manual artificial respiration.' *J. appl. Physiol.*, **4**, 458.

Katz, R. L. and Katz, G. J. (1974). 'Prostaglandins—basic and clinical considerations.' *Anesthesiology*, **40**, 471.

Katz, R. L., Ngai, S. H., Nahas, G. G. and Wang, S. C. (1963). 'Relationship between acid–base balance and the central respiratory mechanisms.' *Am. J. Physiol.*, **204**, 867.

Katz, S. and Horres, A. D. (1972). 'Medullary respiratory neuron response to pulmonary emboli and pneumothorax.' *J. appl. Physiol.*, **33**, 390.

Kaul, S. U., Heath, J. R. and Nunn, J. F. (1973). 'Factors influencing the development of expiratory muscle activity during anaesthesia.' *Br. J. Anaesth.*, **45**, 1013.

Kaye, G. W. C. and Laby, T. H. (1966). *Tables of Physical and Chemical Constants*, 13th edn. London; Longmans.

Kelman, G. R. (1966a). 'Digital computer subroutine for the conversion of oxygen tension into saturation.' *J. appl. Physiol.*, **21**, 1375.

Kelman, G. R. (1966b). 'Calculation of certain indices of cardio-pulmonary function using a digital computer.' *Resp. Physiol.*, **1**, 335.

Kelman, G. R. (1966c). 'Errors in the processing of dye dilution curves.' *Circulation Res.*, **18**, 543.

Kelman, G. R. (1971). *Applied Cardiovascular Physiology.* London and Boston, Mass., Butterworths.

Kelman, G. R. and Nunn, J. F. (1966a). 'Clinical recognition of hypoxaemia under fluorescent lamps.' *Lancet*, **1**, 1400.

Kelman, G. R. and Nunn, J. F. (1966b). 'Nomograms for correction of blood PO_2, PCO_2, pH and base excess for time and temperature,' *J. appl. Physiol.*, **21**, 1484.

Kelman, G. R. and Nunn, J. F. (1968). *Computer Produced Physiological Tables.* London and Boston, Mass.; Butterworths.

Kelman, G. R. and Prys-Roberts C. (1967). 'Circulatory influences of artificial ventilation during nitrous oxide anaesthesia in man. I. Introduction and methods.' *Br. J. Anaesth.*, **39**, 523.

Kelman, G. R., Coleman, A. J. and Nunn, J. F. (1966). 'Evaluation of a microtonometer used with a capillary glass pH electrode.' *J. appl. Physiol.*, **21**, 1103.

Kelman, G. R., Nunn, J. F., Prys-Roberts, C. and Greenbaum, R. (1967). 'The influence of cardiac output on arterial oxygenation.' *Br. J. Anaesth.*, **39**, 450.

Kelman, G. R., Swapp, G. H., Smith, I., Benzie, R. J. and Gordon, N. L. M. (1972). 'Cardiac output and arterial blood-gas tension during laparoscopy.' *Br. J. Anaesth.*, **44**, 1155.

Kemm, J. R. and Kamburoff, P. L. (1970). 'Effort and the forced expiratory volume in one second (FEV₁).' *Clin. Sci.*, **39**, 747.

Kerr, J. H., Smith, A. C., Prys-Roberts, C., Meloche, R. and Foëx, P. (1974). 'Observations during endobronchial anaesthesia. II: Oxygenation.' *Br. J. Anaesth.*, **46**, 84.

Kety, S. S. and Schmidt, C. F. (1948). 'The effects of altered arterial tensions of carbon dioxide and oxygen on cerebral blood flow and cerebral oxygen consumption of normal young men.' *J. clin. Invest.*, **27**, 500.

Khanam, T. and Branthwaite, M. A. (1973). 'Arterial oxygenation during one-lung anaesthesia (2).' *Anaesthesia*, **28**, 280.

Kilburn, K. H. (1974). 'Functional morphology of the distal lung.' *Int. Rev. Cytol.*, **37**, 153.

Killick, E. M. (1935). 'Resistance to inspiration—its effect on respiration in man.' *J. Physiol.*, **84**, 162.

Kilmartin, J. V. and Rossi-Bernardi, L. (1973). 'Interaction of hemoglobin with hydrogen ions, carbon dioxide, and organic phosphates.' *Physiol. Rev.*, **53**, 836.

King, A. J., Cooke, N. J., Leitch, A. G. and Flenley, D. C. (1973). 'The effects of 30% oxygen on the respiratory response to treadmill exercise in chronic respiratory failure.' *Clin. Sci.*, **44**, 151.

King, R. J. (1974). 'The surfactant system of the lung.' *Fedn. Proc.*, **33**, 2238.

King, T. K. C., Weber, B., Okinawa, A., Friedman, S. A., Smith, J. P. and Briscoe, W. A. (1974). 'Oxygen transfer in catastrophic respiratory failure.' *Chest*, **65**, 405.

Kinsman, J. M., Moore, J. W. and Hamilton, W. F. (1929). 'Studies on the circulation. Injection method: physical and mathematical considerations. *Am. J. Physiol.*, **89**, 322.

Kirby, R. R., Downes, J. B. and Civetta, J. M. (1975). 'High level positive end expiratory pressure (PEEP) in acute respiratory insufficiency.' *Chest*, **67**, 156.

Klocke, F. J. and Rahn, H. (1959). 'Breath holding after breathing of oxygen.' *J. appl. Physiol.*, **14**, 689.

Klocke, F. J. and Rahn, H. (1961). 'The arterial—alveolar inert gas ("N₂") difference in normal and emphysematous subjects, as indicated by the analysis of urine.' *J. clin. Invest.*, **40**, 286.

Knowles, J. H., Hong, S. K. and Rahn, H. (1959). 'Possible errors using esophageal balloon in determination of pressure—volume characteristics of the lung and thoracic cage.' *J. appl. Physiol.*, **14**, 525.

Komesaroff, D. and McKie, B. (1972). 'The "Bronchoflator": a new technique for bronchoscopy under general anaesthesia.' *Br. J. Anaesth.*, **44**, 1057.

Krahl, V. E. (1964). 'Anatomy of the mammalian lung.' *Handbk Physiol., section 3*, **1**, 213.

Kuida, H., Hinshaw, L. B., Gilbert, B. P. and Vischer, M. B. (1958). 'Effect of Gram-negative endotoxin on pulmonary circulation.' *Am. J. Physiol.*, **192**, 335.

Kumar, A., Falke, K. J., Geffin, B., Aldredge, C. F., Laver, M. B., Lowenstein, E. and Pontoppidan, H. (1970). 'Continuous positive-pressure ventilation in acute respiratory failure.' *New Engl. J. Med.*, **283**, 1430.

Kumusi, F., Butts, W. C. and Ruff, W. L. (1973). 'Superior analytical performance by electrolytic cell analysis of blood oxygen content.' *J. appl. Physiol.*, **35**, 299.

Lambert, M. W. (1955). 'Accessory bonchiole—alveolar communications.' *J. Path. Bact.*, **70**, 311.

Lambertsen, C. J. (1963). 'Factors in the stimulation of respiration by carbon dioxide.' In: *The Regulation of Human Respiration.* Ed. by D. J. C. Cunningham and B. B. Lloyd. Oxford; Blackwell.

Lambertsen, C. J. (1965). 'Effects of oxygen at high partial pressure.' *Handbk Physiol., section 3*, **2**, 1027.

Lardy, H. A. and Ferguson, S. M. (1969). 'Oxidative phosphorylation in mitochondria.' *A. Rev. Biochem.*, **38**, 991.

Larson, C. P., Eger, E. I. Muallam, M., Buechel, D. R., Munson, E. S. and Eisele, J. H. (1969). 'The effects of diethyl ether and methoxyflurane on ventilation.' *Anesthesiology*, **30**, 174.

Lassen, N. A. (1959). 'Cerebral blood flow and oxygen consumption in man.' *Physiol. Rev.*, **39**, 183.

Lassen, N. A. (1966). 'The luxury perfusion syndrome and its possible relation to acute metabolic acidosis localized within the brain.' *Lancet*, **2**, 1113.

Lassen, N. A. and Ingvar, D. H. (1961). 'The blood flow of the cerebral cortex determined by radioactive krypton[85].' *Experientia*, 17, 42.

Lassen, N. A. and Palvalgyi, R. (1968). 'Cerebral steal during hypercapnia and the inverse reaction during hypocapnia observed by the [133]xenon technique in man.' *Scand. J. clin. Lab. Invest.* suppl. 102.

Laurell, C-B. and Eriksson, S. (1963). 'The electrophoretic α_1-globulin pattern of serum in α_1-antitrypsin deficiency.' *Scand. J. clin. Lab. Invest.*, 15, 132.

Laver, M. B. and Seifen, A. (1965). 'Measurement of blood oxygen tension in anesthesia.' *Anesthesiology*, 26, 73.

Laws, A. K. (1968). 'Effects of induction of anaesthesia and muscle paralysis on functional residual capacity of the lungs.' *Can. Anaesth. Soc. J.*, 15, 325.

Leake, C. D. and Waters, R. M. (1928). 'The anesthetic properties of carbon dioxide. *J. Pharmac. exp. Ther.*, 33, 280.

Leblanc, P., Ruff, F. and Milic-Emili, J. (1970). 'Effects of age and body position on "airway closure" in man.' *J. appl. Physiol.*, 28, 448.

Ledingham, I. McA. and Norman, J. N. (1965). 'Metabolic effects of combined hypothermia and hyperbaric oxygen in experimental total circulatory arrest.' In: *Hyperbaric Oxygenation*. Ed. by I. Ledingham. Edinburgh and London: Churchill Livingstone.

Lee, G. de J. and DuBois, A. B. (1955). 'Pulmonary capillary blood flow in man.' *J. clin. Invest.*, 34, 1380.

Lehmann, H. and Huntsman, R. G. (1966). *Man's Haemoglobin*. Amsterdam; North Holland Publ. (2nd edn., published 1974).

Leigh, J. M. (1973). 'Variation in performance of oxygen therapy devices.' *Ann. R. Coll. Surg.*, 52, 234.

Lenfant, C. and Howell, B. J. (1960). 'Cardiovascular adjustments in dogs during continuous pressure breathing.' *J. appl. Physiol.*, 15, 425.

Lenfant, C., Torrance, J., English, E., Finch, C. A., Reynafarje, C., Ramas, J. and Faura, J. (1968). 'Effect of altitude on oxygen binding by hemoglobin and on organic phosphate levels.' *J. clin. Invest.*, 47, 2652.

Leraand, S. (1962). 'Principles of pressure measurements.' *Acta anaesth. scand.*, suppl. 11, 115.

Leusen, I. R. (1950). 'Influence du pH du liquide cephalo-rachidien sur la respiration.' *Experientia*, 6, 272.

Leusen, I. R. (1954). 'Chemosensitivity of the respiratory center.' *Am. J. Physiol.*, 176, 39.

Leusen, I. (1972). 'Regulation of cerebrospinal fluid composition with reference to breathing.' *Physiol. Rev.*, 52, 1.

Liebow, A. A. (1962). 'Recent advances in pulmonary anatomy.' In: *Pulmonary Structure and Function*. Ed. by A. V. S. de Reuck and M. O'Connor. Edinburgh and London; Churchill Livingstone.

Linden, R. J., Ledsome, J. R. and Norman, J. (1965). 'Simple methods for the determination of the concentrations of carbon dioxide and oxygen in blood.' *Br. J. Anaesth.*, 37, 77.

Lindenberg, R. (1963). 'Patterns of CNS vulnerability in acute hypoxaemia including anaesthetic accidents.' In: *Selective Vulnerability of the Brain in Hypoxaemia*. Ed. by J. P. Schade and W. H. McMenemy. Oxford; Blackwell.

Linton, R. A. F., Poole-Wilson, P. A., Davies, R. J. and Cameron, I. R. (1973). 'A comparison of the ventilatory response to carbon dioxide by steady-state and rebreathing methods during metabolic acidosis and alkalosis.' *Clin. Sci.*, 45, 239.

Lloyd, B. B. (1958). 'A development of Haldane's gas-analysis apparatus.' *J. Physiol.*, 143, 5P.

Lloyd, B. B. and Cunningham, D. J. C. (1963). 'A quantitative approach to the regulation of human respiration ' In: *The Regulation of Human Respiration*. Ed. by D. J. C. Cunningham and B. B. Lloyd. Oxford; Blackwell.

Lloyd, B. B., Jukes, M. G. M. and Cunningham, D. J. C. (1958). 'The relation between alveolar oxygen pressure and the respiratory response to carbon dioxide in man.' *J. exp. Physiol.*, 43, 214.

Loeschcke, H. H. (1965). 'A concept of the role of intracranial chemosensitivity in respiratory control.' In: *Cerebrospinal Fluid and the Regulation of Ventilation*. Ed. by C. McC. Brookes, F. F. Kao and B. B. Lloyd. Oxford; Blackwell.

Loeschcke, H. H., Sweel, A., Kough, R. H. and Lambertsen, C. J. (1953). 'The effect of morphine and of meperidine (dolantin, demerol) upon the respiratory response of normal men to low concentrations of inspired carbon dioxide.' *J. Pharmac. exp. Ther.*, 108, 376.

Loewy, A. (1894). 'Über die Bestimmung der Grösse des "schädlichen Luftraumes" im Thorax und der alveolaren Sauerstoffspannung.' *Pflügers Arch. ges. Physiol.*, 58, 416.

Loh, L., Seed, R. F. and Sykes, M. K. (1973). 'The cardiorespiratory effects of halothane, trichloroethylene and nitrous oxide in the dog.' *Br. J. Anaesth.*, 45, 125.

Longo, L. D. (1970). 'Carbon monoxide in the pregnant mother and fetus and its exchange across the placenta.' *Ann. N. Y. Acad. Sci.*, 174, 313.

Lumsden, T. (1923a). 'Observations on the respiratory centres in the cat.' *J. Physiol.*, 57, 153.

Lumsden, T. (1923b). 'Observations on the respiratory centres.' *J Physiol.*, 57, 354.

Lumsden, T. (1923c). 'The regulation of respiration. Part 1.' *J. Physiol.*, 58, 81.

Lumsden, T. (1923d). 'The regulation of respiration. Part 2.' *J. Physiol.*, 58, 111.

Lundsgaard, C. and Van Slyke D. D. (1923). *Cyanosis.* Baltimore; Williams and Wilkins.

Lurie, A. A., Jones, R. E. Linde, H. W., Price, M. L., Dripps, R. D. and Price, H. L. (1958). 'Cyclopropane anesthesia: cardiac rate and rhythm during steady levels of cyclopropane anesthesia in man at normal and elevated end-expiratory carbon dioxide tensions.' *Anesthesiology*, 19, 457.

Lynch, S., Brand, L. and Levy, A. (1959). 'Changes in lung thorax compliance during orthopedic surgery.' *Anesthesiology*, 20, 278.

McArdle, L. and Roddie, I. C. (1958). 'Vascular responses to carbon dioxide during anaesthesia in man.' *Br. J. Anaesth.*, 30, 358.

McConn, R. and Derrick, J. B. (1972). 'The respiratory function of blood: transfusion and blood storage.' *Anesthesiology* 36, 119.

McDonald, D. M. and Mitchell, R. A. (1975). 'The innervation of glomus cells, ganglion cells and blood vessels in the rat carotid body: a quantitative ultrastructural analysis.' *J. Neurocytol.*, 4, 177.

McDowall, D. G. (1967). 'The effects of clinical concentrations of halothane on the blood flow and oxygen uptake of the cerebral cortex.' *Br. J. Anaesth.*, 39, 186.

McEvoy, J. D. S., Jones, N. L. and Campbell, E. J. M. (1974). 'Mixed venous and arterial PCO_2.' *Br. med. J.* 4, 687.

McHardy, G. J. R. (1972). 'Diffusing capacity and pulmonary gas exchange.' *Br. J. Dis. Chest*, 66, 1.

McIlroy, M. B., Eldridge, F. L., Thomas, J. P. and Christie, R. V. (1956). 'The effect of added elastic and non-elastic resistances on the pattern of breathing in normal subjects.' *Clin. Sci.*, 15, 337.

MacIntosh, R. R., Mushin, W. W. and Epstein, H. G. (1958). *Physics for the Anaesthetist*, 2nd edn. Oxford; Blackwell.

Macklem. P. T. (1971). 'Airway obstruction and collateral ventilation.' *Physiol. Rev.*, 51, 368.

Macklem, P. T. and Mead, J. (1967). 'Resistance of central and peripheral airways measured by a retrograde catheter.' *J. appl. Physiol.*, 22, 395.

Macklem, P. T. and Wilson, N. J. (1965). 'Measurement of intrabronchial pressure in man.' *J. appl. Physiol.*, 20, 653.

Macklem, P. T., Fraser, R. G. and Bates, D. V. (1963). 'Bronchial pressures and dimensions in health and obstructive airway disease.' *J. appl. Physiol.*, 18, 699.

McNicol, M. W. and Campbell, E. J. M. (1965). 'Severity of respiratory failure.' *Lancet*, 1, 336.

Maloney, J. V., Elam, J. O., Handford, S. W., Balla, G. A., Eastwood, D. W., Brown, E. S. and Ten Pas, R. H. (1953). 'Importance of negative pressure phase in mechanical respirators.' *J. Am. med. Ass.*, 152, 212.

Mapleson, W. W. (1954). 'The elimination of rebreathing in various anaesthetic systems.' *Br. J. Anaesth.*, 26, 323.

Mapleson, W. W. (1962). 'The effect of changes of lung characteristics on the functioning of automatic ventilators.' *Anaesthesia*, 17, 300.

Marchand, P., Gilroy, J. C. and Wilson, V. H. (1950). 'An anatomical study of the bronchial vascular system and its variation in disease.' *Thorax*, 5, 207.

Maren, T. H. (1967). 'Carbonic anhydrase: chemistry, physiology, and inhibition.' *Physiol. Rev.*, 47, 595.

Marckwald, M. and Kronecker, H. (1880). 'Die Athembewegungen des Zwerchfells des Kaninchens.' *Arch. Physiol. Leipzig*, p. 441.

Marrubini, M. B., Rossanda, M. and Tretola, L. (1964). 'The role of artificial hyperventilation in the control of brain tension during neurosurgical operations.' *Br. J. Anaesth.*, 36, 415.

Marshall, B. E. and Millar, R. A. (1965). 'Some factors influencing post-operative hypoxaemia.' *Anaesthesia*, 20, 408.

Marshall, B. E. and Wyche, M. Q. (1972). 'Hypoxemia during and after anesthesia.' *Anesthesiology*, 37, 178.

Marshall, B. E., Cohen, P. J., Klingenmaier, C. H. and Aukberg, S. (1969). 'Pulmonary venous admixture before, during, and after halothane: oxygen anesthesia in man.' *J. appl. Physiol.*, 27, 653.

Marshall, R. (1957). 'The physical properties of the lungs in relation to the subdivisions of lung volume.' *Clin. Sci.*, 16, 507.

Marshall, R. and Widdicombe, J. G. (1961). 'Stress relaxation in the human lung.' *Clin. Sci.*, 20, 19.

Mattila, M. A. K. (1974). 'The role of the physical characteristics of the respirator in artificial ventilation of the newborn.' *Acta anaesth. scand.*, suppl. 56, 1974.

Mattson, S. B. and Carlens, E. (1955). 'Lobar ventilation and oxygen uptake in man: influence of body position.' *J. thorac. Surg.*, 30, 676.

Mead, J. (1961). 'Mechanical properties of lungs.' *Physiol. Rev.*, 41, 281.

Mead, J. and Agostoni, E. (1964). 'Dynamics of breathing.' *Handbk Physiol.*, section 3, 1, 1.

Meade, F. and Owen-Thomas, J. B. (1975). 'The estimation of carbon dioxide concentration in the presence of nitrous oxide using a Lloyd–Haldane apparatus.' *Br. J. Anaesth.*, 47, 22.

Meduna, L. J. (1958). *Carbon Dioxide Therapy*, 2nd edn. Springfield, Ill.; Thomas.

Meldrum, N. U. and Roughton, F. J. W. (1933). 'Carbonic anhydrase: its preparation and properties.' *J. Physiol.*, 80, 833.

Mendelson, C. L. (1946). 'Aspiration of stomach contents into the lungs during obstetric anesthesia.' *Am. J. Obstet. Gynec.*, 52, 191.

Menzel, D. B. (1970). 'Toxicity of ozone, oxygen, and radiation.' *A. Rev. Physiol.*, 10, 379.

Merwarth, C. R. and Sieker, H. O. (1961). 'Acid–base changes in blood and cerebrospinal fluid during altered ventilation.' *J. appl. Physiol.*, 16, 1016.

Meyer, B. J., Meyer, A. and Guyton, A. C. (1968). 'Interstitial fluid pressure. V. Negative pressure in the lungs.' *Circulation Res.*, 22, 263.

Meyer, E. C. and Ottaviano, R. (1972). 'Pulmonary collateral lymph flow: detection using lymph oxygen tensions.' *J. appl. Physiol.*, 32, 806.

Michel, C. C. and Milledge, J. S. (1963). 'Respiratory regulation in man during acclimatization to high altitude.' *J. Physiol.*, 168, 631.

Michenfelder, J. D., Fowler, W. S. and Theye, R. A. (1966). 'CO_2 levels and pulmonary shunting in anesthetized man.' *J. appl. Physiol.*, 21, 1471.

Milic-Emili, J., Mead, J. and Turner, J. M. (1964). 'Topography of esophageal pressure as a function of posture in man.' *J. appl. Physiol.*, 19, 212.

Milic-Emili, J., Mead, J., Turner, J. M. and Glauser, E. M. (1964). 'Improved technique for estimating pleural pressure from esophageal balloons.' *J. appl. Physiol.*, 19, 207.

Millar, R. A. (1960). 'Plasma adrenaline and noradrenaline during diffusion respiration.' *J. Physiol.*, 150, 79.

Millar, R. A. and Gregory, I. C. (1972). 'Reduced oxygen content in equilibrated fresh heparinised and ACD-stored blood from cigarette smokers.' *Br. J. Anaesth.*, 44, 1015.

Millar, R. A., Beard, D. J. and Hulands, G. H. (1971). 'Oxyhaemoglobin dissociation curves in vitro with and without the anaesthetics halothane and cyclopropane.' *Br. J. Anaesth.*, 43, 1003.

Milledge, J. S. and Lahiri, S. (1967). 'Respiratory control in lowlanders and Sherpa highlanders at altitude.' *Resp. Physiol.*, 2, 310.

Milledge, J. S. and Nunn, J. F. (1975). 'Criteria of fitness for anaesthesia in patients with chronic obstructive lung disease.' *Br. med. J.*, 3, 670.

Milledge, J. S., Minty, K. B. and Duncalf, D. (1974). 'On-line assessment of ventilatory response to carbon dioxide.' *J. appl. Physiol.*, 37, 596.

Miller, A. H. (1938). 'The role of diaphragmatic breathing in anesthesia and a pneumographic method of recording. *Anesth. Analg.*, 17, 38.

Miller, W. S. (1947). *The Lung*, 2nd ed. Springfield, Ill.; Thomas.

Mills, E. and Jöbsis, F. F. (1972). 'Mitochondrial respiratory chain of carotid body and chemoreceptor response to changes in oxygen tension.' *J. Neurophysiol.*, 35, 405.

Mills, J. E., Sellick, H. and Widdicombe, J. G. (1970). 'Epithelial irritant receptors in the lungs.' In: *Breathing: Hering–Breuer Centenary Symposium*, p. 77. Ed. by R. Porter. Edinburgh and London ; Churchill Livingstone.

Mills, R. J., Cumming, G. and Harris, P. (1963). 'Frequency-dependent compliance at different levels of inspiration in normal adults.' *J. appl. Physiol.*, **18**, 1061.

Mitchell, R. A. (1966). 'Cerebrospinal fluid and the regulation of respiration.' In: *Advances in Respiratory Physiology*. Ed. by C. G. Caro. London; Edward Arnold.

Mitchell, R. A. and Berger, A. J. (1975). 'Neural regulation of respiration.' *Am. Rev. resp. Dis.*, **111**, 206.

Mitchell, R. A. and Herbert, D. A. (1975). 'Potencies of doxapram and hypoxia in stimulating carotid-body chemoreceptors and ventilation in anesthetized cats.' *Anesthesiology*, **42**, 559.

Mitchell, R. A., Loeschcke, H. H., Massion, W. H. and Severinghaus, J. W. (1963). 'Respiratory responses mediated through superficial chemosensitive areas on the medulla.' *J. appl. Physiol.*, **18**, 523.

Mitchell, R. A., Bainton, C. R., Severinghaus, J. W. and Edelist, G. (1964). 'Respiratory response and CSF pH during disturbances in blood acid–base balance in awake dogs with denervated aortic and carotid bodies.' *Physiologist*, **7**, 208.

Mitchell, R. A., Carman, C. T., Severinghaus, J. W., Richardson, B. W., Singer, M. M. and Snider, S. (1965). 'Stability of cerebrospinal fluid pH in chronic acid-base disturbances in blood.' *J. appl. Physiol.*, **20**, 443.

Mitchinson, A. G. and Yoffey, J. M. (1947). 'Respiratory displacement of larynx, hyoid bone and tongue.' *J. Anat.*, **81**, 118.

Morgan, B. C., Crawford, E. W. and Guntheroth, W. G. (1969). The hemodynamic effects of changes in blood volume during intermittent positive-pressure ventilation. *Anesthesiology*, **30**, 297.

Morgan, B. C. Martin, W. E., Hornbein, T. F., Crawford, E. W. and Guntheroth, W. G. (1966). 'Hemodynamic effects of intermittent positive pressure respiration.' *Anesthesiology*, **27**, 584.

Morikawa, S., Safar, P. and DeCarlo, J. (1961). 'Influence of the head–jaw position upon upper airway patency.' *Anesthesiology*, **22**, 265.

Morris, J. G. (1968). *A Biologist's Physical Chemistry*. London; Edward Arnold.

Moser, K. M., Rhodes, P. G. and Kwaan, P. L. (1965). 'Post-hyperventilation apnea.' *Fedn Proc.*, **24**, 273.

Moyer, C. A. and Beecher, H. K. (1942). 'Effects of barbiturate anesthesia (Evipal and pentothal sodium) upon integration of respiratory control mechanisms.' *J. clin. Invest.*, **21**, 429.

Muallam, M., Larson, C. P. and Eger, E. I. (1969). 'The effects of diethyl ether on Pa_{CO_2} in dogs with and without vagal, somatic and sympathetic block.' *Anesthesiology*, **30**, 185.

Munson, E. S. and Merrick, H. C. (1967). 'Effect of nitrous oxide on venous air embolism.' *Anesthesiology*, **27**, 783.

Munson, E. S., Larson, C. P., Babad, A. A., Regan, M. J., Buechel, D. R. and Eger, E. I. (1966). 'The effects of halothane, fluroxene and cyclopropane on ventilation: a comparative study in man.' *Anesthesiology*, **27**, 716.

Mushin, W. W. (1963). *Thoracic Anaesthesia*. Oxford; Blackwell.

Mushin, W. W., Rendell-Baker, L., Thompson, P. and Mapleson, W. W. (1969). *Automatic Ventilation of the Lungs*, 2nd edn. Oxford; Blackwell.

Nahas, G. C., Ligou, J. C. and Mehlman, B. (1960). 'Effects of pH changes on O_2 uptake and plasma catecholamine levels in the dog.' *J. appl. Physiol.*, **198**, 60.

Nahas, R. A., Melrose, D. G., Sykes, M. K. and Robinson, B. (1965a). 'Post-perfusion lung syndrome—role of circulatory exclusion.' *Lancet*, **2**, 251.

Nahas, R. A., Melrose, D. G., Sykes, M. K. and Robinson, B. (1965b). 'Post-perfusion lung syndrome-effect of homologous blood.' *Lancet*, **2**, 254.

Naito, H. and Gillis, C. N. (1973). 'Effects of halothane and nitrous oxide on removal of norepinephrine from the pulmonary circulation.' *Anesthesiology*, **39**, 575.

Nash, G., Blennerhassett, J. B. and Pontoppidan, H. (1967). 'Pulmonary lesions associated with oxygen therapy and artificial ventilation.' *New Engl. J. Med.*, **276**, 368.

Natelson, S. (1951). 'Routine use of ultramicro-methods in the clinical laboratory.' *Am. J. clin. Path.*, **21**, 1153.

Nathan, P. W. and Sears, T. A. (1960). 'Effects of posterior root section on the activity of some muscles in man.' *J. Neurol. Neurosurg. Psychiat.*, **23**, 10.

Naylor, B. A., Welch, M. H., Shafer, A. W. and Guenter, C. A. (1972). 'Blood affinity for oxygen in hemorrhagic shock.' *J. appl. Physiol.*, **32**, 829.

Needham, C. D., Rogan, M. C. and McDonald, I. (1954). 'Normal standards for lung volumes, intrapulmonary gas-mixing, and maximum breathing capacity.' *Thorax*, **9**, 313.

Neergaard, K. von (1929). 'Neue Auffassungen über einen Grundbegriff der Atemmechanik. Die Retraktionskraft der Lunge, abhängig von der Oberflächenspannung in den Alveolen.' *Z. ges. exp. Med.*, **66**, 373.

Neergaard, K. von and Wirz, K. (1927a). 'Uber eine Methode zur Messung der Lungenelastizität am lebenden Menschen, inbesondere beim Emphysem.' *Z. klin. Med.*, **105**, 35.

Neergaard, K. von and Wirz, K. (1927b). 'Die Messung der Strömungswiderstände in der Atemwege des Menschen inbesondere bei Asthma und Emphysem.' *Z. klin. Med.*, **105**, 51.

Neil, E. and Joels, N. (1963). 'The carotid glomus sensory mechanism.' In: *The Regulation of Human Respiration*, p. 163. Ed. by D. J. C. Cunningham and B. B. Lloyd. Oxford; Blackwell.

Nemir, P., Stone, H. H., Mackrell, T. N. and Hawthorne, H. R. (1953). 'Studies on pulmonary function utilizing the method of controlled unilateral bronchovascular occlusion.' *Surg. Forum*, **4**, 234.

Newberg, L. A. and Jones, J. G. (1974). 'A closing volume bolus method using SF_6 enhancement of the nitrogen glow discharge.' *J. appl. Physiol.*, **36**, 488.

Newman, H. C., Campbell, E. J. M. and Dinnick, O. P. (1959). 'A simple method of measuring the compliance and the non-elastic resistance of the chest during anaesthesia.' *Br. J. Anaesth.*, **31**, 282.

Ng, K. K. F. and Vane, J. R. (1967). 'Conversion of Angiotensin I to Angiotensin II.' *Nature*, 216, 762.

Ngai, S. H., Katz, R. L. and Farhie, S. E. (1965). 'Respiratory effects of trichlorethylene, halothane and methoxyflurane in the cat.' *J. Pharmac. exp. Ther.*, **148**, 123.

Newsom Davis, J. and Plum, F. (1972). 'Separation of descending spinal pathways to respiratory motoneurones.' *Expl Neurol.*, **34**, 78.

Niden, A. H. and Aviado, D. M. (1956). 'Effects of pulmonary embolus on the pulmonary circulation with special reference to arteriovenous shunts in the lung.' *Circulation Res.*, **6**, 67.

Nielsen, H. (1932). 'En oplivningsmetode. *Ugeskr. Laeg.*, **94**, 1201.

Nims, R. G., Connor, E. H. and Comroe, J. H. (1955). 'Compliance of the human thorax in anesthetized patients.' *J. clin. Invest.*, **34**, 744.

Noble, M. I. M., Eisele, J. H., Frankel, H. L., Else, W. and Guz, A. (1971). 'The role of the diaphragm in the sensation of holding the breath.' *Clin. Sci.*, **41**, 275.

Nunn, J. F. (1956). 'A new method of spirometry applicable to routine anaesthesia.' *Br. J. Anaesth.*, **28**, 440.

Nunn, J. F. (1958a). 'Ventilation and end-tidal carbon dioxide tension.' *Anaesthesia*, **13**, 124.

Nunn, J. F. (1958b). 'Respiratory measurements in the presence of nitrous oxide.' *Br. J. Anaesth.* **30**, 254.

Nunn, J. F. (1960a). 'Prediction of carbon dioxide tension during anaesthesia.' *Anaesthesia*, **15**, 123.

Nunn, J. F. (1960b). 'The solubility of volatile anaesthetics in oil.' *Br. J. Anaesth.*, **32**, 346.

Nunn, J. F. (1961a). 'The distribution of inspired gas during thoracic surgery.' *Ann. R. Coll. Surg.*, **28**, 223.

Nunn, J. F. (1961b). 'Portable anaesthetic apparatus for use in the Antartic.' *Br. med. J.*, **1**, 1139.

Nunn, J. F. (1962a). 'Predictors for oxygen and carbon dioxide levels during anaesthesia.' *Anaesthesia*, **17**, 182.

Nunn, J. F. (1962b). 'Measurement of blood oxygen tension: handling of samples.' *Br. J. Anaesth.*, **34**, 621.

Nunn, J. F. (1962c). 'Nomenclature and presentation of hydrogen ion regulation data.' In: *Modern Trends in Anaesthesia*, 2. Ed. by F. T. Evans and T. C. Gray. London and Boston, Mass.; Butterworths.

Nunn, J. F. (1962d). 'The effects of hypercapnia.' In: *Modern Trends in Anaesthesia*, 2. Ed. by F. T. Evans and T. C. Gray. London and Boston, Mass.; Butterworths.

Nunn, J. F. (1963). 'Indirect determination of the ideal alveolar oxygen tension during and after nitrous oxide anaesthesia.' *Br. J. Anaesth.*, **35**, 8.

Nunn, J. F. (1964). 'Factors influencing the arterial oxygen tension during halothane anaesthesia with spontaneous respiration.' *Br. J. Anaesth.*, 36, 327.

Nunn, J. F. (1965). 'Influence of age and other factors on hypoxaemia in the postoperative period.' *Lancet*, 2, 466.

Nunn, J. F. (1972). 'Nomograms for calculation of oxygen consumption and respiratory exchange ratio.' *Br. med. J.*, 4, 18.

Nunn, J. F. and Bergman, N. A. (1964). 'The effect of atropine on pulmonary gas exchange.' *Br. J. Anaesth.*, 36, 68.

Nunn, J. F. and Ezi-Ashi, T. I. (1961). 'The respiratory effects of resistance to breathing in anaesthetized man.' *Anesthesiology*, 22, 174.

Nunn, J. F. and Ezi-Ashi, T. I. (1962). 'The accuracy of the respirometer and ventigrator.' *Br. J. Anaesth.*, 34, 422.

Nunn, J. F. and Freeman, J. (1964). 'Problems of oxygenation and oxygen transport during haemorrhage.' *Anaesthesia*, 19, 206.

Nunn, J. F. and Hill, D. W. (1960). 'Respiratory dead space and arterial to end-tidal CO_2 tension difference in anesthetized man ' *J. appl. Physiol.*, 15, 383.

Nunn, J. F. and Matthews, R. L. (1959). 'Gaseous exchange during halothane anaesthesia: the steady respiratory state.' *Br. J. Anaesth.*, 31, 330.

Nunn, J. F. and Newman, H. C. (1964). 'Inspired gas, rebreathing and apparatus dead space.' *Br. J. Anaesth*, 36, 5.

Nunn, J. F. and Payne, J. P. (1962). 'Hypoxaemia after general anaesthesia.' *Lancet*, 2, 631.

Nunn, J. F. and Pincock, A. C. (1957). 'A time-phased end-tidal sampler suitable for use during anaesthesia.' *Br. J. Anaesth.*, 29, 98.

Nunn, J. F. and Pouliot, J. C. (1962). 'The measurement of gaseous exchange during nitrous oxide anaesthesia.' *Br. J. Anaesth.*, 34, 752.

Nunn, J. F., Bergman, N. A. and Coleman, A. J. (1965). 'Factors influencing the arterial oxygen tension during anaesthesia with artificial ventilation.' *Br. J. Anaesth.*, 37, 898.

Nunn, J. F., Campbell, E. J. M. and Peckett, B. W. (1959). 'Anatomical subdivisions of the volume of respiratory dead space and effect of position of the jaw.' *J. appl. Physiol.*, 14, 174.

Nunn, J. F., Bergman, N. A., Coleman, A. J. and Casselle, D. C. (1964). 'Evaluation of the Servomex paramagnetic analyser.' *Br. J. Anaesth.*, 36, 666.

Nunn, J. F., Bergman, N. A., Bunatyan, A. and Coleman, A. J. (1965a). 'Temperature coefficients of PCO_2 and PO_2 of blood in vitro.' *J. appl. Physiol.*, 20, 23.

Nunn, J. F., Coleman, A. J., Sachithanandan, T., Bergman, N. A. and Laws, J. W. (1965b). 'Hypoxaemia and atelectasis produced by forced expiration.' *Br. J. Anaesth.*, 37, 3.

Nunn, J. F., Sturrock, J. E., Wills, E. J., Richmond, J. E. and McPherson, C. K. (1974). 'The effect of inhalational anaesthetics on the swimming velocity of *Tetrahymena pyriformis.*' *J. Cell Sci.*, 15, 537.

Ogilvie, C. M., Forster, R. E., Blakemore, W. S. and Morton, J. W. (1957). 'A standardized breath holding technique for the clinical measurement of the diffusing capacity of the lung for carbon monoxide.' *J. clin. Invest.*, 36, 1.

Otis, A. B. (1954). 'The work of breathing.' *Physiol. Rev.*, 34, 449.

Otis, A. B., Fenn, W. O. and Rahn, H. (1950). 'Mechanics of breathing in man.' *J. appl. Physiol.*, 2, 592.

Otis, A. B., Rahn, H. and Fenn, W. O. (1948). 'Alveolar gas changes during breath holding.' *Am. J. Physiol.* 152, 674.

Otis, A. B., McKerrow, C. B., Bartlett, R. A., Mead, J., McIlroy, M. B., Selverstone, N. J. and Radford, E. P. (1956). 'Mechanical factors in distribution of pulmonary ventilation.' *J. appl. Physiol.*, 8, 427.

Ozanam, C. (1862). 'De l'acide carbonique en inhalations comme agent anesthésique efficace et sans danger pendant les operations chirurgicales.' *C. r. Acad. Sci.*, 54, 1154.

Padmore, G. R. A. and Nunn, J. F. (1974). 'SI units in relation to anaesthesia.' *Br. J. Anaesth.*, 46, 236.

Paintal, A. S. (1970). 'The mechanism of excitation of type J receptors and the J reflex.' In: *Breathing: Hering–Breuer Centenary Symposium*, p. 59. Ed. by R. Porter. Edinburgh and London; Churchill Livingstone.

Palmer, K. N. V. and Diament, M. L. (1967). 'Effect of aerosol isoprenaline on blood-gas tensions in severe bronchial asthma.' *Lancet*, 2, 1232.

Palmer, K. N. V. and Gardiner, A. J. S. (1964). 'Effect of partial gastrectomy on pulmonary physiology.' *Br. med. J.* 1, 347.

Palmer, K. N. V., Gardiner, A. J. S. and McGregor, M. H. (1965). 'Hypoxaemia after partial gastrectomy.' *Thorax*, 20, 73.

Panday, J. and Nunn, J. F. (1968). 'Failure to demonstrate progressive falls of arterial PO_2 during anaesthesia.' *Anaesthesia*, 23, 38.

Pappenheimer, J. R., Comroe, J. H., Cournand, A., Ferguson, J. K. W., Filley, G. F., Fowler, W. S., Gray, J. S., Helmholtz, H. F., Otis, A. B., Rahn, H. and Riley, R. L. (1950). 'Standardization of definitions and symbols in respiratory physiology.' *Fedn Proc.*, 9, 602.

Pappenheimer, J. R., Fencl, V., Heisey, S. R. and Held, D. (1965). 'Role of cerebral fluids in control of respiration as studied in unanesthetized goats.' *Am. J. Physiol.*, 208, 436.

Paterson, G. M., Hulands, G. H. and Nunn, J. F. (1969). 'Evaluation of a new halothane vaporizer: the Cyprane Fluotec mark 3.' *Br. J. Anaesth.*, 41, 109.

Pattle, R. E. (1955). 'Properties, function and origin of the alveolar lining fluid.' *Nature, Lond.*, 175, 1125.

Pattle, R. E., Schock, C. and Battensby, J. (1972). 'Some effects of anaesthetics on lung surfactant.' *Br. J. Anaesth.*, 44, 1119.

Pattle, R. E., Claireaux, A. E., Davies, P. A. and Cameron, A. H. (1962). 'Inability to form a lung lining film as a cause of the respiratory distress syndrome in newborn.' *Lancet*, 2, 469.

Patz, A. (1958). 'Retrolental fibroplasia.' *Pediat. Clins N. Am.*, 239.

Pauling, L., Wood, R. E. and Sturdivant, J. H. (1946). 'Instrument for determining partial pressure of oxygen in gas.' *J. Am. chem. Soc.*, 68, 795.

Pavlin, E. G. and Hornbein, T. F. (1975a). 'Distribution of H^+ and HCO_3^- between CSF and blood during metabolic acidosis in dogs.' *J. Physiol.*, 228, 1134.

Pavlin, E. G. and Hornbein, T. F. (1975b). 'Distribution of H^+ and HCO_3^- between CSF and blood during metabolic alkalosis in dogs.' *J. Physiol.*, 228, 1141.

Payne, J. P. (1958a). 'The influence of carbon dioxide on the neuromuscular blocking activity of relaxant drugs in the cat.' *Br. J. Anaesth.*, 30, 206.

Payne, J. P. (1958b). 'Hypotensive response to carbon dioxide.' *Anaesthesia*, 13, 279.

Payne, J. P. (1962). 'Apnoeic oxygenation in anaesthetized man.' *Acta anaesth. scand.*, 6, 129.

Permutt, S. and Riley, R. L. (1963). 'Hemodynamics of collapsible vessels with tone: the vascular waterfall.' *J. appl. Physiol.* 18, 924.

Pavlin, E. G. and Hornbein, T. F. (1975c). 'Distribution of H^+ and HCO_3^- between CSF and blood during respiratory acidosis in dogs.' *J. Physiol.*, 228, 1145.

Pflüger, E. (1868). 'Ueber die Ursache der Athembewegungen, sowie der Dyspnoë und Apnoë.' *Arch. ges. Physiol.*, 1, 61.

Perutz, M. F. (1969). 'The haemoglobin molecule.' *Proc. R. Soc. B.*, 173, 113.

Pierce, E. C., Lambertsen, C. J., Deutsch, S., Chase, P. E., Linde, H. W., Dripps, R. D. and Price, H. L. (1962). 'Cerebral circulation and metabolism during thiopental anesthesia and hyperventilation in man.' *J. clin. Invest.*, 41, 1664.

Pietak, S., Weenig, C. S., Hickey, R. F. and Fairley, H. B. (1975). 'Anesthetic effects on ventilation in patients with chronic obstructive pulmonary disease.' *Anesthesiology*, 42, 160.

Piiper, J. (1961). 'Variations of ventilation and diffusing capacity to perfusion determining the alveolar–arterial O_2 difference: theory.' *J. appl. Physiol.*, 16, 507.

Piiper, J., Haab, P. and Rahn, H. (1961). 'Unequal distribution of pulmonary diffusing capacity in the anesthetized dog.' *J. appl. Physiol.*, 16, 499.

Piiper, J. P., Dejours, P., Haab, P. and Rahn, H. (1971). 'Concepts and basic quantities in gas exchange physiology.' *Resp. Physiol.*, 13, 292.

Pitts, R. F. (1946). 'Organization of the respiratory center.' *Physiol. Rev.*, 26, 609.

Pitts, R. F., Magoun, H. W. and Ranson, S. W. (1939a). 'Localization of the medullary respiratory centers in the cat.' *Am. J. Physiol.*, 126, 673.

Pitts, R. F., Magoun, H. W. and Ranson, S. W. (1939b). 'Interrelations of the respiratory centers in the cat.' *Am. J. Physiol.*, 126, 689.

Pitts, R. F., Magoun, H. W. and Ranson, S. W. (1939c). 'The origin of respiratory rhythmicity.' *Am. J. Physiol.*, 127, 654.

Polgar, G. and Forster, R. E. (1960). 'Measurement of oxygen tension in unstirred blood with a platinum electrode.' *J. appl. Physiol.*, 15, 706.

Ponte, J. and Purves, M. J. (1974). 'Frequency response of carotid body chemoreceptors in the cat to changes of PaO_2, $PaCO_2$ and pH.' *J. appl. Physiol.*, 37, 635.

Pontoppidan, H., Geffin, B. and Lowenstein, E. (1972). 'Acute respiratory failure in the adult.' *New Engl. J. Med.*, 287, 690, 743 and 799.

Potgieter, S. V. (1959). 'Atelectasis: its evolution during upper urinary tract surgery.' *Br. J. Anaesth.*, 31, 472.

Price, H. L. (1960). 'Effects of carbon dioxide on the cardiovascular system.' *Anesthesiology*, 21, 652.

Price, H. L. and Widdicombe, J. (1962). 'Actions of cyclopropane on carotid sinus baroreceptors and carotid body chemoreceptors.' *J. Pharmac. exp. Ther.*, 135, 233.

Price, H. L., Lurie, A. A., Jones, R. E. and Linde, H. W. (1958). 'Role of catecholamines in the initiation of arrhythmic cardiac contraction by carbon dioxide inhalation in anesthetized man.' *J. Pharmac. exp. Therap.*, 122, 63A.

Price, H. L., Lurie, A. A., Black, G. W., Sechzer, P. H., Linde, H. W. and Price, M. L. (1960). 'Modification by general anesthetics (cyclopropane and halothane) of circulatory and sympathoadrenal responses to respiratory acidosis. *Ann. Surg.*, 152, 1071.

Price, H. L., Deutsch, S., Davidson, I. A., Clement, A. J., Behar, M. G. and Epstein, R. M. (1966). 'Can general anesthetics produce splanchnic visceral hypoxia by reducing regional blood flow.' *Anesthesiology*, 27, 24.

Price, H. L., Cooperman, L. H., Warden, J. C., Morris, J. J. and Smith, T. C. (1969). 'Pulmonary hemodynamics during general anesthesia in man.' *Anesthesiology*, 30, 629.

Priestley, J. (1776). *Experiments and Observations on Different Kinds of Air*, 2nd edn., Vol. 2, p. 101. London; J. Johnson.

Prys, Roberts, C. (1966). 'Applied human pharmacology of analgesic and neuroleptic drugs.' *Proc. 2nd Brit. Symposium on the Use of Neuroleptanalgesia in Anaesthetic Practice.*

Prys-Roberts, C. (1971). 'Hypercapnia.' In *General Anaesthesia*, 3rd edn. Ed. by T. C. Gray and J. F. Nunn. London and Boston, Mass.: Butterworths.

Prys-Roberts, C., Kelman, G. R. and Nunn, J. F. (1966). 'Determination of the *in vivo* carbon dioxide titration curve of anaesthetised man.' *Br. J. Anaesth.*, 38, 500.

Prys-Roberts, C., Smith, W. D. A. and Nunn, J. F. (1967). 'Accidental severe hypercapnia during anaesthesia.' *Br. J. Anaesth.*, 39, 257.

Prys-Roberts, C., Kelman, G. R., Greenbaum, R. and Robinson, R. H. (1967a). 'Circulatory influences of artificial ventilation during nitrous oxide anaesthesia in man. II. Results: the relative influence of mean intrathoracic pressure and arterial carbon dioxide tension.' *Br. J. Anaesth.*, 39, 533.

Prys-Roberts, C., Nunn, J. F., Dobson, R. H., Robinson, R. H., Greenbaum, R. and Harris, R. S. (1967b). 'Radiologically undetectable pulmonary collapse in the supine position.' *Lancet*, 2, 399.

Prys-Roberts, C., Greenbaum, R., Nunn, J. F. and Kelman, G. R. (1970). 'Disturbances of pulmonary function in patients with fat embolism.' *J. clin. Path.*, 23, suppl. (Roy, Coll. Path.), 4, 143.

Pugh, L. G. C. E. (1962). 'Physiological and medical aspects of the Himalayan Scientific and Mountaineering Expedition, 1960–61.' *Br. med. J.*, 2, 621.

Purves, M. J. (1975). *The Peripheral Arterial Chemoreceptors.* Cambridge; Cambridge University Press.

Qvist, J., Pontoppidan, H., Wilson, R. S., Lowenstein, E. and Laver, M. B. (1975). 'Hemodynamic responses to mechanical ventilation with PEEP.' *Anesthesiology*, 42, 45.

Radford, E. P. (1955). 'Ventilation standards for use in artificial respiration.' *J. appl. Physiol.*, 7, 451.

Radford, E. P. (1964). 'The physics of gases.' *Handbk Physiol., section 3*, 2, 125.

Radford, E. P. and Whittenberger, J. L. (1962). In: *Artificial Respiration.* Ed. by J. L. Whittenberger. New York and London; Harper and Row.

Rahn, H. (1964). 'Oxygen stores of man.' In: *Oxygen in the Animal Organism.* Ed. by F. Dickens and E. Neil. Oxford; Pergamon.

Rahn, H. and Farhi, L. E. (1964). 'Ventilation, perfusion, and gas exchange—the $\dot{V}_A/\dot{Q}$ concept.' *Handbk Physiol., section 3*, 1.

Rahn, H. and Otis, A. B. (1949). 'Man's respiratory response during and after acclimatization to high altitude.' *Am. J. Physiol.*, 157, 445.

Rahn, H., Stroud, R. C. and Meier, H. (1952). 'Radiographic anatomy of heart and pulmonary vessels of the dog with observations of the pulmonary circulation time.' *J. appl. Physiol.*, 5, 308.

Rahn, H. Stroud, R. C. and Tobin, C. E. (1952). 'Visualization of arterio-venous shunts by cinefluorography in the lungs of normal dogs.' *Proc. Soc. exp. Biol. Med.*, 80, 239.

Rahn, H., Mohney, J., Otis, A. B. and Fenn, W. O. (1946a). 'A method for the continuous analysis of alveolar air.' *A. Aviat. Med.*, 17, 173.

Rahn, H., Otis, A. B., Chadwick, L. E. and Fenn, W. O. (1946b). 'The pressure–volume diagram of the thorax and lung.' *Am. J. Physiol.*, 146, 161.

Raine, J. M. and Bishop, J. M. (1963). 'A–a difference in O_2 tension and physiological dead space in normal man.' *J. appl. Physiol.*, 18, 284.

Ramwell, P. W. (1958). 'An investigation into the changes in blood gases during anaesthesia.' *PhD Thesis*, University of Leeds.

Ravin, M. B., Epstein, R. M. and Malm, J. R. (1965). 'Contribution of thebesian veins to the physiologic shunt in anesthetized man.' *J. appl. Physiol.*, 20, 1148.

Raymond, L. W. and Standaert, F. G. (1967). 'The respiratory effects of carbon dioxide in the cat.' *Anesthesiology*, 28, 974.

Read, D. J. C. (1967). 'A clinical method for assessing the ventilatory response to carbon dioxide.' *Australas. Ann. Med.*, 16, 20.

Refsum, H. E. (1963). 'Relationship between state of consciousness and arterial hypoxaemia and hypercapnia in patients with pulmonary insufficiency, breathing air.' *Clin. Sci.*, 25, 361.

Rehder, K. and Sessler, A. D. (1973). 'Function of each lung in spontaneously breathing man anesthetized with thiopentalmeperidine.' *Anesthesiology*, 38, 320.

Rehder, K., Sessler, A. D. and Marsh, H. M. (1975). 'General anesthesia and the lung.' *Am. Rev. resp. Dis.*, 112, 541.

Rehder, K., Sittipong, R. and Sessler, A. D. (1972). 'The effects of thiopental–meperidine anesthesia with succinylcholine paralysis on the functional residual capacity and dynamic lung compliance in normal sitting man.' *Anesthesiology*, 37, 395.

Rehder, K. Theye, R. A. and Fowler, W. S. (1961). 'Effect of position and thoracotomy on distribution of air and blood to each lung during intermittent positive pressure breathing.' *Physiologist*, 4, 93.

Rehder, K., Wenthe, F. M. and Sessler, A. D. (1973). 'Function of each lung during mechanical ventilation with ZEEP and with PEEP in man anesthetized with thiopental-meperidine.' *Anesthesiology*, 39, 597.

Rehder, K., Hatch, D. J., Sessler, A. D., Marsh, H. M. and Fowler, W. S. (1971). 'Effects of general anesthesia, muscle paralysis, and mechanical ventilation on pulmonary nitrogen clearance.' *Anesthesiology*, 35, 591.

Rehder, K. Hatch, D. J., Sessler, A. D. and Fowler, W. S. (1972). 'The function of each lung of anesthetized and paralyzed man during mechanical ventilation.' *Anesthesiology*, 37, 16.

Reivich, M. (1964). 'Arterial PCO_2 and cerebral hemodynamics.' *Am. J. Physiol.*, 206, 25.

de Reuck, A. V. S. and O'Connor, M., Eds. (1962). *Pulmonary Structure and Function.* (Ciba Foundation Symposium) Edinburgh and London; Churchill Livingstone.

Richardson, F. J., Chinn, S. and Nunn, J. F. (1976). 'Performance and application of the Quantiflex air/oxygen mixer.' *Br. J. Anaesth.*, 48, 1057.

Riley, R. L. and Cournand, A. (1949). ' "Ideal" alveolar air and the analysis of ventilation/perfusion relationships in the lungs.' *J. app. Physiol.*, 1, 825.

Riley, R. L. and Cournand, A. (1951). 'Analysis of factors affecting partial pressures of oxygen and carbon dioxide in gas and blood of lungs: Theory.' *J. appl. Physiol.*, 4, 77.

Riley, R. L., Campbell, E. J. M. and Shepard, R. H. (1957). 'A bubble method for estimation of PCO_2 and PO_2 in whole blood.' *J. appl. Physiol.*, 11, 245.

Riley, R. L., Cournand, A. and Donald K. W. (1951). 'Analysis of factors affecting partial pressures of O_2 and CO_2 in gas and blood of lungs: Methods.' *J. appl. Physiol.*, 4, 102.

Riley, R. L., Lilienthal., J. L., Proemmel, D. D. and Franke, R. E. (1946). 'On the determination of the physiologically effective pressures of oxygen and carbon dioxide in alveolar air.' *Am. J. Physiol.*, 147, 191.

Riley, R. L., Shepard, R. H., Cohn, J. E., Carroll, D. G. and Armstrong, B. W. (1954). 'Maximal diffusing capacity of lungs.' *J. appl. Physiol.*, 6, 573.

Roberts, J. G., Prys-Roberts, C., Moore, M. A. and Frazer, A. N. L. (1974). 'Cardio-pulmonary function during ether/air/relaxant anaesthesia.' *Anaesthesia*, 29, 4.

Robertson, J. D. and Reid, D. D. (1952). 'Standards for the basal metabolism of normal people in Britain.' *Lancet*, 1, 940.

Robertson, J. D., Swan, A. A. B. and Whitteridge, D. (1956). 'Effect of anaesthetics on systemic baroreceptors.' *J. Physiol.*, 131, 463.

Robinson, J. (1847). *A Treatise on the Inhalation of the Vapour of Ether for the Prevention of Pain in Surgical Operations*. London; Webster and Co.

Robinson, J. S. (1962). 'Hyperventilation'. In: *Modern Trends in Anaesthesia*, 2. Ed. by F. T. Evans and T. C. Gray. London and Boston, Mass.; Butterworths.

Robinson, R. H. (1968). 'Ability to detect changes in compliance and resistance during manual artificial ventilation.' *Br. J. Anaesth.*, 40, 323.

Robson, J. G. (1967). 'The respiratory centres and their responses.' In: *Modern Trends in Anaesthesia*, 3. Ed. by F. T. Evans and T. C. Gray. London and Boston, Mass.; Butterworths.

Robson, J. G., Houseley M. A. and Solis-Quiroga, O. H. (1963). 'The mechanism of respiratory arrest with sodium pentobarbital and sodium thiopental.' *Ann. N. Y. Acad. Sci.*, 109, 494.

Rohrer, F. (1915). 'Der Strömungswiderstand in den menschlichen Atemwegen.' *Pflügers Arch. ges. Physiol.*, 162, 225.

Ross, R. M. and McAllister, T. A. (1965). 'Treatment of experimental bacterial infection with hyperbaric oxygen.' In: *Hyperbaric Oxygenation*. Ed. by I. Ledingham. Edinburgh and London; Churchill Livingstone.

Rossier, P. H. and Méan H. (1943). 'L'insuffisance pulmonaire: ses diverses formes.' *J. suisse Med.*, 11, 327.

Roughton, F. J. W. (1964). 'Transport of oxygen and carbon dioxide.' *Handbk Physiol.*, section 3, 1, 767.

Roughton, F. J. W. and Darling, R. C. (1944). 'The effect of carbon monoxide on the oxyhemoglobin dissociation curve.' *Am. J. Physiol.*, 141, 17.

Roughton, F. J. W. and Forster, R. E. (1957). 'Relative importance of diffusion and chemical reaction rates in determining rate of exchange of gas in the human lung.' *J. appl. Physiol.*, 11, 290.

Roughton, F. J. W. and Severinghaus, J. W. (1973). 'Accurate determination of O_2 dissociation curve of human blood above 98·7% saturation with data on O_2 solubility in unmodified human blood from 0° C to 37° C.' *J. appl. Physiol.*, 35, 861.

Ruben, H. M., Elam, J. O., Ruben, A. M. and Greene, D. G. (1961). 'Investigation of upper airway problems in resuscitation.' *Anesthesiology*, 22, 271.

Safar, P. (1959). 'Failure of manual respiration.' *J. appl. Physiol.*, 14, 84.

Safar, P., Escarraga, L. A. and Chang, F. (1959). 'Upper airway obstruction in the unconscious patient.' *J. appl. Physiol.*, 14, 760.

Safar, P., Brown, T. C., Holtey, W. J. and Wilder, R. J. (1961). 'Ventilation and circulation with closed-chest cardiac massage in man.' *J. Am. med. Ass.*, 176, 574.

Saidman, L. J. and Eger, E. I. (1964). 'Effect of nitrous oxide and of narcotic premedication on the alveolar concentration of halothane required for anesthesia.' *Anesthesiology*, 25, 302.

St John, W. M., Glasser, R. L. and King, R. A. (1972). 'Rhythmic respiration in awake vagotomized cats with chronic pneumotaxic area lesions.' *Resp. Physiol.*, 15, 233.

Salmoiraghi, G. C. (1963). 'Functional organization of brain stem respiratory neurones.' *Ann. N. Y. Acad. Sci.*, 109, 571.

Salmoiraghi, G. C. and von Baumgarten, R. (1961). 'Intracellular potentials from respiratory neurones in the brainstem of the cat and the mechanism of rhythmic respiration.' *J. Neurophysiol.*, 24, 203.

Salmoiraghi, G. C. and Burns, B. D. (1960). 'Localization and patterns of discharge of respiratory neurones in brain stem of cat.' *J. Neurophysiol.*, 23, 2.

Sancetta, S. M. and Rakita, L. (1957). 'Response of pulmonary artery pressure and total pulmonary resistance of untrained, convalescent man to prolonged mild steady state exercise.' *J. clin. Invest.*, 36, 1138.

Sanders, R. D. (1967). 'Two ventilating attachments for bronchoscopes.' *Delaware St. med. J.*, 39, 170.

Schafer, E. A. (1904). 'Description of a simple and efficient method of performing artificial respiration in the human subject.' *Trans. R. med. chir. Soc. London*, 87, 609.

Scholander, P. F. (1947). 'Analyzer for accurate estimation of respiratory gases in one-half cubic centimeter samples.' *J. biol. Chem.*, 167, 235.

Scholfied, E. J. and Williams, N. E. (1974). 'Prediction of arterial carbon dioxide tension using a circle system without carbon dioxide absorption.' *Br. J. Anaesth.*, 46, 442.

Schultz, E. A. Buckley, J. J., Oswald, A. J. and van Bergen, F. H. (1960). 'Profound acidosis in an anesthetized human: report of a case.' *Anesthesiology*, 21, 285.

Scott, D. B., Stephen, G. W. and Davie, I. T. (1972). 'Haemodynamic effects of a negative (subatmospheric) pressure expiratory phase during artificial ventilation.' *Br. J. Anaesth.*, 44, 171.

Scott, J. (1847). 'Etherisation and asphyxia.' *Lancet*, 1, 355.

Scurr, C. F. (1954). 'Carbon dioxide retention simulating curarization.' *Br. med. J.*, 565.

Scurr, C. F. (1956). 'Pulmonary ventilation and carbon dioxide levels.' *Br. J. Anaesth.*, 28, 422.

Sechzer, P. H., Egbert, L. D., Linde, H. W., Cooper, D. Y., Dripps, R. D. and Price, H. L. (1960). 'Effect of CO_2 inhalation on arterial pressure, E. C. G. and plasma catecholamines and 17–OH cortiscosteroids in normal man.' *J. appl. Physiol.*, 15, 454.

Seebohm, P. M. and Hamilton, W. K. (1958). 'A method for measuring nasal resistance without intranasal instrumentation.' *J. Allergy*, 29, 56.

Selman, B. J., White, Y. S. and Tait, A. R. (1975). 'An evaluation of the Lex-O_2-Con oxygen content analyser.' *Anaesthesia*, 30, 206.

Semple, S. J. G. (1965). 'Respiration and the cerebrospinal fluid.' *Br. J. Anaesth.*, 37, 262.

Severinghaus, J. W. (1954). 'The rate of uptake of nitrous oxide in man.' *J. clin. Invest.*, 33, 1183.

Severinghaus, J. W. (1963). 'High temperature operation of the oxygen electrode giving fast response for respiratory gas sampling.' *Clin. Chem.*, 9, 727.

Severinghaus, J. W. (1965). 'Blood gas concentrations.' *Handbk Physiol.*, *section* 3, 2, 1475.

Severinghaus, J. W. (1966). 'Blood gas calculator.' *J. appl. Physiol.*, 21, 1108.

Severinghaus, J. W. (1972). 'Hypoxic respiratory drive and its loss during chronic hypoxia.' *Clin. Physiol.*, 2, 57.

Severinghaus, J. W. and Bradley, A. F. (1958). 'Electrodes for blood PO_2 and PCO_2 determination.' *J. appl. Physiol.*, 13, 515.

Severinghaus, J. W. and Carcelen, B. (1964). 'Cerebrospinal fluid in man native to high altitude.' *J. appl. Physiol.*, 19, 319.

Severinghaus, J. W. and Larson, C. P. (1965). 'Respiration in anesthesia.' *Handbk Physiol.*, *section* 3, 2, 1219.

Severinghaus, J. W. and Mitchell, R. A. (1962). 'Ondine's curse: failure of respiratory center automaticity while awake.' *Clin. Res.*, 10, 122.

Severinghaus, J. W. and Stupfel, M. (1955). 'Respiratory dead space increase following atropine in man, and atropine, vagal or ganglionic blockade and hypothermia in dogs.' *J. appl. Physiol.*, 8, 81.

Severinghaus, J. W. and Stupfel, M. (1957). 'Alveolar dead space as an index of distribution of blood flow in pulmonary capillaries.' *J. app. Physiol.*, 10, 335.

Severinghaus, J. W., Bainton, C. R. and Carcelen, A. (1966). 'Respiratory insensitivity to hypoxia in chronically hypoxic man.' *Resp. Physiol.*, 1, 308.

Severinghaus, J. W., Stupfel, M. and Bradley, A. F. (1956a). 'Accuracy of blood pH and PCO_2 determinations.' *J. appl. Physiol.*, 9, 189.

Severinghaus, J. W., Stupfel, M. and Bradley, A. F. (1956b). 'Variations of serum carbonic acid pK' with pH and temperature.' *J. appl. Physiol.*, 9, 197.

Severinghaus, J. W., Swenson, E. W., Finley, T. N., Lategola, M. T. and Williams, J. (1961). 'Unilateral hypoventilation produced in dogs by occluding one pulmonary artery.' *J. appl. Physiol.*, 16, 53.

Severinghaus, J. W., Mitchell, R. A., Richardson, B. W. and Singer, M. M. (1963). 'Respiratory control at high altitude suggesting active transport regulation of C. S. F. pH.' *J. appl. Physiol.*, 18, 1153.

Shafer, A. W., Tague, L. L., Welch, M. H. and Guenter, C. A. (1971). 2'3-Diphosphoglycerate in red cells stored in acid-citrate-dextrose and citrate-phosphate-dextrose.' *J. Lab. clin. Med.*, 77, 430.

Shah, J., Jones, J. G., Galvin, J. and Tomlin, P. J. (1971). 'Pulmonary gas exchange during induction of anaesthesia with nitrous oxide in seated subjects.' *Br. J. Anaesth.*, 43, 1013.

Shappell, S. D. and Lenfant, C. J. M. (1972). 'Adaptive, genetic and iatrogenic alterations of the oxyhemoglobin-dissociation curve.' *Anesthesiology*, 37, 127.

Sharp, G. R., Ledingham, I. McA. and Norman, J. N. (1962). 'The application of oxygen at 2 atmospheres pressure in the treatment of acute anoxia.' *Anaesthesia*, 17, 136.

Sharpey-Schafer, E. P. (1953). 'Effects of coughing on intra-thoracic pressure, arterial pressure and peripheral blood flow.' *J. Physiol.*, 122, 351.

Shaw, L. A. and Messer, A. C. (1932). 'The transfer of bicarbonate ion between the blood and tissues caused by alterations of the carbon dioxide concentrations in the lungs.' *Am. J. Physiol.*, 100, 122.

Shenkin, H. A. and Bouzarth, W. F. (1970). 'Clinical methods of reducing intracranial pressure.' *New Engl. J. Med.*, 282, 1465.

Shepard, R. H., Campbell, E. J. M., Martin, H. B. and Enns, T. (1957). 'Factors affecting the pulmonary dead space as determined by single breath analysis.' *J. appl. Physiol.*, 11, 241.

Shepard, R. J. (1967). 'The maximum sustained voluntary ventilation in exercise.' *Clin. Sci.*, 32, 167.

Siesjö, B. K. and Nilsson L. (1971). 'The influence of arterial hypoxaemia upon labile phosphates and upon extracellular and intracellular lactate and pyruvate concentrations in the rat brain.' *Scand. J. clin. Lab. Invest.*, 27, 83.

Siggaard-Andersen, O. (1964). *The Acid-Base Status of Blood.* Copenhagen; Munksgaard.

Siggaard-Andersen, O., Engel, K., Jørgensen, K. and Astrup, P. (1960). 'A micro-method for determination of pH, carbon dioxide tension, base excess and standard bicarbonate in capillary blood.' *Scand. J. clin. Lab. Invest.*, 12, 172.

Silvester, H. R. (1857). 'The natural method of treating asphyxia.' *Med. Times Gaz.*, 11, 485.

Singer, M. M., Wright, F., Stanley, L. K., Roe, B. B. and Hamilton, W. K. (1970). 'Oxygen toxicity in man. A prospective study in patients after open-heart surgery.' *New Engl. J. Med.*, 283, 1473.

Slater, E. M., Nilsson, S. E., Leake, D. L., Parry, W. L., Laver, M. B., Hedley-Whyte, J. and Bendixen, H. H. (1965). 'Arterial oxygen tension measurements during nitrous oxide-oxygen anesthesia.' *Anesthesiology*, 26, 642.

Slome, D. (1965). 'Physiology of respiration.' In: *General Anaesthesia*, Vol. 1, 2nd edn. Ed. by F. T. Evans and T. C. Gray. London and Boston, Mass.; Butterworths.

Smith, A. C., Spalding, J. M. K. and Watson, W. E. (1962). 'Ventilation volume as a stimulus to spontaneous ventilation after prolonged artificial ventilation.' *J. Physiol.*, 160, 22.

Smith, A. L. and Wollman, H. (1972). 'Cerebral blood flow and metabolism.' *Anesthesiology*, 36, 378.

Smith, G. and Lawson, D. A. (1958). 'Experimental coronary arterial occlusion: effects of the administration of oxygen under pressure.' *Scott. med. J.*, 3, 346.

Smith, G., Stevens, J., Griffiths, J. C. and Ledingham, I. McA. (1961). 'Near avulsion of foot treated by replacement and subsequent prolonged exposure of patient to oxygen at two atmospheres pressure.' *Lancet*, 2, 1122.

Smith, H. and Pask, E. A. (1959). 'Method for the estimation of oxygen in gas mixtures containing nitrous oxide.' *Br. J. Anaesth.*, 31, 440.

Smith, P., Heath, D. and Moosavi, H. (1974). 'The Clara cell.' *Thorax*, 29, 147.

Smith, W. D. A. (1961). 'The effects of external resistance to respiration. Part II: Resistance to respiration due to anaesthetic apparatus.' *Br. J. Anaesth.*, 33, 610.

Smith, W. D. A. (1964a). 'The measurement of uptake of nitrous oxide by pneumotachography. I: Apparatus, methods and accuracy.' *Br. J. Anaesth.*, 36, 363.

Smith, W. D. A. (1964b). '410 dental anaesthetics.' *Br. J. Anaesth.*, 36, 620 and 633.

Sobin, S. S., Fung, Y. C., Tremer, H. M. and Rosenquist, T. H. (1972). 'Elasticity of the pulmonary alveolar microvascular sheet in the cat.' *Circulation Res.*, 30, 440.

Sørensen, S. C. and Milledge, J. S. (1971). 'Cerebrospinal fluid acid–base composition at high altitude.' *J. appl. Physiol.*, 31, 28.

Spalding, J. M. K. and Smith, A. C. (1963). *Clinical Practice and Physiology of Artificial Respiration.* Oxford; Blackwell.

Spence, A. A. and Ellis, F. R. (1971). 'A critical evaluation of a nitrogen rebreathing method for the estimation of P$\bar{v}_{O_2}$.' *Resp. Physiol.*, 10, 313.

Staněk, V., Widimisky J., Kasalicky, J., Navratil, M., Daum, S. and Levinsky, L. (1967). 'The pulmonary gas exchange during exercise in patients with pulmonary fibrosis.' *Scand. J. resp. Dis.*, 48, 11.

Stanley, T. H., Zikria, B. A. and Sullivan, S. F. (1972). 'The surface tension of tracheobronchial secretions during general anesthesia.' *Anesthesiology*, 37, 445.

Stark, D. C. C. and Smith, H. (1960). 'Pulmonary vascular changes during anaesthesia.' *Br. J. Anaesth.*, 32, 460.

Staub, N. C. (1961). 'A simple small oxygen electrode.' *J. appl. Physiol.*, 16, 192.

Staub, N. C. (1963a). 'Alveolar–arterial oxygen tension gradient due to diffusion.' *J. appl. Physiol.*, 18, 673.

Staub, N. C. (1963b). 'The interdependence of pulmonary structure and function.' *Anesthesiology*, 24, 831.

Staub, N. C. (1971). 'The structural basis of lung function.' In: *General Anaesthesia,* 3rd edn . Ed. by T. C. Gray and J. F. Nunn. London and Boston, Mass.; Butterworths.

Staub, N. C. (1974). 'Pulmonary edema.' *Physiol. Rev.,* 54, 679.

Staub, N. C., Bishop, J. M. and Forster, R. E. (1962). 'Importance of diffusion and chemical blood cells.' *J. appl. Physiol.,* 16, 511.

Staub, N. C., Bishop, J. M. and Forster, R. E. (1962). 'Importance of diffusion and chemical reaction rates in O_2 uptake in the lung.' *J. appl. Physiol.,* 17, 21.

Staub, N. C., Nagano, H. and Pearce, M. L. (1967). 'Pulmonary edema in dogs, especially the sequence of fluid accumulation in lungs.' *J. appl. Physiol.,* 22, 227.

Stein, M., Forkner, C. E., Robin, E. D. and Wessler, S. (1961). 'Gas exchange after autologous pulmonary embolism in dogs.' *J. appl. Physiol.,* 16, 488.

Sugihara, T., Hildebrandt, J. and Martin, C. J. (1972). 'Viscoelastic properties of alveolar wall.' *J. appl. Physiol.,* 33, 93.

Sullivan, S. F., Patterson, R. W. and Papper, E. M. (1966). 'Arterial CO_2 tension adjustment rates following hyperventilation.' *J. appl. Physiol.,* 21, 247.

Sumner, W. and Gurtner, G. H. (1973). 'Evidence for partially carrier mediated CO transfer in the human lung.' *Physiologist,* 16, 466.

Suter, P. M., Fairley, H. B. and Isenberg, M. D. (1975). 'Optimum end-expiratory airway pressure in patients with acute pulmonary failure.' *New Engl. J. Med.,* 292, 284.

Svanberg, L. (1957). 'Influence of posture on lung volumes, ventilation and circulation in normals.' *Scand J. clin. Lab. Invest.,* 9, suppl. 25.

Swartz, H. M. (1973). 'Toxic oxygen effects.' *Int. Rev. Cytol.,* 35, 321.

Sykes, M. K. (1960). 'Observations on a rebreathing technique for the determination of arterial PCO_2 in the apnoeic patient.' *Br. J. Anaesth.,* 32, 256.

Sykes, M. K. and Lumley, J. (1969). 'The effect of varying inspiratory : expiratory ratios during anaesthesia for open-heart surgery.' *Br. J. Anaesth.,* 41, 374.

Sykes, M. K., Young, W. E. and Robinson, B. E. (1965). 'Oxygenation during anaesthesia with controlled ventilation.' *Br. J. Anaesth.,* 37, 314.

Sykes, M. K., Adams, A. P., Finlay, W. E. I., McCormick, P. W. and Economider, A. (1970). 'The effect of variations in end-expiratory inflation pressure on cardiorespiratory function in normo-, hypo-, and hyper-volaemic dogs.' *Br. J. Anaesth.,* 42, 669.

Sykes, M. K., Davies, D. M., Chakrabarti, M. K. and Loh, L. (1973). 'The effect of halothane, trichloroethylene and ether on the hypoxic pressor response and pulmonary vascular resistance in the isolated, perfused cat lung.' *Br. J. Anaesth.,* 45, 655.

Sykes, M. K., Arnot, R. N., Jastrzebski, J., Gibbs, J. M., Obdrzalek, J. and Hurtig, J. B. (1975). 'Reduction of hypoxic pulmonary vasoconstriction during trichloreothylene anesthesia.' *J. appl. Physiol.,* 39, 103.

Szidon, J. P., Pietra, G. G. and Fishman, A. P. (1972). 'The alveolar-capillary membrane and pulmonary edema.' *New Engl. J. Med.,* 286, 1200.

Takahashi, S., Shigematsu, A. and Furukawa, T. (1974). 'Interaction of volatile anesthetics with rat hepatic microsomal cytochrome P-450.' *Anesthesiology,* 41, 375.

Tenney, S. M. (1956). 'Sympatho-adrenal stimulation by carbon dioxide and the inhibitory effect of carbonic acid on epinephrine response.' *Am. J. Physiol.,* 187, 341.

Tenney, S. M. (1960). 'The effect of carbon dioxide on neurohumoral and endocrine mechanisms.' *Anesthesiology,* 21, 674.

Tenney, S. M. and Lamb T. W. (1965). 'Physiological consequences of hypoventilation and hyperventilation.' *Handbk Physiol., section* 3, 2, 979.

Thews, G. (1961). In: *Bad Oeynhausener Gespräche,* IV. Ed. by H. Bartels and E. Witzleb. Berlin; Springer.

Theye, R. A. (1972). 'The contributions of individual organ systems to the decrease in whole-body $\dot{V}O_2$ with halothane.' *Anesthesiology,* 37, 367.

Theye, R. A. and Fowler, W. S. (1959). 'Carbon dioxide balance during thoracic surgery.' *J. appl. Physiol.,* 14, 552.

Theye, R. A. and Tuohy, G. F. (1964b). 'Considerations in the determination of oxygen uptake and ventilatory performance during methoxyflurane anesthesia in man.' *Curr. Res. Anesth. Analg.,* 43, 306.
uptake and ventilatory performance during methoxyflurane anesthesia in man.' *Curr. Res. Anesth. Analg.,* 43, 306.

Thilenius, O. G. and Derenzo, C. (1972). 'Effects of acutely induced changes in arterial pH on pulmonary vascular resistance during normoxia and hypoxia in awake dogs.' *Clin. Sci.,* 42, 277.

Thomas, D. P. and Vane, J. R. (1967). '5-Hydroxytryptamine in the circulation of the dog.' *Nature Lond.*, 216, 335.

Thompson, S. P. (1965). *Calculus Made Easy.* London; Macmillan.

Thornton, J. A. (1960). 'Physiological dead space: changes during general anaesthesia.' *Anaesthesia*, 15, 381.

Thornton, J. A. and Nunn, J. F. (1960). 'Accuracy of determination of PCO_2 by the indirect method.' *Guy's Hosp. Rep.*, 109, 203.

Tierney, D. F. (1974). 'Lung metabolism and biochemistry.' *A. Rev. Physiol.*, 36, 209.

Tobin, C. E. and Zariquiey, M. O. (1950). 'Arteriovenous shunts in the human lung.' *Proc. Soc. exp. Biol. Med.*, 75, 827.

Tomlin, P., Conway, C. M. and Payne, J. P. (1964). 'Hypoxaemia due to atropine.' *Lancet*, 1, 14.

Tomlin, P., Gardner, R., Thung, N. and Finley, T. N. (1961). 'Factors affecting the surface tension of lung extracts.' *Fedn Proc.*, 20, 428.

Torrance, J., Jacobs, P., Restrepo, A., Eschbach, J., Lenfant, C. and Finch, C. A. (1970). 'Intraerythrocytic adaptation to anemia.' *New Engl. J. Med.*, 283, 165.

Trichet, B., Falke, K. Togut, A. and Laver, M. B. (1975). 'The effect of pre-existing pulmonary vascular disease on the response to mechanical ventilation with PEEP following open-heart surgery.' *Anesthesiology*, 42, 56.

Turner, J. E., Lambertsen, C. J., Owen, S. G., Wendel, H. and Chiodi, H. (1957). 'Effects of ·08 and ·8 atmospheres of inspired PO_2 upon cerebral hemodynamics at a "constant" alveolar PCO_2 of 43 mm Hg.' *Fedn Proc.*, 16, 130.

Ullman, E. (1970). 'About Hering and Breuer.' In: *Breathing: Hering–Breuer Centenary Symposium*, p. 3. Ed. by R. Porter. Edinburgh and London; Churchill Livingstone.

Utting, J. (1963). 'pH as a factor influencing plasma concentrations of *d*-tubocurarine. *Br. J. Anaesth.*, 35, 706.

Uzawa, T. and Ashbaugh, D. G. (1969). 'Continuous positive-pressure breathing in acute hemorrhagic pulmonary edema.' *J. appl. Physiol.*, 26, 427.

Valeri, C. R. (1975). 'Blood components in the treatment of acute blood loss, use of freeze-preserved red cells, platelets, and the plasma proteins.' *Anesth. Analg.*, 54, 1.

Van Slyke, D. D. and Neill, J. M. (1924). 'The determination of gases in blood and other solutions by vacuum extraction and manometric measurement.' *J. biol. Chem.*, 61, 523.

Vance, J. P., Brown, D. M. and Smith, G. (1973). 'The effects of hypocapnia on myocardial blood flow and metabolism.' *Br. J. Anaesth.*, 45, 455.

Vane, J. R. (1969). 'The release and fate of vaso-active hormones in the circulation.' *Br. J. Pharmac.*, 35, 209.

Velasquez, T. and Farhi, L. E. (1964). 'Effect of negative pressure breathing on lung mechanics and venous admixture.' *J. appl. Physiol.*, 19, 665.

Verloop, M. C. (1948). 'The arteriae bronchiales and their anastomoses with the arteria pulmonalis in the human lung: a micro-anatomical study.' *Acta anat.*, 5, 171.

Virgil, Publius Vergilius Maro (19 B.C.) *The Aeneid*, Book II, p. 1.

Wade, J. G., Larson, C. P., Hickey, R. F., Ehrenfeld, W. K. and Severinghaus, J. W. (1970). 'Effect of carotid endarterectomy on carotid chemoreceptor and baroreceptor function in man.' *New Engl. J. Med.*, 282, 823.

Wade, O. L. and Bishop, J. M. (1962). *Cardiac Output and Regional Blood Flow.* Oxford; Blackwell.

Wade, O. L. and Gilson, J. C. (1951). 'The effect of posture on diaphragmatic movement and vital capacity in normal subjects.' *Thorax*, 6, 103.

Wagner, P. D., Naumann, P. F. and Laravuso, R. B. (1974). 'Simultaneous measurements of eight foreign gases in blood by gas chromatography.' *J. appl. Physiol.*, 36, 600.

Wagner, P. D., Saltzman, H. A. and West, J. B. (1974). 'Measurement of continuous distribution of ventilation–perfusion ratios: theory.' *J. appl. Physiol.*, 36, 588.

Wagner, P. D., Laravuso, R. B., Uhl, R. R. and West, J. B. (1974). 'Continuous distributions of ventilation–perfusion ratios in normal subjects breathing air and 100% O_2.' *J. clin. Invest.*, 54, 54.

Wagner, P. D., Laravuso, R. B., Goldzimmer, E., Naumann, P. F. and West, J. B. (1975). 'Distribution of ventilation–perfusion ratios in dogs in normal and abnormal lungs.' *J. appl. Physiol.*, 38, 1099.

Wakai, I. (1963). 'Human oxygenation by air during anaesthesia. The relation of ventilatory volume and arterial oxygen saturation.' *Br. J. Anaesth.*, 35, 414.

Walder, D. N. (1965). 'Some dangers of a hyperbaric environment.' In: *Hyperbaric Oxygenation*. Ed. by I. Ledingham. Edinburgh and London; Churchill Livingstone.

Wang, S. C. and Ngai, S. H. (1964). 'General organization of central respiratory mechanisms.' *Handbk Physiol., section* 3, 1, 487.

Wang, S. C., Ngai, S. H. and Frumin, M. J. (1957). 'Organization of central respiratory mechanisms in the brain stem of the cat: genesis of normal respiratory rhythmicity.' *Am. J. Physiol.*, 190, 333.

Wardle, E. N. (1974). 'Post-traumatic respiratory insufficiency: what is "shock lung"?' *J. Jl R. Coll. Phys. Lond.*, 8, 251.

Warrell, D. A., Evans, J. W., Clarke, R. O., Kingaby, G. P. and West, J. B. (1972). 'Pattern of filling in the pulmonary capillary bed.' *J. appl. Physiol.*, 32, 346.

Warren, B. A. (1963). 'Fibrinolytic properties of vascular endothelium.' *Br. J. exp. Path.*, 44, 365.

Waters, D. J. and Mapleson, W. W. (1964). 'Exponentials and the anaesthetist.' *Anaesthesia*, 19, 274.

Watson, W. E. (1961). 'Physiology of artificial respiration.' *PhD Thesis*, University of Oxford.

Watson, W. E. (1962a). 'Some observations on dynamic lung compliance during intermittent positive pressure respiration.' *Br. J. Anaesth.*, 34, 153.

Watson, W. E. (1962b). 'Observations on physiological dead space during intermittent positive pressure respiration.' *Br. J. Anaesth.*, 34, 502.

Wayne, D. J. and Chamney, A. R. (1969). 'Oxygen tents.' *Anaesthesia*, 24, 591.

Webb, S. J. S. (1965). 'A method of recording the minute volume of respiration.' *Br. J. Anaesth.*, 37, 292.

Webb, S. J. S. and Nunn, J. F. (1967). 'A comparison between the effect of nitrous oxide and nitrogen on arterial PO_2.' *Anaesthesia*, 22, 69.

Weibel, E. R. (1962). 'Morphometrische Bestimmung von Zahl, Volumen und Oberfläche der Alveolen und Kapillaren der menschlichen Lunge.' *Z. Zellforsch. mikrosk. Anat.*, 57, 648.

Weibel, E. R. (1963). *Morphometry of the Human Lung.* (1963). Berlin; Springer.

Weibel, E. R. (1964). 'Morphometrics of the lung.' *Handbk Physiol., section* 3, 1, 285.

Weibel, E. R. (1971). 'Oxygen effect on lung cells.' *Archs intern. Med.*, 128, 54.

Weibel, E. R. (1973). 'Morphological basis of alveolar-capillary gas exchange.' *Physiol. Rev.*, 53, 419.

Weibel, E. R. and Gil, J. (1968). 'Electron microscopic demonstration of an extracellular duplex lining layer of alveoli.' *Resp. Physiol.*, 4, 42.

Weibel, E. R. and Gomez, D. M. (1962). 'Architecture of the human lung.' *Science*, 137, 577.

Weil, J. V., Sodal, I. E. and Speck, R. P. (1967). 'A modified fuel cell for the analysis of oxygen concentration of gases.' *J. appl. Physiol.*, 23, 419.

Weil, J. V., Byrne-Quinn, E., Sodal, I. E., Kline, J. S., McCullough, R. E. and Filley, G. F. (1972). 'Augmentation of chemosensitivity during mild exercise in normal man.' *J. appl. Physiol.*, 33, 813.

Weiskopf, R. B. and Severinghaus, J. W. (1972). 'Lack of effect of high altitude on hemoglobin oxygen affinity.' *J. appl. Physiol.*, 33, 276.

Weiskopf, R. B., Nishimura, M. and Severinghaus, J. W. (1971). 'The absence of an effect of halothane on blood hemoglobin O_2 equilibrium *in vitro*.' *Anesthesiology*, 35, 579.

Weiskopf, R. B., Raymond, L. W. and Severinghaus, J. W. (1974). 'Effects of halothane on canine respiratory responses to hypoxia with and without hypercarbia.' *Anesthesiology*, 41, 350.

West, J. B. (1962). 'Regional differences in gas exchange in the lung of erect man.' *J. appl. Physiol.*, 17, 893.

West, J. B. (1963). 'Distribution of gas and blood in the normal lung.' *Br. med. Bull.*, 19, 53.

West, J. B. (1965). *Ventilation: Blood Flow and Gas Exchange*. Oxford; Blackwell (2nd edn., published 1970).

West, J. B. (1974). 'Blood flow to the lung and gas exchange.' *Anesthesiology*, 41, 124.

West, J. B. (1975). 'New advances in pulmonary gas exchange.' *Anesth. Analg.*, 54, 409.

West, J. B. and Dollery, C. T. (1965). 'Distribution of blood flow and the pressure–flow relations of the whole lung.' *J. appl. Physiol.*, 20, 175.

West, J. B., Dollery, C. T. and Naimark, A. (1964). 'Distribution of blood flow in isolated lung; relation to vascular and alveolar pressures.' *J. appl. Physiol.*, 19, 713.

West, J. B., Holland, R. A. B., Dollery, C. T. and Matthews, C. M. E. (1962a). 'Interpretation of radioactive gas clearance rates in the lung.' *J. appl. Physiol.*, 17, 14.

West, J. B., Lahiri, S., Gill, M. B., Milledge, J. S., Pugh, L. G. C. E. and Ward, M. P. (1962b). 'Arterial oxygen saturation during exercise at high altitude.' *J. appl. Physiol.*, 17, 617.

Westbrook, P. R., Stubbs, S. E., Sessler, A. D., Rehder, K. and Hyatt, R. E. (1973). 'Effects of anesthesia and muscle paralysis on respiratory mechanics in normal man.' *J. appl. Physiol.*, 34, 81.

Westlake, E. K., Simpson, T. and Kaye, M. (1955). 'Carbon dioxide narcosis in emphysema.' *Q. Jl Med.*, 24, 155.

Whitelaw, W. A., Derenne, J.-P. and Milic-Emili, J. (1975). 'Occlusion pressure as a measure of respiratory center output in conscious man.' *Resp. Physiol.*, 23, 181.

Whitfield, A. G. W., Waterhouse, J. A. H. and Arnott, W. M. (1950). 'The total lung volume and its subdivisions.' *Br. J. soc. Med.*, 4, 1.

Whittenberg, J. B. (1970). 'Myoglobin-facilitated oxygen diffusion.' *Physiol. Rev.*, 50, 559.

Whittenberger, J. L., McGregor, M., Berglund, E. and Borst, H. G. (1960). 'Influence of state of inflation of the lungs on pulmonary vascular resistance.' *J. appl. Physiol.*, 15, 878.

Whitteridge, D. and Bulbring, E. (1944). 'Changes in activity of pulmonary receptors in anaesthesia and the influence of respiratory behaviour.' *J. Pharmac. exp. Ther.*, 81, 340.

Whyche, M. Q., Teichner, R. L., Kallos, T., Marshall, B. E. and Smith, T. C. (1973). 'Effects of continuous positive-pressure breathing on functional residual capacity and arterial oxygenation during intra-abdominal operations.' *Anesthesiology*, 38, 68.

Widdicombe, J. G. (1961). 'Respiratory reflexes in man and other mammalian species.' *Clin. Sci.*, 21, 163.

Widdicombe, J. G. (1964). 'Respiratory reflexes.' *Handbk Physiol.*, *section* 3, 1, 585.

Wilhjelm, B. J. (1966). 'Protective action of anaesthetics against anoxia.' *Acta anaesth., scand.*, suppl. 25, 318.

Williams, K. G. and Hopkinson, W. I. (1965). 'Small chamber techniques in hyperbaric oxygen therapy.' In: *Hyperbaric Oxygenation*. Ed. by I. Ledingham. Edinburgh and London; Churchill Livingstone.

Wilson, R. S. and Laver, M. B. (1972). 'Oxygen analysis: advances in methodology.' *Anesthesiology* 37, 112.

Winter, P. M. and Smith, G. (1972). 'The toxicity of oxygen.' *Anesthesiology*, 37, 210.

Winterstein, H. (1911). 'Die Regulierun g der Athmung durch das Blut.' *Pflügers Arch. ges. Physiol.*, 138, 167.

Wolfe, W. G. and DeVries, W. C. (1975). 'Oxygen toxicity.' *A. Rev. Med.*, 26, 203.

Woo, S. W., Berlin, D. and Hedley-Whyte, J. (1969). 'Surfactant function and anesthetic agents.' *J. appl. Physiol.*, 26, 571.

Woodbury, J. W. (1965). 'Regulation of pH.' In: *Physiology and Biophysics.* Ed. by T. C. Ruch and H. D. Patton. Philadelphia and London; W. B. Saunders.

Woodbury, D. M. and Karler, R. (1960). 'The role of carbon dioxide in the nervous system.' *Anesthesiology* 21, 686.

Woolcock, A. J., Vincent, N. J. and Macklem, P. T. (1969). 'Frequency dependence of compliance as a test for obstruction in the small airways.' *J. clin. Invest.*, 48, 1097.

Wright, B. M. (1955). 'A respiratory anemometer.' *J. Physiol.*, 127, 25P.

Wright, B. M. and McKerrow, C. B. (1959). 'Maximum forced expiratory flow rate as a measure of ventilatory capacity.' *Br. med. J.*, 2, 1041.

Wright, B. M., Slavin, G., Kreel, L., Callan, K. and Sandin, B. (1974). 'Postmortem inflation and fixation of human lungs.' *Thorax*, 29, 189.

Wulf, R. J. and Featherstone, R. M. (1957). 'A correlation of Van der Waals constants with anesthetic potency.' *Anesthesiology*, 18, 97.

Wulff, K. E. and Aulin, I. (1972). 'The regional lung function in the lateral decubitus position during anesthesia and operation.' *Acta anaesth. scand.*, 16, 195.

Wyke, B. D. (1957). 'Electrographic monitoring of anaesthesia.' *Anaesthesia*, 12, 157.

Zamel, N., Jones, J. G., Bach, S. M. and Newberg, L. (1974). 'Analog computation of alveolar pressure and airway resistance during maximum expiratory flow.' *J. appl. Physiol.*, 36, 240.

Zapol, W. M., Snider, M. T. and Schneider, R. C. (1977). 'Extracorporeal membrane oxygenation for acute respiratory failure.' *Anesthesiology*, 46, 272.

Zechman, F., Hall, F. G. and Hull, W. E. (1957). 'Effects of graded resistance to tracheal air flow in man.' *J. appl. Physiol.*, 10, 356.

Zierler, K. L. (1962). 'Theoretical basis of indicator-dilution methods for measuring flow and volume.' *Circulation Res.*, 10, 393.

Zijlstra, W. G. (1958). *A Manual of Reflection Oximetry.* Assen, Netherlands; van Gorcum's Medical Library.

Zuntz, N. (1882). 'Physiologie der Blutgase und des respiratorischen Gaswechsels.' *Hermann's Handbuch Physiol.*, 4, 1.

Index

507